Professional's Handbook of

PSYCHOTROPIC DRUGS

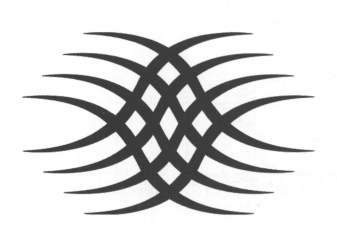

SPRINGHOUSE
Springhouse, Pennsylvania

Staff

Senior Publisher
Donna O. Carpenter

Editorial Director
William J. Kelly

Creative Director
Jake Smith

Art Director
Elaine Kasmer Ezrow

Drug Information Editor
Tracy Roux, RPh, PharmD

Project Editor
Catherine E. Harold

Clinical Project Editor
Eileen Cassin Gallen, RN, BSN

Associate Editor
Raphe Cheli

Clinical Editors
Lori Musolf Neri, RN, MSN, CCRN, CRNP; Margaret Friant Cramer, RN, MSN; Heather Rischel Burcher, RN, BSN(c)

Copy Editor
Beth E. Pitcher

Designers
Arlene Putterman (associate design director), Stephanie Peters, Joseph John Clark, Donald G. Knauss

Typographers
Diane Paluba (manager), Joyce Rossi Biletz

Manufacturing
Deborah Meiris (director), Patricia K. Dorshaw (manager), Otto Mezei (book production manager)

Editorial Assistants
Carol A. Caputo, Arlene P. Claffee

Visit our Web site at eDrugInfo.com

ISBN 1-58255-062-2

PHPD-- D N O S A J J M A M F J
04 03 02 01 10 9 8 7 6 5 4 3 2 1

Library of Congress Cataloging-in-Publication Data

Professional's handbook of psychotropic drugs.
    p. cm.
    Includes bibliographical references and index.
    Psychotropic drugs — Handbooks, manuals, etc. I. Springhouse Corporation.
    [DNLM: 1. Psychotropic Drugs – Handbooks. 2. Mental Disorders – drug therapy – Handbooks. QV 39 P96242 2001]
RM315 .P713 2001
615'.788—dc21
ISBN 1-58255-066-2 (pbk.)
                                    00-047624

Contents

Clinical contributors and consultants — iv

Foreword — vi

How to use this book — vii

A guide to abbreviations — x

Part 1. Principles of psychotropic drug use

1. Understanding psychiatric disorders — 3

2. Working with special populations — 19

3. Managing overdose and withdrawal — 33

Part 2. Psychotropic drugs

4. Antianxiety drugs — 49

5. Anticonvulsants — 87

6. Antidepressants — 143

7. Mood stabilizing drugs — 217

8. Antiparkinsonians — 227

9. Antipsychotics — 269

10. Central nervous system stimulants — 341

11. Drugs for treating alcoholism and substance abuse — 371

12. Sedative-hypnotics — 409

13. Drugs for treating Alzheimer's disease and migraine headaches — 453

Part 3. Appendices and index

Guidelines for monitoring selected psychotropic drugs — 483

Herbs and dietary supplements used for psychotropic effects — 485

Resources — 487

Index — 489

Clinical contributors and consultants

Susan C. Beylotte, PhD, ANP, CS
Clinical Nurse Specialist, Nurse
  Practitioner
Ralph H. Johnson Veterans
  Administration Medical Center
Charleston, SC

Anne E. Braun, RNC, MSN, CEN, CCRN
Clinical Education Consultant
Princeton House
Princeton, NJ

Heather Rishel Burcher, RN, BSN(c)
Staff Nurse, Critical Care Float Pool
Susquehanna Health Systems
Williamsport, Pa

Jill Chappell, PharmD
Clinical Pharmacist
The Mount Sinai Medical Center
New York, NY

Lisa R. Colodny, PharmD, BCNSP
Clinical Coordinator
Broward General Medical Center
Ft. Lauderdale, Fla

Jennifer L. Defilippi, PharmD, BCPP
Clinical Psychiatric Specialist
Central Texas Veterans Health Care
  System
Waco, Tex

Jeff Duffey, MD
Psychiatrist, Private Practice
Milledgeville, Ga

Desiree D. Dunlap, PharmD
Coordinator of Clinical Services
Harris County Hospital District
Houston, Tex

Vincent Elliott, RN, MSN
Clinical Nurse Specialist,
  Gero-psychiatry
Department of Veterans Affairs
Palo Alto Health Care System
San Jose, Calif

Beverly Sigl Felten, RN, PhD(c), CS, APNP
President
Gero-Psych Nursing, SC
Lannon, Wis

Michael J. Gitlin, MD
Professor of Clinical Psychiatry
UCLA School of Medicine
Los Angeles, Calif

Tatyana Gurvich, PharmD
Clinical Pharmacologist
Glendale Adventist Family Practice
  Remedy Program
Glendale, Calif

Donna Iszler, RNC, MA, MSN
Nurse Educator
Fox Valley Technical College
Appleton, Wis

Jennifer H. Justice, PharmD
Clinical Assistant Professor of
  Pharmacy Practice
West Virginia University
Charleston, WVa

Misao M. Kusuda, MD
Psychiatrist
Veterans Administration San Jose
  Outpatient Clinic
San Jose, Calif

John Lauriello, MD
Clinical Vice Chairman
Department of Psychiatry
University of New Mexico
Albuquerque, NM

Jeanette M. Logan, PharmD
Psychiatric Pharmacist
Contra Costa County Mental Health
Martinez, Calif

Pamela M. Mammano, RN, MSN
Instructor of Nursing
Illinois Valley Community College
Ottawa, Ill

John S. Markowitz, PharmD
Assistant Professor
Department of Pharmacy Sciences
Medical University of South Carolina
Institute of Psychiatry
Charleston, SC

Stuart M. Olinsky, MD
Neurologist
Private Practice
Williamsport, Pa

Lorraine Flint Rother, RN, MSN
Psychiatric Clinical Nurse Specialist
Department of Veterans Affairs
Palo Alto Health Care System
San Jose, Calif

Samuel D. Shillcutt, PharmD, PhD
Associate Professor
Department of Psychiatry and
    Behavioral Sciences
Mercer University School of Medicine
Director of Research
Central State Hospital
Milledgeville, Ga

Susan Sonne, PharmD
Medical University of South Carolina
Institute of Psychiatry
Charleston, SC

Phyllis Tipton, RN, MSN
ADN Evening Coordinator
McLennan Community College
Waco, Tex

Andrew R. Topliff, MD
Emergency Physician, Toxicologist
Hennepin County Medical Center
Minneapolis, Minn

Laurie Willhite, PharmD
Pharmacy Department
Fairview University Medical Center
Minneapolis, Minn

Foreword

These days, professionals in virtually every subset of health care need a sound knowledge of psychotropic drugs and the principles of psychotropic therapy. That's because up to 40% of the patients in primary care practices have depression, anxiety, or other mental disorders.

Largely because of the influence of managed health care, a growing number of these patients receive drug treatment not from psychiatrists or other mental health professionals, but from family practice physicians, internists, and advanced practice nurses. As a psychopharmacologist, I find myself interacting ever more often with a broad range of health care professionals who manage mental disorders. Naturally, all such professionals must understand mental disorders and the drugs used to treat them.

Where do you get such an understanding? In part at least, you can get it from a book that combines broad coverage of psychiatric care with detailed, up-to-date coverage of the psychotropic drugs in use today. That's exactly what *Professional's Handbook of Psychotropic Drugs* provides.

The first section of the book reviews important principles that underlie the appropriate use of psychotropic drugs. Chapter 1 gives a valuable overview of the assessment steps needed to diagnose and treat mental disorders. Chapter 2 explores the challenges of managing psychotropic therapy for pregnant and breast-feeding women and for children, adolescents, and elderly patients. And Chapter 3 offers general guidelines for responding to a psychotropic overdose and managing the process of withdrawal.

The second section of the book includes detailed, practical information about more than 100 psychotropic drugs. You'll find them conveniently grouped into 10 chapters arranged by therapeutic function. A special section at the start of each chapter presents important information about each therapeutic class.

After that, you'll find individual drug entries arranged alphabetically by generic drug name. Each entry includes trade names, pharmacologic and therapeutic classifications, pregnancy risk category, controlled substance schedule, indications and dosages, pharmacodynamics, pharmacokinetics, contraindications and precautions, interactions, adverse reactions, and overdose and treatment. Each entry ends with special considerations and patient teaching.

The final section of the book provides handy, quick-reference appendices. You'll find guidelines for monitoring selected psychotropic drugs, a review of herbs and dietary supplements used for their psychotropic effects, and a valuable list of mental health resources for professionals and laypeople alike.

Throughout this book, you'll discover a great deal of information that can help you develop a sound understanding of psychotropic drug therapy. Given the current trends in health care, that understanding will not only help you provide the best possible care for your patients, but it also will stand you in good stead for the future.

Eric Hollander, MD
Professor of Psychiatry
Director of Clinical
Psychopharmacology
Director of Compulsive, Impulsive,
and Anxiety Disorders Program
Mount Sinai School of Medicine
New York

How to use this book

The *Professional's Handbook of Psychotropic Drugs* was designed to provide drug information that zeroes in on precisely what health care professionals need to know. In other words, it emphasizes the clinical aspects of drugs and drug therapy instead of trying to duplicate exhaustive pharmacology texts. The result is a book that's readily accessible and useful in any clinical setting.

The *Professional's Handbook of Psychotropic Drugs* is arranged into three major sections: introductory chapters, therapeutic class chapters, and quick-reference appendices.

Introductory chapters

Chapter 1 explains generally how mental illnesses are assessed, diagnosed, and treated. Chapter 2 explains some of the challenges of managing psychotropic drug therapy for patients in certain "special" populations, such as pregnant women, breast-feeding women, children, adolescents, and elderly patients. And Chapter 3 provides an overview of psychotropic overdose and withdrawal. Together, these chapters give you a basic foundation on which to effectively manage a patient's psychotropic drug therapy.

Therapeutic class chapters

Chapters 4 through 13 present therapeutic classes of psychotropic drugs, specifically antianxiety drugs, anticonvulsants, antidepressants, mood stabilizing drugs, antiparkinsonians, antipsychotics, central nervous system stimulants, drugs used to treat alcoholism and substance abuse, sedative-hypnotic drugs, and drugs used to treat Alzheimer's disease and migraine headaches.

Each chapter begins with an alphabetical list of the generic drugs used for that chapter's therapeutic purpose. Keep in mind that some of the drugs listed may have a different *primary* therapeutic purpose. In that case, you'll see a cross-reference to a different chapter next to the drug's name. To find material specific to that drug, simply turn to the chapter indicated.

Introductory text

Next, you'll find introductory text designed to give you an overview of pertinent disorders and comparative information about the drugs in the chapter.

Drug entries

Next, you'll find generic drugs arranged alphabetically. Each entry includes trade names, pharmacologic and therapeutic classifications, controlled substance schedule (if applicable), pregnancy risk category, how supplied, indications and dosages, pharmacodynamics, pharmacokinetics, contraindications and precautions, interactions, adverse reactions, overdose and treatment, special considerations, and patient teaching.

Trade names

A trade name followed by an open diamond is only available in Canada. A trade name not followed by an open diamond is available in the United States, Canada, and possibly other countries. The mention of a brand name in no way implies endorsement of that product or guarantees its legality.

Pharmacologic and therapeutic classifications

Classification by pharmacologic and therapeutic criteria offers several benefits. It helps you identify an unknown drug by its chemical status and its clinical application. It also helps you quickly identify other drugs that share the same properties and uses. Thus, it may help you compare dosages, anticipate effects, and identify potential alternatives for patients who can't tolerate or don't respond to a certain drug.

Pregnancy risk category

The pregnancy risk categories included here match those assigned by the Food and Drug Administration (FDA). These categories express the relative level of risk that a drug could cause birth defects. Although drugs are best avoided during pregnancy, this rating system permits rapid assessment of the risk-benefit ratio for a pregnant woman. Drugs in category A are usually considered safe during pregnancy; drugs in category X are usually contraindicated.

- **A:** Studies in pregnant women haven't shown a risk to the fetus.
- **B:** Animal studies haven't shown a risk to the fetus, but controlled studies haven't been conducted in pregnant women; or animal studies have shown an adverse effect on the fetus, but adequate studies in pregnant women haven't shown a risk.
- **C:** Animal studies have shown an adverse effect on the fetus, but adequate studies have not been conducted in humans. The benefits may be acceptable despite potential risks.
- **D:** The drug may pose risks to the human fetus, but potential benefits may be acceptable despite the risks.
- **X:** Studies in animals or humans show fetal abnormalities, or reports of adverse reactions indicate evidence of fetal risk. The risks clearly outweigh the potential benefits.
- **NR:** Not rated.

Controlled substance schedules

The controlled substance schedules included here reflect those assigned to drugs regulated under the Controlled Substances Act of 1970. They include schedules I, II, III, IV, and V.

- **I:** High abuse potential, no accepted medical use.
- **II:** High abuse potential, severe dependence liability.
- **III:** Less abuse potential than schedule II drugs, moderate dependence liability.
- **IV:** Less abuse potential than schedule III drugs, limited dependence liability.
- **V:** Limited abuse potential (such as small amounts of narcotics used for antitussive or antidiarrheal purposes). Under federal law, limited quantities of some schedule V drugs may be purchased from a pharmacist by adults without a prescription if allowed by state statute.

How supplied

This section lists the forms and strengths available for each drug.

Indications and dosages

Each drug entry includes dosages for FDA-approved and major off-label uses. Dosage instructions reflect current clinical trends in therapeutics and can't be considered as absolute or universal recommendations. For individual application, dosage instructions must be considered in light of the patient's clinical condition.

A special *Dosage adjustment* feature in pertinent entries details the dosage adjustments you may need to make for certain patients, such as elderly patients, children, or patients with hepatic or renal impairment.

Pharmacodynamics

This section describes the mechanism by which a drug produces its major effects. Naturally, different drugs used to treat a disorder may exert their effects in very different ways.

Pharmacokinetics

In this section, you'll find descriptions of each drug's absorption, distribution, metabolism, and excretion patterns.

Contraindications and precautions

This section lists any conditions, especially diseases, in which the use of a drug is dangerous or undesirable.

Interactions

This section lists each drug's clinically significant interactions. It includes special headings for interactions with other drugs, with herbs, with foods, and with certain lifestyle choices, such as smoking and alcohol use.

Adverse reactions

This section lists adverse reactions. Common reactions (those experienced by at least 10% of people who took the drug in clinical trials) appear in *italic* type. Less common reactions appear in plain type. Life-threatening reactions appear in ***bold italic*** type. And reactions that are common and life-threatening appear in BOLD CAPITAL LETTERS.

Overdose and treatment

This section describes the signs and symptoms usually caused by an overdose of the drug being described. It also provides general guidelines for reversing the effects of the overdose and supporting the patient's recovery.

Special considerations

This section lists preparation instructions, administration instructions, dosing instructions, and monitoring guidelines. It also notes when a drug interferes significantly with a diagnostic test or its result. The section includes separate headings for pregnant patients, breast-feeding patients, pediatric patients, and geriatric patients.

Patient teaching

The patient teaching section focuses on explaining the drug's purpose, promoting compliance, and ensuring proper use of the drug. It also includes instructions for preventing or minimizing adverse reactions.

Quick-reference appendices

The final section of the book provides a convenient location for important reference information. For instance, it includes guidelines for monitoring psychotropic drug therapy. It provides information about herbs and dietary supplements patients commonly use for psychotropic effects. You'll also find a helpful list of resources for you and your patients.

The *Professional's Handbook of Psychotropic Drugs* brings you hands-on, need-to-know information in an informative, easy-to-use format. By knowing how to use this book properly, you can save time and enhance the safety and accuracy of drug administration.

A GUIDE TO ABBREVIATIONS

ACE	angiotensin-converting enzyme	IND	investigational new drug
ADH	antidiuretic hormone	INR	international normalized ratio
AIDS	acquired immunodeficiency syndrome	IPPB	intermittent positive-pressure breathing
ALT	alanine aminotransferase	IU	international unit
aPTT	activated partial thromboplastin time	I.V.	intravenous
		kg	kilogram
AST	aspartate aminotransferase	M	molar
AV	atrioventricular	m^2	square meter
b.i.d.	twice daily	MAO	monoamine oxidase
BUN	blood urea nitrogen	mcg	microgram
cAMP	cyclic adenosine monophosphate	mEq	millequivalent
		mg	milligram
CBC	complete blood count	MI	myocardial infarction
CK	creatine kinase	ml	milliliter
CMV	cytomegalovirus	mm^3	cubic millimeter
CNS	central nervous system	NSAID	nonsteroidal anti-inflammatory drug
COPD	chronic obstructive pulmonary disease	OTC	over-the-counter
CSF	cerebrospinal fluid	PABA	para-aminobenzoic acid
CV	cardiovascular	PCA	patient-controlled analgesia
CVA	cerebrovascular accident	P.O.	by mouth
D_5W	dextrose 5% in water	P.R.	by rectum
DNA	deoxyribonucleic acid	p.r.n.	as needed
ECG	electrocardiogram	PT	prothrombin time
EEG	electroencephalogram	PTT	partial thromboplastin time
EENT	eyes, ears, nose, throat	PVC	premature ventricular contraction
FDA	Food and Drug Administration	q	every
g	gram	q.d.	every day
G	gauge	q.i.d.	four times daily
GABA	gamma-aminobutyric acid	RBC	red blood cell
GFR	glomerular filtration rate	RDA	recommended daily allowance
GI	gastrointestinal	REM	rapid eye movement
gtt	drops	RNA	ribonucleic acid
GU	genitourinary	SA	sinoatrial
G6PD	glucose-6-phosphate dehydrogenase	S.C.	subcutaneous
H_1	histamine$_1$	SIADH	syndrome of inappropriate antidiuretic hormone
H_2	histamine$_2$	S.L.	sublingual
HIV	human immunodeficiency virus	T_3	triiodothyronine
hr	hour	T_4	thyroxine
h.s.	at bedtime	t.i.d.	three times daily
ICU	intensive care unit	U	units
I.D.	intradermal	UTI	urinary tract infection
I.M.	intramuscular	WBC	white blood cell

PART 1

Principles of psychotropic drug use

3 ■ Understanding psychiatric disorders

19 ■ Working with special populations

33 ■ Managing overdose and withdrawal

CHAPTER 1

Understanding psychiatric disorders

Historically, professionals and laypeople alike have thought of psychiatric disorders as emotional rather than physiologic problems. Besides creating a stigma around mental illness that still exists today, this view offered little incentive for scientists to vigorously pursue new drugs and other medical treatments for mental disorders.

Increasingly, however, we're coming to understand that psychiatric disorders commonly do have some physiologic basis. A growing number of scientists and researchers are now examining the physiologic roots of mental illnesses and finding that neurotransmitters, hormones, and other physical and chemical factors can influence or even cause these illnesses.

What's more, we now understand that the interaction between mental illness and the stress it creates can cause physiologic changes that help to perpetuate the illness. Some of the physiologic changes produced by the stress of mental illness include autonomic hyperactivity, disruption of hypothalamic-pituitary-adrenal regulation, and impaired immune function.

Primary care focus

Our growing understanding of the physiology of mental illness holds good news for patients and the professionals who treat them. That's largely because scientists are translating this growing understanding into new and improved drug treatments that can restore normal functioning for many affected patients. To make safe and effective use of these drugs, however, professionals from nearly all avenues of health care—not just psychiatric specialties—must foster a sound understanding of psychiatric disorders and their treatments.

The simple truth is that many psychiatric disorders aren't diagnosed and treated by psychiatrists and other mental health professionals. In fact, up to 40% of patients in primary care settings have anxiety-related or depressive disorders—sometimes in addition to other disorders for which they originally sought treatment. Consequently, family practice physicians, internists, and advanced practice nurses in many settings routinely prescribe psychotropic drugs.

Naturally, this means that health care professionals in all disciplines and practice settings need an understanding of psychiatric care and psychotropic drugs. Because many patients receive care from multidisciplinary teams of professionals, each team member must also know how to fulfill an assigned role.

No matter what your practice setting or specialty, you need to be prepared to render expert care to patients who have psychiatric disorders. That preparation starts with a sound understanding of assessment, diagnosis, and treatment of psychiatric disorders.

ASSESSMENT

As with all health problems, assessing a patient for psychiatric disorders involves taking a history, performing a physical examination, and obtaining diagnostic tests, as directed. Central to your success in assessing a patient for psychiatric disorders is your ability to view the patient holistically, to identify and organize pertinent data, and to communicate well.

Psychiatric history

The most important component of your assessment for psychiatric disorders is the patient history. Because the lingering stigma of mental illness may make your patient reluctant to talk, make sure to convey openness, empathy, and a non-judgmental attitude during your interview. (See *Conducting a psychiatric assessment.*)

By American Psychiatric Association standards, a formal psychiatric assessment takes more than an hour to complete and may require several interview sessions. In a busy physician's office or hospital, however, where the emphasis may not be on psychiatric issues, you can obtain substantial data about a patient's mental health by performing a focused interview that lasts just 5 or 10 minutes.

Naturally, your interview with the patient should be private. Before you start, however, consider talking briefly with both patient and family members. A patient's loved ones may help you validate information, or they may aid the patient's recall of certain events or feelings. After questioning family members generally and briefly, ask them to leave the room so you can be alone with the patient.

During your private interview, ask the patient how he has been feeling. Ask whether he has felt sad or down. In contrast, ask whether he feels wound up or unable to focus. Inquire about changes in his sleeping habits, his eating patterns, and his ability to function normally at work, home, or school. Ask about changes in his leisure activities as well. Other fruitful areas of inquiry may include questions about lack of energy, lack of pleasure, recurring negative thoughts, recent losses, suspicion, panic episodes, odd perceptions, and suicidal, homicidal, or delusional ideas.

Ask about a family history of mental illness, previous psychiatric treatment, drug and alcohol use, head injuries, and past violent behavior. Get a list of the patient's prescribed and over-the-counter (OTC) drugs, including herbal remedies and vitamin supplements.

Also, ask the patient to describe his previous and current performance at his job or school; doing so will give you an idea of the degree to which a psychiatric disorder has affected his daily function—or the degree to which a physical disorder may be affecting his mental health.

Suicide risk

If you think your patient may have a psychiatric disorder, assess his suicide risk. During your assess-

Conducting a psychiatric assessment

Your success at conducting a psychiatric assessment depends greatly on your skill as an empathetic, nonjudgmental interviewer. Use these tips to help set the tone of your interview and build trust with your patient.

Convey respect
Explain that you think emotional issues are an important part of a person's overall health. Tell the patient that you'd like to help with these issues if he has the need. Assure the patient that all information about him will remain confidential within his network of health care providers.

Ask simple, clear questions
Investigate the patient's mental health using open-ended questions when possible.

Let the patient talk
When the patient answers your questions, don't interrupt him. Also, minimize outside interruptions during your session. Give the patient time to tell you what he's thinking and feeling. Ask probing but gentle questions to clarify his statements.

Watch for important side issues
If the patient brings up what seems to be an unrelated issue, consider that it may not be unrelated at all. In fact, it may hold the key to an underlying problem. As appropriate, question the patient about side issues.

Clarify contradictions
If you notice conflicts or contradictions in what the patient says, ask for more information. By doing so, you can help to clarify what he means and resolve these seemingly conflicting points.

Carefully confront
If you feel that the patient has misinterpreted something or that he may benefit from a different view of reality, present a different interpretation of an issue and assess the patient's response.

Be genuine
By your words, your attitude, and your attention to the interview, let your patient know that you're concerned about the issues he has raised.

Repeat important points
To help clarify your assessment findings and convey your involvement in the patient's issues, repeat the main points of your conversation. Encourage the patient to refine or clarify the points as you outline them.

ment, listen for covert suicide messages, subtle death wishes, or outright statements, such as, "I'd be better off dead." Find out whether the patient exhibits suicide warning signs, such as withdrawal, social isolation, making farewells to friends and family, putting his affairs in order, or giving away prized possessions. And consider the applicability of the risk factors included in the suicide-risk mnemonic SAD PERSONS:

- **S**ex male
- **A**ge adolescent or elderly
- **D**epression
- **P**revious attempts
- **R**ational thought lost

- Social support lost
- Organized plan
- No spouse
- Sick.

Mental status examination

Although a mental status examination isn't a standard part of the patient history, it is an appropriate tool to use if you think your patient may have a psychiatric disorder—especially if you practice in a primary care setting. You can use the mental status examination to assess your patient's appearance, behavior, attitude, mood, affect, speech, thought pattern, and cognition.

Appearance

Note the patient's physical attributes, such as grooming, clothing, and posture. Are they appropriate to the setting? Consider the patient's fingernails, hair, and clothes. Are they clean and neat? Overall, does the patient's appearance seem within normal limits?

Behavior

Observe the patient's mannerisms and gestures. Does he fidget? Twitch? Grimace? Does he tremble or startle? Can he participate normally in your conversation?

Attitude

Does the patient's attitude seem appropriately cooperative and interactive? Be especially careful when answering this question because attitude is an attribute that's easy to misinterpret. Attitude norms can vary widely based on cultural influence, so stay particularly alert for cultural bias on your part that could lead you to an erroneous conclusion about your patient's attitude. Assessment of a patient as cooperative, rude, distant, or evasive, for example, must be done in the context of culturally defined, socially acceptable behaviors.

Mood

Mood refers to a sustained emotional state that can strongly influence a person's personality and outlook on life. Try to assess and document your patient's mood as specifically as possible. Does he seem depressed, anxious, angry, elated?

Affect

Affect refers to the expression of emotions. Usually, you'll describe your patient's affect as normal, blunted, or flat. If your patient has a normal affect, you'll observe a normal range of facial expressions, gestures, and voice inflections. If he has a blunted affect, you'll note a diminished emotional response and a reduced range of expressions. And if he has a flat affect, you'll see little or no emotional response to situations in which you'd expect a response.

Speech

Note the manner, rate, and quality of the patient's speech.

Thought pattern

As you converse with the patient, consider whether his thoughts are logical and ordered. Does he describe delusions? Does he have suicidal or homicidal ideas? If possible, ask family members to validate the accuracy of information the patient gives you.

Cognition

Finally, note whether the patient has insight into his situation and can abstract. Document any impairments in registration, recall, and recent or remote memory.

Specialized tools

For certain patients, you may want to consider using specialized assessment tools. For instance, the Folstein Mini-Mental Health State Exam helps to measure cognition in adults. It addresses memory, concentration, judgment, and attention. It doesn't address mood or thought processes. (See *Elements of the Folstein Mini-Mental Health State Exam*, page 8.)

Other tools can help you assess specific disorders, clinical situations, or age groups. For example, the Beck Depression Inventory helps assess patients who may be depressed. The HANDS tool (also known as the Harvard Department of Psychiatry/National Screening Day Scale) allows rapid screening for depression; it's used most often at health fairs and other public events. The History, Clinical and Risk Management tool helps assess a patient who may have an increased risk for violence. And the Child Behavior Checklist helps assess mental status among pediatric patients.

No matter which specialized tool you choose, remember that you first need adequate training in how to administer it properly. Obviously, performing a test incorrectly can lead not only to an inaccurate diagnosis but to ineffective or even harmful treatment. Indeed, you may want to refer selected patients to a clinical psychologist to ensure accurate use of specialized tools.

If you choose to perform specialized tests on your own, always take a moment first to make sure the patient has adequate vision, hearing, and language skills to understand and respond to your questions. In some cases, you may also need to verify that the patient can read and that he understands basic math. If a patient can't read or doesn't speak English, consider administering written tests orally and in the patient's primary language.

Physical examination

When you turn to the physical exam portion of your assessment, keep in mind that psychiatric problems can create or aggravate physical problems, and that physical problems can create or aggravate psychiatric ones. Also, don't forget that drug allergies, reactions, or interactions may lie at the root of some seemingly psychiatric problems, especially if the patient takes multiple drugs.

As you start your exam, briefly explain the steps you'll be taking, so the patient knows what to expect. Make sure to present your explanation in a manner that won't increase anxiety in a patient who may already be anxious or afraid. Throughout your exam, listen and look for issues that could cause or be caused by psychiatric problems, such as headaches, respiratory problems, cardiovascular (CV) disorders, changes in gastrointestinal (GI) function, reproductive ailments, and musculoskeletal discomforts.

Elements of the Folstein Mini-Mental Health State Exam

The Folstein Mini-Mental Health State Exam allows you to quickly assess a patient's cognitive function using standardized questions. You can complete the assessment in just 5 or 10 minutes, and you can use it repeatedly to help track a patient's cognition over time. It includes five major areas: orientation, registration, attention and calculation, recall, and language.

Orientation
This section of the test contains 2 multi-part questions. Give the patient 1 point for each correct answer, for a possible total of 10 points.
- What is the date? The year? The day of the week? The month? The season of the year?
- What state are we in? County? Town? Hospital? Floor?

Registration
For this section, name three unrelated objects. Speak clearly and slowly, taking about 1 second for each one. Then ask the patient to repeat the names, giving him 1 point for each correct answer. If necessary, repeat the three names until he can list them correctly. Document the number of times you had to repeat the list before the patient could do so.

Attention and calculation
Ask the patient to count backward by 7s, starting with 100. Give him 1 point for each of the first 5 correct answers (93, 86, 79, 72, and 65), and then tell him to stop. An alternative approach is to ask him to spell a 5-letter word backwards, giving him 1 point for each letter in the correct location.

Recall
Now ask the patient if he can remember the three objects you named earlier in the test. Give him 1 point for every correct answer.

Language
This section contains 6 commands and a possible total of 9 points.
- Show the patient a wristwatch and ask him what it is. Then show him a pencil and ask what it is. (2 points)
- Ask the patient to repeat a sentence or phrase after you say it, such as, "No ifs, ands, or buts." (1 point)
- Ask the patient to complete a three-stage command, such as, "Pick up a piece of paper, tear it in half, and place the pieces on the floor." (3 points)
- Give the patient a piece of paper on which you've written, "Close your eyes." Ask him to do what it says on the paper. (1 point)
- Give the patient a blank piece of paper, and ask him to write a sentence. (1 point)
- Show the patient a diagram of two intersecting pentagrams, and ask him to copy it exactly. (1 point)

Now add up the patient's score. Normal people average 27 to 30. Depressed people who don't have dementia average about 24 to 27. If the patient scores 20 or below, he probably has dementia, delirium, schizophrenia, or an affective disorder. Finally, document the patient's level of consciousness on a continuum that includes alert, drowsy, stupor, and coma.

Headache

Many people who are depressed or anxious complain of headaches. However, headaches can stem from a myriad of other influences as well. Before making a connection between a patient's headaches and his mental state, consider the other possible causes.

For instance, migraine headaches commonly result from a reaction to sulfites in certain types of wine, beer, cheese, and dried fruits. Certain allergies can trigger headaches as well. If removing some or all of these trigger factors reduces the frequency or severity of the patient's headaches, you can help to reduce the patient's depression or anxiety while ruling out these psychiatric problems as the cause of the headaches.

As you know, headaches can occasionally result from serious medical problems, such as a brain tumor, cranial bleeding, or head injuries. As directed, obtain a computed tomography scan to rule out these problems.

Respiratory problems

Respiratory illnesses provide good examples of physical disorders that associate strongly with psychiatric disorders. For instance, anxiety and depression can lead to hyperventilation. They also raise the likelihood that a patient smokes. Smoking, in turn, raises the risk of chronic obstructive pulmonary disease and asthma. Both of these disorders can cause or worsen anxiety by interfering with the patient's ability to breathe. And both can cause or worsen depression by interfering with the patient's energy level and ability to perform activities of daily living.

Cardiovascular disorders

CV disorders may associate strongly with psychiatric disorders as well. For example, many patients develop depression in the wake of a myocardial infarction, cardiac surgery, or a cerebrovascular accident; it may stem from the patient's enhanced awareness of mortality, from impaired physical function, and probably for other reasons we have yet to understand.

Also, keep in mind that arrhythmias, tachycardia, and palpitations may be related to anxiety. In fact, a screening electrocardiogram may be appropriate to rule out arrhythmias and to provide baseline measurements if the patient receives a prescription for a psychotropic drug that has cardiac effects. Make sure to question the patient about his consumption of caffeine and drugs (prescription, OTC, herbal, and illicit) that could affect his cardiac status.

Gastrointestinal focus

An inordinate focus on body functioning can be a symptom of depression and anxiety. If the patient complains of GI dysfunction, assess whether he really does have a problem or whether his discomfort results from being overly focused on his digestive system.

Make sure to rule out important causes of GI dysfunction, such as diabetes, cancer, and hyperacidity. Also, find out which prescription, OTC, herbal, and illicit drugs the patient takes to help identify possible causes of constipation, diarrhea, gastric upset, and other GI problems.

Reproductive changes
Sexual dysfunction commonly causes or is caused by depression. Likewise, menstrual irregularities may be related to depression. They also may stem from another psychiatric problem more common among girls and young women: anorexia nervosa.

Musculoskeletal discomfort
Aches and pains may result from anxiety and depression, or they may cause anxiety and depression. This result is especially common when the pain of arthritic joints is inadequately controlled.

Laboratory tests
As directed, obtain laboratory tests needed to rule out physical conditions that could be misdiagnosed as psychiatric conditions. Common laboratory tests for this purpose include:
- complete blood count
- blood chemistry with electrolytes
- blood urea nitrogen
- creatinine level
- glucose level
- liver function tests
- thyroid function tests
- B_{12} levels for elderly patients.

DIAGNOSIS

Naturally, the assignment and documentation of a diagnosis sets the course of a patient's care. Keep in mind, however, that a psychiatric diagnosis can have negative consequences as well as the positive ones that result from successful treatment. For example, because of the stigma of mental illness, a psychiatric diagnosis may label a patient as unstable, unfit, even unemployable—for life. It may result in denied health insurance, denied life insurance, and negative publicity if the patient leads a public life. Perhaps more than with any other category of illnesses, you must be absolutely sure of your findings before documenting a psychiatric diagnosis in a patient's permanent medical record.

If you do need to document such a diagnosis, you may do so in several different ways. For instance, you may use the multiaxial system to describe a psychiatric problem. It includes five axes or domains to systematically and comprehensively evaluate a patient and document an illness. (See *Understanding the axial system*.)

You almost certainly will also use the diagnostic standards laid out in the *Diagnostic and Statistical Manual of Mental Disorders*, commonly known as the *DSM-IV*. This system was developed for use in clinical practice, educational settings, and research studies to help clinicians communicate psychiatric diagnostic labels clearly and efficiently.

Historically, many different nomenclatures have been used to classify behavioral and mental conditions and diagnoses, including the Guze, Hamilton, Kielholz, Kraepelin, Leonhard, Robins, Schneider, and Winokur systems. However, little research has been completed to compare these systems with each other. The most common international system of nomenclature for psychiatric disorders (and reimbursement for their treatment) has become the ICD-10. An analogous system is used to describe and justify insurance reimbursement for physical disorders.

TREATMENT

Typically, obtaining treatment for a patient with a psychiatric disorder presents more obstacles than obtaining treatment for a patient with a physical disorder of similar severity—particularly when the proposed treatment involves a costly psychiatric specialist. That's largely because many managed health care plans limit or even exclude psychiatric treatments from their covered benefits.

Health plans that do include coverage for psychiatric disorders usually require that patients meet certain criteria before treatment services are authorized. Unfortunately, these criteria may be designed more to limit plan expenditures than to maximize treatment success. Dollar limits for psychiatric treatment are common in managed care, even when patients meet the plan's criteria for symptoms and intensity levels. Even in states where legislation demands a certain level of covered inpatient and outpatient care for people with mental illnesses, those with chronic conditions usually exhaust their limited benefits.

These restrictions on covered care stem at least in part from our limited success in treating some forms of mental illness in the days before effective psychotropic drugs became available. These days, effective drugs can be prescribed alone or in combination with other

Understanding the axial system

The *Diagnostic and Statistical Manual of Mental Disorders* uses an axial system for describing and documenting psychiatric diagnoses. Each axis addresses a specific area of assessment.

- **Axis I** refers to diagnoses of mood disorders, dementia, eating disorders, sexual disorders, sleep abnormalities, substance abuse, and other psychiatric disorders.
- **Axis II** refers to personality disorders and mental retardation. Personality disorders commonly linked to other mental disorders, such as borderline, schizoid, and paranoid disorders, are reported here.
- **Axis III** refers to general medical conditions. As discussed elsewhere in this chapter, many physical illnesses can be linked with psychiatric disorders.
- **Axis IV** refers to interpersonal relationship problems, psychosocial behavioral difficulties, and environmental issues related to a patient's psychiatric disorders.
- **Axis V** uses the global assessment of functioning (GAF) scale to measure psychological, social, and occupational functional ability. The GAF score can range from 1 to 100.

therapies to maximize the success of treatment. (See *Lighting the way*, page 12.) For example, psychotherapy is a common approach for many types of mental disorders. And certain patients may benefit

Lighting the way

Some of the newest and most successful psychotropic drugs relieve depression by altering levels of serotonin in the brain. For more than a decade, however, physicians have been treating one type of serotonin-related disorder with nothing more than a bright light. Known as seasonal affective disorder, it's a form of depression that develops during the winter, probably from decreased exposure to sunlight. For this disorder, bright light therapy may act something like a psychotropic drug. It probably enhances the action of serotonin; it probably also affects the patient's circadian rhythm.

Recent improvements

In the 1980s, the boxes used to deliver bright light therapy caused such adverse effects as hypomania, irritability, headache, and nausea. Head-mounted units with incandescent lights inside caused eyestrain

and a "wired" feeling. These days, bright light therapy is delivered in clinical settings using a professionally designed, 10,000 lux, ultraviolet shielded, diffused white fluorescent light from a downward-angled box. Patients typically receive 30 minutes twice daily for 14 days or longer.

This redesigned system still causes some adverse effects, including headaches, blurred vision, other vision changes, nausea, and drowsiness. However, these effects are becoming less common as light boxes are improved. And unlike some antidepressant drugs, which have a delayed onset of action, bright light therapy starts lifting the symptoms of depression in just a week. Patients with bipolar disease or nonseasonal depression may benefit from bright light therapy as well; they commonly receive concurrent treatment with a mood stabilizer.

from new techniques in electroconvulsive therapy (ECT).

Psychotherapy

Before psychotropic drugs were available, interpersonal psychotherapy formed the foundation of treatment for psychiatric disorders. Today, it continues to occupy a substantial role in the treatment regimens of many patients with psychiatric disorders.

Psychotherapy includes three phases. In the first phase, which lasts one to three sessions, the therapist does a diagnostic review, takes the patient's history, and details the patient's interpersonal relationships and patterns of social functioning.

In the second phase, which can last a highly variable amount of time, the therapist focuses on resolving problems in one of four interpersonal problem areas: grief, role conflict, role transitions, or interpersonal deficits. In the third phase, which also takes a variable amount of time, the therapist aims to define gains made through treatment and to prevent relapse.

Partly because of pressure from managed care plans, psychotherapy services are limited or denied for the many patients known as the *worried well*—those with relatively mild disorders. For these patients, the health plan may cover brief psychotherapy lasting only six or sometimes only three visits. Naturally, a patient who can afford to pay for treatment out of pocket can have as much psychotherapy as the prescriber recommends; however, many patients are unable or unwilling to bear this financial burden.

Patients with severe chronic mental illnesses who can't afford to pay for psychotherapy sometimes can receive it and other psychiatric treatments from community mental health centers known as community support programs. Their comprehensive model of treatment integrates the services of multidisciplinary team members in the context of the patient's work or home environment. The focus of psychotherapy in this case is to help the patient cope with a severe psychiatric disorder while continuing to be a functional, employed member of the community.

Drug therapy

In recent years, psychotropic drugs have assumed the central role in many psychiatric treatment regimens. Where once these drugs were prescribed almost exclusively by psychiatrists, they now may be prescribed by physicians and advanced practice nurses of all specialties—commonly by family practice and other primary care providers. This wider prescribing pattern results partly from managed care's increased reliance on primary care providers rather than specialists. It also stems from the development of more and better psychotropic drugs that have fewer and milder adverse effects.

Other influences have played a role in the expansion of psychotropic drugs as well. For example, drug makers are now free to advertise their products directly to consumers. Besides raising awareness about the availability of psychotropic drugs, these ads may also make patients more comfortable in seeking medical care for emotional and mental health issues. The Internet provides an even more detailed resource for both patients and professionals. Sources of medical and drug information—some sponsored by drug companies—are expanding almost daily.

This combination of safer and more effective drugs, increased demand driven by consumer advertising, and increased drug information available via the Internet has greatly increased the number of psychotropic drugs being prescribed. Consequently, because more of your patients than ever will be taking these drugs, you'll need to be ever more vigilant about compliance, adverse effects, and drug interactions.

Compliance

As with all drugs, the success of a patient's treatment with a psychotropic drug depends largely on the patient's compliance with therapy. Many factors can influence a patient's compliance, including adverse effects caused by the drug, the patient's perceived need for the drug, the perceived effectiveness of the drug, and any lingering stigma among family and friends about taking a drug for a mental health problem.

Support and encouragement from health care professionals and the patient's family can do much to foster compliance. Remember, however, that you'll need the patient's permission to involve family members in the treatment plan.

Adverse effects

All psychotropic drugs have adverse effects. To help maintain patient compliance, talk about known adverse effects up front, before the patient starts taking a prescribed drug. Discuss ways to manage or minimize the drug's adverse effects. If those effects tend to subside with continued therapy, emphasize that point when talking with the patient.

The key to discussing adverse effects effectively lies in the level of detail you undertake. Don't alarm or confuse the patient with an exhaustive litany of possible effects. In contrast, don't gloss over probable adverse effects that could worry the patient, affect compliance, or indicate a need for follow-up. Make sure you present information at a level the patient can understand. And encourage the patient to call you about any adverse effects that bother or concern him. Finally, document your discussion of adverse effects and the patient's response.

Drug interactions

Interactions are common, especially among patients who take several drugs. At particular risk of drug interactions is the patient who receives prescriptions from several different prescribers without giving each prescriber a complete list of his prescribed, OTC, and herbal medications and dietary supplements.

When assembling such a list for a patient, try to avoid relying on the patient's memory of the drugs he takes. Instead, at the time he makes an appointment, ask him to either bring a list with him or bring the actual drug bottles.

In general, drug interactions occur when one drug enhances or inhibits the activity of another drug or substance in the body. For example, certain drugs, when given with certain psychotropic drugs, may change the metabolic activity of a set of liver enzymes known as cytochrome P-450 (CYP 450) isoenzymes. A range of serious problems may result, such as increased bleeding time, central nervous system toxicity, and life-threatening cardiac arrhythmias.

Because a substantial number of drugs can lead to CYP 450 interactions, you'll need to stay vigilant whenever a patient takes a psychotropic drug along with other drugs. Check with a pharmacist about possible interactions in the patient's drug regimen. Also, stay current with new drug data via written and computerized literature and continuing education. When drugs first come on the market, the only interaction data available about them comes from premarket clinical trials. The longer the drug stays on the market, however, the more data may become available about its performance and its potential for interactions in actual clinical settings.

Also, keep in mind that a drug interaction may result from more than simply the patient's multidrug regimen. For instance, the ability to metabolize CYP 450 isoenzymes has a genetic component; in particular, Asians and Caucasians may have some impairments in metabolizing certain CYP 450 isoenzymes. Smoking can also affect CYP 450 metabolism.

Because CYP 450 and other interactions may have various causes, you'll need to carefully monitor your patient's response to therapy and stay constantly alert for adverse reactions. If they occur, remember that the Food and Drug Administration has a formal procedure for reporting adverse drug reactions. Information gained from these reports is investigated and shared with clinicians. In some cases, drugs have been taken off the market based on new information submitted by clinicians.

Electroconvulsive therapy

For certain patients with depression or rapid-cycling bipolar disorders, ECT can be a safe and effective component of the overall treatment regimen. Some patients may receive it as an outpatient procedure. Typically, it's reserved for patients who haven't responded to drug treatment.

Decades ago, ECT was known as shock therapy and was performed with the patient awake. Now it's performed under general anesthesia in a surgical suite by highly trained doctors and nurses acting under the direct supervision of a psychiatrist. The anesthesia helps to prevent injuries and keeps the patient from consciously experiencing the procedure.

Most patients receive 6 to 12 treatments. Preparation for ECT is similar to that for surgery and includes a preoperative history and laboratory tests. The patient's psychiatrist is responsible for obtaining the patient's informed consent.

To perform ECT, a specially trained psychiatrist (assisted by an anesthesiologist or a nurse anesthetist) produces a controlled unilateral or bilateral seizure by applying electrical current to the anesthetized patient's head. No one knows exactly how ECT works, but the seizure it causes may enhance serotonin production in the brain. The risks of ECT are similar to those of general anesthesia and include CV changes and confusion.

Naturally, virtually all forms of treatment for psychiatric disorders carry some level of risk. But with astute assessment, precise diagnosis, and a well-crafted and carefully monitored treatment regimen, patients with psychiatric disorders can look forward to maximum therapeutic success with minimum risk.

References

Ablon, J. S., and Jones, E. E. "Psychotherapy Process in the National Institute of Mental Health Treatment of Depression Collaborative Research Program," *Journal of Consulting and Clinical Psychology* 67(1):64-75, February, 1999.

Alderman, C. P. "Patient-Oriented Strategies for the Prevention of Drug Interactions," *Drug Safety* 22(2):103-9, February, 1999.

Baer-Jacobs, D., et al. "Development of a Brief Screening Instrument: The HANDS," *Psychotherapy and Psychosomatics* 69(1): 35-41, 2000.

Barkham, M., et al. "Psychotherapy in Two-Plus-One Sessions: Outcomes of a Randomized Controlled Trial of Cognitive-Behavioral and Psychodynamic-Interpersonal Therapy for Subsyndromal Depression," *Journal of Consulting and Clinical Psychology* 67(2):201-11, April, 1999.

Bilenburg, N. "The Child Behavior Checklist (CBCL) and Related Material: Standardization and Validation in Danish Population Based and Clinically Based Samples," *Acta Psychiatrica Scandinavica* 100:2-52, 1999.

Diagnostic and Statistical Manual of Mental Disorders, 4th ed. Washington, D.C.: American Psychiatric Association, 1994.

Diamond, S., and Moore, K. L. "Chronic Headaches and Depression," *Consultations in Primary Care* 40(1):81-93, 2000.

Furukawa, T., et al. "A Polydiagnostic Study of Depressive Disorders According to DSM-IV and 23 Classical Diagnostic Systems," *Psychiatry and Neurosciences* 53:387-96, June, 1999.

The ICD-10 Classification of Mental and Behavioral Disorders: Diagnostic Criteria for Research. Geneva: World Health Organization, 1993.

Jackson, J. L., et al. "Effects of Physician Awareness of Symptom-Related Expectations and Mental Disorders," *Archives of Family Medicine* 8:135-42, March-April, 1999.

Kampman, O., and Lehtinen, K. "Compliance in Psychoses," *Acta Psychiatrica Scandinavica* 100:167-75, September, 1999.

Kates, N., and Craven, M. *Managing Mental Health Problems: A Practical Guide for Primary Care.* Kirkland, Washington: Hogrefe & Huber Publishers, 1998.

Penn, D. L., et al. "Dispelling the Stigma of Schizophrenia: The Impact of Information on Dangerousness," *Schizophrenia Bulletin* 25(3):437-46, 1999.

Sakamoto, A., et al. "Effects of Propofol Anesthesia on Cognitive Therapy of Patients Undergoing Electroconvulsive Therapy," *Psychiatry and Neurosciences* 53:655-60, December, 1999.

Saunders, C. "A Form-Free Evaluation," *Patient Care for the Nurse Practitioner* 2(8):17-33, August, 1999.

Someya, T., et al. "The Effect of Cytochrome P450 2D6 Genotypes on Haloperidol Metabolism: A Preliminary Study in a Psychiatric Population," *Psychiatry and Clinical Neurosciences* 53:593-97, October, 1999.

Spiegel, D. "Healing Words: Emotional Expression and Disease Outcome," *Journal of The American Medical Association* 281:1328-29, April 14, 1999.

Systematic Assessment for Treatment of Emergent Effects (SAFTEE). Rockville, MD: National Institutes of Mental Health, November, 1986.

Terman, M. and Terman J.S. "Bright Light Therapy: Side Effects and Benefits Across the Symptom Spectrum," *Journal of Clinical Psychiatry* 60(11):799-808, 1999.

Wahl, O. "Mental Health Consumer's Experience of Stigma," *Schizophrenia Bulletin* 25(3):467-78, 1999.

Webster, C. D., et al. *The HCR-20 Scheme: The Assessment of Dangerousness and Risk.* Vancouver, British Columbia, Canada: Simon Frazer University and Psychiatric Services Commission of British Columbia, 1995.

Wolpert, E. A., and Berman, V. "Efficacy of Electroconvulsive Therapy in Continuous Rapid Cycling of Bipolar Disorder," *Psychiatric Annals* 29(12):679-83, 1999.

CHAPTER 2

Working with special populations

In theory, psychotropic drugs exert predictable effects on a patient's mental state. In practice, however, you know that the effects of psychotropic drugs—like all drugs—can vary somewhat based on a host of patient characteristics. In that sense, each patient represents her own "special population" because of her unique set of genetic, physiologic, environmental, and therapeutic variables.

In a larger sense, however, you're also wise to think of certain groups of patients as special populations when it comes to drug therapy. Why? Largely because characteristics of the entire group may foster drug effects that vary somewhat from those documented during the original clinical trials.

The fact is that, during clinical testing, researchers have traditionally tried to minimize variables among study subjects as a means to help define a drug's effects. In other words, they tried to keep the study subjects as homogenous as possible. Many such studies involved medical students, who most often were healthy, young, white men. Likewise, many clinical trials intentionally excluded women, people of color, people who already took drugs, and people with chronic illnesses, such as hypertension, heart disease, and renal impairment.

Patient variables

Although clinical drug trials these days tend to include a wider range of patients than they did in the past, the principle still holds. Clinical practice presents a much wider set of patient variables than even a diverse clinical trial. Especially among certain groups of patients—such as pregnant women, unborn children, newborn children, adolescents, and elderly people—the pharmacokinetics, drug effects, and risks of drug therapy may differ from those that occur in a more controlled laboratory setting. (See *Elements of pharmacokinetics*, pages 20 and 21.)

To maximize the safety and effectiveness of psychotropic drug therapy among these special populations, take the following steps:
- Cultivate an up-to-the-minute knowledge of the drugs you administer.
- Carefully study each drug's packaging information and the information presented in reputable drug references.
- Seek out new data specific to the drug's effects on special populations.
- Assess patients frequently enough to quickly detect and respond to unexpected adverse effects.
- Anticipate the possibility of unexpected drug effects or reactions.

Elements of pharmacokinetics

A drug's pharmacokinetics (its effect on physiologic function) stems from four principles: absorption, distribution, metabolism, and excretion.

Absorption

The easier a drug crosses membranes, the faster it can act. In other words, drugs that are absorbed quickly and systemically take effect faster than drugs absorbed topically and locally. It follows, then, that intravenous administration typically yields the fastest drug effects. Transdermal administration typically yields the slowest drug effects.

Keep in mind, however, that most drugs are administered through the gastrointestinal tract. Here, absorption rates can vary widely based on the presence of food or other drugs, such as antacids. Also, remember that women have slower gastric emptying times and lower gastric acid secretion than men.

Distribution

After being absorbed, the drug can be distributed systemically. Some drugs are distributed by binding with a substance that circulates through the body, such as lipid, albumin, or serum. Other drugs—such as lithium—require a certain level of body fluids to work therapeutically. Dehydration can raise lithium levels and may raise the risk of adverse effects.

In certain populations, drug distribution may be altered. For instance, pregnant women and infants have higher amounts of circulating body fluids than elderly patients do. Older adults have lower amounts of albumin than other age groups.

What's more, in infants and elderly people, the blood-brain barrier is less effective than it is in young and middle-aged adults. By allowing indirect access to brain tissue, the increased permeability of the blood-brain barrier may cause difficulty when you're giving psychotropic drugs to elderly patients and infants.

Metabolism

Although some drugs aren't metabolized at all and pass through the body unchanged, others are metabolized (or biotransformed) into metabolites or other chemical forms. In fact, some drugs produce no therapeutic effect until they undergo first-pass transformation into metabolites. The body responds to those metabolites on the second pass, after they recirculate through the body.

Various patient characteristics may alter a drug's effects at the metabolism stage. For instance, consumption of certain foods—such as cabbage, Brussels sprouts, or grapefruit juice—can reduce the bioavailability of beta blockers, calcium antagonist blockers, cyclosporins, and some other drugs before absorption. High levels of dietary salt can increase first-pass elimination of quinidine, resulting in less circulating drug.

Many drugs are metabolized in the liver (or sometimes the intestinal villi) by the cytochrome P-450 (CYP 450) isoenzyme system before being absorbed into systemic circulation. The CYP 450 system is probably the body's way of detoxifying harmful substances. Fluoxetine, paroxetine, sertraline, and numerous other psychotropic drugs are metabolized by the CYP 450 system as well. Metabolism may take place via several pathways, and it may be

Elements of pharmacokinetics *(continued)*

inhibited or enhanced by drug and nondrug substances. Nicotine and caffeine exert a stimulating effect, for example.

Excretion

After some drugs are metabolized, they're excreted into bile, transferred back into the intestine, and then reabsorbed from the intestine back into systemic circulation, a process that extends the drug's half-life. Eventually, however, most drugs are excreted by the kidneys. Thus, safe excretion of drugs depends on adequate kidney function. If kidney function is impaired by advanced age or chronic illness, the level of circulating drug may increase, leading to adverse effects.

- Stress the importance of taking a drug exactly as prescribed.
- Urge patients to talk with you or the prescriber about any worrisome reactions.
- Involve family members in monitoring a patient's response to a drug, if appropriate.
- Report adverse drug reactions, as mandated by the Food and Drug Administration (FDA).

Besides these crucial steps, also work to understand important characteristics particular to each of the special populations included in this chapter—characteristics that could affect or be affected by psychotropic drug therapy. By doing so, you can maximize the effectiveness of psychotropic drug therapy while safeguarding your patients from predictable adverse effects.

WOMEN

As a group, women experience more mental health disorders than men, including depression, anxiety, panic disorder, bipolar disorder, and eating disorders. Evidence also suggests that women have higher rates of schizophrenia, sensitivity to alcohol, and dementia of the Alzheimer's type.

Besides developing more mental illnesses than men, women tend to face more socioeconomic stresses than men—stresses that can worsen mental illness. For instance, women are more likely to live in poverty than men, largely because more women bear the responsibility of raising children.

Women of color face perhaps the highest risk levels. Although this group represents about 27% of the female population in the United States, it made up about half of the 19 million uninsured people in the U.S. in 1995. Lack of health insurance and barriers to health care can leave these women unable or unwilling to obtain health care in a timely manner, which allows diseases—and stress levels—to progress in them and their children.

Pregnancy

Several pregnancy-related issues can affect women who need psychotropic drug therapy. For one thing, certain psychotropic drugs can reduce fertility. For another, these drugs may harm a developing fetus. Pregnancy may also correlate with increased levels of substance abuse among women with mental illnesses.

Fertility rates

Fertility rates among schizophrenic women who take traditional phenothiazine antipsychotics are reduced to 30% to 80% of the general population. That's probably because these drugs block the action of dopamine and increase prolactin levels, which may inhibit ovulation and stop menses.

However, women who take newer antipsychotics face no such risk of decreased fertility. And women who switch from older antipsychotics to newer ones may face an increased and possibly unwanted risk of getting pregnant. These effects of the newer, atypical antipsychotics (such as clozapine, olanzapine, and quetiapine, which are commonly called "novel" antipsychotics) stem from the fact that these drugs don't seem to change prolactin levels. Consequently, they don't reduce fertility levels.

When caring for a female patient of childbearing age who takes an antipsychotic drug, urge her to use a reliable form of birth control. Warn her that the antipsychotic drug could harm a fetus—especially during the earliest stages of pregnancy.

Also, keep in mind that certain mental illnesses—particularly schizophrenia—are linked to a higher risk of exposure to human immunodeficiency virus (HIV) in women of childbearing age. Women with schizophrenia also have higher rates of induced abortions, sponta-

neous abortions, and stillbirths. And they have an increased risk of child custody problems, a situation that can increase the risk of psychotic symptoms.

Fetal risk

A fetus is most vulnerable to teratogenic drug effects during the first three months of gestation. Typically, the risk of these harmful effects relates largely to dose size and the stage at which the drug is given. Fetal exposure to drugs can cause intrauterine death, impaired growth, behavioral abnormalities, and neonatal toxicity. Teratogenic neurotoxic effects can continue even after birth, altering the child's learning ability, activity levels, and problem-solving ability.

Many psychotropic drugs affect fetuses and neonates. For example, if a pregnant woman takes a drug that causes physical dependence, such as a benzodiazepine, her infant will go through withdrawal shortly after birth and may develop irritability, seizures, and lethargy. If a woman takes a selective serotonin reuptake inhibitor during pregnancy, her newborn has an increased risk of serotonin syndrome. And drugs commonly prescribed in psychiatric practice, such as lithium, depakote, and older tricyclic antidepressants, have been strongly linked to teratogenic effects. (See *Depression in pregnancy: Tough treatment choices.*)

Substance abuse

Women with mental illnesses may be more likely to smoke, drink excessive amounts of alcohol, and take illicit drugs during pregnancy. Smoking and excessive alcohol

Depression in pregnancy: Tough treatment choices

As a group, women of childbearing age face a high risk of depression. This risk rises especially high during and after pregnancy, a time of tremendous psychological, physiologic, and endocrine shifts. About 80% of women report mood fluctuations during the perinatal period. About 10% to 20% meet diagnostic criteria for major depression, and a lesser number develop signs of psychosis. These disorders, in order of increasing severity, are known as postpartum blues, postpartum depression, and postpartum psychosis.

To make these problems even worse, treatment can be tricky. Despite a high frequency of depression during childbearing years, treatment guidelines are sparse. Researchers disagree about which antidepressants are safe to use during pregnancy. And they disagree about what to do if a woman who takes an antidepressant gets pregnant. In fact, many women report having trouble getting drug treatment of any kind during pregnancy.

Obviously, we need more research to help establish the safety and efficacy of psychotropic drug use during pregnancy, particularly with the newer "novel" antipsychotics and antidepressants. In the meantime, however, women who choose not to take these drugs during pregnancy will have to rely on alternative treatment options, such as intensive psychotherapy, family therapy, therapeutic massage, biofeedback, and bright light therapy. As a clinician, you'll need to help balance the risks of drug therapy with the severity of the patient's symptoms and the efficacy of alternative treatments.

---

consumption may lead to low birth weights, reduced cognitive abilities, and behavioral effects in children.

The use of illicit drugs, such as cocaine, during pregnancy has produced decreased head circumference, decreased coping skills, and an impaired attention span in offspring. Fetuses exposed to the illicit drug known as ecstasy may develop congenital defects, cardiovascular anomalies, and musculoskeletal deformities.

Breast-feeding

Little research exists on the effects of psychotropic drugs during breast-feeding. But although no evidence exists to support the use of psychotropic drugs while breast-feeding, scientists are convinced that breast-feeding holds emotional benefits for both mother and child. That's why the American Academy of Pediatrics doesn't preclude the use of psychotropic drugs in nursing mothers.

The idea is to choose a psychotropic drug that helps to restore or maintain the mother's well-being, an effect that presumably will yield benefits for the newborn as well. When weighing the probable effects of a psychotropic drug during breast-feeding, evaluate all available research and information, discuss the pros and cons of the proposed drug with your patient, and make sure that the patient can make a fully informed choice.

CHILDREN

Caring for a child with a mental or behavioral disorder is highly complex and requires expertise in dealing with issues of normal development, developmental delays, family dynamics, unique responses to environmental toxins (such as lead), learning disabilities, and much more. As for all patients with psychiatric disorders, care for a child must be provided by a carefully chosen team of collaborating professionals. It may include a public health nurse, psychiatric nurse specialist, clinical psychologist, social worker, occupational therapist, pediatrician, neurologist, child psychiatrist, and others to thoroughly assess the child and intervene in a behavioral disorder.

One of the most common psychiatric diagnoses in children is attention deficit hyperactivity disorder (ADHD). The drug commonly prescribed to treat it is methylphenidate (Ritalin), an amphetamine and controlled substance. The drug has a stimulating effect on adults but a calming, sedating effect on children.

However, giving psychotropic drugs for childhood behavioral disorders is a topic of growing debate and a host of as yet unanswered questions. For example: Can and should school officials be charged with administering a controlled substance to someone else's children? What dosage is appropriate when evidence-based research has yet to establish dosing standards for children? What's the role of informed consent when the patient has yet to reach adolescence and receives a drug outside the home? Will adolescent siblings of a child who takes a psychotropic drug have an increased risk of abusing it or another psychotropic drug? Indeed, pop culture songs have advocated methylphenidate abuse.

Partly because of these questions and the lack of answers from evidence-based research, treatment patterns for ADHD vary widely. Primary care practitioners tend to prescribe stimulants, perform fewer mental health tests, and recommend fewer office visits. Psychiatrists tend to prescribe multiple drugs, perform more mental health tests, and recommend more office visits.

Besides methylphenidate, a child with ADHD may receive a tricyclic antidepressant, clonidine, or an antipsychotic. However, safe, standardized dosages haven't been established for children who take psychotropic drugs. Consequently, you should use extreme caution when giving such a drug to a child because you may not know its full range of effects.

For instance, a child with a bedwetting problem may receive a tricyclic antidepressant because one of its effects—bladder neck spasm—can cause urine retention and an improvement in bed-wetting symptoms. However, tricyclic antidepressants can also cause sedation, an effect that can worsen bedwetting by allowing the child to sleep through the urge to urinate. These drugs also raise the risk of cardiac arrhythmias and have been linked to sudden deaths in children, even with electrocardiogram monitoring and long-term therapy.

ADOLESCENTS

Adolescence is a time of turbulent physiologic and psychological change. It's so turbulent, in fact, that violent and unnatural acts are the chief causes of death. (See *Adolescence: Dangerous times.*) Some of the most common psychological problems that plague this developmental period are eating disorders and sexual risk-taking.

Eating disorders

The models and celebrities displayed in magazines, movies, and television have created an American definition of beauty that relies on exceeding thinness. As a result, most American girls (and a small percentage of boys) believe that they'll be attractive only if they can achieve a runway-model physique. In an effort to do so, they may diet relentlessly; some develop eating disorders, such as anorexia nervosa or bulimia nervosa.

Besides fostering emotional disorders, anorexia and bulimia may promote dangerous electrolyte changes and other physical problems. That's because patients with eating disorders may vomit repeatedly, exercise excessively, restrict fluids, and abuse diuretics and laxatives in an effort to control their weight. They have an increased likelihood of anxiety and depression. They may even raise their risk of diabetes by manipulating insulin levels to lose weight.

If a patient has depressive symptoms and an eating disorder, she'll likely receive an antidepressant along with psychotherapy to address her underlying issues. Keep in mind, however, that several selective serotonin reuptake inhibitors cause appetite suppression. For example, bupropion significantly enhances weight loss and shouldn't be prescribed for a patient with anorexia.

Sexual risk-taking

The blooming sexuality that marks adolescence may become entangled with a teenager's psychological problems. For instance, substance abuse, early sexual activity, sexual risk-taking, and alcohol use are all linked. The use of illicit drugs may also correlate with sexual behavior—and psychological health.

Euphoriant drugs, such as ecstasy and dextromethorphan, may be readily available at parties and may increase sexual risk-taking. Dextromethorphan (commonly called rave) has opioid properties and is a common ingredient in over-the-counter cough medicine. Ingestion of large amounts can cause ataxia, nystagmus, altered mental status, and seizures. Another drug that may be available at certain parties

---

Adolescence: Dangerous times

Each year in the United States, more adolescents die from violent or unnatural causes than from any other single cause. More than 2,000 children between ages 10 and 19 die by suicide every year. Conduct disorders, eating disorders, and concerns about body image and sexual orientation substantially increase the risk of suicide in adolescents and young adults.

is the illegal gamma-hydroxybutyric acid, also known as the "date rape" drug.

As you know, the use of alcohol and illicit drugs raises the risk not only of sexual behavior but also of sexually transmitted diseases and the emotional problems that commonly follow. Even HIV infection is becoming more common in younger people, particularly minorities, usually as a result of heterosexual sex. HIV-positive adolescents have a high lifetime risk of depression, substance abuse, and behavioral disorders.

Issues of sexual orientation also raise major risk factors for mental health disorders in adolescents and young adults. They may also increase the risk of substance abuse and unprotected sex among gay and bisexual young men. Amyl nitrite, amphetamines, cocaine, inhalants, and benzodiazepines have all been linked with unprotected homosexual intercourse.

Before administering any psychotropic drug to an adolescent, make sure to get an accurate list of all the patient's drugs, including allergy medications, vitamins, supplements, and herbal remedies. Find out if the patient takes illicit drugs or drinks alcohol regularly or excessively. And remember that drug dosages for early teens typically are calculated based on weight. Dosages for older teens typically follow adult guidelines.

ELDERLY PATIENTS

The elderly population in the U.S. is growing rapidly and is projected to continue doing so for some time into the future. Consequently, you can expect this special population to become an ever larger focus for virtually all health care professionals. (See *Who are the elderly?*)

Elderly patients are more prone to certain types of psychological problems than younger patients, such as substance abuse (usually involving prescribed drugs or alcohol), depression, agitation, and possibly psychosis. In general, the psychological problems of aging are those experienced by older women. A significant exception to this generality, however, is that older men have much higher rates of suicide compared with older women.

Elderly patients also are prone to changes in their metabolism of, reactions to, and interactions with drugs. In fact, impairments in drug metabolism, distribution, and excretion require altered dosages for many elderly patients. Plus, many older patients take several drugs at once, which raises the risk of interactions and may require changes to the patient's overall regimen. The general rule when prescribing for the elderly is "start low and go slow." Usually, elderly patients start at one-third to one-half the recommended adult dosage.

Substance abuse

Although older women have a lower risk of substance abuse than older men, they tend to turn to alcohol as the abused substance. When drinking becomes a problem with older women, it commonly does so because the person can no longer metabolize enough alcohol to maintain social drinking patterns established earlier in life. Besides typical physiologic changes, this decreased metabolism level may stem from chronic illness. It also may stem from interactions with other prescribed drugs. Older women tend to take more prescribed drugs than older men. Mixing alcohol and drugs can have serious physiologic and psychological results.

Depression

Depression is common among elderly people. Indeed, up to 31% of ill older adults who live in nursing homes or other clinical settings have signs of major depression. Even among community-dwelling older adults, about 15% have clinically significant signs of a depressed mood, about 4% have signs of major depression, and about 6.5% have a physical illness with signs of depression.

Depression may be more common when an elderly person has an additional psychiatric disorder, such as agitation or cognitive loss. In all cases, a depressed elderly patient is more likely to develop decreased functional ability, dependency, changes in lifestyle, and an accelerated need for assistive care.

Physical illnesses can cause depression as well. For example, illnesses such as Alzheimer's disease, Parkinson's disease, and cerebrovascular accidents can cause physical, mental, and financial devastation, possibly resulting in serious, even overwhelming coping problems. Untreated depression can seriously impair rehabilitation efforts, which can in turn reduce the patient's access to resources.

Identifying depression in elderly people can be a challenge because the signs and symptoms may not

> ## Who are the elderly?
>
> Because old age now has the potential to span more than 30 years of a person's life, most health care professionals have begun to think of older adults as belonging to one of three age-based categories: young old, old, or oldest old. People ages 65 to 74 are considered the young old. People ages 75 to 84 are the old. And people over age 85 are the oldest old.
>
> In this century, the group made up of the oldest old—the people most likely to need substantial health care and physical support—is projected to be the fastest growing segment of the elderly population. Further, by the year 2050, ethnic minorities will make up about one-third of the elderly population.

be as clear-cut as those in younger patients. What's more, these patients may be less willing to verbalize feelings of depression than younger patients. And elderly patients are more likely to have other illnesses and the effects of a multidrug regimen to consider.

Treatment

Treating depression in the elderly can be a challenge as well because of their coexisting illnesses and drug therapies. Thus, treatment for depression must be modified to fit the patient's medical condition, existing drug therapies, and ability to safely tolerate an added psychotropic drug.

Treatment typically lasts longer for elderly patients than for younger ones. With each episode of depression—as age, physical impairments, and functional losses accumulate—the treatment is less likely to restore the patient to her previous level of functioning. Plus, when symptoms return after a successful round of treatment ends, elderly patients may have increasing trouble responding positively to repeated treatment. For this reason, once a depressed elderly patient starts treatment, many clinicians simply plan to keep the person on antidepressant therapy long-term, unless doing so creates financial or reimbursement difficulties. Meticulous documentation and justification can help to maintain appropriate antidepressant therapy.

Keep in mind that tricyclic antidepressants have fallen out of favor for treating depression in the elderly because of these particularly hazardous adverse effects:

- Tricyclic antidepressants can cause cardiac arrhythmias.
- The tertiary amine group (which includes amitriptyline, doxepin, and imipramine) can cause oversedation, orthostasis, and significant anticholinergic effects, such as urine retention and confusion.
- Monoamine oxidase inhibitors can cause serious drug and food interactions.
- Bupropion can cause agitation and seizures in elderly patients and must be given in low doses.
- Even the new selective serotonin reuptake inhibitors and nefazodone can cause serious adverse effects, particularly cytochrome P-450 isoenzyme interactions that can be serious among elderly patients.

Agitation

Frequently, the inability of family members or caregivers to manage agitation in the home is the primary reason given for placing an elderly adult in a long-term care facility. Agitation commonly results from a combination of biological and environmental factors, and it influences the quality of life for the patient, caregivers, and other residents of the home or facility.

Treatment for agitation and anxiety in elderly people commonly involves phenothiazine-based neuroleptics, atypical neuroleptics, buspirone, trazodone, selective serotonin reuptake inhibitors, mood stabilizers, benzodiazepines, beta blockers, or cholinergic drugs. The Omnibus Budget Reconciliation Act of 1987 regulates the use of psychotropics—such as hypnotics, benzodiazepines, and antipsychotics—in long-term care facilities. Although many psychotropic drugs are available for treating agitation and anxiety, the actual drug chosen for a particular patient typically is influenced by the need to comply with regulatory guidelines.

Alzheimer's disease

Although not officially considered a psychiatric disorder, Alzheimer's disease is linked to mood disorders, psychosis, agitation, and cognitive loss. It is a nonreversible form of dementia that eventually impairs all levels of function and leads to the patient's death. (See *How Alzheimer's progresses*.) Usually, death results from an infection, such as pneumonia.

Researchers suspect that the behavioral disturbances of Alzheimer's disease may stem from increased cholinergic activity. Indeed, acetylcholinesterase inhibitors and physostigmine seem to decrease agitation and improve patients' abilities to perform activities of daily living. These two classes of drugs also showed great promise in experiments designed to test their ability to slow the progression of Alzheimer's disease. When given early in the disease, when patients have only mild cognitive impairment, the drugs preserved the patients' functional ability significantly over the results of a placebo.

Tacrine—one of the original cholinesterase inhibitors—is rarely used today because it may greatly increase liver transaminase levels. Donepezil, a second-generation cholinesterase inhibitor, doesn't seem to affect liver enzymes and is a more common choice. Other drugs that may slow the progress of Alzheimer's disease include nonsteroidal anti-inflammatory drugs, estrogen, and antioxidants, such as vitamin E. Many of these alternative drugs aren't approved by the FDA for treating Alzheimer's disease and thus can be used only on an experimental basis. Naturally, prescribing a drug for an unlabeled use has little or no research backing and may carry considerable risk for the patient.

Psychosis

Newly diagnosed psychosis is rare among elderly patients. However, patients in the later stages of Parkinson's disease or Alzheimer's disease may develop certain psychotic events, such as hallucinations and delusions.

How Alzheimer's progresses

Early stage
- Impaired memory
- Altered personality
- Difficulty recalling words
- Deterioration in judgment
- Depression or anxiety

Middle stage
- Loss of motor abilities
- Deterioration in speech
- Wandering
- Decline in social skills
- Aggression when frustrated

Late stage
- Loss of bowel and bladder function
- Hallucinations
- Shuffling gait
- Inability to follow simple commands

Elderly patients with long-standing schizophrenia or bipolar disorders probably have been taking traditional phenothiazine antipsychotics. Keep in mind that, with increased age and added chronic illnesses, the adverse effects of these drugs will increase. If so, the patient may need to switch to a newer atypical or novel antipsychotic, such as olanzapine, quetiapine, or risperidone. For safety in older patients, administer low doses as directed.

One final influence on psychological disorders among elderly patients isn't a health issue at all; it's the Health Care Financing Administration, the government agency that administers Medicare—the major source of health care reimbursement for the elderly. In short, at a time in life when psychological disorders may be more likely than ever, the resources to pay for treatment may be less available than ever.

Medicare doesn't pay for drugs, and it places severe limits on reimbursement for inpatient and outpatient psychiatric treatment. Even reimbursement for home-based care has been seriously curtailed, resulting in the closure of many home care agencies.

Because of Medicare's limited reimbursement, elderly patients may not be able to afford psychotropic drugs, which tend to be costly, even though these drugs may help to keep them more functional and out of assistive care. Plus, few Medicare-reimbursed resources are available to help monitor patients' responses to drugs in the community. These limitations in resources narrow the safety margins when treating older adults with psychiatric disorders.

For all special populations, managing psychotropic drug therapy requires clinical expertise, a wide-ranging knowledge of multiple health risks, and an up-to-date familiarity with popular culture and health policy issues. Every age group faces particular risks. By recognizing them and responding appropriately, you can help maximize the success of psychotropic drug therapy for patients of all ages.

References

Biederman, J., et al. "Pharmaco-therapy of Attention-Deficit/Hyperactivity Disorder Reduces Risk for Substance Use Disorder," *Pediatrics* 104(2):e20, August, 1999.

Birnbaum, C., et al. "Serum Concentrations of Antidepressants and Benzodiazepines in Nursing Infants: A Case Series," *Pediatrics* 104(1):11, July, 1999.

Brody, T. "Absorption, Distribution, Metabolism, and Elimination," in *Human Pharmacology: Molecular to Clinical.* Edited by Brody, T., et al. St. Louis: Mosby, 1994.

Dorian, B., and Garfinkel, P. "The Contributions of Epidemiologic Studies to the Etiology and Treatment of the Eating Disorders," *Psychiatric Annals* 29(4):187-92, 1999.

Duncan, S., et al. "Exploring Associations in Developmental Trends of Adolescent Substance Use and Risky Sexual Behavior in a High-Risk Population," *Journal of Behavioral Medicine* 22(1):21-34, 1999.

Eliason, M. J. "Identification of Alcohol-Related Problems in Older Women," *Journal of Gerontological Nursing* 24(10):8-15, October, 1998.

Empfield, M. "Pregnancy and Schizophrenia," *Psychiatric Annals* 30(1):61-66, 2000.

Felten, B. S. "Resilience in a Multicultural Sample of Community Dwelling Women Over Age 85," *Clinical Nursing Research* 9(2), May, 2000.

Frankenfield, D., et al. "Adolescent Patients-Healthy or Unhealthy," *Archives of Pediatric and Adolescent Medicine* 154(2):162-68, February, 2000.

Halbreich, U. "Evaluation of Women's Mental Health: Delineation of the Field, and Needs and Steps Toward a Consensus," *Psychopharmacology Bulletin* 34(3):247-49, 1998.

Hay, D., et al. "Use of the Newer Antidepressants in the Elderly," *Nursing Home Medicine* 5(2):28, February, 1997.

Hay, D., et al. "Treatment of Depression," *Clinics in Geriatric Medicine* 14(1):33, February, 1998.

Iqbal, M. "Effects of Antidepressants During Pregnancy and Lactation," *Annals of Clinical Psychiatry* 11(4):237-56, December, 1999.

Leigh, W., and Lindquist, M. *Women of Color Health Data Book: Adolescents to Seniors* (98-4247). Washington, DC: Office of Research on Women's Health, 1998.

McElhatton, P., et al. "Congenital Anomalies After Prenatal Ecstasy Exposure," *Lancet* 354(9188):1441-42, October, 1999.

McFee, R., et al. "Dextromethorphan: Another 'Ecstasy'?" *Archives of Family Medicine* 9(2):123, February, 2000.

Mintzer, J., et al. "Treatment of Agitation in Patients with Dementia," *Clinics in Geriatric Medicine* 14(1):147-75, February, 1998.

Pao, M., et al. "Psychiatric Diagnoses in Adolescents Seropositive for the Human Immunodeficiency Virus," *Archives of Pediatrics and Adolescent Medicine* 154(3):240-44, March, 2000.

Schwartz, J. B. "Gender and Dietary Influences on Drug Clearance," *The Journal of Gender-Specific Medicine* 3(2), March-April, 2000.

Sontheimer, D., and Ables, A. "Safety of Antidepressant Medications During Pregnancy," *JAMA* 283(9):1139, March, 2000.

Steiner, M. "Perinatal Mood Disorders," *Psychopharmacology Bulletin* 34(3):301-306, 1998.

Walker, A., et al. "Neurodevelopmental and Neurobehavioral Sequelae of Selected Substances of Abuse and Psychiatric Medications in Utero," *Child and Adolescent Psychiatry Clinics of North America* 8(4):845-67, October, 1999.

Wisner, K., et al. "Pharmocologic Treatment of Depression During Pregnancy," *JAMA* 282(13):1264-69, October, 1999.

Zito, J., et al. "Psychotherapeutic Medication Patterns for Youths with Attention Deficit/Hyperactivity Disorder," *Archives of Pediatrics and Adolescent Medicine* 153(12):1257-63, December, 1999.

CHAPTER 3

Managing overdose and withdrawal

The development of new psychotropic drugs has broadened the options available for managing psychiatric disorders. In general, these newer drugs are more effective and have fewer adverse effects than older drugs. Despite these improvements, however, you still need to be prepared to act promptly and correctly in case of overdose or withdrawal.

OVERDOSE

Patients can overdose on may different types of drugs, including prescribed drugs, over-the-counter (OTC) drugs, illicit drugs, herbal remedies, or a combination of these substances. In fact, any drug can cause toxicity and overdose if taken in extreme amounts.

A history of a psychiatric illness doesn't, in itself, predispose a patient to drug overdose. However, certain psychotropic drugs are linked to overdose relatively often. They include tricyclic antidepressants, benzodiazepines, barbiturates, opiate narcotics, and amphetamines. Overdose with these or other drugs may be accidental or intentional.

Accidental overdose

Although many people assume that psychotropic drug overdoses are usually intentional, that isn't necessarily the case. Indeed, an overdose may result from impaired hepatic or renal function. Or it may result from drug interactions or from characteristics unique to the patient—particularly if the patient is a child or an older adult.

Drug interactions

New psychotropic drugs have entirely different, more tolerable, adverse effects profiles compared with some older generations of psychotropic drugs. (See *Understanding extrapyramidal symptoms*, page 34.) However, the newer drugs also raise new complexities based on how they're metabolized and how they may interact—possibly seriously—with other drugs. Because elderly patients and those with psychiatric disorders commonly take multiple drugs, they have a high risk for toxic effects and interactions.

Proactive approach

Many classes of drugs interact with each other, especially psychotropics. Consequently, your most prudent approach for a patient who takes a psychotropic drug is to assume the possibility of an interaction and take proactive steps to prevent it. For example, if the patient receives prescriptions from more than one prescriber, you can help to reduce the risk of toxic effects by urging the patient to fill

Understanding extrapyramidal symptoms

Some of the first psychotropic drugs to be developed were neuroleptic-based antipsychotics. Besides quieting the symptoms of psychosis and schizophrenia, however, these drugs also raised a risk of serious adverse effects known as extrapyramidal symptoms (EPS).

Neuroleptic-induced EPS probably stem from an increased cholinergic response caused by blockade of nigrostriatal dopamine tracts. It may result in several movement disorders, such as tardive dyskinesia, tardive dystonia, and neuroleptic malignant syndrome. These adverse effects result not so much from overdose as from each drug's action.

Tardive dyskinesia

Poorly understood, tardive dyskinesia is probably a hypersensitivity response to chronic dopamine blockade. It results from long-term use of dopamine receptor antagonists and causes sustained abnormal muscle contractions, twisting or repetitive movements, or abnormal postures. The patient also may seem to make continuous chewing motions.

These abnormal movements represent a distortion or impairment of voluntary movement. They may resolve a few months after therapy stops, or they may continue indefinitely.

Tardive dystonia

About 3% of patients on long-term neuroleptic antipsychotic treatment develop this variation of tardive dyskinesia. It's most likely to affect young male patients. The distinguishing diagnostic feature of tardive dystonia is that it occurs during the first three months of antipsychotic drug treatment. The abnormal movements result from disordered muscle tonicity.

Neuroleptic malignant syndrome

Neuroleptic malignant syndrome is a rare, possibly life-threatening reaction to antipsychotic therapy. It may include a high fever, dystonia, diaphoresis, tachycardia, and muscle rigidity. Treatment involves administration of a dopamine agonist or possibly dantrolene (a skeletal muscle relaxant), fluids, and benzodiazepines. Changing to one of the newer atypical or novel antipsychotics—such as olanzapine or clozapine—will probably help, along with the use of propranolol to control fever.

In general, the new atypical antipsychotics have a much smaller risk of causing EPS and neuroleptic malignant syndrome than older drugs. However, they're much more expensive than the older drugs and may cause their own set of adverse effects. Clozapine, for example, may raise the risk of agranulocytosis; patients who take this drug will require frequent monitoring of their white blood cells. And in white male patients who smoke, olanzapine is metabolized more quickly via the cytochrome P-450 system, a difference that requires a dosage adjustment. For patients who still take the older antipsychotics, vitamin E may help reduce the risk of EPS.

every prescription through the same pharmacist.

Also, suggest that the patient ask the pharmacist to run a computerized drug interaction screen before filling each new prescription. For some patients, you may want to call the pharmacist personally. That way, you can obtain warnings and suggestions directly from another professional.

Finally, do your best to make sure that you know about all substances that the patient takes—or starts taking—during psychotropic drug therapy. The addition of alcohol, an OTC diet pill, or a dose of a family member's prescription drug can have profound clinical implications. Any action or substance that alters drug absorption or metabolism may increase the risk of toxicity and the risk of overdose.

Expanding knowledge
Keep in mind that new drug interactions are being identified every day. You must be vigilant about watching your patients' responses to drugs—even to well-known drugs. Be suspicious about emerging clinical signs, even if they aren't linked to drug interactions on the package insert. The fact is that new clinical observations about drugs and their interactions are constantly being reported and compiled.

One of the areas in which researchers' knowledge is expanding rapidly is in cytochrome chemistry. Drugs metabolized via the cytochrome P-450 (CYP 450) pathways can inhibit excretion of other drugs, resulting in a buildup of those drugs and an increased risk of toxicity.

Scientists and clinicians continue to learn about factors that increase the risk of interaction for other drugs as well. For instance, when lithium, a salt, is given with a diuretic, reduced levels of body fluid cause reduced elimination of lithium from the body. This problem, which occurs most often in elderly patients and in psychiatric patients with hypertension, can lead to serious cardiac arrhythmias and other toxic adverse effects.

Overdose in children
The risk of unintentional overdose is heightened among children. That's in part because a child may accidentally ingest too much of his own or an adult family member's psychotropic drug. It's also because drug pharmacokinetics differ between children and adults.

In fact, we don't know a great deal about how psychotropic drugs act in children's bodies. Drug makers usually don't include children in clinical trials for many reasons, including issues of informed consent. Because this group is excluded, we don't have much research regarding the safe use of psychotropic drugs in children. Consequently, you must administer these drugs with extreme caution, staying fully aware of the possibility of unknown long-term effects.

This approach is especially important because the use of psychotropic drugs is increasing among pediatric patients. Because drugs can achieve relatively rapid short-term results, managed care plans tend to foster the use of psychotropic drugs for children rather than pursuing extended counseling and parental assistance. What's more, certain disorders responsive to psychotropic drug treatment seem to be ever more common. The prime example of this trend is the growing number of children diagnosed with attention deficit hyperactivity disorder, for which they usually receive methylphenidate (Ritalin).

Professionals who prescribe psychotropics for children usually do so based on the child's weight. However, without adequate clinical research to establish safe and effective dosing patterns, you should follow each child—especially a young child—closely to quickly detect any adverse reactions before they become serious.

Overdose in elderly patients

The risk of accidental overdose is also heightened among elderly patients. That's in part because elderly people take more drugs than people in other age groups, which puts them at higher risk for adverse effects and interactions. It's also because drug pharmacokinetics differ between elderly adults and middle-aged adults. And it's because the physical and emotional challenges common to older adults also raise the risk of accidental overdose.

Physical challenges commonly stem from chronic illnesses that cause declining levels of independent function. These changes may lead to an accidental overdose by impairing the person's vision or memory. And declining dexterity may make it more difficult for the patient to handle, cut, or count pills.

Intentional overdose

Although many cases of psychotropic drug overdose are acciden-

tal, a fair number are intentional. The patient may seek increased mood-altering effects, or he may seek death.

Mood-altering effects

Certain patients intentionally take too much of a psychotropic drug to obtain mood-altering effects, especially elderly patients and those who struggle with substance abuse.

Elderly patients have an increased risk of intentional overdose because the hallmarks of adulthood that others take for granted—such as driving a car, holding a job, or chewing food with real teeth—may gradually be taken away. These changes may create a deep sense of loss that younger people may not recognize or understand. Not only must the older adult cope with the actual loss, but also with the loss of symbolic meaning that society assigns to certain abilities of independent adults. The older adult may seek to ease the pain of loss by manipulating the drug regimen.

For other patients, the mood-altering effects of a psychotropic drug are enough to encourage intentional overdose. In effect, the patient thinks, "If one works this well, two will be even better." Even among the safest psychotropic drugs, the chemical properties of a drug's metabolites can result in a serious or lethal overdose if the patient takes too much.

Suicide

When most people think of psychotropic drug overdose, they think suicide attempt. That's with good reason; there's a clear link between suicide and drug overdose. Some of the characteristics of increased suicide risk include mental health problems (such as depression), domestic problems, physical illness, family dysfunction, social isolation, unemployment, and stressful life situations. Another characteristic of an increased risk for suicide is drug misuse, in which a person takes a prescribed drug in ways other than the prescriber intended.

Profile

Although no one can create an absolute demographic profile of the person at highest risk of suicide, some groups and influences can be identified.

For example, we know that men are at higher risk of illicit drug overdose than women. Unemployed people have a higher risk of overdose as well. Low-skilled workers have a higher risk. People with access to a means of self-harm (such as a psychotropic drug) have a higher risk. And those who abuse drugs have a higher risk. Other predisposing characteristics include poor coping skills and a history of physical abuse, sexual abuse, or psychosis.

Behaviors

Many behaviors can offer clues to a patient's suicidal thoughts. These behaviors can range from vague suicidal "gesturing" to frank expressions of wishing to die. Between these two extremes is a wide range of clues to a risk of suicide. The patient may express thoughts, intentions, and plans. He may seem ambivalent, confused, or angry, leading you to suspect a potential for spontaneous self-harm.

The patient also may express a desire for pain, escape from an unbearable life situation, desperation, or vengeance. He may speak of wanting to frighten or influence others. Or he may intimate an overwhelming need for attention.

Prevention

One way to help prevent intentional overdose is to help prevent the misuse of drugs. For example, try to avoid administering a psychotropic drug prescription that has automatic refills. In fact, the higher the patient's risk, the more important it is to administer small quantities of drug, such as a 2-week supply or less.

Make sure the patient has to call the prescriber's office for refills, which gives you an opportunity to monitor the patient's compliance with dosing patterns and frequency of drug use. For some patients, this brief phone contact for a refill may provide a life-saving opportunity for the patient to get help if he needs it. Remember that patients at risk of drug overdose are emotionally vulnerable; they may reach out for assistance if they believe that assistance is accessible.

Symptoms and treatment

A drug overdose—either accidental or intentional—may be a life-threatening emergency. You or other emergency personnel must try to find out which drug or drugs the patient took, how much he took, and how long ago he took it. The specific treatment he receives will depend on this information. Also, keep in mind that a patient who survives a life-threatening drug overdose will need long-term psychological care to address the causes of overdose and to prevent a recurrence. Family support is especially important after a drug overdose.

As you know, the results of an overdose can be profoundly serious even from a relatively benign drug. For instance, an overdose of acetaminophen, a common drug found in many homes, can cause hepatic failure and multiple organ damage. Because of the increased risk of overdose with psychotropic drugs, you should also make a point of knowing the symptoms and treatments of overdose from these drugs, especially benzodiazepines, amphetamines, barbiturates, opiates, and antidepressants. (See *Recognizing signs and symptoms of drug overdose.*)

Benzodiazepine overdose

Benzodiazepines are used to produce sedation, induce sleep, relieve anxiety, treat panic disorders, relieve depression, manage somatopsychic disorders, decrease muscle spasms, and treat seizures. This group of psychotropics has low toxicity and, usually, is tolerated well. These characteristics have made benzodiazepines the most widely prescribed drugs in the United States. According to the Drug Enforcement Administration of the U.S. Department of Justice, however, they're also the most frequently abused drugs. Many people who abuse benzodiazepines do so by obtaining prescriptions from several legitimate prescribers at once.

Even typical benzodiazepine dosage levels can produce fatigue, drowsiness, reduced concentration, and impaired motor function, especially at the start of treatment. Benzodiazepines that have long half-lives can impair diurnal vigilance, especially in elderly people, and can have a hangover effect from accumulated drug. Benzodiazepine overdose can also cause numbness, dizziness, poor coordination, and ataxia. If the patient combines a benzodiazepine with alcohol or other sedatives, these toxicities are greatly increased. Indeed, a patient with an acute overdose may need mechanical ventilation and blood pressure support.

Amphetamine overdose

Amphetamines are stimulants. They may be prescribed, or they may be produced for illegal sale in clandestine laboratories. Methamphetamine is an example of an illicit amphetamine produced in this way. These illicit drugs contain varying, unquantified components.

The symptoms of amphetamine overdose vary with the specific drug taken and the route of administration. They include hyperpyrexia, aggressiveness, tremor, arrhythmias, changes in blood pressure, restlessness, seizures, and coma. (See *Managing aggression*, pages 40 and 41.) Acute pulmonary edema has been reported after amphetamine overdose. Occasionally, methamphetamine abuse may be fatal.

Treatment for amphetamine overdose is symptomatic and supportive. Give the patient a sedative, such as a short-acting barbiturate. Also, keep the patient's environment quiet and calm to help manage his excitability. To help slow absorption of the drug, perform gastric lavage or induce emesis if

Recognizing signs and symptoms of drug overdose

The following lists give you key signs and symptoms of benzodiazepine, amphetamine, barbiturate, opiate, and antidepressant overdoses—at a glance.

Benzodiazepines

- numbness
- dizziness
- poor coordination
- ataxia.

Amphetamines

- hyperpyrexia
- aggressiveness
- tremor
- cardiac arrhythmias
- changes in blood pressure
- restlessness
- seizures
- coma.

Barbiturates

- slurred speech
- confusion
- unsteady gait
- respiratory depression
- hypotension
- tachycardia
- coma.

Opiates

- urinary retention
- muscle spasm
- hyperpyrexia
- itching
- pinpoint pupils
- hypotension
- hypothermia
- respiratory depression
- pulmonary edema
- seizures
- bradycardia
- cardiac arrest.

Antidepressants

Tricyclic antidepressants

- cardiac arrhythmias
- seizures
- hypotension
- sedation.

Selective serotonin reuptake inhibitors

- dizziness
- nausea
- vomiting
- tremor.

he took the drug orally. Apply a tourniquet and ice packs if he injected the drug.

Barbiturate overdose

Barbiturates are depressants. Like benzodiazepines, they have properties that can lead to physical dependence. Barbiturate overdose causes slurred speech, confusion, an unsteady gait, respiratory depression, and coma. Alcohol amplifies these symptoms. Patients in

barbiturate overdose may be found in shock—hypotensive, tachycardic, and with respiratory depression.

Treatment for barbiturate overdose is mainly supportive. The patient may need mechanical ventilation for respiratory support. If the patient took the drug during the previous 30 minutes, activated charcoal may help to absorb it. If he took the drug within the previous 4 hours, gastric lavage may be helpful.

Managing aggression

Besides their increased risk of self-harm, people who misuse amphetamines and certain other psychotropic drugs may develop an increased risk of aggression and violence. These behaviors may be especially likely if the patient takes a combination of prescription and illicit substances. They also may stem from overdose, withdrawal, or drug-seeking behavior. And they may be spurred on by environmental or lifestyle characteristics.

Assessment

The patients most likely to exhibit aggressive, violent behaviors tend to have these characteristics:

- anger
- childhood abuse
- family dysfunction
- history of previous violence
- impulsiveness
- lack of community support
- male gender
- psychopathology
- psychotic symptoms
- stress
- substance abuse
- suicidality
- treatment noncompliance
- young age.

Remember that assessing a patient's risk of violence is a complex task. One tool you can use to help judge it is the Historical, Clinical and Risk Management Scale, commonly called the HRC-20. Use this tool only after receiving training in how to do so properly.

Especially in elderly patients, aggressive behavior may result from delirium. This sudden, acute change in mental status may stem from drug effects or from the effects of a physiologic process, such as infection, dehydration, pain, electrolyte imbalance, toxic levels of nonpsychotropic drugs, or organ system failure.

If you're caring for an older adult, make sure your patient has had a thorough physical evaluation, basic laboratory screenings (such as a urinalysis with culture and sensitivity, if indicated), a complete blood count, an electrolyte panel that includes blood urea nitrogen and creatinine levels, and tests of blood drug levels, such as digoxin. Some patients may need a computed tomography scan of the brain.

Management

Drug therapy for aggressive patients typically involves short- and middle-range care planning and safety goals. Several groups of drugs can be used for short-term aggression management, including antipsychotics and benzodiazepines. Seclusion and, as a last resort, restraints may be needed in inpatient settings.

Middle-range mood stabilization can be achieved with lithium and some anticonvulsants, such as valproic acid. Because lithium levels are closely related to body fluid levels, a patient who receives lithium must be monitored closely because this drug has been linked to permanent thyroid and kidney damage. Valproic acid doesn't require such strict monitoring, but it can cause liver damage and blood dyscrasias.

Long-term management of aggressive patients is difficult. These patients need close monitoring and anger-management counseling. Keep good lines of communication open among the patient, family,

Managing aggression (continued)

school officials, and community agencies. Always follow facility safety policies when a patient is deemed at risk to self or others. As needed, make an immediate referral to appropriate agencies.

Many of these patients end up in the criminal justice system or the state mental health system because they pose a continuing danger to themselves or others. Many are too difficult to manage in less structured community settings. For these and all patients, remember the goals of aggression management: Keep the patient safe, in the least restrictive environment possible, while protecting the rights and privacy of both patient and those around him.

Opiate overdose

A patient with an opiate overdose typically has miosis, or pinpoint pupils, possibly together with such life-threatening problems as hypotension, hypothermia, respiratory depression, pulmonary edema, seizures, bradycardia, and cardiac arrest.

Treatment of opiate overdose depends on the time elapsed between the time of drug use and time of treatment, as well as the route by which the patient took the drug. Priorities of treatment include respiratory support, administration of a narcotic antagonist (such as naloxone), monitoring of vital signs, and correction of electrolyte imbalances.

Antidepressant overdose

With the advent of selective serotonin reuptake inhibitors, researchers and clinicians alike hoped that their worries about antidepressant overdose would be all but over. These drugs were heralded as being much safer than the older tricyclic antidepressants, an overdose of which could cause life-threatening cardiac arrhythmias, seizures, hypotension, and sedation.

However, evidence is beginning to suggest that even the safer, newer drugs have a risk of possibly fatal effects from overdose, especially among vulnerable, already depressed patients. Fluoxetine, one of the older selective serotonin reuptake inhibitors, has a long half-life of seven days, which can increase the risk of overdose. What's more, the new drugs can interact with many drugs metabolized in the CYP 450 system.

Although this interaction may not always pose a significant clinical threat, you must always stay alert for an increased risk of toxic overdose. The safety profile of selective serotonin reuptake inhibitors is indeed better than that of the tricyclic antidepressants. However, as with all classes of drugs, this class of psychotropic drugs requires vigilance in prescribing and patient monitoring. Treatment for an overdose of a selective serotonin reuptake inhibitor is symptomatic and supportive.

WITHDRAWAL

Certain psychotropic drugs can cause dependence and withdrawal symptoms. In particular, benzodiazepines and narcotics can lead to physical dependence. That's why they're categorized as controlled substances.

The risk of dependence and withdrawal rises with the length of treatment, the amount of drug taken, an increasing need for the drug over time, unrealistic expectations of the drug's effects, and the intensity of stressful life events. Patients may have a particular risk of dependence based on certain types of problems:

- a history of addiction
- a chronic painful physical condition
- long-term depression
- a personality disorder
- a sleep disorder.

Benzodiazepine dependence creates a particularly dangerous withdrawal scenario. Patients with benzodiazepine dependence may have one of two distinct problems: low-dose dependence, which commonly results from low-dose treatment of chronic anxiety or a sleep disorder, or high-dose dependence, which commonly results from a steadily increasing dosage over time.

Symptoms

Withdrawal symptoms may occur when any drug that causes physical dependence is abruptly stopped. If the patient took a short-acting benzodiazepine, the most severe withdrawal symptoms occur two to three days after abrupt discontinuation; if he took a long-acting benzodiazepine, the worst symptoms occur after four to seven days.

A patient in withdrawal from a benzodiazepine may develop life-threatening problems, including seizures, arrhythmias, and electrolyte imbalances. (See *Benzodiazepines: Adverse effects and withdrawal symptoms.*)

Symptoms of narcotic withdrawal may appear within hours of the last dose. They peak at 36 to 72 hours for morphine, 8 to 12 hours for meperidine. A patient in withdrawal from a narcotic may initially develop restlessness, tearing, yawning, gooseflesh, and mydriasis. As withdrawal progresses, symptoms may intensify into muscle spasms, severe back and abdominal pain, insomnia, nausea, vomiting, and diarrhea. The patient may experience hot and cold flashes as his body temperature, blood pressure, pulse, and respiratory rate rise. Usually, the effects of meperidine withdrawal are milder than those of morphine withdrawal.

Treatment

Withdrawal from benzodiazepines, narcotics, and many other drugs should be accomplished under close medical supervision. Traditionally, withdrawal from benzodiazepines was performed on an inpatient basis, although these days insurers—particularly managed care plans—pressure clinicians to try outpatient and community-based treatment for withdrawal. Because of limited mental health care coverage in some insurance plans, outpatient and day treatment can be a cost-effective way to help some patients withdraw from an addictive psychotropic drug.

Keep in mind, however, that an outpatient dependent on a drug may be taking multiple legal and illegal substances that could alter the typical withdrawal scenario. Alcohol is one such complicating factor. Also, people who abuse benzodiazepines are more likely to abuse heroin. And government officials report that about half the people who seek treatment for a narcotic addiction are also addicted to a benzodiazepine.

When weaning a patient from a benzodiazepine, taper the drug gradually, reducing the dosage by no more than one-fourth of the daily dose per week. Anticipate that elderly patients and patients with panic disorders may have more difficulty reducing the dose of long-term benzodiazepines. Consider the patient's overall medical condition when planning to stop a drug, including personality factors and the type of psychiatric illness he has. Some patients benefit from a sedative antidepressant to help them cope with the dosage reduction period.

Besides physical monitoring of the patient's response, counseling is also especially important during withdrawal. The patient may need help with managing anger, reducing stress, and finding new ways to deal with everyday problems. A support group may be helpful for some patients in avoiding dependence and the lifestyle that fostered it.

Sound management of psychotropic drug therapy requires you to have a thorough knowledge of your patient's mental health, his baseline physical health, and the combination of drugs he takes. By applying a team approach to these

Benzodiazepines: Adverse effects and withdrawal symptoms

Adverse effects

- Addiction
- Depressive mood swings with prolonged use
- Dizziness
- Dysphoria with prolonged use
- Excitement
- Loss of drive with prolonged use
- Memory disorders
- Muscle weakness
- Respiratory depression, especially when taken with alcohol
- Restlessness
- Sedation
- Speech difficulties

Withdrawal symptoms

- Acute psychosis
- Agitation
- Anorexia
- Anxiety
- Delirium
- Diarrhea
- Distorted reality
- Distraction
- Dysphoria
- Hallucinations
- Optical distortions
- Photosensitivity
- Seizures
- Sleep disorders
- Sweating
- Tachycardia
- Tremor
- Vomiting

typically complex situations, you can help to protect your patient from the possibly life-threatening effects of overdose and withdrawal.

References

Bond, G., and Hite, L. "Population-Based Incidence and Outcome of Acetaminophen Poisoning by Type of Ingestion," *Academic Emergency Medicine* 6(11):1115-20, November, 1999.

Catalano, G., et al. "Olanzapine Overdose in an 18-Month Old Child," *Journal of Child and Adolescent Psychopharmacology* 9(4):267-71, 1999.

Coumbaros, J., et al. "Application of Solid-Phase Microextraction to the Profiling of an Illicit Drug: Manufacturing Impurities in Illicit 4-methoxyamphetamine," *Journal of Forensic Science* 44(6):1237-42, November, 1999.

Douglas, K. S., et al. "Assessing Risk of Violence Among Psychiatric Patients: The HCR-20 Violence Risk Assessment Scheme and the Psychopathology Checklist Screening Version," *Journal of Consulting and Clinical Psychology* 67(6):917-30, December, 1999.

Dyer, K., and Woolf, A. "Use of Phenothiazines as Sedatives in Children: What are the Risks?" *Drug Safety* 21(2):81-90, August, 1999.

Ferguson, J., and Smith, A. "Aggressive Behavior on an Inpatient Geriatric Unit," *Journal of Psychosocial Nursing* 34(3):27-32, March, 1996.

Gill, M., et al. "Serotonin Syndrome in a Child After a Single Dose of Fluvoxamine," *Annals of Emergency Medicine* 33(4):457-59, April, 1999.

Glazer, W. "Extrapyramidal Side Effects, Tardive Dyskinesia, and the Concept of Atypicality" *Journal of Clinical Psychiatry* 61(suppl 3):16-21, 2000.

Gonner, F., et al. "Neuroleptic Malignant Syndrome During Low Dosed Neuroleptic Drug in First Episode Psychosis: A Case Report," *Psychopharmacology* 144(4):416-18, June, 1999.

Greenblatt, D. J., et al. "Human Cytochromes and Some Newer Antidepressants: Kinetics, Metabolism, and Drug Interactions," *Journal of Clinical Psychopharmacology* 19(5 suppl 1):23s-34s, October, 1999.

Harrigan, R., and Brady, W. "ECG Abnormalities in Tricyclic Antidepressant Ingestion," *American Journal of Emergency Medicine* 17(4):387-93, July, 1999.

Lee, E. "Overview: The Assessment and Treatment of Asian American Families" in *Working with Asian Americans.* Edited by Lee, E. New York: The Guilford Press, 1997.

Massello, W., and Carpenter, D. "A Fatality Due to the Intranasal Abuse of Methylphenidate (Ritalin)," *Journal of Forensic Science* 44(1):220-21, January, 1999.

Matsumura, et al. "Electrolyte Disorders Following Massive Insulin Overdose in a Patient with Type 2 Diabetes," *Internal Medicine* 39(1):55-57, January, 2000.

Maury, E., et al. "Acute Pulmonary Edema Following Amphetamine Ingestion," *Intensive Care Medicine* 25(3):332-33, March, 1999.

Moller, H. "Effectiveness and Safety of Benzodiazepines," *Journal of Clinical Psychopharmacology* 19(6 suppl 2):2s-11s, December, 1999.

Neale, J. "Suicidal Intent and Non-Fatal Illicit Drug Overdose," *Addiction* 95(1):85-93, January, 2000.

Pope, H., et al. "Effects of Supraphysiologic Doses of Testosterone on Mood and Aggression in Normal Men: A Randomized Trial," *Archives of General Psychiatry* 57(2):133-40, February, 2000.

Sachdev, P., et al. "The Preventative Role of Antioxidants (Selegiline and Vitamin E) in a Rat Model of Tardive Dyskinesia," *Biologic Psychiatry* 46(12):1672-81, December, 1999.

Saltz, B., et al. "Side Effects of Antipsychotic Drugs. Avoiding and Minimizing Their Impact on Elderly Patients," *Postgraduate Medicine* 107(2):169-72, February, 2000.

Shrier, M., and Diaz, J. "Cardiotox-icity Associated with Bupropion Overdose," *Annals of Emergency Medicine* 35(1):100, January, 2000.

Van Harten, P., and Kahn, R. "Tardive Dystonia," *Schizophrenia Bulletin* 25(4):741-48, 1999.

Wilkinson, R., et al. "Neuroleptic Malignant Syndrome Induced by Haloperidol Following Traumatic Brain Injury," *Brain Injury* 13(12):1025-31, December, 1999.

PART 2

Psychotropic drugs

49 ■ **Antianxiety drugs**

87 ■ **Anticonvulsants**

143 ■ **Antidepressants**

217 ■ **Mood stabilizing drugs**

227 ■ **Antiparkinsonians**

269 ■ **Antipsychotics**

341 ■ **Central nervous system stimulants**

371 ■ **Drugs for treating alcoholism and substance abuse**

409 ■ **Sedative-hypnotics**

453 ■ **Drugs for treating Alzheimer's disease and migraine headaches**

CHAPTER 4

Antianxiety drugs

51 ■ **Introduction**

58 ■ **Generic drugs**

■ alprazolam

■ amitriptyline hydrochloride (See Chapter 6, ANTIDEPRESSANTS)

■ buspirone hydrochloride

■ chlordiazepoxide, chlordiazepoxide hydrochloride

■ clorazepate dipotassium

■ diazepam

■ doxepin hydrochloride (See Chapter 6, ANTIDEPRESSANTS)

■ fluoxetine hydrochloride (See Chapter 6, ANTIDEPRESSANTS)

■ fluvoxamine maleate (See Chapter 6, ANTIDEPRESSANTS)

■ hydroxyzine hydrochloride, hydroxyzine pamoate

■ imipramine hydrochloride, imipramine pamoate (See Chapter 6, ANTIDEPRESSANTS)

■ lorazepam

■ meprobamate

■ midazolam hydrochloride

■ oxazepam

■ paroxetine hydrochloride (See Chapter 6, ANTIDEPRESSANTS)

■ propranolol hydrochloride (See Chapter 13, DRUGS FOR TREATING ALZHEIMER'S DISEASE AND MIGRANE HEADACHES)

■ sertraline hydrochloride (See Chapter 6, ANTIDEPRESSANTS)

■ venlafaxine hydrochloride (See Chapter 6, ANTIDEPRESSANTS)

For virtually everyone, feelings of anxiety arise in response to stressful life events or crises. After a crisis passes, however, the anxiety gradually subsides on its own. In contrast to this normal response, a person with an anxiety disorder has pronounced, persistent anxiety that usually arises without warning, making the person's simplest routine the source of unbearable discomfort, even terror.

UNDERSTANDING ANXIETY DISORDERS

Anxiety disorders affect more than 20 million Americans, making them the most common of all emotional disorders. Symptoms of an anxiety disorder include:
- overwhelming feelings of fear and panic
- uncontrollable obsessive thoughts
- recurring nightmares
- painful, disruptive memories
- unpleasant physical reactions, such as nausea, sweating, and muscle tension.

Naturally, if persistent anxiety interferes with daily life, the affected person needs medical attention and possible drug treatment. Examples of disorders that produce this persistent, overwhelming anxiety include generalized anxiety disorder, phobias, panic disorder, post-traumatic stress disorder, and obsessive-compulsive disorder.

Generalized anxiety disorder
A person with generalized anxiety disorder is consumed by unrealistic or excessive worrying about life's circumstances, although she typically doesn't take steps to avoid specific situations. Commonly, the patient has trouble relaxing, difficulty concentrating, and a tendency to become easily irritable or tired. She may experience insomnia, muscle tension, fatigue, and headaches. She may feel shaky or on edge. And she has an increased risk of such concurrent problems as depression and substance abuse.

Phobias
Phobias are persistent, irrational fears of certain objects or situations. A person may have one of three types of phobia: a specific phobia, a social phobia, or agoraphobia.

A specific phobia is an excessive fear of an object or activity that isn't dangerous or harmful under normal conditions. Examples include a fear of cats, spiders, getting in an elevator, or entering a dark room.

A social phobia, also called social anxiety disorder, is an inordinate fear of being embarrassed or ridiculed in a social situation. A person with a social phobia may avoid the feared situation or she may manage to tolerate it—but not without severe discomfort.

Agoraphobia is a marked fear of being alone or in a public situation from which escape may be embarrassing or difficult if something alarming were to occur. Untreated, the condition worsens over time until, eventually, the person may be unable to leave her home.

Panic disorder
A person with a panic disorder develops sudden, intense, overwhelming fright for seemingly no reason. Called a panic attack, this reaction is anxiety in its most severe form.

Picture of a panic attack

A patient having a panic attack will abruptly develop at least four of the following symptoms, and they'll peak within 10 minutes:
- chest pain or discomfort
- depersonalization or derealization
- dizziness or faintness
- fear of losing control or "going crazy"
- fear of dying
- feeling of choking
- hot or cold flashes
- nausea or abdominal distress
- numbness or tingling sensations
- palpitations, pounding heart, or tachycardia
- shortness of breath or smothering sensation
- sweating
- trembling or shaking.

Indeed, the attack may be so abrupt and severe that the person may think she's having a heart attack.

By definition, a panic attack is a discrete period of intense fear or discomfort in which certain types of symptoms begin abruptly and peak rapidly. (See *Picture of a panic attack.*) The disorder that causes panic attacks is equally common among men and women. However, panic attacks that occur together with agoraphobia affect women about twice as often as men.

A person with a panic disorder has a high risk for substance abuse because she may turn to alcohol or anxiolytics in an attempt to ease her anxiety. Without treatment, she may become despondent and suicidal.

Post-traumatic stress disorder

Psychological changes that persist for a month or more after a traumatic event may indicate that a person has post-traumatic stress disorder. This disorder can follow almost any distressing event that's outside the range of usual human experience. For example, the disorder may stem from a natural or man-made disaster, from physical or sexual abuse, or from an assault or a rape.

When the traumatic event occurs at the hands of another person, the resulting disorder is typically more severe. Psychological trauma accompanies the physical trauma and involves intense fear and feelings of helplessness and loss of control.

Post-traumatic stress disorder can be acute, chronic, or delayed. The disorder may be delayed because avoidance can keep symptoms from developing until months or years after the traumatic event. Indeed, onset can occur at any age. Common symptoms include:
- pangs of painful emotions and unwelcome thoughts
- intrusive memories
- dissociative episodes
- a traumatic reexperiencing of the event
- difficulty falling or staying asleep, frequent nightmares of the traumatic event, and aggressive outbursts on awakening
- emotional numbing, with a diminished or constricted response
- chronic anxiety or panic attacks.

Obsessive-compulsive disorder

A person with obsessive-compulsive disorder develops severe anxi-

Defining compulsions

Compulsions contain all of the following elements:

- Repetitive behaviors or mental acts performed by a person who feels driven to perform them in response to an obsession or according to rules that must be applied rigidly.
- Behaviors or mental acts that are aimed at preventing or reducing distress or preventing a dreaded event or situation. However, either the activity is clearly excessive or it's not connected in a realistic way with what the person wants to neutralize or prevent.
- The person recognizes that her behavior is excessive or unreasonable. Exceptions include young children and patients whose obsessions have evolved into overvalued ideas.

ety from frequent, intrusive, irrational thoughts (obsessions) that can't be controlled through reasoning. Instead, to ease the obsessive thoughts, the person engages in repetitive rituals (compulsions) to reduce the distress caused by the obsession. (See *Defining compulsions*.)

Roughly 2.4 million people in the United States have obsessive-compulsive disorders. Although people with obsessive disorders don't always have compulsive behaviors, most people with compulsions also have obsessions.

TREATING ANXIETY DISORDERS

Anxiety can accompany many physiologic conditions, such as angina, myocardial infarction, pulmonary disease, peptic ulcer disease, ulcerative colitis, and thyroid disorder. It also may be a symptom of depression or dementia. Because anxiety can stem from such a varied range of physiologic and psychological disorders, you'll need to make sure that other disorders

have been ruled out before treating a patient for an anxiety disorder.

Even with a firm diagnosis, treatment for an anxiety disorder can be complex. That's in part because our understanding of anxiety disorders and what causes them has been developing rapidly. In recent years, researchers have gained considerable knowledge about the influence of neurotransmitters on brain function and mental health. As a consequence, they've developed and continue to develop drugs that alter the brain's production, storage, and release of certain neurotransmitters.

As we gain a greater understanding of neurotransmitters and their effects on mental health, the drugs available for treating anxiety disorders will continue to evolve. For now, however, several drug classes can be used to treat anxiety disorders, including benzodiazepines, azapirones, antihistamines, beta blockers, and antidepressants. Keep in mind that drugs in all of these classes can produce adverse effects. To minimize them, start with low doses and gradually adjust the dosage upward. In many cases, adverse effects become less severe after several weeks of treatment.

Benzodiazepines

The benzodiazepines form the mainstay of drug therapy for anxiety, particularly for generalized anxiety disorder. This class includes such drugs as alprazolam (Xanax), diazepam (Valium), and lorazepam (Ativan).

Benzodiazepines tend to be highly effective and fast-acting. Because they relieve anxiety quickly, benzodiazepines are a common first choice for patients who need rapid control of their symptoms.

The main disadvantage of benzodiazepines is that they can lead to dependence. For this reason, they're usually inappropriate for patients with a history of substance abuse. Another drawback of benzodiazepines is that abrupt discontinuation can cause withdrawal symptoms and symptomatic rebound after as little as 6 weeks of therapy.

Withdrawal may be more severe in patients being treated for panic disorder than for generalized anxiety disorder. To minimize withdrawal symptoms, the benzodiazepine dosage must be tapered slowly. Because withdrawal symptoms may be most pronounced toward the end of the taper, experts suggest reducing the dosage over 2 to 4 months by no more than 10% of the dosage each week.

Drug effects

Benzodiazepines exert an anxiolytic effect by potentiating the inhibitory neurotransmitter gamma-aminobutyric acid in the brain. Although two benzodiazepine receptors have been recently identified (BZD_1 and BZD_2), binding at BZD_2 seems to produce the anxiolytic effect. Besides their anxiolytic activity, benzodiazepines also have sedative-hypnotic, muscle relaxant, and anticonvulsant effects.

Pharmacokinetics

Benzodiazepines are readily absorbed in the gastrointestinal tract and are highly lipid soluble. The most lipid-soluble drugs in the class penetrate the blood-brain barrier the fastest and therefore have the fastest onset of action.

All benzodiazepines are highly protein-bound (70% to 99%), and all are metabolized in the liver. Long-acting benzodiazepines are metabolized into several active metabolites, which explains their prolonged action. Short-acting benzodiazepines have no clinically significant active metabolites and therefore have a significantly shorter duration of action.

Because of the drugs' significant biotransformation in the liver, benzodiazepine doses must be adjusted in patients who have liver impairment. Most benzodiazepines are excreted in the urine after biotransformation.

Overdose and treatment

Usually, benzodiazepine overdose is relatively benign. Deaths have been reported only after benzodiazepines were ingested with alcohol.

Azapirones

The class of drugs known as azapirones thus far contains but a single drug: buspirone hydrochloride (BuSpar). Several studies comparing buspirone to benzodiazepines have shown them to be equally effective. However, buspirone's effects typically take 2 to 4 weeks to occur, which may be too long for patients with acute, severe anxiety.

Buspirone possesses no cross-tolerance with benzodiazepines, and it won't prevent benzodiazepine withdrawal symptoms. Therefore, if a patient is switching from a benzodiazepine to buspirone, the benzodiazepine should be withdrawn gradually, especially if the patient has received prolonged or high-dose therapy.

Drug effects

Unlike benzodiazepines, buspirone exerts only anxiolytic effects, although its mechanism of action is largely unknown. In vitro, it has no binding affinity for benzodiazepine receptors. However, it has a high affinity for serotonin and acts as a dopamine agonist. Buspirone has a relatively short half-life of 2 to 11 hours, which explains the need for multiple daily doses. (See *Comparing half-lives of antianxiety drugs,* page 56.)

Antihistamines

First-generation antihistamines, such as hydroxyzine (Vistaril, Atarax) and diphenhydramine (Benadryl), are occasionally prescribed for anxiety. Although they tend to be less effective than benzodiazepines in relieving anxiety, they have the advantage of producing no physical dependence. Antihistamines probably exert anxiolytic effects via their sedative properties.

Beta blockers

Beta blockers (particularly propranolol) are probably most useful as adjunctive therapy for patients who continue to have cardiovascular (CV) symptoms, such as tachycardia or palpitations, despite otherwise successful treatment of their anxiety. The drug may be especially useful in stressful situations, such as public speaking. However, most experts agree that a beta blocker will most likely yield inadequate results when given alone to treat generalized anxiety.

Drug effects

The exact mechanism by which propranolol exerts its anxiolytic effect is unknown. It probably relieves such symptoms as palpitations, tremulousness, and tachycardia through $beta_1$-blockade in the heart.

Antidepressants

Several types of antidepressants may help to ease anxiety disorders, including tricyclic antidepressants, selective serotonin reuptake inhibitors, and venlafaxine.

Tricyclic antidepressants—such as amitriptyline hydrochloride (Elavil) and imipramine hydrochloride (Tofranil)—may be especially helpful for patients who have underlying depression along with their anxiety. However, elderly or mentally impaired patients may have trouble adapting to the adverse effects caused by this class of drugs.

Some professionals consider the selective serotonin reuptake inhibitors—fluoxetine, sertraline, paroxetine, and fluvoxamine—drugs of choice for treating gener-

Comparing half-lives of antianxiety drugs

DRUG	HALF-LIFE OF PARENT DRUG	HALF-LIFE OF METABOLITE
LONG-ACTING BENZODIAZEPINES		
chlordiazepoxide	5-30 hr	36-200 hr
clorazepate dipotassium	40-50 hr	36-200 hr
diazepam	20-80 hr	36-200 hr
SHORT-ACTING BENZODIAZEPINES		
alprazolam	12-15 hr	none
lorazepam	10-20 hr	none
midazolam hydrochloride	6 min to 4 hr (biphasic)	60-80 min
oxazepam	5-20 hr	none
AZAPIRONES		
buspirone hydrochloride	2-11 hr	none
BETA BLOCKERS		
propranolol	3-5 hr	none
ANTIDEPRESSANTS		
amitriptyline hydrochloride	31-46 hr	none
doxepin hydrochloride	8-24 hr	none
fluoxetine hydrochloride	24-144 hr	24-144 hr
imipramine hydrochloride	11-25 hr	none
paroxetine hydrochloride	10-24 hr	none
sertraline hydrochloride	1-4 hr	1-4 hr
venlafaxine hydrochloride	5-11 hr	5-11 hr

alized anxiety. Although they have a risk of adverse sexual effects, these drugs don't produce significant anticholinergic and CV effects. Plus, they don't cause physical dependence and withdrawal. Some of these drugs are approved for treating panic disorder with or without agoraphobia, obsessive-compulsive disorder, and noncombat post-traumatic stress disorder.

Venlafaxine hydrochloride (Effexor XR) is a relatively new antidepressant that's structurally unrelated to the tricyclic antidepressants. It can be helpful for treating generalized anxiety disorder.

Drug effects

Antidepressants probably exert an anxiolytic effect via the same mechanism as their antidepressant effect: by increasing levels of certain neurotransmitters.

Adverse effects

The most common adverse effects of tricyclic antidepressants stem from their anticholinergic action. Discontinue a tricyclic antidepressant if the patient develops symptoms of esophageal reflux.

Typically, venlafaxine produces milder adverse effects than tricyclic antidepressants, and patients find it easier to tolerate.

Overdose and treatment

An overdose of a tricyclic antidepressant is very serious and may be fatal. Cardiac toxicity may be fatal in as little as 6 hours. Hospitalize and observe the patient for ECG changes and respiratory depression for at least 6 hours or until her cardiac status returns to normal.

Remember that concurrent use of tricyclic antidepressants and sympathomimetic drugs—such as isoproterenol, phenylephrine, norepinephrine, epinephrine, or amphetamines—may increase sympathetic activity so much that it threatens the patient's life. Use these drugs together only with extreme caution.

Patients who receive an overdose of venlafaxine will most likely develop somnolence, although they may have no adverse effects at all. The overdose may be life-threatening if the patient takes venlafaxine together with other drugs and alcohol.

PATIENT TEACHING

If your patient takes a benzodiazepine, tell her to do so on an as-needed basis. Explain that the drug works quickly and typically eases symptoms within about an hour. However, because this group of drugs remains effective for a limited time (usually 8 to 12 weeks), emphasize that she shouldn't exceed the prescribed dosage without first consulting the prescriber. Prolonged therapy may require regular dosage adjustments.

If the patient takes any other drug besides a benzodiazepine for anxiety, urge her to take it on a specific schedule each day. Warn her not to expect immediate results; in fact, mention that the full effect of the drug may take up to a month to occur. Also, explain that adverse effects may subside as her body becomes accustomed to the drug. Encourage her to call the prescriber about bothersome or persistent adverse effects.

No matter which drug the patient takes for anxiety, urge her to make regular appointments so the prescriber can check for improvement in her symptoms or the development of adverse effects. Also, warn her not to drink alcohol while taking a drug for anxiety. And suggest that she wait until the full effects of the drug are apparent before driving a car or performing other hazardous tasks. Finally, warn her not to suddenly stop taking her medication.

alprazolam
Alprazolam Intensol, Apo-Alpraz◇, Novo-Alprazol◇, Xanax

Pharmacologic classification:
benzodiazepine

Therapeutic classification:
antianxiety drug

Controlled substance schedule IV

Pregnancy risk category D

How supplied
Available by prescription only
Oral solution: 0.1 mg/1 ml, 1 mg/1 ml
Tablets: 0.25 mg, 0.5 mg, 1 mg, 2 mg

Indications and dosages
Anxiety
Adults: initially, 0.25 to 0.5 mg P.O. t.i.d. Increase dosage p.r.n. q 3 to 4 days. Maximum, 4 mg daily in divided doses.

▶ **DOSAGE ADJUSTMENT.** In elderly or debilitated patients or those with hepatic impairment, initial dosage is 0.25 mg P.O. b.i.d. or t.i.d.

Panic disorder
Adults: initially, 0.5 mg P.O. t.i.d. Increase as needed and tolerated q 3 to 4 days in increments of 1 mg daily. Dosages from 1 to 10 mg daily have been reported; most patients need more than 4 mg daily.

Agoraphobia with social phobia*
Adults: 2 to 8 mg/day P.O.

Depression, premenstrual syndrome*
Adults: 0.25 mg P.O. t.i.d.

Pharmacodynamics
Anxiolytic action: Alprazolam depresses the CNS at the limbic and subcortical levels of the brain. It reduces anxiety by enhancing the effect of gamma-aminobutyric acid on its receptor in the ascending reticular activating system, which increases inhibition and blocks both cortical and limbic arousal.

Pharmacokinetics
Absorption: Alprazolam is well absorbed by oral route. Drug action begins in 15 to 30 minutes and peaks in 1 to 2 hours.
Distribution: Drug is distributed widely throughout the body. About 80% to 90% of the dose is bound to plasma protein.
Metabolism: Alprazolam is metabolized in the liver, equally to alpha-hydroxyalprazolam and inactive metabolites.
Excretion: Alpha-hydroxyalprazolam and other metabolites are excreted in urine. Alprazolam's half-life is 12 to 15 hours.

Contraindications and precautions
Contraindicated in patients with acute angle-closure glaucoma or hypersensitivity to alprazolam or other benzodiazepines.

Use cautiously in patients with hepatic, renal, or pulmonary disease.

Interactions
Drug-drug
Antidepressants, antihistamines, barbiturates, general anesthetics, MAO inhibitors, narcotics, phenothiazines: potentiated CNS depres-

---

Reactions may be *common,* uncommon, *life-threatening,* or COMMON AND LIFE-THREATENING.

sant effects. Avoid concomitant use.

Cimetidine, possibly disulfiram: decreased hepatic metabolism of alprazolam, increasing its plasma level. Avoid concomitant use.

Digoxin: may increase plasma digoxin levels. Check serum drug levels, and monitor patient closely for evidence of digoxin toxicity.

Haloperidol: may decrease serum haloperidol levels. Monitor patient closely.

Rifampin: may decrease alprazolam's effects. Monitor patient closely.

Theophylline: may increase alprazolam's sedative effects. Monitor patient closely.

Drug-herb
Kava kava: may cause coma. Avoid concomitant use.

Drug-lifestyle
Alcohol use: potentiated CNS depressant effects. Avoid concomitant use.

Heavy smoking: accelerated alprazolam metabolism and decreased effectiveness. Discourage smoking during therapy.

Adverse reactions
CNS: confusion, *depression,* dizziness, *drowsiness,* headache, insomnia, *light-headedness,* tremor, syncope, nervousness.
CV: hypotension, tachycardia.
EENT: blurred vision, nasal congestion.
GI: *constipation, diarrhea, dry mouth,* nausea, vomiting.
Hepatic: elevated liver function test results.
Metabolic: weight gain or loss.

Musculoskeletal: muscle rigidity.
Skin: dermatitis.

Overdose and treatment
Overdose may cause bradycardia, confusion, coma, dyspnea, hypoactive reflexes, hypotension, impaired coordination, labored breathing, slurred speech, somnolence, and an unsteady gait.

Monitor patient's vital signs, and support blood pressure and respirations until drug effects subside. Flumazenil, a specific benzodiazepine antagonist, may be useful. Mechanical ventilation via endotracheal tube may be needed to maintain a patent airway and oxygenation.

Give I.V. fluids and vasopressors, such as dopamine and phenylephrine, for hypotension as needed. If patient is conscious, induce emesis. Perform gastric lavage if ingestion was recent, but only if an endotracheal tube is in place to prevent aspiration. After emesis or lavage, give a single dose of activated charcoal with a cathartic.

Dialysis is of limited value. Don't give barbiturates if excitation occurs because of possible increase in excitation or CNS depression.

Special considerations
■ Alprazolam may be used to treat anxiety with depression, but patient may need more frequent dosing than normal.
■ Provide the smallest prudent quantity of drug if patient has suicidal tendencies or a history of increasing the dosage without permission.
■ Carefully monitor patient for signs of drug abuse.

■ Obtain liver function tests, kidney function tests, and blood counts regularly during therapy.
■ After prolonged therapy with high doses, wean patient gradually to prevent withdrawal symptoms. A 2- to 3-month withdrawal may be needed.
■ Store drug in a cool, dry place away from direct light.

Breast-feeding patients
■ A breast-fed infant of a woman taking alprazolam may become sedated, have feeding difficulties, or lose weight. Avoid use in breast-feeding women.

Pediatric patients
■ Closely observe neonate for withdrawal symptoms if mother took alprazolam during pregnancy. Use of alprazolam during labor may cause neonatal flaccidity.
■ Safety has not been established in children or adolescents.

Geriatric patients
■ Give lower doses to elderly patients and those with renal or hepatic dysfunction.
■ At the start of therapy or after a dosage increase, elderly patients who receive drug may need assistance with ambulation and activities of daily living.

Patient teaching
■ Stress the possibility of physical and psychological dependence with long-term therapy. If patient has a history of previous substance abuse, consider developing a contract to enhance compliance.
■ Warn patient to take drug exactly as prescribed and not to stop therapy abruptly. Explain that seizures may result.
■ Tell patient to promptly notify prescriber about behavioral or mental changes that occur after therapy starts, including disturbing thoughts.
■ Caution patient that sudden position changes can cause dizziness. Suggest that she dangle her legs for a few minutes before getting out of bed.

---

buspirone hydrochloride
BuSpar

Pharmacologic classification: **azaspirodecanedione derivative**

Therapeutic classification: **antianxiety drug**

Pregnancy risk category B

How supplied
Available by prescription only
Tablets: 5 mg, 10 mg

Indications and dosages
Anxiety disorders
Adults: initially, 5 mg P.O. t.i.d. Increase at 3-day intervals p.r.n. Usual maintenance dosage is 20 to 30 mg daily in divided doses. Maximum, 60 mg/day.

Symptoms of premenstrual syndrome, including aches, pains, fatigue, cramps, irritability*
Adults: 25 mg P.O. daily.

Pharmacodynamics
Anxiolytic action: Buspirone suppresses conflict and aggressive be-

havior and inhibits conditioned avoidance responses. Its precise mechanism of action is unknown, but it seems to exert simultaneous effects on several neurotransmitters and receptor sites, thus decreasing serotonin neuronal activity, increasing norepinephrine metabolism, and acting as a presynaptic dopamine antagonist. It may have an indirect effect on benzodiazepine gamma-aminobutyric acid (GABA)-chloride receptor complex, GABA receptors, or other neurotransmitter systems.

Buspirone isn't pharmacologically related to benzodiazepines, barbiturates, or other sedative and anxiolytic drugs. It has a nontraditional clinical profile and is only anxiolytic, with no anticonvulsant action, muscle relaxant action, physical dependence, or significant sedation.

Pharmacokinetics
Absorption: Drug is absorbed rapidly and completely after oral administration, but extensive first-pass metabolism limits absolute bioavailability to 1% to 13% of an oral dose. Food slows absorption but increases the amount of unchanged drug in systemic circulation.
Distribution: Drug is 95% protein-bound; it doesn't displace other highly protein-bound drugs, such as warfarin. Onset of therapeutic effect may take 1 to 2 weeks.
Metabolism: Drug is metabolized in the liver by hydroxylation and oxidation, resulting in at least one pharmacologically active metabolite: 1, pyrimidinylpiperazine (1-PP).

Excretion: 29% to 63% is excreted in urine in 24 hours, primarily as metabolites; 18% to 38% is excreted in feces.

Contraindications and precautions
Contraindicated in patients hypersensitive to drug or within 14 days of taking an MAO inhibitor.

Avoid giving drug to breast-feeding women or to patients with severe renal or hepatic impairment.

Interactions
Drug-drug
CNS depressants: sedation may result, especially with dosages above 30 mg/day. Avoid concomitant use.
Digoxin: may be displaced from serum-binding sites by buspirone. Monitor serum digoxin levels, and watch for signs of toxicity.
Haloperidol: serum haloperidol levels may increase. Monitor patient closely.
MAO inhibitors: buspirone may raise blood pressure. Avoid concomitant use.

Drug-herb
Kava kava, valerian root: sedation may result. Avoid concomitant use.

Drug-lifestyle
Alcohol use: drug doesn't increase alcohol-induced impairments, but CNS effects aren't predictable. Discourage alcohol use during therapy.

Adverse reactions
CNS: *dizziness, drowsiness,* fatigue, headache, insomnia, light-headedness, nervousness, numbness.

EENT: blurred vision.
GI: abdominal distress, diarrhea, dry mouth, nausea.

Overdose and treatment
Overdose may cause drowsiness, nausea, severe dizziness, unusual pupillary constriction, and vomiting.

Treatment is symptomatic and supportive. Perform gastric lavage immediately to empty patient's stomach. Monitor patient's respirations, pulse, and blood pressure. No specific antidote is known. Effect of dialysis is unknown.

Special considerations
■ Expect that a patient who previously received a benzodiazepine may not respond well to buspirone.
■ Monitor patient's hepatic and renal function. Hepatic and renal impairment impedes metabolism and excretion of drug and may lead to toxic accumulation; dosage reduction may be needed.
■ Although buspirone doesn't seem to cause tolerance or dependence, patients prone to drug abuse may experience these effects.
■ Because buspirone doesn't block withdrawal symptoms caused by other benzodiazepines, taper the benzodiazepine gradually before replacing it with buspirone.

Patient teaching
■ Urge patient to take drug exactly as prescribed. Explain that improvement may occur after 7 to 10 days, but that full therapeutic effect may take 2 to 4 weeks to occur.
■ Tell patient to take a missed dose as soon as she remembers it unless the next dose is almost due; warn against doubling the dose.
■ Recommend regular follow-up visits to check progress, and encourage patient to report adverse effects immediately.
■ Caution patient to avoid hazardous tasks until full CNS effects of drug are known.
■ Tell patient to avoid substances that worsen sedation and drowsiness caused by buspirone, such as alcohol, antihistamines, sedatives, tranquilizers, sleeping aids, prescription pain medication, barbiturates, seizure medicine, muscle relaxants, anesthetics, valerian root, kava kava, and medicines for colds, coughs, hay fever, or allergies.
■ Tell patient to store drug away from heat and light, safely out of the reach of children.

---

chlordiazepoxide
Libritabs

chlordiazepoxide hydrochloride
Librium, Mitran, Reposans-10

Pharmacologic classification:
benzodiazepine

Therapeutic classification:
antianxiety drug, anticonvulsant, sedative-hypnotic

Controlled substance schedule IV

Pregnancy risk category D

How supplied
Available by prescription only
Capsules: 5 mg, 10 mg, 25 mg
Powder for injection: 100 mg/ampule

Tablets: 5 mg, 10 mg, 25 mg

Indications and dosages
Mild to moderate anxiety and tension
Adults: 5 to 10 mg P.O. t.i.d. or q.i.d.
Children over age 6 and elderly or debilitated patients: 5 mg P.O. b.i.d. to q.i.d. Maximum, 10 mg P.O. b.i.d. or t.i.d.

Severe anxiety and tension
Adults: 20 to 25 mg P.O. t.i.d. or q.i.d.

Withdrawal symptoms from acute alcoholism
Adults: 50 to 100 mg P.O., I.M., or I.V. Maximum, 300 mg/day.

Preoperative apprehension and anxiety
Adults: 5 to 10 mg P.O. t.i.d. or q.i.d. the day before surgery; or 50 to 100 mg I.M. 1 hour before surgery.

▶ **DOSAGE ADJUSTMENT.** Reduce dosage if patient has renal or hepatic dysfunction. Closely monitor patient's renal and hepatic studies.

Pharmacodynamics
Anxiolytic action: Chlordiazepoxide depresses the CNS at the limbic and subcortical levels of the brain. It produces an anxiolytic effect by influencing the effect of gamma-aminobutyric acid on its receptor in the ascending reticular activating system, which increases inhibition and blocks cortical and limbic arousal after stimulation of the reticular formation.
Anticonvulsant action: Drug suppresses the spread of seizure activi-

ty produced by epileptogenic foci in the cortex, thalamus, and limbic structures by enhancing presynaptic inhibition.

Pharmacokinetics
Absorption: When given orally, drug is absorbed well through the GI tract. Action begins in 30 to 45 minutes and peaks in 1 to 3 hours. I.M. administration yields erratic absorption; onset usually takes 15 to 30 minutes. After I.V. administration, onset occurs in 1 to 5 minutes.
Distribution: Drug is distributed widely throughout the body; 90% to 98% is protein-bound.
Metabolism: Chlordiazepoxide is metabolized in the liver to several active metabolites.
Excretion: Most metabolites are excreted in urine as glucuronide conjugates. Drug half-life is 5 to 30 hours.

Contraindications and precautions
Contraindicated in patients hypersensitive to drug. Don't give drug to breast-feeding women.
  Use cautiously if patient has impaired renal or hepatic function, mental depression, or porphyria.

Interactions
Drug-drug
Antacids: may delay chlordiazepoxide absorption. Separate administration times.
Antidepressants, antihistamines, barbiturates, general anesthetics, MAO inhibitors, narcotics, phenothiazines: chlordiazepoxide potentiates CNS depressant effects. Monitor patient closely.

---

*Unlabeled use

Cimetidine, possibly disulfiram: decreased hepatic metabolism of chlordiazepoxide, which increases its plasma level. Monitor patient closely.

Digoxin, phenytoin: serum digoxin or phenytoin levels may be increased. Monitor patient for toxic effects.

Haloperidol: serum haloperidol levels may decrease. Monitor patient closely.

Levodopa: therapeutic effects of levodopa may decrease. Monitor patient closely.

Oral contraceptives: may impair chlordiazepoxide metabolism. Urge patient to use another form of contraception.

Drug-lifestyle
Alcohol use: potentiated CNS depressant effects of alcohol. Discourage alcohol use during therapy.

Heavy smoking: increased chlordiazepoxide metabolism, which decreases effectiveness. Discourage tobacco use, and monitor patient for reduced drug effect.

Adverse reactions
CNS: ataxia, confusion, *drowsiness,* EEG changes, extrapyramidal symptoms, *lethargy.*
GI: constipation, nausea.
GU: increased or decreased libido, menstrual irregularities.
Hematologic: *agranulocytosis.*
Hepatic: jaundice.
Skin: edema, pain at injection site, skin eruptions, swelling.

Overdose and treatment
Overdose may cause bradycardia, coma, confusion, dyspnea, hypoac-

tive reflexes, hypotension, impaired coordination, labored breathing, slurred speech, somnolence, and an unsteady gait.

To treat an overdose, support the patient's blood pressure and respirations until drug effects subside; monitor her vital signs throughout. Flumazenil, a specific benzodiazepine antagonist, may be useful. Mechanical ventilatory assistance via endotracheal tube may be required to maintain a patent airway and oxygenation. Give I.V. fluids and vasopressors, such as dopamine and phenylephrine, for hypotension as needed. Induce emesis if the patient is conscious. Or, if ingestion was recent and the patient has an endotracheal tube in place, perform gastric lavage. After emesis or lavage, give a single dose of activated charcoal with a cathartic. Don't give barbiturates if excitation occurs. Expect dialysis to provide limited assistance.

Special considerations
■ Prepare I.V. and I.M. solutions immediately before use. Discard unused portions.
■ Avoid I.M. administration because of slow, erratic absorption. If you must use I.M. route, reconstitute with special diluent only. Don't use hazy diluent. Inject deep into large muscle mass.
■ For I.V. use, reconstitute with sterile water or normal saline solution and infuse slowly, directly into a large vein, at 50 mg/minute or less for adults. Don't infuse drug into small veins. Observe infusion site for phlebitis, and avoid extravasation. Keep resuscitation

---

Reactions may be *common,* uncommon, *life-threatening,* or COMMON AND LIFE-THREATENING.

equipment nearby in case of emergency.
■ Keep patient in bed under observation for at least 3 hours after parenteral administration.
■ Chlordiazepoxide may cause false-positive results in pregnancy test, depending on method used. It may also alter urine 17-keto-steroids (Zimmerman reaction), urine alkaloid determination (Frings thin layer chromatography method), and urine glucose determinations (Chemstrip uG and Diastix, but not glucose enzymatic test strip).

Pediatric patients
■ Safety of oral form hasn't been established in children under age 6. Safety of parenteral form has not been established in children under age 12. Avoid parenteral form for children under age 12.

Geriatric patients
■ Reduced dosages are usually effective in elderly patients because of decreased elimination.
■ Expect elderly patients to show greater CNS depressant effects. Some may need help with ambulation and activities of daily living when therapy starts or dosage increases.
■ Parenteral administration of drug is more likely to cause apnea, hypotension, and bradycardia in elderly patients.

Patient teaching
■ Warn patient about possible dizziness with sudden position changes. Tell her to dangle her legs for a few minutes before getting out of bed to prevent falls and injury.
■ Tell patient to avoid hazardous activities until drug's CNS effects are clear.
■ Urge patient to avoid alcohol.
■ Tell patient to promptly notify prescriber about behavioral or mental changes that occur after therapy starts, including disturbing thoughts.

---

clorazepate dipotassium
Novoclopate◊, Tranxene, Tranxene-SD, Tranxene-SD Half Strength

Pharmacologic classification: **benzodiazepine**

Therapeutic classification: **antianxiety drug, anticonvulsant, sedative-hypnotic**

Controlled substance schedule IV

Pregnancy risk category NR

How supplied
Available by prescription only
Capsules: 3.75 mg, 7.5 mg, 15 mg
Tablets: 3.75 mg, 7.5 mg, 11.25 mg, 15 mg, 22.5 mg

Indications and dosages
Acute alcohol withdrawal
Adults: on day 1, 30 mg P.O. followed by 30 to 60 mg P.O. in divided doses. On day 2, 45 to 90 mg P.O. in divided doses. On day 3, 22.5 to 45 mg P.O. in divided doses. On day 4, 15 to 30 mg P.O. in divided doses. On day 5 and after, gradually reduce to 7.5 to 15 mg daily.

Anxiety
Adults: 15 to 60 mg P.O. daily.

Partial seizures (adjunct)
Adults and children over age 12: Maximum recommended initial dosage is 7.5 mg P.O. t.i.d. Dosage increases should not exceed 7.5 mg/week. Maximum, 90 mg daily.
Children ages 9 to 12: Maximum recommended initial dosage is 7.5 mg P.O. b.i.d. Dosage increases should not exceed 7.5 mg/week. Maximum, 60 mg daily.

Pharmacodynamics
Anxiolytic and sedative actions: Clorazepate depresses the CNS at the limbic and subcortical levels of the brain. It produces an anxiolytic effect by enhancing the action of gamma-aminobutyric acid on its receptor in the ascending reticular activating system, which increases inhibition and blocks cortical and limbic arousal.
Anticonvulsant action: Drug suppresses the spread of seizure activity produced by epileptogenic foci in the cortex, thalamus, and limbic structures by enhancing presynaptic inhibition.

Pharmacokinetics
Absorption: After oral administration, clorazepate is hydrolyzed in the stomach to desmethyldiazepam, which is absorbed completely and rapidly. Serum levels peak after 1 to 2 hours.
Distribution: Drug is distributed widely throughout the body. About 80% to 95% of a dose is bound to plasma protein.

Metabolism: Desmethyldiazepam is metabolized in the liver to conjugated oxazepam.
Excretion: Inactive glucuronide metabolites are excreted in urine. The half-life of desmethyldiazepam ranges from 30 to 100 hours.

Contraindications and precautions
Contraindicated in patients hypersensitive to drug or other benzodiazepines and in patients with acute angle-closure glaucoma.

Use cautiously if patient has suicidal tendencies, a history of drug abuse, or impaired renal or hepatic function. Avoid use in pregnant patients, especially during the first trimester.

Interactions
Drug-drug
Antacids: may delay clorazepate absorption and reduce total amount absorbed. Separate administration times.
Antidepressants, antihistamines, barbiturates, general anesthetics, MAO inhibitors, narcotics, phenothiazines: clorazepate potentiates CNS depressant effects. Monitor patient closely.
Cimetidine, possibly disulfiram: reduces hepatic metabolism of clorazepate, which increases plasma levels. Monitor patient closely.
Haloperidol: decreased serum haloperidol levels. Monitor for loss of drug effect.
Levodopa: clorazepate may decrease levodopa's effectiveness. Monitor patient closely.

Drug-lifestyle
Alcohol use: clorazepate potentiates CNS depression. Discourage alcohol use during therapy.
Heavy smoking: accelerates clorazepate's metabolism, thus lowering its effectiveness. Monitor patient closely.

Adverse reactions
CNS: confusion, depression, dizziness, *drowsiness,* headache, insomnia, irritability, nervousness, tremor.
CV: hypotension, minor changes in EEG patterns.
EENT: blurred vision, diplopia.
GI: abdominal discomfort, dry mouth, nausea, vomiting.
GU: incontinence, urine retention.
Hepatic: elevated liver function test results.
Skin: rash.

Overdose and treatment
Overdose may cause bradycardia, coma, confusion, dyspnea, hypoactive reflexes, hypotension, impaired coordination, labored breathing, slurred speech, somnolence, and an unsteady gait.

To treat an overdose, support the patient's blood pressure and respirations until drug effects subside; monitor her vital signs throughout. Flumazenil, a specific benzodiazepine antagonist, may be useful. Mechanical ventilatory assistance via endotracheal tube may be required to maintain a patent airway and oxygenation. Give I.V. fluids and vasopressors, such as dopamine and phenylephrine, for hypotension as needed. Induce emesis if the patient is conscious. Or, if ingestion was recent and the patient has an endotracheal tube in place, perform gastric lavage. After emesis or lavage, give a single dose of activated charcoal with a cathartic. Don't give barbiturates because they may worsen CNS effects.

Special considerations
■ Provide the smallest prudent quantity of drug if patient has suicidal tendencies or a history of increasing the dosage without permission.
■ Store in a cool, dry place away from direct light.

Breast-feeding patients
■ Avoid use in breast-feeding woman because infant may become sedated, have feeding difficulties, or lose weight.

Pediatric patients
■ Safety has not been established in children under age 9.

Geriatric patients
■ Reduced doses are usually effective in elderly patients because of decreased elimination.
■ Elderly patients may need help with ambulation and activities of daily living when therapy starts or dosage increases.

Patient teaching
■ Caution patient about possible physical and psychological dependence with long-term use of clorazepate.
■ If patient takes an antacid, tell her to do so 1 hour before or after taking clorazepate.
■ Tell patient to take drug exactly as prescribed and not to change without consulting prescriber.

■ Caution patient about possible dizziness with sudden position. Urge her to dangle her legs for a few minutes before getting out of bed to prevent falls and injury.
■ Warn patient not to suddenly stop taking drug.
■ Tell patient to promptly notify prescriber about behavioral or mental changes that occur after therapy starts, including disturbing thoughts.
■ Tell women of childbearing age to use reliable contraception and to notify prescriber about suspected or known pregnancy.

---

diazepam
Apo-Diazepam◇, Diastat, Novodipam◇, Valium, Vivol◇, Zetran

Pharmacologic classification: benzodiazepine

Therapeutic classification: amnesic, antianxiety drug, anticonvulsant, sedative-hypnotic, skeletal muscle relaxant

Controlled substance schedule IV

Pregnancy risk category D

How supplied
Available by prescription only
Capsules (extended-release): 15 mg
Disposable syringe: 2-ml Tel-E-Ject
Injection: 5 mg/ml in 2-ml ampules or 10-ml vials
Oral solution: 5 mg/ml, 5 mg/5 ml
Oral suspension: 5 mg/5 ml
Rectal gel: 2.5 mg, 5 mg, 10 mg, 15 mg, 20 mg
Tablets: 2 mg, 5 mg, 10 mg

Indications and dosages
Anxiety
Adults: depending on severity, 2 to 10 mg P.O. b.i.d. to q.i.d. or 15 to 30 mg extended-release capsules P.O. once daily. Alternatively, 2 to 10 mg I.M. or I.V. q 3 to 4 hours, p.r.n.
Children age 6 months and older: 1 to 2.5 mg P.O. t.i.d. or q.i.d. Increase gradually as needed and tolerated.

Acute alcohol withdrawal
Adults: 10 mg P.O. t.i.d. or q.i.d. for the first 24 hours; then reduce to 5 mg t.i.d. or q.i.d., p.r.n. Or 10 mg I.M. or I.V. initially, followed by 5 to 10 mg q 3 to 4 hours, p.r.n.

Seizure disorders (adjunct)
Adults: 2 to 10 mg P.O. b.i.d. to q.i.d.
Children age 6 months and older: initially, 1 to 2.5 mg P.O. t.i.d. or q.i.d., increased as needed and tolerated.

Status epilepticus
Adults: initially, 5 to 10 mg I.V. (preferred) or I.M., repeated at 10- to 15-minute intervals to a maximum of 30 mg. Repeat q 2 to 4 hours, p.r.n.
Children age 5 and older: 1 mg I.V. q 2 to 5 minutes to a maximum of 10 mg. Repeat in 2 to 4 hours, p.r.n.
Infants over age 30 days to children age 5: 0.2 to 0.5 mg I.V. q 2 to 5 minutes to a maximum of 5 mg.

Reactions may be *common,* uncommon, *life-threatening,* or COMMON AND LIFE-THREATENING.

Acute repetitive seizure activity in patients already taking antiepileptic drugs

Children age 12 and older: 0.2 mg/kg P.R. using applicator. A second dose may be given 4 to 12 hours after the first dose, if needed.
Children ages 6 to 11: 0.3 mg/kg P.R. using applicator. A second dose may be given 4 to 12 hours after the first dose, if needed.
Children ages 2 to 5: 0.5 mg/kg P.R. using applicator. A second dose may be given 4 to 12 hours after the first dose, if needed.

Pharmacodynamics

Anxiolytic and sedative-hypnotic actions: Diazepam depresses the CNS at the limbic and subcortical levels of the brain. It produces an anxiolytic effect by influencing the effect of gamma-aminobutyric acid on its receptor in the ascending reticular activating system, which increases inhibition and blocks cortical and limbic arousal.
Anticonvulsant action: Diazepam suppresses the spread of seizure activity produced by epileptogenic foci in the cortex, thalamus, and limbic structures by enhancing presynaptic inhibition.
Amnesic action: Unknown.
Skeletal muscle relaxant action: The exact mechanism is unknown, but it probably involves inhibiting polysynaptic afferent pathways.

Pharmacokinetics

Absorption: When administered orally, drug is absorbed through the GI tract. Action starts in 30 to 60 minutes and peaks in 1 to 2 hours. I.M. administration results in erratic absorption; onset usually takes 15 to 30 minutes. Onset of action occurs 1 to 5 minutes after I.V. administration. Drug is well absorbed rectally and reaches peak plasma levels in 1½ hours in adults.
Distribution: Drug is distributed widely throughout the body. About 85% to 95% of a dose is bound to plasma protein.
Metabolism: Drug is metabolized in the liver to the active metabolite desmethyldiazepam.
Excretion: Most metabolites of diazepam are excreted in urine, with only small amounts excreted in feces. Half-life of desmethyldiazepam is 30 to 200 hours. Duration of sedative effect is 3 hours but may be prolonged up to 90 hours in elderly patients and those with hepatic or renal dysfunction. Anticonvulsant effect occurs 15 to 60 minutes after I.V. administration.

Contraindications and precautions

Contraindicated in patients hypersensitive to drug; patients with angle-closure glaucoma; patients experiencing shock, coma, or acute alcohol intoxication (parenteral form); and children under age 6 months (oral form).

Use cautiously in elderly patients, debilitated patients, and patients with impaired hepatic or renal function, depression, or chronic open-angle glaucoma. Avoid use in pregnant women, especially during the first trimester.

Interactions

Drug-drug

Antacids: may decrease diazepam absorption rate. Separate administration times.

Antidepressants, antihistamines, barbiturates, general anesthetics, MAO inhibitors, narcotics, phenothiazines: diazepam potentiates CNS depressant effects. Monitor patient closely.

Cimetidine, possibly disulfiram: diminished hepatic metabolism of diazepam, which increases its plasma levels. Monitor patient closely.

Digoxin: diazepam may decrease digoxin clearance. Monitor patient for digoxin toxicity.

Haloperidol: may change seizure patterns of patients who take diazepam. Benzodiazepines may reduce serum haloperidol levels. Monitor patient closely.

Levodopa: diazepam may inhibit levodopa's effect. Monitor patient for reduced effect.

Nondepolarizing neuromuscular blockers, such as pancuronium and succinylcholine: intensified and prolonged respiratory depression. Avoid concomitant use.

Oral contraceptives: may impair diazepam metabolism. Have patient use another contraceptive method.

Drug-lifestyle

Alcohol use: diazepam potentiates CNS depressant effects. Discourage concomitant use.

Heavy smoking: accelerates diazepam metabolism, thus lowering effectiveness. Discourage concomitant use.

Adverse reactions

CNS: ataxia, changes in EEG patterns, *drowsiness,* fatigue, hallucinations, headache, insomnia, paradoxical anxiety, slurred speech, transient amnesia, tremor.

CV: *bradycardia, CV collapse,* hypotension.

EENT: blurred vision, diplopia, nystagmus.

GI: constipation, nausea.

GU: altered libido, incontinence, urine retention.

Hematologic: *neutropenia.*

Hepatic: elevated liver function test results, *jaundice.*

Musculoskeletal: *dysarthria.*

Respiratory: *respiratory depression.*

Skin: rash.

Other: *acute withdrawal syndrome* after sudden discontinuation in physically dependent person, *pain or phlebitis* at injection site, physical or psychological dependence.

Overdose and treatment

Overdose may cause bradycardia, coma, confusion, dyspnea, hypoactive reflexes, hypotension, impaired coordination, labored breathing, slurred speech, somnolence, and an unsteady gait.

To treat an overdose, support the patient's blood pressure and respirations until drug effects subside; monitor her vital signs throughout. Flumazenil, a specific benzodiazepine antagonist, may be useful but shouldn't be administered during status epilepticus. Mechanical ventilatory assistance via endotracheal tube may be required to maintain a patent airway and oxygenation. Give I.V. fluids and vaso-

---

Reactions may be *common,* uncommon, *life-threatening,* or COMMON AND LIFE-THREATENING.

pressors, such as dopamine and phenylephrine, for hypotension as needed. Induce emesis if the patient is conscious. Or, if ingestion was recent and the patient has an endotracheal tube in place, perform gastric lavage. After emesis or lavage, give a single dose of activated charcoal with a cathartic. Dialysis is of limited value.

Special considerations
■ Consider a different therapy if patient has COPD or sleep apnea.
■ Provide the smallest prudent quantity of drug if patient has suicidal tendencies or a history of increasing the dosage without permission.
■ Monitor patient for signs of abuse or misuse of drug during therapy.
■ Have patient swallow extended-release capsules whole; don't crush or allow patient to chew them.
■ Shake oral suspension well immediately before giving it.
■ To improve taste, mix oral solution with liquids or semisolid foods, such as applesauce or pudding, just before administration.
■ Give Diastat rectal gel to treat no more than 5 episodes per month and one episode every 5 days.
■ Parenteral forms of diazepam may be diluted in normal saline solution. Solution can be used even if a slight precipitate forms.
■ Don't mix diazepam with other drugs in a syringe or infusion container.
■ Because diazepam interacts with plastic, don't store it in plastic syringes or administer it in plastic administration sets. Doing so will decrease drug availability.

■ I.V. route is preferred because of rapid and more uniform absorption, but continuous I.V. infusion isn't recommended.
■ During I.V. administration, infuse drug slowly, directly into a large vein, at no more than 5 mg/minute for adults (0.25 mg/kg over 3 minutes for children). Don't inject drug into small veins to avoid extravasation. Observe infusion site for phlebitis.
■ If direct I.V. administration isn't possible, inject drug into I.V. tubing at point closest to venous insertion site to prevent extravasation.
■ Use I.M. route only if I.V. or oral routes are unavailable. Inject I.M. dose deep into deltoid muscle. Aspirate for backflow to prevent inadvertent arterial administration.
■ Keep patient in bed under observation for at least 3 hours after parenteral administration to minimize hazards; keep resuscitation equipment nearby.
■ During prolonged therapy, periodically monitor the patient's blood counts and liver function studies.
■ Don't discontinue drug suddenly; instead, decrease dosage slowly over 8 to 12 weeks after long-term therapy.
■ When using diazepam as adjunctive therapy for a seizure disorder, anticipate a possible transient increase in frequency or severity of seizures. Take seizure precautions.
■ Besides standard indications, drug may be used for muscle spasms, tetanus, and adjunct to anesthesia and cardioversion.

- When administering with opiates for endoscopic procedures, reduce opiate dose by at least one-third.
- Assess patient's gag reflex after endoscopy and before resuming oral intake to prevent aspiration.

Pregnant patients
- Use of diazepam during labor may cause neonatal flaccidity.
- Closely observe neonate whose mother took diazepam for a prolonged period during pregnancy; infant may show withdrawal symptoms.

Breast-feeding patients
- Because diazepam enters breast milk, the breast-fed infant may become sedated, have feeding difficulties, or lose weight. Avoid use of drug in breast-feeding women.

Pediatric patients
- Safe use of oral diazepam in infants under age 6 months has not been established.
- Safe use of parenteral diazepam in infants under age 30 days has not been established.

Geriatric patients
- Lower doses are effective in patients with renal or hepatic dysfunction and in elderly patients.
- Elderly patients are more sensitive to CNS depressant effects and may need help with ambulation and activities of daily living when therapy starts or dosage increases. Parenteral administration is more likely to cause apnea, hypotension, and bradycardia in elderly patients.

Patient teaching
- Urge patient to take diazepam exactly as prescribed and not to change dosage or discontinue drug without consulting prescriber.
- Caution patient about possible physical and psychological dependence with long-term use.
- Warn patient about possible dizziness with sudden position changes. Advise patient to dangle her legs for a few minutes before getting out of bed to prevent falls and injury.
- Encourage patient to avoid or limit smoking to prevent interference with drug action.
- Tell patient to avoid alcohol while taking diazepam.
- Tell patient to promptly notify prescriber about behavioral or mental changes that occur after therapy starts, including disturbing thoughts.
- Warn women to immediately notify prescriber about planned, suspected, or known pregnancy.
- Teach patient's caregiver how and when to administer rectal gel and how to monitor and record patient's response.

hydroxyzine hydrochloride
**Anxanil, Apo-Hydroxyzine◇,
Atarax, Hydroxacen, Hyzine-50,
Multipax◇, Novo-Hydroxyzin◇,
Quiess, Vistacon-50, Vistazine 50**

hydroxyzine pamoate
Vistaril

Pharmacologic classification:
**antihistamine (piperazine
derivative)**

Therapeutic classification:
**antianxiety drug, antiemetic,
antispasmodic, antipruritic,
sedative**

*Pregnancy risk category X (in
early pregnancy)*

How supplied
Available by prescription only
hydroxyzine hydrochloride
Capsules: 10 mg, 25 mg, 50 mg
Injection: 25 mg/ml, 50 mg/ml
Syrup: 10 mg/5 ml
Tablets: 10 mg, 25 mg, 50 mg,
100 mg
hydroxyzine pamoate
Capsules: 25 mg, 50 mg, 100 mg
Oral suspension: 25 mg/5 ml

Indications and dosages
Anxiety, tension, hyperkinesia
Adults: 50 to 100 mg P.O. q.i.d.
Children over age 6: 50 to 100 mg
P.O. daily in divided doses.
Children under age 6: 50 mg P.O.
daily in divided doses.

Pharmacodynamics
Anxiolytic and sedative actions:
Hydroxyzine produces sedative and
anxiolytic effects by suppressing
activity at subcortical levels; analgesia occurs with high doses.
Antipruritic action: Drug competes
directly with histamine for binding
at cellular receptor sites.

Pharmacokinetics
Absorption: Drug is absorbed
rapidly and completely after oral
administration. Serum levels peak
in 2 to 4 hours. Sedation and other
effects are usually noticed in 15 to
30 minutes.
Distribution: Not well understood.
Metabolism: Drug is metabolized
almost completely in the liver.
Excretion: Drug metabolites are
excreted primarily in urine; small
amounts of drug and metabolites
appear in feces. Drug has 3-hour
half-life. Sedative effects can last 4
to 6 hours; antihistaminic effects
can persist up to 4 days.

Contraindications and precautions
Contraindicated in patients hypersensitive to drug and during early
pregnancy.
Use cautiously in elderly or debilitated patients.

Interactions
Drug-drug
Anticholinergic drugs: additive anticholinergic effects. Monitor patient
closely.
*Barbiturates, CNS depressants, opi-
oids, tranquilizers:* hydroxyzine
may add to or potentiate effects of
these drugs; reduce CNS depressant dose by 50%.
Epinephrine: hydroxyzine may
block epinephrine's vasopressor
action. If patient needs a vasocon-

strictor, use norepinephrine or metaraminol.

Drug-lifestyle
Alcohol use: hydroxyzine may add to or potentiate alcohol effects. Discourage concomitant use.

Adverse reactions
CNS: confusion, *drowsiness*, involuntary motor activity.
GI: *constipation, dry mouth.*
GU: urine retention.
Other: *hypersensitivity reactions* (wheezing, dyspnea, chest tightness), marked discomfort at I.M. injection site.

Overdose and treatment
Overdose may cause excessive sedation and hypotension; seizures may occur.

To treat overdose, provide supportive care. For recent oral ingestion, empty gastric contents through induced emesis or lavage. Correct hypotension with fluids and vasopressors (norepinephrine or metaraminol). Don't give epinephrine because hydroxyzine may counteract its effect.

Special considerations
■ Anticipate that hydroxyzine may be used as a preoperative and postoperative adjunct for its sedative, antihistaminic, and anticholinergic activity. Drug is also prescribed to control emesis and as an adjunct to asthma treatment.
■ Don't give drug by intra-arterial, I.V., or S.C. route. Give only by deep I.M. injection. Aspirate carefully to prevent inadvertent intravascular administration.

■ Watch for excessive sedation, especially if patient receives other CNS depressants.
■ Expect drug to falsely elevate urine 17-hydroxycorticosteroid levels. It also may cause false-negative skin allergen tests by attenuating or inhibiting cutaneous response to histamine.

Breast-feeding patients
■ No data exist to demonstrate whether drug is excreted in breast milk. Safe use hasn't been established in breast-feeding women.

Geriatric patients
■ Elderly patients may experience greater CNS depression and anticholinergic effects; give reduced doses.

Patient teaching
■ Caution patient to avoid hazardous activities until drug's full CNS effects are known. Urge patient to avoid additional CNS depressants (such as alcohol) unless prescribed.
■ Instruct patient to consult prescriber before taking OTC antihistamines, such as cold or allergy medications, because they may increase the effects of hydroxyzine.
■ If patient complains of dry mouth, suggest sugarless gum or candy. Also, suggest drinking plenty of water to minimize dry mouth and constipation.

Reactions may be *common,* uncommon, *life-threatening,* or COMMON AND LIFE-THREATENING.

lorazepam
Apo-Lorazepam◊, Ativan, Novo-Lorazem◊

Pharmacologic classification:
benzodiazepine

Therapeutic classification:
antianxiety drug, sedative-hypnotic

Controlled substance schedule IV

Pregnancy risk category D

How supplied
Available by prescription only
Injection: 2 mg/ml, 4 mg/ml
Tablets: 0.5 mg, 1 mg, 2 mg
Tablets (S.L.)◊: 1 mg, 2 mg

Indications and dosages
Anxiety, tension, agitation, irritability, especially in anxiety neuroses or organic (especially GI or CV) disorders
Adults: 2 to 6 mg P.O. daily in divided doses. Maximum, 10 mg/day.

Insomnia
Adults: 2 to 4 mg P.O. h.s.

Pharmacodynamics
Anxiolytic and sedative actions:
Lorazepam depresses the CNS at the limbic and subcortical levels of the brain. It produces an anxiolytic action by influencing the effect of gamma-aminobutyric acid on its receptor in the ascending reticular activating system, which increases inhibition and blocks both cortical and limbic arousal after stimulation of the reticular formation.

Pharmacokinetics
Absorption: When administered orally, drug is well absorbed through the GI tract. Levels peak in 2 hours. Half-life is 10 to 20 hours.
Distribution: Drug is distributed widely throughout the body. It's about 85% protein-bound.
Metabolism: Drug is metabolized in the liver to inactive metabolites.
Excretion: The metabolites of lorazepam are excreted in urine as glucuronide conjugates.

Contraindications and precautions
Contraindicated in patients with acute angle-closure glaucoma and in patients hypersensitive to drug, to its vehicle (parenteral form), or to other benzodiazepines.

Use cautiously in patients with pulmonary, renal, or hepatic impairment and in elderly, acutely ill, or debilitated patients. Avoid use in pregnant patients, especially during the first trimester.

Interactions
Drug-drug
Antidepressants, antihistamines, barbiturates, general anesthetics, MAO inhibitors, narcotics, phenothiazines: lorazepam potentiates CNS depressant effects. Monitor patient closely.
Cimetidine, possibly disulfiram: diminishes hepatic metabolism of lorazepam, which increases its plasma levels. Monitor patient closely.
Scopolamine: combined use with parenteral lorazepam may increase the risk of hallucinations, irrational behavior, and sedation. Monitor patient closely.

Drug-food
Caffeine-containing products: may interfere with drug's effectiveness. Discourage concomitant use.

Drug-lifestyle
Alcohol use: lorazepam potentiates CNS depressant effects. Discourage concomitant use.
Heavy smoking: accelerates lorazepam's metabolism, thus lowering its effectiveness. Advise against smoking and concomitant use.

Adverse reactions
CNS: agitation, amnesia, depression, disorientation, dizziness, *drowsiness,* headache, insomnia, *sedation,* unsteadiness, weakness.
EENT: visual disturbances.
GI: abdominal discomfort, change in appetite, nausea.
Other: *acute withdrawal syndrome* after sudden discontinuation in physically dependent person.

Overdose and treatment
Overdose may cause bradycardia, coma, confusion, dyspnea, hypoactive reflexes, hypotension, impaired coordination, labored breathing, slurred speech, somnolence, and an unsteady gait.

To treat an overdose, support the patient's blood pressure and respirations until drug effects subside; monitor her vital signs throughout. Flumazenil, a specific benzodiazepine antagonist, may be useful. Mechanical ventilatory assistance via endotracheal tube may be required to maintain a patent airway and oxygenation. Give I.V. fluids and vasopressors, such as dopamine and phenylephrine, for hypotension as needed. Induce emesis if the patient is conscious. Or, if ingestion was recent and the patient has an endotracheal tube in place, perform gastric lavage. After emesis or lavage, give a single dose of activated charcoal with a cathartic. Dialysis is of limited value.

Special considerations
■ Lorazepam is a preferred choice of benzodiazepine if the patient has hepatic disease. Periodically assess liver function studies to ensure adequate drug metabolism and detect cumulative effects.
■ To avoid oversedation, use the lowest effective dosage.
■ Consider a different therapy if patient has COPD or sleep anea.
■ Provide the smallest prudent quantity of drug if patient has suicidal tendencies or a history of increasing the dosage without permission.
■ Parenteral lorazepam appears to possess potent amnestic effects.
■ Give oral drug in divided doses, with the largest dose at bedtime.
■ For I.V. administration, dilute drug with an equal volume of a compatible diluent, such as D_5W, sterile water for injection, or normal saline solution. Give diluted solution immediately. Don't use discolored or precipitated solution.
■ Inject drug directly into a vein or into the tubing of a compatible I.V. infusion, such as normal saline solution or D_5W. Don't exceed 2 mg/minute of lorazepam. Keep emergency resuscitative equipment nearby during I.V. administration.
■ Administer I.M. dose undiluted and deep into a large muscle mass.

Reactions may be *common,* uncommon, *life-threatening,* or COMMON AND LIFE-THREATENING.

■ Lorazepam injection has also been used to manage status epilepticus, nausea and vomiting caused by chemotherapy, acute alcohol withdrawal, and psychogenic catatonia.

Breast-feeding patients
■ Drug may be excreted in breast milk. Don't administer to breast-feeding women.
■ Closely observe neonate for withdrawal symptoms if mother took lorazepam for a prolonged period during pregnancy.

Pediatric patients
■ Safe use of oral lorazepam in children under age 12 hasn't been established.
■ Safe use of S.L. or parenteral lorazepam in children under age 18 hasn't been established.

Geriatric patients
■ Elderly patients are more sensitive to lorazepam's CNS depressant effects and may need help with ambulation and activities of daily living when therapy starts or dosage increases.
■ Parenteral administration is more likely to cause apnea, hypotension, bradycardia, and cardiac arrest in elderly patients.

Patient teaching
■ Caution patient about possible physical and psychological dependence with long-term use.
■ Warn patient to avoid hazardous activities until full CNS effects of drug are known.
■ Teach safety measures, as appropriate, to minimize the risk of injury. For example, advise gradual

position changes and assisted walking.
■ Tell patient to avoid large amounts of caffeine-containing products because caffeine may reduce drug's effectiveness.
■ Tell patient that drug must be discontinued gradually, over 8 to 12 weeks, after long-term therapy. Caution patient not to alter drug regimen without consulting prescriber.
■ Advise patient about possible retrograde amnesia after I.V. or I.M. delivery.

meprobamate
Apo-Meprobamate◇, Equanil, Meprospan, Miltown, Neuramate

Pharmacologic classification: carbamate

Therapeutic classification: antianxiety drug

Controlled substance schedule IV

Pregnancy risk category D

How supplied
Available by prescription only
Capsules (sustained-release): 200 mg, 400 mg
Tablets: 200 mg, 400 mg, 600 mg

Indications and dosages
Anxiety and tension
Adults: 1.2 to 1.6 g P.O. daily in three or four equal doses. Maximum, 2.4 g daily. Sustained-release capsules, 400 to 800 mg b.i.d.
Children ages 6 to 12: 100 to 200 mg P.O. b.i.d. or t.i.d. Not recommended for children under age 6.

Sustained-release capsules, 200 mg b.i.d.

Pharmacodynamics
Anxiolytic action: Cellular mechanism is unknown, but drug causes nonselective CNS depression similar to that of barbiturates. Meprobamate acts at multiple CNS sites, including the thalamus, hypothalamus, limbic system, and spinal cord, but not the medulla or reticular activating system.

Pharmacokinetics
Absorption: After oral administration, drug is well absorbed; serum levels peak in 1 to 3 hours. Sedation usually occurs within 1 hour.
Distribution: Meprobamate is distributed throughout the body; 20% is protein-bound. Drug is excreted in breast milk at two to four times the serum level. Meprobamate also crosses the placenta.
Metabolism: Drug is metabolized rapidly in the liver to inactive glucuronide conjugates. Drug's half-life is 6 to 17 hours.
Excretion: Metabolites are excreted in urine along with 10% to 20% of a single dose as unchanged drug.

Contraindications and precautions
Contraindicated in patients hypersensitive to meprobamate or related compounds (such as carbromal, carisoprodol, mebutamate, and tybamate) and in those with porphyria. Avoid giving drug during first trimester of pregnancy.

Use cautiously in patients with seizure disorders or suicidal tendencies, in elderly or debilitated patients, and in those with impaired renal or hepatic function.

Interactions
Drug-drug
Antihistamines, barbiturates, other CNS depressants, narcotics, tranquilizers: meprobamate may add to or potentiate CNS effects. Monitor patient closely.

Drug-lifestyle
Alcohol use: meprobamate may add to or potentiate CNS effects. Discourage concomitant use.

Adverse reactions
CNS: ataxia, dizziness, *drowsiness,* headache, ***seizures,*** slurred speech, syncope, vertigo.
CV: ***arrhythmias,*** hypotension, palpitations, tachycardia.
GI: diarrhea, nausea, vomiting.
Hematologic: ***agranulocytosis, aplastic anemia, thrombocytopenia.***
Skin: erythematous maculopapular rash, ***hypersensitivity reactions,*** pruritus, urticaria.

Overdose and treatment
Overdose may cause ataxia, coma, drowsiness, hypotension, lethargy, respiratory depression, and shock. Serum levels above 100 mcg/ml may be fatal.

To treat overdose, give supportive care for symptoms. Maintain a patent airway with mechanical ventilation if necessary. Give fluids and vasopressors as needed for hypotension. If ingestion was recent, empty patient's gastric contents by inducing emesis or performing gastric lavage (if patient has an endotracheal tube in place to prevent aspiration). Then give activated charcoal and a cathartic. Treat seizures with parenteral diazepam. Peritoneal dialysis and hemodialysis may remove drug.

Special considerations
■ Assess patient's level of consciousness and vital signs often.
■ Evaluate patient's CBC periodically during long-term therapy to detect adverse hematologic effects.
■ Drug may falsely elevate urine 17-ketosteroids, 17-ketogenic steroids (Zimmerman reaction), and 17-hydroxycorticosteroid levels (Glenn-Nelson technique).
■ Avoid prolonged use, especially in alcoholics and patients prone to substance abuse. Carefully monitor dosage. Dispense the smallest amount of drug feasible at a time.
■ Monitor patient for signs of drug abuse or misuse.
■ Withdraw drug gradually after long-term therapy to prevent withdrawal symptoms. Abrupt withdrawal of long-term therapy may cause severe, generalized, tonic-clonic seizures.

Breast-feeding patients
■ Drug appears in breast milk at two to four times the serum level. Don't give to breast-feeding women.

Pediatric patients
■ Safety hasn't been established in children under age 6.

Geriatric patients
■ Elderly patients may have more pronounced CNS effects. Use lowest dose possible. Impose such safety precautions as raised bed rails, when starting treatment or increasing dosage. Patient may need assistance with walking or performing activities of daily living.

Patient teaching
■ Warn patient about potential for physical or psychological dependence with chronic use.
■ Urge patient to take drug exactly as prescribed, not to alter dose or frequency, and not to abruptly discontinue drug.
■ Tell patient to avoid alcohol and other CNS depressants, such as antihistamines, narcotics, and tranquilizers, while taking drug.
■ Caution patient to avoid hazardous activities until full CNS effects of drug are known.
■ If patient complains of a dry mouth, recommend ice chips or sugarless candy or gum.
■ Tell patient to notify prescriber about a sore throat, fever, or unusual bleeding or bruising.

midazolam hydrochloride
Versed

Pharmacologic classification: **benzodiazepine**

Therapeutic classification: **adjunct for inducing general anesthesia, amnesic, conscious sedative, preoperative sedative**

Controlled substance schedule IV

Pregnancy risk category D

How supplied
Available by prescription only

Injection: 1 mg/ml in 2-ml, 5-ml, and 10-ml vials; 5 mg/ml in 1-ml, 2-ml, 5-ml, and 10-ml vials; 5 mg/ml in 2-ml disposable syringe
Syrup: 2 mg/ml in 118-ml bottle

Indications and dosages
Preoperative sedation (to induce sleepiness or drowsiness and relieve apprehension)
Adults under age 60: 0.07 to 0.08 mg/kg I.M. about 1 hour before surgery. May be administered with atropine or scopolamine and reduced doses of narcotics.
▶ **DOSAGE ADJUSTMENT.** Reduce dosage in patients over age 60, those with COPD, and those considered surgical high-risk. If narcotic premedication or other CNS depressants are used, decrease dose by about 30%.

Sedation, anxiolysis, and amnesia before diagnostic, therapeutic, or endoscopic procedures or before induction of anesthesia in pediatric patients
Children: (syrup only) single dose of 0.25 to 1 mg/kg P.O. Maximum, 20 mg. Lower doses may provide adequate therapeutic effect for children ages 6 to 16 or cooperative patients.

Pharmacodynamics
Amnesic action: Unknown.
Sedative and anesthetic actions: Although its exact mechanism is unknown, midazolam, like other benzodiazepines, is thought to facilitate the action of gamma-aminobutyric acid to provide short-acting CNS depression.

Pharmacokinetics
Absorption: Absorption after I.M. administration appears to be 80% to 100%. Serum levels peak in 45 minutes and are about half of those after I.V. administration. Sedation begins within 15 minutes after an I.M. dose, 2 to 5 minutes after I.V. injection. After I.V. administration, induction of anesthesia occurs in 1½ to 2½ minutes. After oral doses of syrup in children ages 6 months to 2 years, serum levels peak in 10 to 15 minutes; in children ages 2 to 12, serum levels peak in 45 to 60 minutes. Absorption is slower and peak levels lower after oral doses of syrup in children ages 12 to 16.
Distribution: Drug has a large volume of distribution and is about 97% protein-bound. It crosses the placenta and enters fetal circulation.
Metabolism: Midazolam is metabolized in the liver.
Excretion: Metabolites of midazolam are excreted in urine. Drug's half-life is 1¼ to 12¼ hours. Duration of sedation is usually 1 to 4 hours. Patients with heart failure have a twofold increase in the elimination half-life. In alcoholic patients and those with hepatic impairment, the mean half-life may increase 2.5 times, reducing clearance by 50%.

Contraindications and precautions
Contraindicated in patients hypersensitive to drug and those with acute angle-closure glaucoma, shock, coma, or acute alcohol intoxication.

Reactions may be *common,* uncommon, *life-threatening,* or COMMON AND LIFE-THREATENING.

Use cautiously in patients with uncompensated acute illnesses and in elderly or debilitated patients.

Interactions
Drug-drug
Antidepressants, antihistamines, barbiturates, CNS depressants, narcotics, respiratory depressants, tranquilizers: midazolam may add to or potentiate effects of these drugs. Monitor patient closely.

Azole antifungals, cimetidine, droperidol, fentanyl, fluvoxamine, indinavir, narcotics, oral contraceptives, ritonavir, valproic acid, verapamil: may potentiate midazolam's hypnotic effect. Monitor patient closely.

Erythromycin: may decrease plasma clearance of midazolam. Monitor patient closely.

Inhaled anesthetics: midazolam may decrease the anesthetic dose needed by depressing the respiratory drive. Monitor patient closely.

Isoniazid: may decrease midazolam metabolism. Monitor patient closely.

Rifamycins, theophylline: may decrease midazolam's sedative effects. Monitor patient for lack of effect.

Drug-lifestyle
Alcohol use: midazolam may add to or potentiate alcohol effects. Discourage concomitant use.

Adverse reactions
CNS: amnesia, drowsiness, headache, oversedation.
CV: *cardiac arrest,* hypotension, irregular pulse.
GI: *nausea,* vomiting.

Respiratory: *apnea, decreased respiratory rate, hiccups, **respiratory arrest.***
Other: *pain at injection site.*

Overdose and treatment
Overdose may cause coma, confusion, hypotension, respiratory depression, and stupor.
   Treatment is supportive. Maintain a patent airway, and ensure adequate ventilation with mechanical support, if necessary. Monitor the patient's vital signs. Give I.V. fluids or ephedrine for hypotension. Give flumazenil, a specific benzodiazepine-receptor antagonist, for complete or partial reversal of sedative effects.

Special considerations
■ Consider a different therapy if patient has COPD or sleep anea.
■ Individualize the dosage to the smallest effective amount.
■ Provide the smallest prudent quantity of drug if patient has suicidal tendencies or a history of increasing the dosage without permission.
■ If you administer midazolam, make sure you're familiar with airway management procedures. Close monitoring of cardiopulmonary function is required. Continuously monitor any patient receiving midazolam to detect potentially life-threatening respiratory depression.
■ Laryngospasm and bronchospasm occur on occasion; keep countermeasures available.
■ Give syrup form only to patients being visually monitored by health care professionals.

■ Midazolam is compatible with D_5W, normal saline solution, and lactated Ringer's solution.

■ Don't use a discolored or precipitated solution.

■ Before I.V. administration, ensure the immediate availability of oxygen and resuscitative equipment. Administer an I.V. dose slowly to prevent respiratory depression. Apnea and death have been reported with rapid I.V. administration. Avoid intra-arterial injection because of its unknown hazards. Avoid extravasation.

■ Administer I.M. dose deep into a large muscle mass to prevent tissue injury.

■ As needed, mix midazolam in the same syringe with atropine, meperidine, morphine, and scopolamine.

■ Hypotension occurs more frequently in patients premedicated with narcotics. Monitor patient closely.

■ Drug is also used for sedation of intubated and mechanically ventilated patients as a component of anesthesia or during treatment in the critical care setting.

■ Drug has been used to treat epileptic seizures and as an alternative for the termination of refractory status epilepticus.

Breast-feeding patients

■ No data exist to demonstrate whether drug passes into breast milk; use caution when giving drug to breast-feeding women.

Pediatric patients

■ Because benzyl alcohol may cause adverse effects in neonates (hypotension, metabolic acidosis, kernicterus), consider the amount of benzyl alcohol when giving midazolam and other drugs that contain this preservative.

■ Safety and efficacy have been established in children only for oral dose forms.

Geriatric patients

■ Elderly or debilitated patients, especially those with COPD, have a significantly increased risk of respiratory depression and hypotension. Reduce doses and use with caution. Oral forms aren't recommended for elderly patients.

Patient teaching

■ Urge patient to avoid hazardous activities until full CNS effects of drug are known.

■ As needed, teach safety measures, such as assisted walking and gradual position changes, to prevent injury.

■ Caution patient to consult prescriber before taking other prescribed drugs, OTC medications, or herbal remedies.

■ Tell patient to promptly notify prescriber about behavioral or mental changes that occur after therapy starts, including disturbing thoughts.

Reactions may be *common*, uncommon, ***life-threatening***, or COMMON AND LIFE-THREATENING.

oxazepam
Apo-Oxazepam◇ , Novoxapam◇ ,
Serax

Pharmacologic classification:
benzodiazepine

Therapeutic classification:
antianxiety drug, sedative-
hypnotic

Controlled substance schedule IV

Pregnancy risk category D

How supplied
Available by prescription only
Capsules: 10 mg, 15 mg, 30 mg
Tablets: 15 mg

Indications and dosages
**Alcohol withdrawal, severe
anxiety**
Adults: 15 to 30 mg P.O. t.i.d. or
q.i.d.

**Tension, mild to moderate
anxiety**
Adults: 10 to 15 mg P.O. t.i.d. or
q.i.d.
▶ DOSAGE ADJUSTMENT. Start with
10 mg P.O. t.i.d. for elderly patients; then increase to 15 mg t.i.d.
or q.i.d., p.r.n.

Pharmacodynamics
*Anxiolytic and sedative-hypnotic ac-
tions:* Oxazepam depresses the
CNS at the limbic and subcortical
levels of the brain. It produces an
anxiolytic effect by enhancing the
effect of GABA on its receptor in
the ascending reticular activating
system, which increases inhibition
and blocks cortical and limbic
arousal.

Pharmacokinetics
Absorption: When administered
orally, oxazepam is well absorbed
through the GI tract. Onset of action occurs at 1 to 2 hours. Levels
peak in 3 hours.
Distribution: Drug is distributed
widely throughout the body. It's
85% to 95% protein-bound.
Metabolism: Drug is metabolized
in the liver to inactive metabolites.
Excretion: Metabolites of oxazepam are excreted in urine as
glucuronide conjugates. Drug's
half-life is 5.7 to 10.9 hours.

Contraindications and
precautions
Contraindicated in patients with
psychosis or hypersensitivity to
drug. Also, contraindicated in patients with aspirin sensitivity because oxazepam contains tartrazine.
　　Use cautiously in elderly or debilitated patients, in those with a
history of drug abuse, and in those
for whom decreased blood pressure could cause cardiac problems.

Interactions
Drug-drug
Antacids: may decrease the rate of
oxazepam absorption. Separate administration times.
*Antidepressants, antihistamines,
barbiturates, general anesthetics,
MAO inhibitors, narcotics, phenothiazines:* oxazepam potentiates
CNS depressant effects. Monitor
patient for increased sedation.
*Fosphenytoin, oral contraceptives,
phenytoin:* may increase oxazepam's clearance. Monitor patient for reduced drug effect.

Levodopa: oxazepam may inhibit levodopa's therapeutic effects. Avoid concomitant use.
Theophylline: may reverse sedative effects of oxazepam. Monitor patient closely.

Drug-food
Caffeine: may reverse the sedative effects of oxazepam. Discourage concomitant use.

Drug-lifestyle
Alcohol use: oxazepam potentiates CNS depressant effects. Discourage concomitant use.
Heavy smoking: accelerates oxazepam metabolism, thus lowering effectiveness. Urge patient to stop smoking or avoid concomitant use.

Adverse reactions
CNS: dizziness, *drowsiness,* headache, *lethargy,* vertigo, slurred speech, syncope, tremor.
CV: edema.
EENT: increased intraocular pressure.
GI: nausea.
GU: altered libido.
Hepatic: *hepatic dysfunction.*
Skin: rash.

Overdose and treatment
Overdose may cause somnolence, coma, confusion, hypoactive reflexes, dyspnea, labored breathing, hypotension, bradycardia, slurred speech, and unsteady gait or impaired coordination.

To treat an overdose, support the patient's blood pressure and respirations until drug effects subside; monitor her vital signs throughout. Flumazenil, a specific benzodiazepine antagonist, may be useful. Mechanical ventilatory assistance via endotracheal tube may be required to maintain a patent airway and oxygenation. Give I.V. fluids and vasopressors, such as dopamine and phenylephrine, for hypotension as needed. Induce emesis if the patient is conscious. Or, if ingestion was recent and the patient has an endotracheal tube in place, perform gastric lavage. After emesis or lavage, give a single dose of activated charcoal with a cathartic. Dialysis is of limited value.

Special considerations
■ Oxazepam tablets contain tartrazine dye; check patient's history for allergy to this substance.
■ Provide the smallest prudent quantity of drug if patient has suicidal tendencies or a history of increasing the dosage without permission.
■ Monitor patient's hepatic and renal function studies during therapy to ensure normal function.
■ Changes in EEG patterns—usually low-voltage, fast activity—may occur during and after oxazepam therapy.
■ Consider a different therapy if patient has COPD or sleep anea.
■ Reduce dosage gradually over 8 to 12 weeks after long-term use.
■ Oxazepam has been used to for narcotic detoxification, insomnia, and pruritus during pregnancy.
■ Store drug in a cool, dry place away from light.

Breast-feeding patients
■ The breast-fed infant of a mother who takes oxazepam may become sedated, have feeding diffi-

culties, or lose weight; avoid use in breast-feeding women.

Pediatric patients
■ If mother took oxazepam for a prolonged period during pregnancy, observe neonate closely for withdrawal symptoms.
■ Safe use in children under age 12 hasn't been established.

Geriatric patients
■ Elderly patients are more susceptible to CNS depressant effects. As needed, help with ambulation and activities of daily living when therapy starts or dosage increases. Lower doses are usually effective.

Patient teaching
■ Warn patient about potential physical and psychological dependence with long-term use.
■ Tell patient to take drug exactly as prescribed and not to alter dosage or discontinue drug without consulting prescriber.
■ Tell patient to promptly notify prescriber about behavioral or mental changes that occur after therapy starts, including disturbing thoughts.
■ Teach safety measures, such as gradual position changes and assisted ambulation, to prevent injury.
■ Caution patient that sleepiness may occur up to 2 hours after taking oxazepam.

CHAPTER 5

Anticonvulsants

89 ■ **Introduction**

101 ■ **Generic drugs**

- ■ acetazolamide, acetazolamide sodium
- ■ carbamazepine
- ■ clonazepam
- ■ clorazepate dipotassium (See Chapter 4, ANTIANXIETY DRUGS)
- ■ diazepam (See Chapter 4, ANTIANXIETY DRUGS)
- ■ ethosuximide
- ■ fosphenytoin sodium
- ■ gabapentin
- ■ lamotrigine
- ■ levetiracetam
- ■ lorazepam (See Chapter 4, ANTIANXIETY DRUGS)
- ■ magnesium sulfate
- ■ mephenytoin
- ■ oxcarbazepine
- ■ pentobarbital sodium (See Chapter 12, SEDATIVE-HYPNOTICS)
- ■ phenobarbital, phenobarbital sodium (See Chapter 12, SEDATIVE-HYPNOTICS)
- ■ phenytoin, phenytoin sodium
- ■ primidone
- ■ tiagabine hydrochloride
- ■ topiramate
- ■ valproic acid, divalproex sodium, valproate sodium

About 2.5 million Americans have a seizure disorder, making it the most common chronic neurologic disorder in the country. Its primary symptom is the unpredictable recurrence of seizures, which vary greatly in their etiology, clinical features, treatment, and prognoses.

UNDERSTANDING SEIZURES

A seizure is an intermittent central nervous system (CNS) derangement usually caused by a sudden, excessive, chaotic discharge of neurons. Most seizures occur in response to hypoxia, toxins, fever, or stress. Seizures caused by these types of physiologic and psychogenic causes are classified as nonepileptic. Treatment for nonepileptic seizures is based on the on the underlying cause and usually doesn't involve anticonvulsants.

Epileptic seizures result from a primary dysfunction in the biochemical mechanisms of the CNS. The normal balance of inhibition and excitation in the neurons becomes imbalanced, which results in neuronal hyperexcitability. Many underlying causes contribute to the development of this imbalance, including metabolic defects, congenital malformation, genetic predisposition, perinatal injury, postnatal trauma, motor syndromes, infection, brain tumors, and cerebrovascular disease.

The clinical manifestations of a seizure depend on the location at which abnormal electrical activity occurs in the brain. During or around the time of the seizure (the ictal state) the person may lose awareness or consciousness and may show disturbances of movement, sensation (such as vision, hearing, or taste), autonomic function, mood, and mental function. After the seizure (in the postictal period), the person typically feels confused and may have memory impairment. The postictal period may last for minutes, hours, or even days.

Seizure types

The International League Against Epilepsy (ILAE) classifies seizures as either partial or generalized. A partial seizure arises from a distinct region—or focal area—in the brain. Partial seizures are further subdivided based on whether the affected person has impaired consciousness; that is, whether he can understand or remember the seizure.

Generalized seizures stem from extensive dysfunction in both sides of the brain, although a generalized seizure can sometimes start in a focal area and then spread to other brain areas. This type of seizure is called a secondarily generalized seizure. Generalized seizures may be convulsive or nonconvulsive.

Status epilepticus, the third major category of seizures, is a life-threatening emergency in which a seizure of any type fails to spontaneously stop or else it recurs so often that the patient doesn't return to full consciousness between episodes.

The classification of seizures is based primarily on an accurate, detailed history from the patient, someone who has witnessed the seizures, or both. Sometimes you can't distinguish between a partial and a generalized seizure from the clinical description alone. In these cases, an electroencephalogram (EEG) can help in making a diagnosis.

Simple partial seizures

Simple partial seizures begin with motor, somatosensory, sensory, autonomic, or psychic changes, depending on the area of the brain that's affected. Motor changes may involve clonic movements of any muscle group. Somatosensory changes may involve an aura. Sensory changes may include visual, auditory, and olfactory events. Autonomic changes may include sweating, flushing, piloerection, and pupil dilation. Psychic changes may include fear, anger, a dreamy state, and a feeling of déjà vu.

Most simple partial seizures last only a few seconds and don't cause impaired consciousness or postictal confusion. A seizure type characterized by clonic movements of the hand that commonly progresses to a generalized tonic-clonic seizure is called a Jacksonian seizure.

Complex partial seizures

Complex partial seizures usually consist of a vague stare accompanied by some impairment in responsiveness, cognitive function, and recall. Automatic movements, called automatisms, are common and involve the mouth (lip smacking, chewing, swallowing), arms (fumbling, picking), vocalizations (grunts, repeating a phrase), or complex acts (such as shuffling cards). More dramatic automatisms occasionally occur and may include such actions as urination, disrobing, or other socially embarrassing behaviors.

Complex partial seizures may last from 5 seconds to 5 minutes. Postictal confusion usually lasts less than 15 minutes, although other symptoms, such as fatigue, may persist for hours.

Primary generalized convulsive seizures

These seizures, known as generalized tonic-clonic seizures, can occur without warning, although the initial tonic contraction of respiratory muscles may produce a cry with exhalation. The tongue contracts and may be injured as the affected person falls to the ground. This tonic phase is followed by a clonic phase of symmetrical limb jerking caused by alternating muscle contraction and relaxation.

These movements stop after 1 or 2 minutes, and the person lies still and limp, in a deep coma. In some cases, the person's mouth may froth with saliva. Relaxation of the bowel and bladder muscles may cause incontinence. Usually, the person regains consciousness in 10 or 15 minutes, but postictal confusion and fatigue may last for hours or days.

Other types of generalized convulsive seizures include myoclonic, clonic, and tonic seizures. Myoclonic seizures can stem from several rare hereditary neurodegenerative disorders. They're characterized by quick muscle jerks that may be localized to a few muscles or to one or more limbs. Consciousness usually isn't impaired. Clonic seizures occur most commonly in children and produce repetitive clonic jerking movements and a loss of consciousness. Tonic seizures are characterized by continuing contraction of muscles in the arms and legs, leading to falls.

Primary generalized nonconvulsive seizures

Two types of primary generalized nonconvulsive seizures are absence seizures and atonic seizures.

Absence seizures begin in childhood. They cause a brief, 5- to 10-second, loss of consciousness, and they may cause eye blinking, staring, or a slight head turning. Full consciousness returns immediately after the seizure. These seizures can occur many times a day, disrupting the child's school performance; indeed, absence seizures are commonly recognized first by a teacher. Initially, the child may be misdiagnosed with mental retardation before the diagnosis of epilepsy is made. Differences in ictal and interictal EEG patterns determine whether the child has atypical or typical absence seizures.

Atonic seizures, which cause the person to fall abruptly to the floor, are also known as drop attacks. They result from a sudden loss of tone in postural muscles. They typically last only a few seconds and cause no loss of consciousness. Atonic seizures most commonly occur in children with Lennox-Gastaut syndrome.

Once thorough physical and neurologic examinations, laboratory testing, and imaging studies (such as magnetic resonance imaging and computed tomography) have helped to classify the type of seizures a patient is having, therapy with anticonvulsant drugs can help to control the seizures and establish a more normal life for the patient. Selecting the most appropri-

ate therapy requires extensive interaction between the prescriber and the patient. The patient's seizure type, personal characteristics, lifestyle, and ability to adhere to a drug regimen are important considerations when designing the treatment plan. To decrease the likelihood of seizures, the patient's CNS must contain therapeutic levels of anticonvulsant drugs. For this reason, and because seizures occur unpredictably, compliance with the medication regimen is essential.

TREATING SEIZURE DISORDERS

The goal of antiepileptic therapy is to prevent or decrease seizure frequency while avoiding adverse effects. Just a decade ago, only a few anticonvulsants were available to treat patients with seizure disorders. Among them were benzodiazepines (clonazepam, clorazepate, diazepam), carbamazepine, ethosuximide, phenobarbital, phenytoin, primidone, and valproate. These drugs are still in use today and may provide effective therapy for many patients. For about 20% of patients, however, they fail to control the seizures. What's more, they may cause significant adverse effects.

During the last decade, newer second-generation drugs have become available, such as gabapentin, lamotrigine, levetiracetam, tiagabine, and topiramate. These drugs tend to have more specific sites of action and fewer adverse effects. However, until adequate studies demonstrate that they're cost-effective compared to the older anticonvulsant drugs, most experts recommend using the more expensive second-generation drugs only after therapy with the first-generation drugs has failed.

All in all, about two-thirds of patients with seizure disoders have their seizures completely or almost completely controlled by anticonvulsant therapy. In another 20% to 25% of patients, the frequency and severity of attacks are significantly reduced.

Selecting a regimen

Classifying seizures according to the ILAE system—and following the tried-and-true principles of therapy for seizure disorders—enables a rational approach to anti-epileptic therapy and a reasonable ability to predict the patient's response. (See *Principles of managing seizure disorders.*) Based on their clinical efficacy and actions, we know that certain drugs are more effective at treating certain types of seizures.

For instance, carbamazepine and phenytoin seem to be better than phenobarbital and primidone at controlling partial and secondarily generalized tonic-clonic seizures. They also produce fewer toxic effects. What's more, although valproate and carbamazepine seem to be equally effective in decreasing tonic-clonic seizures, carbamazepine is better at decreasing complex-partial seizures and has fewer adverse effects.

If a patient has absence seizures, phenytoin, phenobarbital, and carbamazepine will all be ineffective. In some cases, they may even increase the patient's seizure activity. For a patient with absence seizures alone, ethosuximide may be effective. If he has a combination of absence and other generalized or partial seizures, or he can't tolerate ethosuximide, valproic acid is the preferred choice.

In 40% to 75% of patients with a seizure disorder, a single drug can satisfactorily control their seizures. For patients whose seizures aren't controlled despite adequate anticonvulsant blood levels, an increased dosage could produce unacceptable adverse effects. In that case, an additional drug may be helpful. However, the combination of two drugs should continue only until the second drug has reached therapeutic levels. The original drug can then be discontinued gradually.

If the first drug partially controls the patient's seizures, it may be continued along with the second drug. Keep in mind, however, that using drugs with different pharmacologic and toxicologic characteristics can raise the risk of adverse effects and drug interactions. This risk can be minimized by choosing drugs that have different mechanisms of action and drugs that have few or no drug interactions and few adverse effects. Naturally, a patient who takes two drugs to control seizures requires frequent close follow-up.

Drug effects

A seizure results when the electrical activity of neurons is pathologically altered so that excitation overwhelms the inhibitory pathways. Anticonvulsants act by altering this seizure-causing imbalance. Although we commonly don't know exactly how these drugs exert

Principles of managing seizure disorders

Use these four key principles to guide drug therapy for seizure disorders:
- Establish the diagnosis.
- Select the best drug for the type of seizures the patient is having. Consider contraindications and coexisting diagnoses (multiple seizure types or mood disorders, for example).
- Adjust the dosage based on how well the patient's seizures are controlled.
- Evaluate one drug at a time.

Besides adhering to these main principles, you'll also want to monitor the therapeutic and toxic effects of the drug, teach the patient about seizure disorders and the prescribed drug therapy, and discontinue the therapy when appropriate.

their effect, we do know that they interact with ion channels and neurotransmitter receptors, and that they affect neurotransmitter metabolism. (See *Quick guide to anticonvulsants*, pages 94 to 97.)

The main inhibitory neurotransmitter in the brain is gamma-aminobutyric acid (GABA). GABA is formed in neurons and released into the synaptic space between neurons. It then acts on the GABA$_A$ receptor. Activation of this receptor allows negatively charged chloride ions to flow into the postsynaptic neuron, thus decreasing its excitability.

Gabapentin, a GABA analog, acts presynaptically to promote GABA release into the synapse. Benzodiazepines and barbiturates enhance the flow of chloride ions into the cell by acting directly on the GABA$_A$ receptor. Tiagabine increases GABA levels in the synapse by blocking postsynaptic reuptake.

Carbamazepine and phenytoin work by a different mechanism. Normally, a neuron has a negative resting membrane potential. Excitatory processes make the intracellular potential less negative by mediating the passage of ions through pores in the cell membrane. Sodium and calcium, both positively charged ions, pass into the cell, making the intracellular potential less negative. When the pores stay open, the intracellular potential becomes more positive, which makes the neuron hyperexcitable. Carbamazepine and phenytoin block voltage-gated sodium channels during rapid neuronal discharge. Lamotrigine and topiramate also act at least in part by this mechanism. Topiramate also inhibits glutamate, the main excitatory neurotransmitter in the CNS.

Glutamate acts on sodium and calcium ion channels by binding to N-methyl-D-aspartate (NMDA), receptors which control the movement of ions into cells. As with the sodium channel blockers, these NMDA receptor antagonists decrease the excitability of rapidly firing neurons. Ethosuximide exerts its effect in a similar manner by reducing the flow of calcium through channels found mainly in the thalamus (T-type calcium

Quick guide to anticonvulsants

DRUG	MAIN MECHANISM OF ACTION
acetazolamide	Inhibits carbonic anhydrase
carbamazepine	Inhibits sodium channels
clonazepam	Enhances action of gamma-aminobutyric acid (GABA)
clorazepate dipotassium	Enhances action of GABA
diazepam	Enhances action of GABA
ethosuximide	Reduces T-calcium channel
fosphenytoin sodium	Inhibits sodium channels
gabapentin	Inhibits sodium channels
lamotrigine	Enhances action of GABA
levetiracetam	Inhibits sodium channels
lorazepam	Mixed mechanisms
magnesium sulfate	Enhances action of GABA
mephenytoin	Blocks neuromuscular transmission of acetylcholine
oxcarbazepine	Inhibits sodium channels
pentobarbital	Enhances action of GABA

USES	THERAPEUTIC SERUM LEVEL
■ Tonic-clonic seizures ■ Simple and complex partial seizures ■ Myoclonic seizures	Not applicable
■ Tonic-clonic seizures ■ Simple and complex partial seizures ■ Mixed seizure disorders	4–12 mcg/ml
■ Tonic-clonic seizures ■ Simple and complex partial seizures ■ Absence seizures ■ Myoclonic seizures ■ Lennox-Gastaut syndrome ■ Atonic seizures	20-80 ng/ml
■ Simple and complex partial seizures (adjunctive)	Not applicable
■ Status epilepticus (adjunctive) ■ Acute convulsive episodes	Not applicable
■ Absence seizures	40-100 mcg/ml
■ Tonic clonic seizures ■ Simple and complex partial seizures ■ Sustained control of status epilepticus	phenytoin metabolite: 10-20 mcg/ml (40-80 micromoles/L)

■ Simple and complex seizures in adults,
  with and without secondary generalization
  (adjunctive)
	Not applicable

■ Simple and complex partial seizures ■ Lennox-Gastaut syndrome	Not applicable
■ Simple and complex partial seizures in adults (adjunctive)	Not applicable
■ Status epilepticus (adjunctive)	Not applicable
■ Pre-eclamptic and eclamptic seizures of pregnancy ■ Convulsions from acute nephritis in children	4-7 mEq/L (2-3.5 mmol/L)
■ Tonic-clonic seizures ■ Simple (Jacksonian) and complex partial seizures ■ Focal seizures	Not applicable
■ Partial seizures	Not applicable
■ Acute convulsive episodes ■ Status epilepticus	Not applicable

(continued)

Quick guide to anticonvulsants (continued)

DRUG	MAIN MECHANISM OF ACTION
phenobarbital	Enhances action of GABA
phenytoin	Inhibits sodium channels
primidone	Enhances action of GABA
tiagabine hydrochloride	Enhances action of GABA
topiramate	Inhibits sodium channels
valproic acid derivatives	Unknown but may enhance action of GABA

channels.) The rate-dependent action of these drugs is important because inhibition of all excitatory activity would yield a coma.

Valproic acid may act by all three of these mechanisms, and it may have other, less understood, actions as well. This may explain the usefulness of valproate in treating partial, generalized, and absence seizures. The potential for synergistic effects with multiple mechanisms of action may account for the broad clinical spectrum of activity for some of the newer antiepileptic drugs.

Pharmacokinetics

A number of factors can influence the absorption, distribution, metabolism, and elimination of anticonvulsant drugs. For example, although most oral anticonvulsant drugs undergo complete or nearly complete absorption, the presence of food in the patient's stomach can slow that absorption. Indeed, giving an anticonvulsant with food is commonplace as a way to intentionally slow absorption and increase tolerability. The drug's formulation, patient characteristics, and the co-administration of antacids or other drugs can also af-

USES	THERAPEUTIC SERUM LEVEL
■ Tonic-clonic seizures ■ Cortical focal seizures ■ Simple partial seizures ■ Acute convulsive episodes ■ Status epilepticus	10-40 mcg/ml
■ Tonic-clonic seizures ■ Simple and complex partial seizures ■ Sustained control of status epilepticus ■ Seizure prophylaxis	10-20 mcg/ml free phenytoin: 0.8-2 mcg/ml
■ Tonic-clonic seizures ■ Focal seizures ■ Myoclonic seizures ■ Simple and complex partial seizures	primidone: 5-12 mcg/ml phenobarbital metabolite: 20-40 mcg/ml
■ Simple and complex partial seizures (adjunctive)	Not applicable
■ Tonic-clonic seizures ■ Simple and complex partial seizures (adjunctive)	Not applicable
■ Tonic-clonic seizures ■ Simple and complex partial seizures ■ Absence seizures ■ Myoclonic seizures ■ Mixed seizure disorders (adjunctive)	total valproate: 50-100 mcg/ml

fect the rate and extent of absorption.

The distribution of anticonvulsant drugs into the CNS is the basis for their efficacy. Therapeutic blood levels have been determined for many anticonvulsants to give prescriber's a reasonable assurance that enough drug is present to penetrate the blood-brain barrier. An important consideration when monitoring blood levels is the degree to which the drug binds to proteins in the blood. Various diseases and drug interactions can alter protein-binding, which can alter blood levels and, possibly,

seizure control. Valproate and phenytoin are highly protein-bound and are therefore the most affected by these alterations.

Drug metabolism also influences the pharmacokinetics of anticonvulsants. Cytochrome P-450 (CYP 450) microsomal enzymes are involved in inactivating most anticonvulsant drugs, although some, such as carbamazepine and primidone, also have active metabolites. The stable epoxide metabolite of carbamazepine has some therapeutic effect, but it also has more toxicity than the parent compound. Primidone is converted to phenobarbital and to phenylethylmalon-amide, which is also highly active.

Many anticonvulsant drugs also induce (phenytoin, carbamazepine, phenobarbital, primidone) or inhibit (valproate) CYP 450 enzymes, resulting in a high risk of drug interactions. Gabapentin has fewer drug interactions because it's almost entirely eliminated in the urine. Primidone, phenobarbital, and levetiracetam also have a component of renal elimination. Patients who take these drugs need periodic follow-up to assess their renal function and the need to adjust their doses.

Adverse effects

Routine follow-up of anticonvulsant therapy should include an assessment not only of seizure control but also of adverse effects. In general, anticonvulsants may cause acute dose-related effects, acute idiosyncratic effects, adverse effects from long-term use, and teratogenicity.

Acute dose-related effects

The object of anticonvulsant therapy is to keep blood levels between the low level (where seizure risk rises) and the high level (where the patient develops nonspecific symptoms of neural toxicity). For most anticonvulsants, this therapeutic range between efficacy (seizure control) and toxicity is small. Even at moderately high levels, some patients may experience sedation, involuntary movements, and nystagmus; others may be able to tolerate high levels without significant adverse effects.

In general, however, as the level of a drug increases, the risk of severe toxic reactions—such as ataxia, confusion, and even seizure—also increases. Phenytoin is especially likely to cause toxic dose-related effects because of its saturable pharmacokinetics, in which the highest levels occur in the brain, the liver, and the salivary glands. The autoinduction of CPY 450 enzymes by carbamazepine may also be problematic if the dose size increases too quickly. Because of the CNS effects of anticonvulsants, changes in cognitive function and behavior may occur with any of these drugs, although carbamazepine and valproate are probably least likely to cause them.

Acute idiosyncratic effects

Some idiosyncratic reactions caused by anticonvulsants can be severe and life-threatening. In particular, carbamazepine has been linked with fatal aplastic anemia, valproate with hepatotoxicity, and lamotrigine with Stevens-Johnson syndrome. For this reason, baseline laboratory tests should be obtained that include CBC and platelet counts, liver function tests, and renal function tests. These tests should be repeated regularly as the patient becomes stabilized on his drug regimen.

Adverse effects from long-term use

Although some patients may be able to stop taking their anticonvulsant after remaining seizure-free for 2 to 5 years, most will continue taking an anticonvulsant indefinitely. Certain adverse effects can result from this long-term use despite the successful maintenance of therapeutic drug levels. Adverse effects from long-term use are most likely with carbamazepine, phenobarbital, phenytoin, and valproic acid. They may include ataxia, mental dullness, nystagmus, and vertigo.

Teratogenicity

Long-term therapy with an anticonvulsant also raises concerns for women who are contemplating pregnancy. Some controversy exists regarding the effect of pregnancy on seizure frequency; current thinking is that pregnancy may cause no major change in the frequency of seizures, but it may increase the risk of status epilepticus. This increased risk must be balanced against the possibility of teratogenic effects from most anticonvulsants.

Phenytoin and the barbiturates increase the risk of fetal malformation twofold to threefold. Valproate and carbamazepine slightly increase the occurrence of neural tube defects. In women whose seizures have been well-controlled, it may be worth trying to withdraw these anticonvulsants. However, the newer anticonvulsants may cause less risk of fetal harm. And in general, if an anticonvulsant has effectively controlled a patient's seizures before pregnancy, and its benefits outweigh its risks, the patient probably doesn't need to change to another drug before or during her pregnancy.

Drug interactions

Because the established anticonvulsants are metabolized mainly through the CYP 450 hepatic enzyme system (as are many other common drugs), this mechanism underlies a majority of the significant drug interactions that involve anticonvulsants. Enzyme inducers (such as carbamazepine, phenobarbital, and phenytoin,) and enzyme inhibitors (such as valproate) can affect the levels of other anticonvulsants as well as many other drugs when used concurrently.

Overdose and treatment

Because of the narrow therapeutic range of many anticonvulsants and the significant dose-related toxicities they cause, an anticonvulsant overdose can have serious consequences. In fact, anticonvulsants are one of the most common drug classes that result in death after overdose. Treating an anticonvulsant overdose resembles routine poison management.

Besides the serious problems anticonvulsants can cause after an overdose, these drugs also have a role in treating overdoses caused by other drugs. That's because overdoses of other drugs can cause seizures. Benzodiazepines are commonly used to control seizures in these acute situations.

PATIENT TEACHING

To achieve an optimal outcome from their anticonvulsant therapy, patients must understand both their seizure disorder and their drug regimen. Noncompliance, which may result from a lack of understanding or lack of tolerance for the drug or its adverse effects, is the most common reason why anticonvulsant therapy fails. Therefore, patient education should be continuous and compliance stressed at every visit. Make sure to emphasize these points along with information specific to the patient's regimen.

■ Discuss the risks and benefits of stopping or starting any new drug.

■ Discuss the risks and benefits of anticonvulsant therapy in particular, especially if the patient is female and might contemplate pregnancy.

■ Tell the patient to take the drug exactly as prescribed.

■ Caution the patient not to stop the drug abruptly or change its dosage without first consulting the prescriber.

■ Urge the patient to take a missed dose as soon as possible after remembering it, unless it's almost time for the next dose. Warn against doubling doses.

■ Recommend that the patient avoid alcohol.

■ Suggest that the patient wear or carry medical identification that describes the seizure disorder and drug regimen.

By carefully determining the type of seizures a patient is having, making the best choice in a drug regimen, and following up appropriately as the patient becomes established on an anticonvulsant regimen, you can help to give the patient a more normal life that's free from the dangers and difficulties inherent in having seizures.

acetazolamide
Dazamide, Diamox, Diamox
Sequels

acetazolamide sodium
Diamox

Pharmacologic classification:
carbonic anhydrase inhibitor

Therapeutic classification:
altitude sickness prevention and
treatment, anticonvulsant,
antiglaucoma drug, diuretic

Pregnancy risk category C

How supplied
Available by prescription only
Capsules (extended-release): 500 mg
Injection: 500 mg
Tablets: 125 mg, 250 mg

Indications and dosages
***Myoclonic seizures, refractory
generalized tonic-clonic or
absence seizures, mixed seizures***
Adults: 375 mg P.O. or I.V. daily up
to 250 mg q.i.d. Usual initial
dosage is 250 mg daily when given
with other anticonvulsants.
Children: 8 to 30 mg/kg P.O. or I.V.
daily, divided t.i.d. or q.i.d.

Pharmacodynamics
Anticonvulsant action: Inhibition of
carbonic anhydrase in the CNS appears to slow abnormal paroxysmal
discharge from neurons.
Antiglaucoma action: By decreasing
the formation of aqueous humor,
acetazolamide and acetazolamide
sodium lower intraocular pressure.
Diuretic action: Acetazolamide and
acetazolamide sodium noncom-
petitively, reversibly inhibit car-

bonic anhydrase, an enzyme that
forms hydrogen and bicarbonate
ions from carbon dioxide and water. This inhibition decreases the
hydrogen concentration in renal
tubules, thus promoting excretion
of bicarbonate, sodium, potassium,
and water. Because carbon dioxide
isn't eliminated as rapidly, systemic
acidosis may develop.
*Altitude sickness prevention and
treatment:* Acetazolamide shortens
the period of high-altitude ac-
climatization; by inhibiting conversion of carbon dioxide to bicarbonate, it may increase carbon
dioxide tension in tissues and decrease it in the lungs. The resulting
metabolic acidosis may also increase oxygenation during hypoxia.

Pharmacokinetics
Absorption: Acetazolamide is well
absorbed from the GI tract after
oral administration.
Distribution: Drug is distributed
throughout body tissues.
Metabolism: None.
Excretion: Drug is excreted primarily in urine via tubular secretion and passive reabsorption.

Contraindications and
precautions
Contraindicated in patients hypersensitive to the drug, patients in
long-term therapy for chronic
noncongestive angle-closure glaucoma, and patients with hyponatremia, hypokalemia, renal or hepatic dysfunction, adrenal gland
failure, or hyperchloremic acidosis.
  Use cautiously in patients receiving other diuretics and those
with respiratory acidosis, emphysema, diabetes, or COPD.

Interactions
Drug-drug
Amphetamines, flecainide, procainamide, quinidine: acetazolamide alkalinizes urine and thus may decrease excretion of these drugs. Monitor patient closely.
Lithium, phenobarbital, salicylates: excretion of these drugs may increase, lowering their plasma levels. Dosage adjustment may be necessary.

Adverse reactions
CNS: confusion, drowsiness, paresthesia.
EENT: hearing dysfunction, tinnitus, transient myopia.
GI: anorexia, altered taste, diarrhea, nausea, vomiting.
GU: hematuria, polyuria.
Hematologic: *aplastic anemia, hemolytic anemia, leukopenia.*
Metabolic: asymptomatic hyperuricemia, hyperchloremic acidosis, hypokalemia.
Skin: rash.

Overdose and treatment
Overdose may cause exaggerated adverse effects. Treatment is supportive and symptomatic. Induce emesis or perform gastric lavage. Don't induce catharsis because doing so may worsen electrolyte disturbances, including hypokalemia and hyperchloremic acidosis. Monitor patient's fluid and electrolyte levels.

Special considerations
■ Suspensions that contain 250 mg in 5 ml of syrup are the most palatable and can be made by a pharmacist. (Tablets won't dissolve in fruit juice.) The suspension remains stable for about 1 week.
■ If drug must be given parenterally, use direct I.V. administration.
■ Reconstitute powder by adding at least 5 ml of sterile water for injection.
■ Because it alkalinizes urine, drug may cause false-positive results (proteinuria) in Albustix or Albutest. It also may decrease thyroid iodine uptake.
■ Besides standard indications, drug is used for preoperative management of acute angle-closure glaucoma and for open-angle glaucoma, edema, and mountain sickness. Unlabeled uses include prevention of uric acid or cystine nephrolithiasis, and promotion of diuresis and urine alkalization when treating toxicity caused by weakly acidic drugs.

Breast-feeding patients
■ Safety in breast-feeding women hasn't been established.

Geriatric patients
■ Assess elderly and debilitated patients frequently because they have an increased risk of drug-induced diuresis, which may lead to rapid dehydration, hypovolemia, hypokalemia, hyponatremia, and possible circulatory collapse. Consider reduced dosages for these patients.

Patient teaching
■ Warn patient to avoid hazardous activities until full effects of drug are clear.
■ Encourage patient to wear or carry medical identification that

---

Reactions may be *common*, uncommon, *life-threatening*, or COMMON AND LIFE-THREATENING.

describes the seizure disorder and the drug regimen.

---

carbamazepine
Atretol, Carbatrol, Epitol, Tegretol

Pharmacologic classification: iminostilbene derivative, chemically related to tricyclic antidepressants

Therapeutic classification: analgesic, anticonvulsant

Pregnancy risk category D

How supplied
Available by prescription only
Capsules (extended-release):
200 mg, 300 mg
Oral suspension: 100 mg/5 ml
Tablets: 200 mg
Tablets (chewable): 100 mg
Tablets (extended-release): 100 mg, 200 mg, 400 mg

Indications and dosages
Generalized tonic-clonic, complex-partial, mixed seizures
Adults and children over age 12: initially, 200 mg P.O. b.i.d. or 100 mg P.O. q.i.d. of suspension. Increase by 200 mg/day at weekly intervals, in divided doses q 6 to 8 hours. Adjust to minimum effective level when seizures are controlled. Don't exceed 1,000 mg/day in children ages 12 to 15 or 1,200 mg/day in those over age 15. Some adults may need up to 1,600 mg/day. For extended-release forms, initial dosage is 200 mg P.O. b.i.d. Increase at weekly intervals by up to 200 mg/day until optimal response occurs. Maintenance dosage is usually 800 to 1,200 mg/day. Don't exceed 1,000 mg/day in children ages 12 to 15 or 1,200 mg/day in those over 15. Some adults may need up to 1,600 mg/day.
Children ages 6 to 12: initially, 100 mg P.O. b.i.d. or 50 mg P.O. q.i.d. of suspension. Increase at weekly intervals by adding 100 mg P.O. daily, first t.i.d. and then q.i.d. if needed. Adjust dosage to patient response. In general, dosage should not exceed 1,000 mg/day. Children who are taking 400 mg or more daily of immediate-release form may be converted to an extended-release form using a b.i.d. regimen.
Children under age 6: initially, 10 to 20 mg/kg/day P.O. b.i.d. or t.i.d. as tablets or q.i.d. as suspension. Increase weekly and administer t.i.d. or q.i.d. to achieve optimal response. If optimal response hasn't occurred at a dose below 35 mg/kg/day, check to see whether plasma levels are within therapeutic range. There's no recommendation for safe administration above 35 mg/kg/day.

Oral loading dose for rapid seizure control
Adults and children over age 12: 8 mg/kg of oral suspension.

Bipolar affective disorder*, intermittent explosive disorder*
Adults: initially, 200 mg P.O. b.i.d., increased p.r.n. q 3 to 4 days. Maintenance dosage may range from 600 to 1,600 mg/day.

Trigeminal neuralgia
Adults: initially, 100 mg P.O. b.i.d. with meals. Increase by 100 mg q 12 hours until pain is relieved.

Maintenance dosage is 200 to 1,200 mg P.O. daily. Don't exceed 1,200 mg daily. For extended-release forms, 200 mg P.O. on day 1, increased p.r.n. by up to 200 mg/day q 12 hours to relieve pain. Maintenance dosage is typically 400 to 800 mg/day.

Chorea*
Children: 15 to 25 mg/kg/day.

Restless leg syndrome*
Adults: 100 to 300 mg h.s.

Pharmacodynamics

Analgesic action: In trigeminal neuralgia, carbamazepine reduces specific pain by reducing synaptic neurotransmission.
Anticonvulsant action: Carbamazepine is chemically unrelated to other anticonvulsants and its mechanism of action is unknown. It probably limits seizure propagation by reducing post-tetanic potentiation of synaptic transmissions.

Pharmacokinetics

Absorption: Carbamazepine is absorbed slowly from the GI tract; plasma levels peak at 1½ hours after giving suspension, 4 to 6 hours after giving tablets, or 6 hours after giving extended-release tablets.
Distribution: Drug is distributed widely throughout the body. About 75% is protein-bound. Therapeutic serum levels in adults are 4 to 12 mcg/ml. Nystagmus can occur above 4 mcg/ml and ataxia, dizziness, and anorexia at or above 10 mcg/ml. Serum levels may be misleading because an unmeasured active metabolite also can cause toxicity. Carbamazepine crosses the placenta and accumulates in fetal tissue. Levels in breast milk approach 60% of serum levels. Plasma levels and dosage correlate poorly in children.
Metabolism: Drug is metabolized by the liver to an active metabolite. It may also induce its own metabolism; over time, higher doses are needed to maintain plasma levels. Half-life is initially 25 to 65 hours and then 12 to 17 hours with multiple dosing.
Excretion: Drug is excreted in urine (70%) and feces (30%).

Contraindications and precautions

Contraindicated in patients with a history of bone marrow suppression, hypersensitivity to drug or tricyclic antidepressants, or use of an MAO inhibitor within 14 days.

Use cautiously in patients with mixed-type seizure disorders.

Interactions

Drug-drug
Calcium channel blockers (verapamil, possibly diltiazem): may significantly increase serum carbamazepine levels. Decrease carbamazepine dosage by 40% to 50% when given with verapamil, and monitor patient closely.
Cimetidine, clarithromycin, erythromycin, fluoxetine, fluvoxamine, isoniazid, propoxyphene, valproic acid: may increase serum carbamazepine levels. Monitor patient and drug levels closely.
Ethosuximide, haloperidol, phenytoin, valproic acid, warfarin: carbamazepine may increase metabo-

lism and reduce effects of these drugs.

Felbamate: may reduce serum levels of either drug. Avoid concomitant use.

MAO inhibitors: may cause hypertensive crisis. Avoid concomitant use.

Oral contraceptives: induction of hepatic microsomal enzymes increases metabolism of oral contraceptive, thus decreasing its reliability. Avoid concurrent use.

Phenobarbital, phenytoin, primidone: reduces serum carbamazepine levels. Monitor levels closely.

Theophylline: induces metabolism of both drugs, altering half-lives and serum levels. Monitor levels closely.

Drug-herb

Psyllium seed: may inhibit GI absorption of carbamazepine. Avoid concomitant use.

Adverse reactions

CNS: *ataxia,* confusion, *dizziness, drowsiness,* fatigue, headache, syncope, *vertigo, **worsening of seizures.***

CV: aggravation of coronary artery disease, ***arrhythmias, AV block, heart failure,*** hypertension, hypotension.

EENT: blurred vision, conjunctivitis, diplopia, dry mouth and pharynx, nystagmus.

GI: abdominal pain, anorexia, diarrhea, glossitis, *nausea,* stomatitis, *vomiting.*

GU: albuminuria, elevated BUN, glycosuria, impotence, urinary frequency, urine retention.

Hematologic: ***aplastic anemia, agranulocytosis,*** eosinophilia, leukocytosis, ***thrombocytopenia.***

Hepatic: abnormal liver function test results, ***hepatitis.***

Metabolic: decreased thyroid function test results, SIADH.

Respiratory: pulmonary hypersensitivity.

Skin: erythema multiforme, rash, ***Stevens-Johnson syndrome,*** urticaria.

Other: Chills, excessive diaphoresis, fever.

Overdose and treatment

Overdose may cause anuria, arrhythmias, blood pressure changes, drowsiness, impaired consciousness (ranging to deep coma), irregular breathing, nausea, oliguria, psychomotor disturbances, respiratory depression, restlessness, seizures, shock, tachycardia, or vomiting.

Treat an overdose with repeated gastric lavage, especially if the patient also ingested alcohol. Oral charcoal and laxatives may hasten excretion. Carefully monitor patient's vital signs, ECG, and fluid and electrolyte balance. Diazepam may control seizures but can worsen respiratory depression.

Special considerations

■ For administering via nasogastric tube, mix with an equal volume of diluent (D_5W or normal saline solution) and administer; then flush with 100 ml of diluent.

■ Adjust drug dosage based on individual response. Obtain blood levels regularly to monitor compliance.

◇ Available in Canada only   *Unlabeled use

■ Hematologic toxicity is rare but serious. Routinely monitor patient's hematologic and liver functions.

■ Worsening of seizures usually occurs only in patients with mixed-type seizure disorders, including atypical absence seizures.

■ Drug has also been used to treat hypophyseal diabetes insipidus.

Breast-feeding patients

■ Significant amounts of drug appear in breast milk; recommend an alternate feeding method during therapy.

Pediatric patients

■ Safety and efficacy haven't been established for children under age 6 in doses above 35 mg/kg/day.

■ Chewable tablets are available for children.

Geriatric patients

■ Drug may activate latent psychosis, confusion, or agitation in elderly patients.

Patient teaching

■ As needed, tell patient that Carbatrol capsules can be opened and contents sprinkled over food (such as a teaspoon of applesauce). Caution against crushing or chewing capsules or their contents.

■ Remind patient to shake suspension well before using it.

■ Tell patient that drug may cause GI distress and should be taken with food at equally spaced intervals.

■ Warn patient that drug may cause drowsiness, dizziness, and blurred vision. Caution against hazardous activities, especially during first week of therapy and increases in dosage.

■ Emphasize the importance of follow-up laboratory tests and continued medical supervision.

■ Urge patient to have periodic eye examinations.

■ Encourage patient to promptly report unusual bleeding, bruising, jaundice, dark urine, pale stools, abdominal pain, impotence, fever, chills, sore throat, mouth ulcers, edema, or disturbances in mood, alertness, or coordination.

■ Warn patient not to stop drug abruptly.

■ Remind patient to store drug in a cool, dry place—not in the bathroom. Improper storage has been linked to reduced bioavailability.

■ Encourage patient to wear or carry medical identification that describes the seizure disorder and the drug regimen.

---

clonazepam
Klonopin, Rivotril◇

Pharmacologic classification:
benzodiazepine

Therapeutic classification:
anticonvulsant

Controlled substance schedule IV

Pregnancy risk category C

How supplied
Available by prescription only
Tablets: 0.5 mg, 1 mg, 2 mg

Indications and dosages
Panic disorder
Adults: initially, 0.25 mg P.O. b.i.d.
Increase to a target of 1 mg/day af-

ter 3 days. Some patients may benefit from up to 4 mg/day, the maximum. To achieve 4 mg/day, increase in increments of 0.125 to 0.25 mg b.i.d. q 3 days as tolerated until panic disorder is controlled. Discontinue gradually by decreasing 0.125 mg b.i.d. q 3 days until drug is stopped.

Absence and atypical absence seizures, akinetic and myoclonic seizures, generalized tonic-clonic seizures*

Adults: Initial dosage shouldn't exceed 1.5 mg P.O. daily, divided into three doses. May be increased by 0.5 to 1 mg q 3 days until seizures are controlled. Maximum recommended daily dose, 20 mg.
Children up to age 10 or who weigh 30 kg (66 lb) or less: 0.01 to 0.03 mg/kg P.O. daily (maximum 0.05 mg/kg daily), divided q 8 hours. Increase dosage by 0.25 to 0.5 mg q third day to a maximum maintenance dosage of 0.1 to 0.2 mg/kg daily.

Acute manic episodes*
Adults: 0.75 to 16 mg P.O. daily.

Adjunct treatment of schizophrenia*, leg movements during sleep*
Adults: 0.5 to 2 mg P.O. h.s.

Parkinsonian dysarthria*
Adults: 0.25 to 0.5 mg P.O. daily.

Multifocal tic disorders*
Adults: 1.5 to 12 mg P.O. daily.

Neuralgia*
Adults: 2 to 4 mg P.O. daily.

Pharmacodynamics
Anticonvulsant action: Mechanism of anticonvulsant activity is unknown; drug appears to act in the limbic system, thalamus, and hypothalamus.

Pharmacokinetics
Absorption: Clonazepam is well absorbed from the GI tract. Action begins in 20 to 60 minutes and persists for 6 to 8 hours in infants and children, up to 12 hours in adults.
Distribution: Drug is distributed widely throughout the body and is about 85% protein-bound.
Metabolism: Clonazepam is metabolized by the liver to several metabolites. Drug half-life is 18 to 39 hours.
Excretion: Drug is excreted in urine.

Contraindications and precautions
Contraindicated in patients with significant hepatic disease, hypersensitivity to benzodiazepines, or acute angle-closure glaucoma.

Use cautiously in children and in patients with mixed-type seizures, respiratory disease, or glaucoma.

Interactions
Drug-drug
CNS depressants (anticonvulsants, antidepressants, antipsychotics, anxiolytics, barbiturates, narcotics): produces additive CNS depressant effects. Monitor patient closely.
Ritonavir: may significantly increase clonazepam levels. Monitor patient closely, and adjust dosage as needed.

Valproic acid: may induce absence seizures. Monitor patient closely.

Drug-lifestyle
Alcohol use: produces additive CNS depressant effects. Avoid concurrent use.

Adverse reactions
CNS: agitation, *ataxia, behavioral disturbances,* confusion, *drowsiness,* psychosis, slurred speech, tremor.
CV: palpitations.
EENT: abnormal eye movements, nystagmus, sore gums.
GI: anorexia, change in appetite, constipation, diarrhea, gastritis, nausea.
GU: dysuria, enuresis, nocturia, urine retention.
Hematologic: eosinophilia, *leukopenia, thrombocytopenia.*
Hepatic: increased liver function test results.
Respiratory: chest congestion, *respiratory depression,* shortness of breath.
Skin: rash.

Overdose and treatment
Overdose may cause ataxia, coma, confusion, decreased reflexes, and hypotension.

Treat an overdose with gastric lavage and supportive therapy. Flumazenil, a specific benzodiazepine antagonist, may be useful. Give vasopressors for hypotension. Carefully monitor patient's vital signs, ECG, and fluid and electrolyte balance. Clonazepam isn't removed by dialysis.

Special considerations
■ Give drug to treat myoclonic, atonic, and absence seizures that are resistant to other anticonvulsants and to suppress or eliminate attacks of sleep-related nocturnal myoclonus (restless legs syndrome).
■ Monitor patient's CBC and liver function tests periodically.
■ Abrupt withdrawal may precipitate status epilepticus; after long-term use, taper dosage gradually.
■ Avoid concomitant use with barbiturates or other CNS depressants because patient's ability to perform tasks that require alertness may be impaired.

Breast-feeding patients
■ Breast-feeding isn't recommended during clonazepam therapy.

Pediatric patients
■ Long-term safety hasn't been established for children.
■ Long-term use may increase the risk of behavioral disturbances.

Geriatric patients
■ Elderly patients may require lower doses because of diminished renal function. Such patients also face a greater risk of falls and oversedation from CNS depressants.

Patient teaching
■ Explain the rationale for therapy and its risks and benefits.
■ Review signs and symptoms of adverse reactions; urge patient to report them promptly.
■ Tell patient to avoid alcohol and other sedatives to prevent added CNS depression.
■ Urge patient to avoid hazardous tasks until full effects of drug are clear.

Reactions may be *common,* uncommon, *life-threatening,* or COMMON AND LIFE-THREATENING.

■ Warn patient not to stop drug or change dosage unless prescribed.
■ Encourage patient to wear a medical identification bracelet or necklace that identifies the seizure disorder and the drug regimen.

ethosuximide
Zarontin

Pharmacologic classification: succinimide derivative

Therapeutic classification: anticonvulsant

Pregnancy risk category NR

How supplied
Available by prescription only
Capsules: 250 mg
Syrup: 250 mg/5 ml

Indications and dosages
Absence seizures refractory to other drugs
Adults and children age 6 and older: initially, 250 mg P.O. b.i.d. May increase by 250 mg q 4 to 7 days up to 1.5 g daily.
Children ages 3 to 6: 250 mg P.O. daily. Optimal dosage is 20 mg/kg/day.

Pharmacodynamics
Anticonvulsant action: Ethosuximide raises the seizure threshold. It suppresses the characteristic spike-and-wave pattern by depressing neuronal transmission in the motor cortex and basal ganglia.

Pharmacokinetics
Absorption: Ethosuximide is absorbed from the GI tract; steady-state plasma levels occur in 4 to 7 days.
Distribution: Ethosuximide is distributed widely throughout the body; protein binding is minimal.
Metabolism: Drug is metabolized extensively in the liver to several inactive metabolites.
Excretion: Drug is excreted mainly in urine, with small amounts in bile and feces. Plasma half-life is about 60 hours in adults, 30 hours in children.

Contraindications and precautions
Contraindicated in patients hypersensitive to succinimide derivatives.
   Use with extreme caution in patients who have hepatic or renal disease.

Interactions
Drug-drug
Barbiturates: may decrease serum barbiturate levels. Monitor patient closely; adjust therapy as needed.
CNS depressants (anticonvulsants, antidepressants, antipsychotics, anxiolytics, barbiturates, narcotics): additive CNS depression and sedation. Monitor patient closely.
Phenytoin: may increase serum phenytoin levels. Monitor patient closely; adjust therapy as needed.
Valproic acid: may increase or decrease serum ethosuximide levels. Monitor patient closely, and adjust therapy as needed.

Drug-lifestyle
Alcohol use: may cause additive CNS depression and sedation. Discourage concomitant use.

Adverse reactions

CNS: *ataxia, depression, dizziness, drowsiness, euphoria, fatigue, headache, hiccups, irritability, lethargy, psychosis.*
EENT: gingival hyperplasia, myopia, tongue swelling.
GI: *abdominal cramps, anorexia, diarrhea, epigastric and abdominal pain, nausea, vomiting, weight loss.*
GU: abnormal renal function test results, urinary frequency, vaginal bleeding.
Hematologic: *agranulocytosis,* eosinophilia, *leukopenia, pancytopenia.*
Hepatic: elevated liver enzymes.
Skin: hirsutism, pruritic and erythematous rash, *Stevens-Johnson syndrome,* urticaria.

Overdose and treatment

Overdose from ethosuximide alone or combined with other anticonvulsants may cause ataxia, CNS depression, coma, stupor.

Treatment for an overdose is symptomatic and supportive. Carefully monitor patient's vital signs and fluid and electrolyte balance.

Special considerations

■ Observe patient for dermatologic reactions, joint pain, unexplained fever, or unusual bruising or bleeding (which may signal hematologic or other severe adverse reactions).
■ Don't stop drug abruptly because doing so may precipitate absence seizures.
■ Therapeutic plasma levels range from 40 to 100 mcg/ml.
■ Obtain CBC, liver function tests, and urinalysis periodically.
■ Give ethosuximide with food to minimize GI distress.

■ Anticipate that ethosuximide may cause false-positive results on Coombs' test.

Breast-feeding patients

■ Advise breast-feeding mother to use alternative feeding method during therapy with ethosuximide.

Pediatric patients

■ Don't give drug to a child under age 3.

Geriatric patients

■ Use cautiously in elderly patients.

Patient teaching

■ Urge patient to avoid hazardous activities until full effects of drug are clear. It may cause drowsiness, dizziness, or blurred vision.
■ Tell patient to report rash, joint pain, fever, sore throat, or unusual bleeding or bruising.
■ Tell patient to take drug with food or milk to prevent GI distress.
■ Explain that drug may color urine pink to reddish-brown.
■ Caution patient to avoid alcohol during therapy.
■ Advise patient to immediately report planned, suspected, or known pregnancy.
■ Encourage patient to wear or carry medical identification that describes the seizure disorder and the drug regimen.

Reactions may be *common*, uncommon, *life-threatening*, or COMMON AND LIFE-THREATENING.

fosphenytoin sodium
Cerebyx

Pharmacologic classification:
hydantoin derivative

Therapeutic classification:
anticonvulsant

Pregnancy risk category D

How supplied
Available by prescription only
Injection: 2 ml (150 mg fosphenytoin sodium equivalent to 100 mg phenytoin sodium), 10 ml (750 mg fosphenytoin sodium equivalent to 500 mg phenytoin sodium)

Indications and dosages
Status epilepticus
Adults: 15 to 20 mg phenytoin sodium equivalent (PE)/kg I.V. at 100 to 150 PE/minute as a loading dose. Then 4 to 6 mg PE/kg/day I.V. as a maintenance dose. (Phenytoin may be used instead of fosphenytoin as maintenance using the appropriate dosage.)

Prevention and treatment of seizures during neurosurgery
Adults: 10 to 20 mg PE/kg I.M. or I.V. infused at no more than 150 mg PE/minute as a loading dose. Maintenance dosage is 4 to 6 mg PE/kg/day I.V.

Short-term substitution for oral phenytoin therapy
Adults: Same total daily dosage as oral phenytoin sodium therapy given as a single daily dose I.M. or I.V. infused at no more than 150 mg PE/minute. (Some patients may need more frequent dosing.)

Pharmacodynamics
Anticonvulsant action: Because fosphenytoin is a prodrug of phenytoin, its anticonvulsant action is the same as phenytoin. Phenytoin stabilizes neuronal membranes and limits seizure activity by modulating voltage-dependent neuronal sodium and calcium channels, inhibiting calcium flux across neuronal membranes, and enhancing sodium-potassium adenosine triphosphatase activity in neurons and glial cells.

Pharmacokinetics
Absorption: Plasma fosphenytoin levels peak about 30 minutes after I.M. administration or at the end of I.V. infusion.
Distribution: About 95% to 99% is bound to plasma proteins, primarily albumin. The volume of distribution increases with dose and rate and ranges from 4.3 to 10.8 L.
Metabolism: Conversion half-life of fosphenytoin to phenytoin is about 15 minutes. Phosphatases are believed to play a major role in the conversion.
Excretion: Unknown, although it isn't excreted in urine.

Contraindications and precautions
Contraindicated in patients hypersensitive to fosphenytoin, phenytoin, other hydantoins, or their components. Also contraindicated in patients with sinus bradycardia, SA block, second- or third-degree AV block, or Adams-Stokes syndrome because of the effect of parenteral phenytoin on ventricular automaticity.

Use cautiously in patients with hypotension, severe myocardial insufficiency, impaired renal or hepatic function, hypoalbuminemia, porphyria, diabetes mellitus, or a history of hypersensitivity to similarly structured drugs, such as barbiturates and succinimides.

Interactions
Drug-drug
Amiodarone, chloramphenicol, chlordiazepoxide, cimetidine, diazepam, dicumarol, disulfiram, estrogens, ethosuximide, fluoxetine, H₂-antagonists, halothane, isoniazid, methylphenidate, phenothiazines, phenylbutazone, salicylates, succinimides, sulfonamides, tolbutamide, trazodone: increased plasma phenytoin levels and increased therapeutic effects. Dosage adjustment may be needed.

Carbamazepine, reserpine: plasma phenytoin levels may be decreased. Dosage adjustment may be needed.

Coumarin, digitoxin, doxycycline, estrogens, furosemide, oral contraceptives, quinidine, theophylline: efficacy of these drugs may be decreased from increased hepatic metabolism. Monitor patient closely.

Dilantin, phenobarbital, rifampin, sodium valproate, tegretol, valproic acid: may increase or decrease plasma phenytoin levels. Similarly, phenytoin may affect levels of these drugs. Dosage adjustment may be needed.

Lithium: increased risk of lithium toxicity. Monitor patient closely.

Tricyclic antidepressants: may lower seizure threshold. Adjustment of phenytoin dosage may be needed.

Drug-lifestyle
Acute alcohol use: may increase plasma phenytoin levels and therapeutic effects. Discourage alcohol use.

Long-term alcohol use: may decrease plasma phenytoin levels. Discourage alcohol use.

Adverse reactions
CNS: agitation, asthenia, *ataxia,* brain edema, ***cerebral hemorrhage,*** confusion, *dizziness,* dysarthria, extrapyramidal symptoms, headache, hypesthesia, incoordination, increased or decreased reflexes, ***intracranial hypertension,*** nervousness, *nystagmus,* paresthesia, speech disorders, *somnolence,* stupor, thinking abnormalities, tremor, vertigo.

CV: atrial flutter, ***bundle branch block, cardiac arrest,*** cardiomegaly, ***heart failure,*** hypertension, hypotension, orthostatic hypotension, palpitations, prolonged QT interval, ***pulmonary embolus, sinus bradycardia,*** tachycardia, thrombophlebitis, vasodilation, ventricular extrasystoles.

EENT: amblyopia, conjunctivitis, deafness, diplopia, ear pain, epistaxis, eye pain, hyperacusis, mydriasis, parosmia, pharyngitis, photophobia, rhinitis, sinusitis, taste loss, taste perversion, tinnitus, visual field defect.

GI: anorexia, constipation, diarrhea, dry mouth, dyspepsia, dysphagia, flatulence, gastritis, GI hemorrhage, ileus, increased salivation, nausea, tenesmus, tongue edema, vomiting.

GU: albuminuria, dysuria, genital edema, kidney failure, oliguria, polyuria, urethral pain, urine retention, urinary incontinence, vaginal candidiasis, vaginitis.

Hematologic: *agranulocytosis,* anemia, ecchymosis, *granulocytopenia,* hypochromic anemia, leukocytosis, *leukopenia,* megaloblastic anemia, *pancytopenia, thrombocytopenia.*

Hepatic: elevated liver enzymes.

Metabolic: acidosis, alkalosis, dehydration, diabetes insipidus, hyperglycemia, hyperkalemia, hypokalemia, hypophosphatemia, ketosis.

Musculoskeletal: arthralgia, back pain, leg cramps, myalgia, myasthenia, myopathy, pelvic pain.

Respiratory: *apnea,* aspiration pneumonia, asthma, atelectasis, bronchitis, cyanosis, dyspnea, hemoptysis, hyperventilation, hypoxia, increased cough, increased sputum, pneumonia, pneumothorax.

Skin: contact dermatitis, maculopapular rash, petechia, *pruritus,* pustular rash, rash, skin discoloration, skin nodule, sweating, urticaria.

Other: lymphadenopathy.

Overdose and treatment

There have been no reports of fosphenytoin overdose. However, because it's a prodrug of phenytoin, overdose may be similar. Early phenytoin overdose may cause ataxia, drowsiness, dysarthria, nausea, nystagmus, slurred speech, tremor, and vomiting. Hypotension, respiratory depression, and coma may follow. Death may result from respiratory and circulatory depression. The estimated lethal phenytoin dose is 2 to 5 g in adults.

Formate and phosphate are metabolites of fosphenytoin and therefore may contribute to signs of toxicity following overdose. Signs of formate toxicity are similar to those of methanol toxicity and accompany severe anion-gap metabolic acidosis. Large amounts of phosphate, delivered rapidly, could cause hypocalcemia with paresthesia, muscle spasms, and seizures. Ionized free calcium levels can be measured and, if low, used to guide treatment.

Treatment involves gastric lavage or emesis followed by supportive measures. Monitor patient's vital signs and fluid and electrolyte balance. Forced diuresis has little or no value. Hemodialysis or peritoneal dialysis may be helpful.

Special considerations

■ Fosphenytoin should always be prescribed and dispensed in PE units. Therefore, don't adjust recommended doses when substituting fosphenytoin for phenytoin and vice versa.

■ I.M. administration generates systemic phenytoin levels similar enough to oral phenytoin sodium to allow essentially interchangeable use.

■ If rapid phenytoin loading is a primary goal, give fosphenytoin I.V. rather than I.M.

■ Before I.V. infusion, dilute fosphenytoin in D_5W or normal saline solution for injection to yield 1.5 to 25 mg PE/ml. Don't exceed a rate of 150 mg PE/minute.

■ A dose of 15 to 20 mg PE/kg of fosphenytoin infused at 100 to 150 mg PE/minute yields plasma-free phenytoin levels over time that approximate those achieved when an equivalent dose of phenytoin

sodium is administered at 50 mg/minute I.V.
- Monitor patient's ECG, blood pressure, and respirations continuously during period of maximal serum phenytoin levels, about 10 to 20 minutes after the end of fosphenytoin infusion.
- Expect patients who receive fosphenytoin at 20 mg PE/kg and 150 mg PE/minute to experience some discomfort, usually in the groin. The occurrence and intensity of discomfort can be reduced by slowing or temporarily stopping the infusion.
- Interpret total phenytoin plasma levels cautiously in patients who have renal or hepatic disease or hypoalbuminemia because of an increased fraction of unbound phenytoin. Unbound phenytoin levels may be a better measurement in these patients. Also, these patients have an increased risk of more frequent, more severe adverse reactions (especially hypotension) when fosphenytoin is given I.V.
- Discontinue drug if rash appears. If rash is exfoliative, purpuric, or bullous, or if lupus erythematosus, Stevens-Johnson syndrome, or toxic epidermal necrolysis is suspected, don't resume drug, and seek alternative therapy. If the rash is mild (measleslike or scarlatiniform), therapy may be resumed after the rash has completely disappeared. If it recurs when therapy resumes, further fosphenytoin or phenytoin administration is contraindicated.
- The phosphate load provided by fosphenytoin (0.0037 mmol phosphate/mg PE fosphenytoin) must be taken into consideration when treating patients who need phosphate restriction, such as those with severe renal impairment.
- Fosphenytoin may produce artificially low results in dexamethasone or metyrapone tests.
- When treating status epilepticus with I.V. fosphenytoin, use a maximum rate of 150 mg PE/minute. Typical infusion takes 5 to 7 minutes for a 50-kg patient. Delivery of an identical molar dose of phenytoin takes 15 to 20 minutes, possibly more, because of the adverse CV effects that accompany direct I.V. delivery of phenytoin at more than 50 mg/minute. Don't give fosphenytoin by I.M. route because therapeutic phenytoin levels may not occur as rapidly as with I.V. delivery.
- Following drug administration, don't monitor phenytoin levels until conversion to phenytoin is essentially complete—about 2 hours after the end of an I.V. infusion or 4 hours after I.M. administration.
- Severe CV complications are most likely among elderly or gravely ill patients. Reduce the rate of administration or stop drug as needed.

Breast-feeding patients
- Because it isn't known whether fosphenytoin is excreted in breast milk, breast-feeding isn't recommended.

Pediatric patients
- Safety and effectiveness in children have not been established.

Geriatric patients
■ Elderly patients metabolize and excrete phenytoin slowly; therefore, give fosphenytoin cautiously to elderly patients.

Patient teaching
■ Warn patient that sensory disturbances may occur with I.V. administration.
■ Tell patient to immediately report adverse reactions, especially rash.
■ Stress the importance of monthly follow-up appointments to monitor CBC results, especially at start of treatment.
■ Encourage patient to wear or carry medical identification that describes the seizure disorder and the drug regimen.

---

gabapentin
Neurontin

Pharmacologic classification: 1-amino-methyl cyclohexoneacetic acid

Therapeutic classification: anticonvulsant

Pregnancy risk category C

How supplied
Available by prescription only
Capsules: 100 mg, 300 mg, 400 mg

Indications and dosages
Adjunctive treatment of partial seizures with and without secondary generalization
Adults: 300 mg P.O. on day 1, 300 mg P.O. b.i.d. on day 2, and 300 mg P.O. t.i.d. on day 3. Increase dosage as needed and tolerated to 1,800 mg daily in three divided doses. Usual dosage is 300 to 600 mg P.O. t.i.d., although dosages up to 3,600 mg/day have been well tolerated.
▶ DOSAGE ADJUSTMENT. In adult patients with renal failure, give 400 mg P.O. t.i.d. if creatinine clearance is above 60 ml/minute, 300 mg P.O. b.i.d. if creatinine clearance is between 30 and 60 ml/minute, 300 mg P.O. daily if creatinine clearance is between 15 and 30 ml/minute, or 300 mg P.O. every other day if creatinine clearance is less than 15 ml/minute. Patients on hemodialysis should receive a loading dose of 300 to 400 mg P.O., then 200 to 300 mg P.O. 4 hours after hemodialysis.

Pharmacodynamics
Anticonvulsant action: Gabapentin's mechanism of action is unknown. Although it is structurally related to GABA, it doesn't interact with GABA receptors, isn't metabolically converted into GABA or a GABA agonist, and doesn't inhibit GABA uptake or degradation. It also exhibits no affinity for other common receptor sites.

Pharmacokinetics
Absorption: Drug bioavailability is not dose proportional. A 400-mg dose, for example, is about 25% less bioavailable than a 100-mg dose. Over the recommended dose range of 300 to 600 mg t.i.d., however, bioavailability is about 60% and differences in bioavailability aren't large. Food has no effect on the rate or extent of absorption.
Distribution: Gabapentin circulates largely unbound (less than

---

3%) to plasma protein. It crosses the blood-brain barrier; about 20% of corresponding plasma levels appear in CSF.
Metabolism: Drug is not metabolized appreciably.
Excretion: Gabapentin is eliminated from systemic circulation by renal excretion as unchanged drug. Its elimination half-life is 5 to 7 hours. It can be removed from plasma by hemodialysis.

Contraindications and precautions
Contraindicated in patients hypersensitive to drug.

Interactions
Drug-drug
Antacids: decrease the absorption of gabapentin. Separate administration by at least 2 hours.

Adverse reactions
CNS: abnormal thinking, amnesia, *ataxia,* depression, *dizziness,* dysarthria, *fatigue,* incoordination, nervousness, *somnolence, tremor,* twitching.
CV: peripheral edema, vasodilation.
EENT: *amblyopia,* dental abnormalities, *diplopia,* dry throat, *nystagmus,* pharyngitis, *rhinitis.*
GI: constipation, dry mouth, dyspepsia, nausea, vomiting.
GU: impotence.
Hematologic: decreased WBC count, *leukopenia.*
Metabolic: increased appetite, weight gain.
Musculoskeletal: back pain, fractures, myalgia.
Respiratory: coughing.
Skin: abrasion, pruritus.

Overdose and treatment
Acute overdose may cause diarrhea, double vision, drowsiness, lethargy, and slurred speech.
　　Supportive care is recommended. Gabapentin can be removed by hemodialysis if the patient's clinical state warrants it or patient has significant renal impairment.

Special considerations
■ Routine monitoring of plasma drug levels isn't needed. Drug doesn't appear to alter plasma levels of other anticonvulsants.
■ Don't use Ames N-Multistix SG dipstick to test for urine protein because false-positive results can occur. Instead, use the more specific sulfosalicylic acid precipitation procedure to detect urine protein.
■ Discontinue drug therapy or substitute alternative medication gradually over at least 1 week to minimize risk of precipitating seizures. Don't suddenly withdraw other anticonvulsant drugs in patients starting gabapentin therapy.

Breast-feeding patients
■ It isn't known whether drug is excreted in breast milk. Use in breast-feeding patients only if drug's benefits clearly outweigh its risks.

Pediatric patients
■ Safety and effectiveness in children under age 12 haven't been established.

Patient teaching
■ Inform patient that drug can be taken without regard to meals.

- Instruct patient to take first dose at bedtime to minimize drowsiness, dizziness, fatigue, and ataxia.
- Warn patient to avoid hazardous activities until drug's adverse CNS effects are fully known.
- Encourage patient to wear a medical identification bracelet or necklace that identifies the seizure disorder and the drug regimen.

lamotrigine
Lamictal

Pharmacologic classification: phenyltriazine

Therapeutic classification: anticonvulsant

Pregnancy risk category C

How supplied
Available by prescription only
Chewable tablets: 5 mg, 25 mg
Tablets: 25 mg, 100 mg, 150 mg, 200 mg

Indications and dosages
Adjunct therapy for partial seizures caused by epilepsy
Adults and children age 16 and older: 50 mg P.O. daily for 2 weeks, followed by 100 mg daily in two divided doses for 2 weeks. Thereafter, usual maintenance dose is 300 to 500 mg P.O. daily in two divided doses. For patients who also take valproic acid, give 25 mg of lamotrigine P.O. every other day for 2 weeks followed by 25 mg P.O. daily for 2 weeks. Thereafter, maximum is 150 mg P.O. daily in two divided doses.

Adjunct therapy for generalized seizures of Lennox-Gastaut syndrome
Adults and children age 12 and older: 50 mg P.O. daily for 2 weeks, followed by 100 mg daily in two divided doses for 2 weeks. Thereafter, usual maintenance dose is 300 to 500 mg P.O. daily in two divided doses. For patients who also take valproic acid, give 25 mg of lamotrigine P.O. every other day for 2 weeks followed by 25 mg P.O. daily for 2 weeks. Thereafter, usual maintenance dosage is 100 to 400 mg P.O. daily in one or two divided doses.
Children ages 2 to 12: 0.6 mg/kg (rounded down to the nearest 5 mg) P.O. daily in two divided doses for 2 weeks, followed by 1.2 mg/kg (rounded down to the nearest 5 mg) P.O. daily in two divided doses. Increase q 1 to 2 weeks by 1.2 mg/kg/day (rounded down to the nearest 5 mg) until you reach an effective maintenance dosage of 5 to 15 mg/kg/day (maximum 400 mg/day). For patients who also take valproic acid, give 0.15 mg/kg (rounded down to the nearest 5 mg) P.O. daily in one dose or two divided doses for 2 weeks. If the initial calculated dose is 2.5 to 5 mg, give a 5-mg dose on alternate days for the first 2 weeks. During the next 2 weeks, give 0.3 mg/kg (rounded down to the nearest 5 mg) P.O. daily in one dose or two divided doses. Increase dose every 1 to 2 weeks by 0.3 mg/kg/day (rounded down to the nearest 5 mg) until you reach an effective maintenance dosage of 1 to 5 mg/kg/day. Maximum 200 mg/

day in one dose or divided into two doses.

Pharmacodynamics
Anticonvulsant action: Unknown. May be related to inhibited release of glutamate and aspartate in the brain, possibly from drug action on voltage-sensitive sodium channels.

Pharmacokinetics
Absorption: Drug is rapidly and completely absorbed from the GI tract with negligible first-pass metabolism. Absolute bioavailability is 98%.
Distribution: About 55% is bound to plasma proteins.
Metabolism: Drug is metabolized predominantly by glucuronic acid conjugation. The major metabolite is an inactive 2-N-glucuronide conjugate.
Excretion: Drug is excreted primarily in urine with only a small portion being excreted in feces.

Contraindications and precautions
Contraindicated in patients hypersensitive to drug.

Use cautiously in patients with impaired renal, hepatic, or cardiac function.

Interactions
Drug-drug
Acetaminophen: decreases serum lamotrigine levels. Monitor patient closely.
Carbamazepine, phenobarbital, phenytoin, primidone: decrease in lamotrigine's steady state levels. Monitor patient closely.

Folate inhibitors (co-trimoxazole, methotrexate): may be affected because lamotrigine inhibits dihydrofolate reductase, an enzyme involved in the synthesis of folic acid. Monitor patient closely because drug may have an additive effect.
Valproic acid: decreases lamotrigine clearance, which increases drug's steady state levels. Monitor patient's response.

Adverse reactions
CNS: anxiety, *ataxia,* concentration disturbance, decreased memory, depression, *dizziness,* emotional lability, *headache,* incoordination, insomnia, irritability, malaise, mind racing, **seizures,** sleep disorder, *somnolence,* speech disorder, *suicide attempts,* tremor, vertigo.
CV: palpitations.
EENT: *blurred vision, diplopia,* nystagmus. pharyngitis, rhinitis, vision abnormality.
GI: abdominal pain, anorexia, constipation, diarrhea, dry mouth, dyspepsia, *nausea,* tooth disorder, *vomiting.*
GU: amenorrhea, dysmenorrhea, vaginitis.
Musculoskeletal: dysarthria, muscle spasm, neck pain.
Respiratory: cough, dyspnea.
Skin: acne, alopecia, epidermal neurolysis, hot flashes, photosensitivity, pruritus, *rash,* **Stevens-Johnson syndrome.**
Other: chills, fever, flulike syndrome, infection.

Overdose and treatment
Limited information available about the effects of overdose. One patient became comatose for 8 to 12 hours. A second patient experi-

enced dizziness, headache, and somnolence. Both patients recovered without sequelae.

Following a suspected overdose, give supportive treatment. Induce emesis or perform gastric lavage, if needed. It isn't known whether hemodialysis is effective.

Special considerations
■ Evaluate patient for reduced frequency and duration of seizures. Obtain periodic evaluation of adjunct anticonvulsant's serum levels.
■ Don't discontinue drug abruptly because doing so may increase seizure frequency. Instead, taper drug over at least 2 weeks.
■ Stop drug immediately if drug-induced rash occurs.
■ If you add lamotrigine to a multidrug regimen that includes valproate, reduce the lamotrigine dosage.
■ Reduce the maintenance dosage in patients with severe renal impairment.

Breast-feeding patients
■ Drug use in breast-feeding women isn't recommended.

Pediatric patients
■ Recommended use for children ages 2 to 12 is very limited. Administer drug carefully and follow detailed guidelines provided with drug. Severe, potentially life-threatening rash is much more common in children than in adults.

Geriatric patients
■ Safety and effectiveness in patients over age 65 haven't been established.

Patient teaching
■ Warn patient not to perform hazardous activities until drug's CNS effects are known.
■ Advise patient to take protective measures against photosensitivity reactions until tolerance is known.
■ Inform patient that rash may occur, especially during first 6 weeks of therapy and especially in children. Combination therapy with valproic acid and lamotrigine may cause a serious rash. Although the rash may resolve with continued therapy, tell patient to report it immediately in case drug needs to be discontinued.
■ Warn patient not to stop drug abruptly because seizures may occur.
■ Encourage patient to wear or carry medical identification that describes the seizure disorder and the drug regimen.

---

levetiracetam
Keppra

Pharmacologic classification: anticonvulsant

Therapeutic classification: anticonvulsant

Pregnancy risk category C

How supplied
Tablets: 250 mg, 500 mg, 750 mg

Indications and dosages
Partial seizures (adjunct)
Adults: initially, 500 mg P.O. b.i.d. May increase by 500 mg b.i.d. at 2-week intervals, as needed for

---

seizure control, to a maximum of 1,500 mg b.i.d.

▶ **DOSAGE ADJUSTMENT.** If patient has renal failure, give 500 to 1,500 mg q 12 hours if creatinine clearance is more than 80 ml/ minute, 500 to 1,000 mg q 12 hours if clearance is 50 to 80 ml/ minute, 250 to 750 mg q 12 hours if clearance is 30 to 50 ml/minute, or 250 to 500 mg q 12 hours if clearance is less than 30 ml/ minute. If patient receives dialysis, give 500 to 1,000 mg q 24 hours and a 250- to 500-mg dose after each dialysis treatment.

Pharmacodynamics
Unknown. Drug is thought to inhibit kindling activity in hippocampus, thus preventing the simultaneous neuronal firing that leads to seizure activity.

Pharmacokinetics
Absorption: Drug is rapidly absorbed in the GI tract, and serum levels peak in about 1 hour. Although drug can be taken with food, doing so delays time to reach peak levels by about 1½ hours and yields slightly lower serum levels. Serum levels reach steady state in about 2 days.
Distribution: Protein binding is minimal.
Metabolism: No active metabolites. Drug isn't metabolized through the cytochrome P-450 system.
Excretion: Elimination half-life is about 7 hours in patients with normal renal function. About 66% of drug is eliminated unchanged by glomerular filtration and tubular reabsorption.

Adverse reactions
CNS: amnesia, anxiety, *asthenia,* ataxia, depression, dizziness, emotional lability, *headache,* hostility, paresthesia, nervousness, *somnolence,* vertigo.
EENT: diplopia infection, pharyngitis, rhinitis, sinusitis.
GI: anorexia.
Respiratory: cough.
Musculoskeletal: pain.
Hematologic: *leukopenia, neutropenia.*

Contraindications and precautions
Contraindicated in patients hypersensitive to drug.

Use cautiously in immunocompromised patients and in those with poor renal function.

Interactions
Drug-drug
Drugs known to cause drowsiness (antihistamines, benzodiazepines, narcotics, tricyclic antidepressants): may lead to severe sedation. Avoid concomitant use.
Drugs known to cause leukopenia or neutropenia (carbamazepine, clozapine): increases the risk of these disorders. Use only when benefit outweighs risks or when no alternative drugs are available.

Drug-lifestyle
Alcohol use: may lead to severe sedation. Discourage concomitant use.

Overdose and treatment
Drowsiness has been reported with doses of up to 6,000 mg.

Supportive care and observation are recommended. Induced emesis or gastric lavage may be helpful in the early stages of treatment. Hemodialysis removes about 50% of drug if performed within 4 hours of overdose. No antidote is available.

Special considerations
■ Drug is approved only as an adjunct for treating partial seizures and isn't recommended for monotherapy. Use only with other anticonvulsants.
■ For patients with poor renal function, base dosage reduction on creatinine clearance.
■ If patient is immunocompromised, obtain baseline CBC and periodic follow-ups because of reports of leukopenia and neutropenia.
■ Taper drug when discontinuing it.
■ Drug can be taken with or without food.

Breast-feeding patients
■ It isn't known whether drug appears in breast milk. Determine risks and benefits before giving it to breast-feeding women.

Patient teaching
■ Caution patient not to stop drug abruptly.
■ Tell patient to notify prescriber about adverse effects.
■ Warn patient about an increased risk of falling and the need to take safety precautions to prevent injury.
■ Tell patient to take drug with other seizure drugs as prescribed.
■ Inform patient that drug can be taken with or without food.

■ Encourage patient to wear or carry medical identification that describes the seizure disorder and the drug regimen.

magnesium sulfate

Pharmacologic classification: mineral, electrolyte

Therapeutic classification: anticonvulsant

Pregnancy risk category A

How supplied
Available by prescription only
Injectable solutions: 4%, 8%, 10%, 12.5%, 20%, 50% in 2-ml, 5-ml, 8-ml, 10-ml, 20-ml, 30-ml, and 50-ml ampules, vials, and prefilled syringes

Indications and dosages
Hypomagnesemic seizures
Adults: 1 to 2 g (as 10% solution) I.V. over 15 minutes, then 1 g I.M. q 4 to 6 hours, based on patient's response and magnesium blood levels.

Hypomagnesemic seizures in acute nephritis
Children: 0.2 ml/kg of 50% solution I.M. q 4 to 6 hours, p.r.n., or 100 mg/kg of 10% solution I.V. given slowly. Adjust dosage according to magnesium blood levels and seizure response.

Prevention or control of seizures in preeclampsia or eclampsia
Adults: initially, 4 g I.V. in 250 ml D$_5$W and 4 to 5 g deep I.M. in each

buttock; then 4 g deep I.M. into alternate buttock q 4 hours, p.r.n. Alternatively, 4 g I.V. as a loading dose followed by 1 to 2 g hourly as an I.V. infusion. Maximum daily dose, 40 g I.V. over 3 hours.

Pharmacodynamics

Anticonvulsant action: Magnesium sulfate has CNS and respiratory depressant effects. It acts peripherally, causing vasodilation. Moderate doses cause flushing and sweating; high doses cause hypotension. It prevents or controls seizures by blocking neuromuscular transmission.

Pharmacokinetics

Absorption: I.V. magnesium sulfate acts immediately; effects last about 30 minutes. After I.M. injection, it acts within 60 minutes and lasts for 3 to 4 hours. Effective anticonvulsant serum levels are 2.5 to 7.5 mEq/L.
Distribution: Magnesium sulfate is distributed widely throughout the body.
Metabolism: None.
Excretion: Drug is excreted unchanged in urine; some is excreted in breast milk.

Contraindications and precautions

Parenteral administration contraindicated in patients with heart block or myocardial damage. Do not give drug to patient with toxemia of pregnancy during the two hours preceding delivery.

Use cautiously in patients with impaired renal function and in women in labor.

Interactions
Drug-drug

Antidepressants, antipsychotics, anxiolytics, barbiturates, general anesthetics, hypnotics, narcotics: may increase CNS depressant effects. Reduced dosages may be required.
Cardiac glycosides: changes in cardiac conduction in digitalized patients may lead to heart block if I.V. calcium is administered to treat magnesium toxicity. Use extreme caution when giving concurrently.
Succinylcholine, tubocurarine: potentiates and prolongs neuromuscular blocking action of these drugs. Use with caution.

Drug-lifestyle

Alcohol use: may increase CNS depressant effects. Discourage concomitant use.

Adverse reactions

CNS: drowsiness, *depressed reflexes,* flaccid paralysis, hypothermia.
CV: *hypotension, flushing, **circulatory collapse,*** depressed cardiac function.
Metabolic: hypocalcemia.
Respiratory: *respiratory paralysis.*
Skin: diaphoresis.

Overdose and treatment

Overdose of magnesium sulfate may cause a sharp drop in blood pressure, asystole, ECG changes (increased PR, QRS, and QT intervals), heart block, and respiratory paralysis.

Treatment requires artificial ventilation and I.V. calcium salt to reverse respiratory depression and heart block. Usual dose is 5 to 10

Reactions may be *common,* uncommon, *life-threatening,* or COMMON AND LIFE-THREATENING.

mEq of calcium (10 to 20 ml of a 10% calcium gluconate solution).

Special considerations
■ For I.V. administration, avoid concentrations above 20% and rates above 150 mg/minute (1.5 ml of a 10% concentration or equivalent). For I.M. administration in adults, anticipate using 25% or 50% concentration; for infants and children, levels shouldn't exceed 20%.
■ To calculate grams of magnesium in a percentage of solution, use following equation: $x\% = x$ g/ 100 ml (for example, 25% = 25 g/ 100 ml = 250 mg/ml).
■ To avoid respiratory or cardiac arrest, I.V. bolus must be injected slowly.
■ Administer by constant infusion pump, if possible, at a maximum infusion rate of 150 mg/minute. Rapid drip causes feeling of heat.
■ When giving repeated doses, test knee jerk reflex before each dose; if it's absent, discontinue the drug. Continued use risks respiratory center failure.
■ Respiratory rate must be 16 breaths per minute or more before each dose. Keep I.V. calcium salts on hand.
■ Monitor serum magnesium load and clinical status to avoid overdose.
■ Maintain at least 100 ml of urine output every 4 hours.
■ Discontinue drug as soon as needed effect is achieved.
■ In patients with normal renal function, all magnesium sulfate is excreted within 24 hours of discontinuing drug.

■ Drug is also used to treat life-threatening arrhythmias, barium poisoning, preterm labor management, and mild hypomagnesemia. May be used (unlabeled) for patients with asthma who respond poorly to beta agonists.

Breast-feeding patients
■ Drug is excreted in breast milk. An alternative feeding method is recommended during therapy.

Patient teaching
■ Teach patient about purpose of drug and its risks and benefits.
■ Encourage patient to wear or carry medical identification that describes the seizure disorder and the drug regimen.

---

mephenytoin
Mesantoin

Pharmacologic classification: **hydantoin derivative**

Therapeutic classification: **anticonvulsant**

Pregnancy risk category NR

How supplied
Available by prescription only
Tablets: 100 mg

Indications and dosages
Generalized tonic-clonic or complex-partial seizures
Adults: 50 to 100 mg P.O. daily; may increase by 50 to 100 mg at weekly intervals up to 200 mg P.O. q 8 hours. Doses up to 800 mg/day may be needed.

Children: initially, 50 to 100 mg P.O. daily. May increase by 50 to 100 mg at weekly intervals up to 200 mg P.O. t.i.d., divided q 8 hours. Dosage must be adjusted individually. Usual maintenance dosage is 100 to 400 mg/day (or 3 to 15 mg/kg/day or 100 to 450 mg/m²/day) administered in three equally divided doses.

Pharmacodynamics
Anticonvulsant action: Like other hydantoin derivatives, mephenytoin stabilizes the neuronal membranes and limits seizure activity either by increasing efflux or by decreasing influx of sodium ions across cell membranes in the motor cortex during generation of nerve impulses. Like phenytoin, mephenytoin appears to have antiarrhythmic effects.

Pharmacokinetics
Absorption: Mephenytoin is absorbed from the GI tract. Onset of action occurs in 30 minutes and persists for 24 to 48 hours.
Distribution: Drug is distributed widely throughout the body; good seizure control without toxicity occurs when serum levels of drug and major metabolite reach 25 to 40 mcg/ml.
Metabolism: Mephenytoin is metabolized by the liver.
Excretion: Drug and its metabolites are excreted in urine.

Contraindications and precautions
Contraindicated in patients hypersensitive to hydantoin.

Interactions
Drug-drug
Antihistamines, chloramphenicol, cimetidine, diazepam, diazoxide, disulfiram, isoniazid, phenylbutazone, salicylates, sulfamethizole, valproate: mephenytoin's therapeutic effects and toxicity may be increased. Monitor patient closely.
Folic acid: mephenytoin's therapeutic effects may be decreased. Monitor patient closely.
Oral contraceptives: mephenytoin's therapeutic effects and toxicity may be increased. Monitor patient closely. Also, mephenytoin may decrease oral contraceptive effects. Alternative method of birth control should be used.

Drug-lifestyle
Alcohol use: may reduce therapeutic effects of mephenytoin. Discourage alcohol consumption.

Adverse reactions
CNS: ataxia, choreiform movements, depression, dizziness, *drowsiness,* fatigue, insomnia, irritability, tremor.
EENT: conjunctivitis, diplopia, gingival hyperplasia, nystagmus.
GI: nausea, vomiting.
Hematologic: *agranulocytosis,* eosinophilia, leukocytosis, *leukopenia, neutropenia, thrombocytopenia.*
Musculoskeletal: polyarthropathy.
Respiratory: *pulmonary fibrosis.*
Skin: rash, *exfoliative dermatitis, Stevens-Johnson syndrome, fatal dermatitides.*
Other: edema, lymphadenopathy.

Reactions may be *common,* uncommon, *life-threatening,* or COMMON AND LIFE-THREATENING.

Overdose and treatment

Acute mephenytoin toxicity may cause ataxia, dizziness, drowsiness, dysarthria, nausea, nystagmus, restlessness, slurred speech, tremor, and vomiting. Hypotension, respiratory depression, and coma may follow. Death may result from respiratory and circulatory depression.

Treat a mephenytoin overdose with gastric lavage or induced emesis and follow with supportive care. Carefully monitor the patient's vital signs and fluid and electrolyte balance. Forced diuresis is of little or no value. Hemodialysis or peritoneal dialysis may be helpful.

Special considerations

- Mephenytoin is usually prescribed for patients refractory to less toxic drugs and is usually combined with phenytoin, phenobarbital, or primidone. Phenytoin is preferred because it causes less sedation than barbiturates.
- Mephenytoin also is used with succinimides to control combined absence and tonic-clonic disorders.
- Combined use with oxazolidinediones, paramethadione, or trimethadione isn't recommended because of the increased hazard of blood dyscrasias.
- CBC and platelet counts should be performed before therapy, after 2 weeks of therapy, and after 2 weeks on maintenance dose. Tests should be repeated every month for 1 year and, subsequently, at 3-month intervals.

- Decreased alertness and coordination are most pronounced at the start of treatment. Patient may need help with walking and activities of daily living for the first few days.
- Nausea, vomiting and gingival hyperplasia is more commonly associated with prolonged use.
- Don't discontinue drug abruptly. The transition from mephenytoin to other anticonvulsant drug should progress over 6 weeks.

Pregnant patients

- Safe use of mephenytoin during pregnancy hasn't been established. Give drug to pregnant patients only when clearly needed.

Breast-feeding patients

- Safe use of mephenytoin during breast-feeding hasn't been established. An alternative feeding method is recommended during therapy.

Pediatric patients

- Children usually require 100 to 400 mg/day.

Patient teaching

- Warn patient never to discontinue drug or change dosage except as prescribed.
- Caution patient to avoid alcohol because it decreases drug effectiveness and increases sedative effects.
- Explain that follow-up laboratory tests are essential for safe use.
- Instruct patient to report unusual changes immediately, such as cutaneous reactions, a sore throat,

fever, or swelling of lymph nodes or mucous membranes.
- Encourage patient to wear or carry medical identification that descibes the seizure disorder and the drug regimen.

oxcarbazepine
Trileptal

Pharmacologic classification: **carboxamide derivative**

Therapeutic classification: **antiepileptic**

Pregnancy risk category C

How supplied
Available by prescription only
Tablets (film-coated): 150 mg, 300 mg, 600 mg

Indications and dosages
Partial seizures in patients with epilepsy (adjunct)
Adults: initially, 300 mg P.O. b.i.d. Increase by a maximum of 600 mg/day (300 mg P.O b.i.d.) at weekly intervals. Recommended daily dose is 1,200 mg P.O. divided b.i.d.
Children ages 4 to 16: initially, 8 to 10 mg/kg/day P.O. divided b.i.d., not to exceed 600 mg/day. Target maintenance dosage depends on patient's weight, and should be divided b.i.d. If patient weighs 20 to 29 kg (44 to 63 lb), then the target maintenance dosage is 900 mg/day. If patient weighs 29.1 to 39 kg (64 to 86 lb), target maintenance dosage is 1,200 mg/day. If patient weighs more than 39 kg, target maintenance dosage is 1,800 mg/

day. Target dosages should be achieved over 2 weeks.

Conversion to monotherapy in treatment of partial seizures in patients with epilepsy
Adults: initially, 300 mg P.O. b.i.d., with simultaneous reduction in dose of concomitant antiepileptics. Increase oxcarbazepine by a maximum of 600 mg/day at weekly intervals over 2 to 4 weeks. Recommended daily dose is 2,400 mg P.O. divided b.i.d. Concomitant antiepileptics should be withdrawn over 3 to 6 weeks.

Initiation of monotherapy for treatment of partial seizures in patients with epilepsy
Adults: initially, 300 mg P.O. b.i.d. Increase by 300 mg/day every third day to 1,200 mg/day divided b.i.d.
⊠ **DOSAGE ADJUSTMENT.** If patient's creatinine clearance is less than 30 ml/minute, start therapy at 150 mg P.O. b.i.d. (half the usual starting dose) and increase slowly to achieve the desired response.

Pharmacodynamics
Anticonvulsant action: Activity of oxcarbazepine is primarily in response to its active 10-monohydroxy (MHD) metabolite. The antiseizure activity of oxcarbazepine and MHD is thought to result from blockade of voltage-sensitive sodium channels, which stabilizes hyperexcited neural membranes, inhibits repetitive neuronal firing, and diminishes propagation of synaptic impulses. This activity is thought to prevent the spread of seizures in the brain.

Anticonvulsant effects may also be attributed to increased potassium conductance and modulation of high-voltage activated calcium channels.

Pharmacokinetics
Absorption: Oxcarbazepine is completely absorbed after oral administration.
Distribution: About 40% of MHD is bound to serum proteins, mostly to albumin.
Metabolism: Oxcarbazepine is rapidly metabolized in the liver to MHD, which is primarily responsible for the pharmacological effects. Minor amounts (4% of the dose) are oxidized to the pharmacologically inactive 10,11-dihydroxy metabolite.
Excretion: Oxcarbazepine and its metabolites are primarily excreted by the kidneys. More than 95% of a dose appears in the urine, with less than 1% as unchanged oxcarbazepine. Fecal excretion accounts for less than 4% of the administered dose. The half-life of the parent compound is about 2 hours; the half-life of MHD is about 9 hours. Children under age 8 have about 30% to 40% increased clearance of drug.

Adverse reactions
CNS: abnormal coordination, *abnormal gait, **aggravated seizures,** agitation, amnesia, anxiety, asthenia, *ataxia*, confusion, *dizziness,* emotional lability, *fatigue,* feeling abnormal, *headache,* hypoesthesia, impaired concentration, insomnia, nervousness, *somnolence,* speech disorder, *tremor, vertigo.*

CV: chest pain, edema, hypotension.
EENT: abnormal accommodation, *abnormal vision, diplopia,* epistaxis, *nystagmus,* pharyngitis, rhinitis, sinusitis, toothache.
GI: *abdominal pain,* anorexia, constipation, diarrhea, dry mouth, dyspepsia, gastritis, *nausea,* rectal hemorrhage, taste perversion, thirst, *vomiting.*
GU: urinary frequency, urinary tract infection, vaginitis.
Metabolic: decreased thyroxine level, hyponatremia, weight increase.
Musculoskeletal: back pain, muscle weakness.
Respiratory: bronchitis, chest infection, coughing, *upper respiratory tract infection.*
Skin: acne, bruising, hot flushes, increased diaphoresis, purpura, rash.
Other: allergy, fever, lymphadenopathy.

Interactions
Drug-drug
Carbamazepine, valproic acid, verapamil: decreased serum levels of the active metabolite of oxcarbazepine. Monitor patient and serum levels closely.
Felodipine: decreased felodipine level. Monitor patient closely.
Hormonal contraceptives: decreased plasma levels of ethinylestradiol and levonorgestrel, decreasing effectiveness of oral contraceptive. Women of childbearing age should use alternative forms of contraception.
Phenobarbital: decreased serum levels of the active metabolite of oxcarbazepine and increased phe-

nobarbital level. Monitor patient closely.

Phenytoin: decreased serum levels of the active metabolite of oxcarbazepine. May increase phenytoin level in adults who receive high doses of oxcarbazepine. Monitor phenytoin levels closely when initiating therapy in these patients.

Drug-lifestyle
Alcohol use: increased CNS depression. Avoid concomitant use.

Overdose and treatment
If patient experiences an overdose of oxcarbazepine, give symptomatic and supportive treatment as appropriate. There is no specific antidote. Remove the drug by gastric lavage, inactivate it via activated charcoal, or both, as appropriate.

Contraindications and precautions
Contraindicated in patients hypersensitive to oxcarbazepine or its components.

Use cautiously in patients who have had hypersensitivity reactions to carbamazepine.

Special considerations
■ Ask patient about a history of hypersensitivity reaction to carbamazepine, because 25% to 30% of these patients may develop hypersensitivities to oxcarbazepine. Discontinue drug immediately if signs or symptoms of hypersensitivity occur.
■ Monitor patient's serum sodium levels during maintenance therapy, especially if patient receives other therapies that may decrease serum sodium levels.
■ Watch for evidence of hyponatremia, such as nausea, malaise, headache, lethargy, confusion, or decreased sensation.
■ Oxcarbazepine raises the risk of psychomotor slowing, lack of concentration, speech or language problems, somnolence, fatigue, and coordination abnormalities, including ataxia and gait disturbances.
■ Withdraw drug gradually to minimize potential for increased seizure frequency.

Breast-feeding patients
■ Drug and its active metabolite appear in breast milk. Because of the risk of serious adverse reactions in the infant, either discontinue therapy or discontinue breast-feeding.

Geriatric patients
■ Dosage may need to be adjusted in elderly patients to compensate for age-related decreases in creatinine clearance.

Patient teaching
■ Tell patient that drug can be taken with or without food.
■ Advise patient not to interrupt therapy or stop drug without consulting prescriber.
■ Urge patient to notify prescriber about nausea, malaise, headache, lethargy, or confusion—evidence of hyponatremia.
■ Caution patient to avoid hazardous activities until the full CNS effects of the drug are known.
■ If patient takes an oral contraceptive, advise her to use another

---

Reactions may be *common*, uncommon, *life-threatening*, or COMMON AND LIFE-THREATENING.

form of birth control during therapy.

■ Discourage alcohol consumption during therapy.

■ Tell patient to notify prescriber about any previous hypersensitivity reactions to carbamazepine.

■ Encourage patient to wear or carry medical identification that describes the seizure disorder and the drug regimen.

phenytoin
Dilantin-30◊, Dilantin Infatab, Dilantin-125

phenytoin sodium
Dilantin

phenytoin sodium (extended)
Dilantin Kapseals

phenytoin sodium (prompt)

Pharmacologic classification: hydantoin derivative

Therapeutic classification: anticonvulsant

Pregnancy risk category D

How supplied
Available by prescription only
phenytoin
Oral suspension: 30 mg/5 ml◊, 125 mg/5 ml
Tablets (chewable): 50 mg
phenytoin sodium
Injection: 50 mg/ml
phenytoin sodium (extended)
Capsules: 30 mg, 100 mg
phenytoin sodium (prompt)
Capsules: 30 mg, 100 mg

Indications and dosages
Generalized tonic-clonic seizures, status epilepticus, nonepileptic seizures (post-head trauma, Reye's syndrome)
Adults: I.V. loading dose, 10 to 15 mg/kg at no more than 50 mg/minute; oral loading dose, 1 g divided into three doses (400 mg, 300 mg, 300 mg) and given at 2-hour intervals. Maintenance dosage, once controlled, is 300 mg P.O. divided t.i.d. Consider using 300 mg daily in extended capsules; don't use prompt form for once-daily dosing.
Children: loading dose, 15 to 20 mg/kg I.V. at 50 mg/minute or P.O. divided and given q 8 to 12 hours. Then start maintenance dosage of 4 to 8 mg/kg P.O. or I.V. daily, divided q 12 hours.

Neuritic pain (migraine, trigeminal neuralgia, Bell's palsy)
Adults: 200 to 600 mg P.O. daily in divided doses.

Skeletal muscle relaxant
Adults: 200 to 600 mg P.O. daily, p.r.n.

Prophylaxis of seizures during neurosurgery
Adults: 100 to 200 mg I.V. at intervals of about 4 hours during perioperative and postoperative periods.

Pharmacodynamics
Anticonvulsant action: Like other hydantoin derivatives, phenytoin stabilizes neuronal membranes and limits seizure activity by either increasing efflux or decreasing influx

of sodium ions across cell membranes in the motor cortex during generation of nerve impulses.

Antiarrhythmic action: Phenytoin exerts antiarrhythmic effects by normalizing sodium influx to Purkinje's fibers in patients with cardiac glycoside–induced arrhythmias.

Other actions: Phenytoin inhibits excessive collagenase activity in patients with epidermolysis bullosa.

Pharmacokinetics

Absorption: Phenytoin is absorbed slowly from the small intestine; absorption is formulation-dependent and bioavailability may differ among products. Extended-release capsules give peak serum levels at 4 to 12 hours; prompt-release products peak at 1½ to 3 hours. I.M. doses are absorbed erratically; about 50% to 75% of an I.M. dose is absorbed in 24 hours.

Distribution: Drug is distributed widely throughout the body. Therapeutic plasma levels are 10 to 20 mcg/ml, although in some patients, they occur at 5 to 10 mcg/ml. At levels above 20 mcg/ml, lateral nystagmus may occur; above 30 mcg/ml, ataxia usually occurs; at 40 mcg/ml, mental capacity decreases significantly. Phenytoin is about 90% protein-bound, less so in uremic patients. Following oral administration, steady state achieved in 7 to 10 days.

Metabolism: Drug is metabolized by the liver to inactive metabolites.

Excretion: Drug is excreted in urine and exhibits dose-dependent (zero-order) elimination kinetics; above a certain dosage level, small increases in dosage disproportionately increase serum levels.

Contraindications and precautions

Contraindicated in patients with hydantoin hypersensitivity, sinus bradycardia, SA block, second- or third-degree AV block, or Adams-Stokes syndrome.

Use cautiously in elderly or debilitated patients, patients receiving hydantoin derivatives, and patients with hepatic dysfunction, hypotension, myocardial insufficiency, diabetes, uremic patients, or respiratory depression.

Interactions

Drug-drug

Acetaminophen, amiodarone, carbamazepine, corticosteroids, cyclosporine, dicumarol, digitoxin, disopyramide, dopamine, doxycycline, estrogens, furosemide, haloperidol, levodopa, mebenazole, meperidine, methadone, metyrapone, oral contraceptives, phenothiazines, quinidine, sulfonylureas: phenytoin may decrease the effects of these drugs by stimulating hepatic metabolism. Monitor patient closely.

Allopurinol, amiodarone, benzodiazepines, chloramphenicol, chlorpheniramine, cimetidine, diazepam, disulfiram, fluconazole, fluoxetine, ibuprofen, imipramine, isoniazid, metrodiazole, miconazole, omeprazole, phenacemide, phenylbutazone, salicylates, succinimides, trimethoprim, valproic acid: phenytoin's therapeutic effects may be increased. Check serum levels when drug regimen is altered, and monitor patient for toxicity.

Antacids, antineoplastics, antipsychotics, barbiturates, calcium, calcium gluconate, carbamazepine, charcoal, diazoxide, drugs that lower the seizure threshold, folic acid, ketorolac, loxapine, nitrofurantoin, pyridoxine, rifampin, sucralfate, theophylline: phenytoin's therapeutic effects may be decreased. Monitor closely.

Felodipine, nimodipine, verapamil: phenytoin may decrease serum levels of these drugs. Monitor patient closely.

Influenza vaccine: may increase phenytoin levels. Monitor patient closely.

Drug-lifestyle
Alcohol use: therapeutic effects of phenytoin may be decreased. Discourage concomitant use.

Adverse reactions
CNS: *ataxia,* chorea, *decreased coordination,* dizziness, headache, insomnia, *mental confusion,* nervousness, *slurred speech,* twitching.
CV: *bradycardia,* hypotension, periarteritis nodosa.
EENT: blurred vision, *diplopia, gingival hyperplasia, nystagmus.*
GI: constipation, *nausea, vomiting.*
Hematologic: *agranulocytosis, leukopenia,* macrocythemia, *megaloblastic anemia, pancytopenia, thrombocytopenia.*
Hepatic: *toxic hepatitis.*
Metabolic: hyperglycemia.
Musculoskeletal: osteomalacia.
Skin: bullous or purpuric dermatitis, discoloration of skin ("purple glove syndrome") if given by I.V. push in back of hand, *exfoliative dermatitis, hirsutism,* lupus erythematosus, necrosis at injection site, pain and inflammation at injection site, photosensitivity, scarlatiniform or morbilliform rash, *Stevens-Johnson syndrome, toxic epidermal necrolysis.*
Other: gynecomastia, hypertrichosis, lymphadenopathy.

Overdose and treatment
Early overdose may cause ataxia, drowsiness, dysarthria, nausea, nystagmus, slurred speech, tremor, and vomiting. Hypotension, arrhythmias, respiratory depression, and coma may follow. Death may result from respiratory and circulatory depression. Estimated lethal dose in adults is 2 to 5 g.

Treat overdose with gastric lavage or induced emesis, and follow with supportive care. Carefully monitor patient's vital signs and fluid and electrolyte balance. Forced diuresis is of little or no value. Hemodialysis or peritoneal dialysis may be helpful.

Special considerations
■ Phenytoin interacts with many drugs. Therapeutic effects and toxic reactions commonly result from recent changes in drug therapy.
■ Monitoring of serum levels is essential because of dose-dependent excretion. Therapeutic serum level is 10 to 20 mcg/ml.
■ Mix I.V. doses in normal saline solution; mixtures with D_5W will precipitate. Don't refrigerate solution, and don't mix with other drugs. Use it within 30 minutes. An in-line filter is recommended.
■ When giving phenytoin I.V., continuous monitoring of patient's ECG, blood pressure, and respiratory status is essential.

- If giving an I.V. bolus, use slow (50 mg/minute) I.V. push or constant infusion; too-rapid I.V. injection may cause hypotension and circulatory collapse.
- Don't use veins on back of hand for I.V. push; instead, use larger veins to prevent discoloration from purple glove syndrome.
- Avoid I.M. administration; it's painful and drug absorption is erratic.
- Only extended-release capsules are approved for once-daily dosing; give all other forms in divided doses every 8 to 12 hours.
- Shake oral suspension well before use.
- Oral or nasogastric feeding may interfere with absorption of oral suspension; separate doses as much as possible from feedings and by at least 1 hour. During continuous tube feeding, flush tube before and after giving dose.
- Abrupt withdrawal may cause status epilepticus.
- Phenytoin may raise blood glucose levels by inhibiting pancreatic insulin release. It also may decrease serum levels of protein-bound iodine and may interfere with the 1-mg dexamethasone suppression test.
- Besides its labeled uses, phenytoin has been used for ventricular arrhythmias unresponsive to lidocaine or procainamide, for arrhythmias induced by cardiac glycosides, for preeclampsia, and for refractory epilepsy.

Pregnant patients
- Dosage requirements may be higher in pregnancy.

Breast-feeding patients
- Drug is excreted in breast milk; recommend an alternative feeding method during therapy.

Pediatric patients
- A pediatric-strength suspension (30 mg/5 ml) is available in Canada only. Take extreme care to use the correct strength and to avoid confusion with the adult strength (125 mg/5 ml).

Geriatric patients
- Elderly patients metabolize and excrete phenytoin slowly; therefore, they may need lower doses.

Patient teaching
- Instruct patient to take drug with food or milk to minimize GI distress.
- Tell patient to use one brand of phenytoin consistently. Changing brands may change therapeutic effects.
- Tell patient to avoid hazardous activities until drug's full CNS effect is clear.
- Warn patient to avoid alcoholic beverages because they can decrease the drug's effectiveness and increase adverse reactions.
- Stress good oral hygiene to minimize overgrowth and sensitivity of gums.
- Warn patient not to discontinue drug without consulting prescriber.
- Urge patient to wear or carry medical identification that describes the seizure disorder and the drug regimen.

primidone
Myidone, Mysoline, Sertan ◇

Pharmacologic classification:
barbiturate analogue

Therapeutic classification:
anticonvulsant

Pregnancy risk category NR

How supplied
Available by prescription only
Suspension: 250 mg/5 ml
Tablets: 50 mg, 250 mg

Indications and dosages
Generalized tonic-clonic seizures,
focal seizures, complex-partial
(psychomotor) seizures
Adults and children age 8 and over:
100 to 125 mg P.O. h.s. on days 1 to
3, b.i.d. on days 4 to 6, and t.i.d. on
days 7 to 9. Begin maintenance
dosage of 250 mg P.O. t.i.d. on day
10. May require up to 2 g/day.
Children under age 8: 50 mg P.O.
h.s. on days 1 to 3, b.i.d. on days 4
to 6, and 100 mg P.O. t.i.d. on days
7 to 9. Begin maintenance dosage
of 125 to 250 mg P.O. t.i.d. on day
10.

Benign familial tremor
(essential tremor)*
Adults: 750 mg P.O. daily.

Pharmacodynamics
Anticonvulsant action: Primidone
acts as a nonspecific CNS depressant when used alone or with other
anticonvulsants to control refractory tonic-clonic seizures and to
treat psychomotor or focal
seizures. Mechanism of action is
unknown; some activity may be
from phenobarbital, an active
metabolite.

Pharmacokinetics
Absorption: Primidone is absorbed
readily from the GI tract; serum
levels peak at about 3 hours.
Phenobarbital appears in plasma
after several days of continuous
therapy. Most laboratory assays detect both phenobarbital and primidone. Therapeutic levels are 5 to
12 mcg/ml for primidone and 15
to 40 mcg/ml for phenobarbital.
Distribution: Primidone is distributed widely throughout the body.
Metabolism: Primidone is metabolized slowly by the liver to
phenylethylmalonamide (PEMA)
and phenobarbital. PEMA is the
major metabolite.
Excretion: Primidone is excreted in
urine, and substantial amounts are
excreted in breast milk.

Contraindications and precautions
Contraindicated in patients with
phenobarbital hypersensitivity or
porphyria.

Interactions
Drug-drug
Acetazolamide, succinimides: may
decrease primidone levels. Monitor
patient closely.
Carbamazepine, phenytoin: may
decrease effects of primidone and
increase its conversion to phenobarbital. Monitor patient's serum
levels to prevent toxicity.
*CNS depressants, including narcotic
analgesics:* excessive depression
may result. Monitor patient closely.

◇ Available in Canada only   *Unlabeled use

Isoniazid, nicotinamide: may increase serum primidone levels. Monitor patient closely.

Drug-lifestyle
Alcohol use: may cause depression in patients taking primidone. Discourage concurrent use.

Adverse reactions
CNS: *ataxia, drowsiness,* emotional disturbances, fatigue, hyperirritability, paranoia, vertigo.
EENT: *diplopia,* nystagmus.
GI: anorexia, nausea, vomiting.
GU: impotence, polyuria.
Hematologic: *megaloblastic anemia, thrombocytopenia.*
Hepatic: abnormal liver function test results.
Skin: morbilliform rash.

Overdose and treatment
Overdose may resemble barbiturate intoxication; it may cause areflexia, CNS and respiratory depression, coma, hypotension, hypothermia, oliguria, shock, and tachycardia.

Treat an overdose supportively. If the patient is conscious with an intact gag reflex, induce emesis with ipecac. Follow in 30 minutes with repeated doses of activated charcoal. Use gastric lavage if emesis isn't feasible. Alkalinization of urine and forced diuresis may hasten excretion. Hemodialysis may be needed. Monitor patient's vital signs and fluid and electrolyte balance throughout.

Special considerations
■ Obtain a CBC and liver function tests every 6 months.

■ Watch for evidence of anticonvulsant-induced reactions, such as cutaneous lesions, high fever, severe headache, stomatitis, conjunctivitis, rhinitis, or urethritis.
■ To discontinue drug, taper dosage gradually; abrupt withdrawal may cause status epilepticus.

Breast-feeding patients
■ A significant amount of drug is excreted in breast milk; recommend an alternative feeding method during therapy.

Pediatric patients
■ Primidone may cause hyperexcitability in children under age 6.

Geriatric patients
■ Reduce dosage in elderly patients; many have decreased renal function.

Patient teaching
■ Explain the rationale for therapy and the potential risks and benefits.
■ Tell patient to shake oral suspension well before use.
■ Tell patient to avoid alcohol and other sedatives to prevent added CNS depression.
■ Warn patient to avoid hazardous tasks until drug's full effects are clear. Explain that dizziness and incoordination are common at first but will disappear.
■ Teach patient signs and symptoms of adverse reactions.
■ Instruct patient not to discontinue drug or to alter dosage without consulting prescriber.
■ Explain that barbiturates may render oral contraceptives ineffec-

---

Reactions may be *common,* uncommon, *life-threatening,* or **COMMON AND LIFE-THREATENING.**

tive; advise patient to use a different or additional birth control method during therapy.
■ Suggest that the patient wear or carry medical identification that describes the seizure disorder and the drug regimen.

tiagabine hydrochloride
Gabitril

Pharmacologic classification: gamma-aminobutyric acid (GABA) enhancer

Therapeutic classification: anticonvulsant

Pregnancy risk category C

How supplied
Available by prescription only
Tablets: 4 mg, 12 mg, 16 mg, 20 mg

Indications and dosages
Partial seizures (adjunct)
Adults: initially, 4 mg P.O. once daily. May increase daily dose by 4 to 8 mg at weekly intervals until adequate response occurs or you reach maximum of 56 mg/day. Give total daily dose in divided doses b.i.d. to q.i.d.
Adolescents ages 12 to 18: initially, 4 mg P.O. once daily. May increase total daily dose by 4 mg beginning of week 2 and thereafter by 4 to 8 mg/week at weekly intervals until clinical response is seen or up to maximum of 32 mg/day. Give total daily dose in divided doses b.i.d. to q.i.d.
▶ DOSAGE ADJUSTMENT. Patients with impaired liver function may need reduced initial and maintenance doses or longer dosing intervals.

Pharmacodynamics
Anticonvulsant action: Exact mechanism is unknown. Tiagabine probably acts by enhancing the activity of GABA, the major inhibitory neurotransmitter in the CNS. It binds to recognition sites for the GABA uptake carrier and may thus permit more GABA to be available for binding to receptors on postsynaptic cells.

Pharmacokinetics
Absorption: Drug is rapidly and nearly completely absorbed (over 95%). Plasma levels peak 45 minutes after an oral dose in the fasting state. Absolute bioavailability is about 90%.
Distribution: About 96% is bound to human plasma proteins, mainly to serum albumin and alpha-1 acid glycoprotein.
Metabolism: Drug is likely to be metabolized by cytochrome P-450 3A isoenzymes.
Excretion: About 2% is excreted unchanged, with 25% and 63% of dose excreted into the urine and feces, respectively. Approximate half-life is 7 to 9 hours.

Contraindications and precautions
Contraindicated in patients hypersensitive to drug or its ingredients.
Use cautiously in breast-feeding patients.

◊ Available in Canada only   *Unlabeled use

Interactions
Drug-drug
Carbamazepine, phenobarbital, phenytoin: increased tiagabine clearance. Monitor patient closely.
CNS depressants: enhanced effects of these drugs. Monitor patient for oversedation.
Valproate: valproate levels may decrease slightly. Monitor patient for loss of effect.

Drug-lifestyle
Alcohol use: may produce enhanced CNS effects. Discourage concomitant use.

Adverse reactions
CNS: abnormal gait, agitation, *asthenia,* ataxia, confusion, depression, difficulty with concentration and attention, difficulty with memory, *dizziness,* emotional lability, hostility, insomnia, language problems, *nervousness,* paresthesia, *somnolence,* speech disorder, tremor.
CV: vasodilation.
EENT: amblyopia, nystagmus, pharyngitis.
GI: abdominal pain, diarrhea, increased appetite, mouth ulceration, *nausea,* vomiting.
GU: urinary tract infection.
Musculoskeletal: myalgia, myasthenia.
Respiratory: increased cough.
Skin: rash, pruritus.
Other: flulike syndrome.

Overdose and treatment
Overdose may cause agitation, confusion, depression, hostility, impaired consciousness, impaired speech, myoclonus, somnolence, and weakness.

There's no specific antidote for tiagabine. If indicated, elimination of unabsorbed drug should be achieved by induced emesis or gastric lavage. Observe the usual precautions to maintain patient's airway, and provide general supportive care. Dialysis is unlikely to be beneficial.

Special considerations
■ Status epilepticus and sudden unexpected death have occurred in epileptic patients who receive tiagabine.
■ Patients not already receiving at least one other enzyme-inducing antiepilepsy drug when tiagabine therapy starts may need lower doses or a slower dose titration.
■ A therapeutic range for plasma drug levels hasn't been established.
■ Because tiagabine may interact with drugs that induce or inhibit hepatic metabolizing enzymes, obtain plasma tiagabine levels before and after changing the regimen.
■ Never withdraw drug suddenly because seizure frequency may increase. Withdraw tiagabine gradually unless safety concerns require a more rapid withdrawal.

Breast-feeding patients
■ Give drug to breast-feeding women only if benefits clearly outweigh risks.

Pediatric patients
■ Drug has not been adequately investigated in patients under age 12.

Patient teaching
■ Caution patient to take drug only as prescribed.

Reactions may be *common,* uncommon, ***life-threatening,*** or COMMON AND LIFE-THREATENING.

- Tell patient to take drug with food.
- Warn patient to avoid hazardous activities until drug's full CNS effects are clear; it may cause dizziness, somnolence, and other evidence of CNS depression.
- Tell women to notify prescriber about suspected or known pregnancy.
- Encourage patient to wear or carry medical identification that describes the seizure disorder and the drug regimen.

topiramate
Topamax

Pharmacologic classification: sulfamate-substituted monosaccharide

Therapeutic classification: antiepileptic

Pregnancy risk category C

How supplied
Available by prescription only
Sprinkle capsules: 15 mg, 20 mg
Tablets: 25, 100, 200 mg

Indications and dosages
Adjunctive therapy of partial onset seizures
Adults: Adjust up to maximum daily dose of 400 mg in two divided doses. Adjustment schedule is as follows.
Week 1: 50 mg P.O. in the evening.
Week 2: 50 mg P.O. b.i.d.
Week 3: 50 mg P.O. in the morning and 100 mg P.O. in the evening.
Week 4: 100 mg P.O. b.i.d.

Week 5: 100 mg P.O. in the morning and 150 mg P.O. in the evening.
Week 6: 150 mg P.O. b.i.d.
Week 7: 150 mg P.O. in the morning and 200 mg P.O. in the evening
Week 8: 200 mg P.O. b.i.d.
▶ DOSAGE ADJUSTMENT. In patients with moderate to severe renal impairment, reduce dosage by 50%. A supplemental dose may be required during hemodialysis.

Pharmacodynamics
Antiepileptic action: Mechanism of action is unknown. Drug is thought to block action potential, suggestive of a state-dependent sodium channel blocking action. Drug may increase the frequency at which GABA activates GABA receptors and may enhance the ability of GABA to induce a flux of chloride ions into neurons, suggesting that topiramate potentiates the activity of the inhibitory neurotransmitter. Drug may also antagonize the ability of kainate to activate the kainate/AMPA subtype of excitatory amino acid (glutamate) receptor. Topiramate also has weak carbonic anhydrase inhibitor activity, which is unrelated to its antiepileptic properties.

Pharmacokinetics
Absorption: Drug is rapidly absorbed. Plasma levels peak about 2 hours after 400-mg oral dose. Relative bioavailability of drug is about 80% and is not affected by food.
Distribution: Plasma levels increase proportionately with dose. Steady state is reached in 4 days in patients with normal renal func-

tion. Drug is 13% to 17% bound to plasma proteins.

Metabolism: Drug is not extensively metabolized.

Excretion: Drug is primarily eliminated unchanged in urine (about 70% of an administered dose). Mean plasma half-life is 21 hours.

Contraindications and precautions

Contraindicated in patients with a history of hypersensitivity to any component of the preparation.

Use cautiously in patients with hepatic or renal impairment because drug clearance may be decreased.

Interactions
Drug-drug

Carbamazepine: decreases topiramate levels. Monitor patient carefully.

Carbonic anhydrase inhibitors (acetazolamide, dichlorphenamide): may increase the risk of renal calculi. Avoid concomitant use.

Oral contraceptives: contraceptive effectiveness may be decreased. Tell patient to report changes in menstrual patterns and to use another form of contraception.

Phenytoin: increases phenytoin levels while decreasing topiramate levels. Monitor serum levels closely, and monitor patient for signs of toxicity.

Drug-lifestyle

Alcohol use: may cause topiramate-induced CNS depression and other adverse cognitive and neuropsychiatric events. Discourage concomitant use.

Adverse reactions

CNS: abnormal coordination, agitation, apathy, asthenia, *ataxia, confusion,* depression, difficulty with concentration or attention, difficulty with language or memory, *dizziness,* emotional liability, euphoria, *fatigue,* **generalized tonic-clonic seizures,** hallucinations, hyperkinesia, hypertonia, hypoaesthesia, hypokinesia, insomnia, malaise, mood problems, *nervousness, paresthesia,* personality disorder, *psychomotor slowing,* psychosis, *somnolence, speech disorders,* stupor, **suicide attempts,** *tremor,* vertigo.

CV: chest pain, edema, palpitations.

EENT: *abnormal vision,* conjunctivitis, *diplopia,* eye pain, epistaxis, hearing or vestibular problems, *nystagmus,* pharyngitis, sinusitis, taste perversion, tinnitus.

GI: abdominal pain, anorexia, constipation, diarrhea, dry mouth, dyspepsia, flatulence, gastroenteritis, gingivitis, *nausea,* vomiting.

GU: amenorrhea, dysmenorrhea, dysuria, hematuria, impotence, intermenstrual bleeding, leukorrhea, menorrhagia, menstrual disorder, renal calculi, urinary frequency, urinary incontinence, urinary tract infection, vaginitis.

Hematologic: anemia, *leukopenia.*

Metabolic: increased or decreased weight.

Musculoskeletal: arthralgia, back pain, leg pain, muscle weakness, myalgia.

Respiratory: bronchitis, coughing, dyspnea, *upper respiratory infection.*

Skin: acne, alopecia, aggressive reaction, increased sweating, pruritus, rash.
Other: body odor, fever, flulike symptoms, hot flashes, rigors.

Overdose and treatment
In acute overdose after recent ingestion, perform gastric lavage or induce emesis. Activated charcoal is not recommended. Provide supportive treatment. Hemodialysis is an effective method for removing drug and may be needed.

Special considerations
■ Because of their bitter taste, tablets should not be broken.
■ If necessary, withdraw antiepileptic drugs (including topiramate) gradually to minimize risk of increased seizure activity.

Breast-feeding patients
■ It is not known whether drug is excreted in breast milk; use with caution.

Pediatric patients
■ Safety and effectiveness in children have not been established.

Patient teaching
■ Carefully review dosing schedule with patient to avoid undermedication or overmedication.
■ Tell patient that drug may be taken without regard to meals.
■ Caution patient to maintain adequate fluid intake during therapy because of increased risk of renal calculi.
■ Tell patient to avoid hazardous activities until drug's full effects are known.

■ Encourage patient to wear or carry medical identification that describes the seizure disorder and the drug regimen.

valproic acid
Depakene, Epival ◊

divalproex sodium
Depakote, Depakote Sprinkle

valproate sodium
Depacon

Pharmacologic classification:
carboxylic acid derivative

Therapeutic classification:
anticonvulsant

Pregnancy risk category D

How supplied
Available by prescription only
valproic acid
Capsules: 250 mg
Syrup: 250 mg/5 ml
divalproex sodium
Capsules (sprinkle): 125 mg
Tablets (enteric-coated): 125 mg, 250 mg, 500 mg
valproate sodium
Injection: 500 mg/5 ml single-dose vials

Indications and dosages
Simple and complex absence seizures and mixed seizure types Tonic-clonic seizures *
Adults and children: initially, 10 to 15 mg/kg daily (15 mg/kg for simple or complex absence seizures) P.O. b.i.d. or t.i.d. or as a 60-minute I.V. infusion at 20 mg/minute or less. May increase by 5 to 10 mg/kg daily at weekly inter-

vals to a maximum of 60 mg/kg daily, divided b.i.d. or t.i.d. The b.i.d. dosage is recommended for the enteric-coated tablets.
Note: Doses of divalproex sodium (Depakote) are expressed as valproic acid.

Mania
Adults: 750 mg P.O. daily in divided doses (divalproex sodium).

Status epilepticus refractory to I.V. diazepam*
Adults: 400 to 600 mg P.R. q 6 hours.

Pharmacodynamics
Anticonvulsant action: Valproic acid's mechanism of action is unknown; effects may be from increased brain levels of GABA, an inhibitory transmitter. Valproic acid also may decrease GABA's enzymatic catabolism. Onset of therapeutic effects may require a week or more.

Pharmacokinetics
Absorption: Valproate sodium and divalproex sodium quickly convert to valproic acid after administration of oral dose. Plasma levels peak in 1 to 4 hours with uncoated tablets, 3 to 5 hours with enteric-coated tablets, 15 minutes to 2 hours with syrup, and immediately after a 60-minute I.V. infusion. Bioavailability of drug is same for all dose forms.
Distribution: Valproic acid is distributed rapidly throughout the body; drug is 80% to 95% protein-bound.
Metabolism: Valproic acid is metabolized by the liver.

Excretion: Valproic acid is excreted mainly in urine, although some drug is excreted in feces and exhaled air. Breast milk levels are 1% to 10% of serum levels.

Contraindications and precautions
Contraindicated in patients hypersensitive to drug. Don't administer valproate sodium injection to patients with hepatic disease or significant hepatic dysfunction.
   Use cautiously in patients with history of hepatic dysfunction.

Interactions
Drug-drug
Clonazepam: may cause absence seizures. Avoid concomitant use.
CNS depressants, MAO inhibitors, oral anticoagulants: valproic acid may potentiate effects of these drugs. Monitor patient closely.
Ethosuximide, phenobarbital, phenytoin, primidone: may increase serum levels causing excessive somnolence. Careful monitoring may be required.
Felbamate, salicylates: may increase valproate levels. Monitor patient closely.
Lamotrigine: may increase valproate levels or decrease lamotrigine levels. Monitor patient closely and check serum levels of both drugs.

Drug-lifestyle
Alcohol use: may decrease valproic acid effectiveness and increase adverse CNS effects. Discourage concomitant use.
Sunlight: photosensitivity reaction may occur. Urge patient to avoid

unprotected or extensive exposure to sunlight.

Adverse reactions

CNS: abnormal thinking, aggressiveness, amnesia, asthenia, ataxia, behavioral deterioration, depression, dizziness, emotional upset, headache, hyperactivity, incoordination, muscle weakness, psychosis, *sedation,* tremor.
EENT: diplopia, nystagmus, pharyngitis, rhinitis, tinnitus.
GI: abdominal cramps, anorexia, constipation, diarrhea, increased appetite and weight gain, *indigestion, nausea,* **pancreatitis,** *vomiting.*
Hematologic: *bone marrow suppression,* bruising, eosinophilia, **hemorrhage,** increased bleeding time, *leukopenia,* petechiae, **thrombocytopenia.**
Hepatic: *elevated liver enzymes,* **toxic hepatitis.**
Respiratory: bronchitis, dyspnea, infection.
Skin: rash, alopecia, erythema multiforme, photosensitivity, pruritus, **Stevens-Johnson syndrome.**
Other: edema, flulike symptoms.

Overdose and treatment

Overdose may cause heart block, somnolence, and coma.

Give supportive treatment for an overdose. Maintain adequate urinary output, and monitor patient's vital signs and fluid and electrolyte balance carefully. Naloxone reverses CNS and respiratory depression but also may reverse anticonvulsant effects of valproic acid. Hemodialysis and hemoperfusion have been used. Benefits of gastric lavage depends on amount of time since drug was ingested.

Special considerations

■ Drug can be used as an alternative to lithium, especially if patient can't comply with frequent monitoring required for lithium therapy.
■ Monitor plasma level and make dose adjustments as needed. Tremors may indicate need for dose reduction.
■ Therapeutic range is 50 to 100 mcg/ml.
■ Evaluate patient's liver function, platelet count, and PT at baseline and monthly, especially during first 6 months of therapy.
■ For I.V. use, dilute drug in at least 50 ml of compatible diluent.
■ Administer I.V. as 60-minute infusion at no more than 20 mg/minute.
■ Use of valproate sodium injection for periods longer than 14 days hasn't been studied.
■ Switch patient to oral route as soon as clinically feasible. When switching from I.V. to oral therapy or from oral to I.V. therapy, the total daily dose should be equivalent with the same frequency.
■ Administer oral form with food to minimize GI irritation. Enteric-coated formulation may be better tolerated.
■ Because drug usually is used with other anticonvulsants, adverse reactions may not be caused by valproic acid alone.
■ Don't withdraw drug abruptly.
■ Drug may cause false-positive test results for urinary ketones.
■ Valproate is also used for migraine prophylaxis.

Breast-feeding patients
- Valproic acid is excreted in breast milk in serum levels from 1% to 10%. Alternate feeding method is recommended during therapy.

Pediatric patients
- Valproic acid is not recommended for children under age 2 because these patients are at highest risk for hepatotoxicity.
- Hyperexcitability and aggressiveness have occurred in a few children.

Geriatric patients
- Elderly patients eliminate drug more slowly; lower doses are recommended.

Patient teaching
- Tell patient to swallow tablets or capsules whole to avoid local mucosal irritation. If necessary, suggest taking drug with food but not with a carbonated beverage because tablet may dissolve before swallowing, causing irritation and an unpleasant taste.
- Warn patient not to stop drug suddenly, not to alter dose without consulting prescriber, and not to change brands or use a generic drug without consulting prescriber.
- Caution patient to avoid alcohol during therapy because it may decrease drug's effectiveness and increase CNS adverse effects.
- Tell patient to avoid hazardous activities until drug's full effects are clear. Explain that drowsiness and dizziness may occur. Suggest bedtime administration of drug to help minimize CNS depression.
- Review signs and symptoms of hypersensitivity and adverse effects, and tell patient to report them to prescriber.
- Encourage patient to wear a medical identification bracelet or necklace that identifies the seizure disorder and the drug regimen.
- Encourage patient to wear or carry medical identification that describes the seizure disorder and the drug regimen.

CHAPTER 6

Antidepressants

145 ■ **Introduction**

153 ■ **Generic drugs**

■ amitriptyline hydrochloride

■ amoxapine

■ bupropion hydrochloride

■ citalopram hydrobromide

■ clomipramine hydrochloride

■ desipramine hydrochloride

■ doxepin hydrochloride

■ fluoxetine hydrochloride

■ fluvoxamine maleate

■ imipramine hydrochloride, imipramine pamoate

■ maprotiline hydrochloride

■ mirtazapine

■ nefazodone hydrochloride

■ nortriptyline hydrochloride

■ paroxetine hydrochloride

■ phenelzine sulfate

■ protriptyline hydrochloride

■ sertraline hydrochloride

■ tranylcypromine sulfate

■ trazodone hydrochloride

■ trimipramine maleate

■ venlafaxine hydrochloride

Major depression is the most common of all the psychiatric disorders. Nearly 1 person in 5 has a major depressive episode at some point in their lives. The rate of depression is particularly high among older adults.

What's more, the stakes may be rising. Experts estimate that, by 2020, depression may be the second most common cause of disability worldwide. Some evidence suggests that the disability caused by depression may be more severe than that caused by other chronic conditions, such as hypertension, diabetes, arthritis, and back pain.

These days, primary care practitioners are the ones most likely to diagnose and treat depression. Indeed, depression has become more common in primary care practices than any other condition except hypertension. Clearly, the ability to identify and treat depression is crucial in all areas of health care.

UNDERSTANDING DEPRESSION

Depression is a complex phenomenon diagnosed based on a variable set of persistent mental, physical, and behavioral changes. (See *Defining depression*, page 146.) This condition affects much more than mood. Indeed, it disrupts circadian rhythms, psychomotor function, appetite, sleep patterns, and cognitive functioning. It can cause fatigue, morbid thoughts, poor concentration, lack of motivation, and more.

Depression has been linked to negative thinking patterns, genetic predisposition, some prescribed drugs, and certain types of medical illnesses, such as heart disease, cancer, cerebrovascular accident, Parkinson's disease, Alzheimer's disease, diabetes, and some hormonal disorders. Ischemic heart disease has a particularly strong link to depression. Depressed people have a 7- to 10-fold increase in the risk of ischemic heart disease, possibly because of increased platelet aggregation. The reciprocal is also true: Almost half of the people who have a myocardial infarction also develop depression.

Although any or all of these problems can contribute to depression, the most commonly cited cause of depression is altered neurotransmitter levels in the brain, particularly decreased levels of serotonin, serotonin metabolites, dopamine, and corticotropin-releasing factor. This change may be the most discussed of all the underlying causes of depression because, so far, it offers the most opportunities for successful treatment.

TREATING DEPRESSION

In general, depression is readily treatable. Most patients return to their predepression state, although they have an increased risk of relapse or recurrence. Usually, treatment for depression involves evaluating the patient's suicide risk, teaching the patient, and treating the patient's symptoms with antidepressants, psychotherapy, or both. Some patients may receive other therapies, such as electroconvulsive therapy, light therapy, and exercise.

Many antidepressants are available in several drug categories, in-

Defining depression

Before deciding that your patient should be diagnosed with depression, make sure she has at least five of the following symptoms and at least one of the first two. They must be prominent and relatively persistent, occurring for most of every day for at least 2 weeks.

- Depressed mood
- A greatly diminished interest or pleasure in all or almost all activities
- Significant weight loss or gain even though not dieting, or a decrease or increase in appetite
- Insomnia or hypersomnia
- Psychomotor agitation or retardation
- Fatigue or loss of energy
- Feelings of worthlessness, or excessive or inappropriate guilt
- Diminished ability to think or concentrate, or indecisiveness
- Recurrent thoughts of death or suicide, or a suicide attempt not in conjunction with a medical condition, substance abuse, or the death of a loved one.

cluding tricyclic antidepressants, selective serotonin reuptake inhibitors, and monoamine oxidase (MAO) inhibitors. Newer, more receptor-specific drugs include mirtazapine, nefazodone, and venlafaxine. Even an herb may eventually prove to have effects rivaling those of some antidepressant drugs. (See *Investigating St. John's wort.*) Often, choosing among antidepressants has more to do with their adverse effects profiles than with differences in their effectiveness.

The goals of treatment are to reduce the symptoms of depression, to prevent relapse and recurrence, and to restore the patient to normal function. The starting treatment commonly proves inadequate, which means that you may have to try different drugs before obtaining the desired antidepressant effect.

If a particular drug fails to produce an adequate response, the patient may need to switch to a different drug. Usually, you'll accomplish this switch by cross-tapering, in which you give an increasing amount of the replacement drug while giving a decreasing amount of the failed drug. In some cases, you may give a second drug to enhance the patient's response to an antidepressant. Commonly, the second drug is one of the following: buspirone, lithium, thyroid hormone, a tricyclic antidepressant, a dopaminergic drug, estrogen (in perimenopausal women), pindolol, or an anticonvulsant.

Eventually, 60% to 80% of patients with major depression show a 50% or greater reduction in depression. Keep in mind, however, that 10% to 25% of patients relapse during the first year despite continued treatment. More than half relapse within 16 weeks of stopping therapy. And 50% to 85% have a recurrence of their depression at some point in the future.

Investigating St. John's wort

European studies involving more than 1,700 people suggest that extracts of the herb St. John's wort (*Hypericum perforatum*) may help to ease the symptoms of mild to moderate depression. What's more, it may do so without causing as many adverse effects as standard antidepressant drugs.

However, because the European studies used varying doses, differing extracts, and independent study protocols, officials at the National Institutes of Health have launched a study of their own. This controlled U.S. trial will involve more than 300 people over 3 years, with the goal of determining whether standardized amounts of St. John's wort do indeed have an antidepressant effect—and how potent it is. The study also will look at how safe the herb is and what types of adverse effects it causes.

We already know that St. John's wort has adverse effects. For instance, we know it can adversely affect the function of indinavir, an antiviral drug prescribed for some HIV-infected patients. It also may cause adverse effects when combined with cyclosporine. What's more, it may activate the cytochrome P-450 pathway, which can adversely affect other drugs metabolized by this route. Finally, St. John's wort may cause a dry mouth, dizziness, gastrointestinal upset, photosensitivity, fatigue, and confusion.

Especially because St. John's wort isn't regulated as a drug by the U.S. Food and Drug Administration, its increasing popularity among American consumers creates an increased responsibility for health care professionals to explain what we know—and still don't know—about the effects of this wild-growing plant.

Drug effects

Antidepressant drugs exert their effects through several different mechanisms of action, all of which affect levels of dopamine, serotonin, norepinephrine, or some combination of these and possibly other neurotransmitters in the brain. Even within drug classes, individual drugs exert varying effects on closely related substances. For instance, the selective serotonin reuptake inhibitors influence several different types of serotonin receptors by varying amounts, which helps to explain the variation in adverse effects produced by these drugs. MAO inhibitors slow the breakdown of amines by MAO.

Most antidepressants inhibit the reuptake of norepinephrine and serotonin at the presynaptic neuron. They also inhibit histamine and acetylcholine receptors to varying degrees, causing some sedative and anticholinergic effects as a result. Newer antidepressants tend to have less affinity for muscarinic, gamma-aminobutyric acid, benzodiazepine, and histamine receptors, which yields a lesser amount of the corresponding adverse effects.

Pharmacokinetics

As a rule, antidepressants are well absorbed from the gastrointestinal tract and reach peak levels in about 2 to 12 hours. These drugs are widely distributed into the tissues and the central nervous system (CNS). Most undergo significant first-pass hepatic metabolism by demethylation, hydroxylation, and glucuronidation. They're typically metabolized into inactive and active metabolites. Most are eliminated mainly via the kidneys, with a lesser percentage eliminated via the feces. Dosages may need to be adjusted for patients with hepatic or renal impairment.

Some antidepressants move through the body in a different pattern. Maprotiline is excreted in bile, for example. Tricyclic antidepressants are secreted into the hepatobiliary circulation and the stomach, and then reabsorbed and excreted into the urine. They're about 85% to 88% bound to plasma proteins, and metabolism takes place in the liver to both active and inactive metabolites. Some selective serotonin reuptake inhibitors have even higher protein binding, which can produce adverse effects if they displace drugs that are bound more loosely to their carrier proteins.

Adverse effects

In general, antidepressants—especially the older ones—are known for causing a wide range of adverse effects. (See *Comparing antidepressants*, pages 150 and 151.) Some of the effects patients find most objectionable include disrupted sleep, weight gain, and sexual dysfunction.

Disrupted sleep

People with depression commonly have disturbed sleep, probably from decreased serotonin neurotransmission. The problem is, however, that antidepressants can also disrupt sleep. Nefazodone may be the only antidepressant that actually improves sleep, possibly because it antagonizes the serotonin receptor 5-HT$_2$. If a patient still has trouble sleeping after about 12 weeks of antidepressant therapy, you may need to decrease the dosage or try a benzodiazepine, an antihistamine, another hypnotic, mirtazapine, or trazodone.

Weight gain

Except for bupropion, which tends to cause weight loss, most antidepressants tend to increase the patient's weight. To help minimize weight gain, suggest increased exercise and a reduced calorie diet. Ensure adequate hydration. Consider an appetite suppressant or a fat blocker. If all else fails, you may want to consider a different antidepressant. Why? Because unless the weight gain is helping to compensate for depression-related weight loss, it can upset the patient and lead to noncompliance with therapy.

Keep in mind that most selective serotonin reuptake inhibitors cause little weight gain early in therapy. Paroxetine may cause more weight gain than fluoxetine or sertraline.

With mirtazapine, a lack of early weight gain suggests that this adverse effect won't cause problems later either. Usually, patients who gain weight while taking mirtazapine do so early in therapy. Women are more likely than men to gain weight, with older women more likely than younger women.

Sexual dysfunction

Sexual dysfunction is a common adverse effect of tricyclic antidepressants (especially clomipramine), MAO inhibitors, selective serotonin reuptake inhibitors, and venlafaxine. These drugs may affect all phases of the sexual cycle, including desire, arousal, orgasm, and resolution. For instance, the patient may experience reduced sexual excitement, reduced genital sensation, delayed orgasm, impotence, premature ejaculation, or inadequate vaginal lubrication.

Antidepressants affect sexual function because neurotransmitters affect sexual function. Specifically, dopamine enhances desire and arousal. Serotonin inhibits them. And norepinephrine seems to have no effect. Keep in mind, however, that many problems can interfere with sexual functioning, including depression itself. Others include substance abuse, concurrent medical problems, and stressful or difficult life situations. Naturally, you'll need to rule out such problems before concluding that a patient's sexual dysfunction results from an antidepressant.

If the patient's depression responds to a drug that causes adverse sexual effects, and those effects continue even after the patient's body adjusts to the drug, consider decreasing the dosage, using an antidote (such as an anxiolytic, another antidepressant, a stimulant, or a cholinergic enhancer), or switching to another antidepressant. Antidepressants with a relatively low risk of adverse sexual effects include bupropion, mirtazapine, and nefazodone. Women may benefit from estrogen creams and vaginal lubricants.

Overdose and treatment

Early signs of CNS toxicity include confusion, agitation, hallucinations, drowsiness, and stupor. Respiratory depression, cyanosis, shock, diaphoresis, and aspiration may occur in severe overdoses. Rhabdomyolysis and renal failure may result from prolonged seizures or coma.

Any patient who overdoses on an antidepressant needs hospitalization and close observation with electrocardiogram monitoring. Watch for CNS, cardiac, and respiratory effects for at least 6 hours, regardless of the amount of drug ingested. Maintain adequate respiratory exchange, but avoid respiratory stimulants. Prevent water intoxication by using normal or half-normal saline solution.

If the patient ingested the drug within the previous hour and she's intubated, consider giving an activated charcoal slurry after gastric lavage to help decrease drug absorption. Avoid inducing emesis unless the patient took bupropion, venlafaxine, or a selective serotonin reuptake inhibitor. For these drugs, you may use ipecac syrup. Because most antidepressants undergo rapid fixation in the tissues, hemodialysis, peritoneal dialysis, exchange transfusions, and diuresis rarely help to remove the drug.

Cardiovascular toxicity is the leading cause of death in tricyclic antidepressant overdose because these drugs have anticholinergic activity and a quinidine-like effect that decreases myocardial contraction, heart rate, and coronary blood flow. The resulting arrhythmias may include tachycardia, intraventricular block, and complete atrioventricular block.

Cardiac effects may be aggressively treated with hypertonic sodium bicarbonate. Give a 50-mEq bolus I.V., repeated to keep the pa-

Comparing antidepressants

Drug	Therapeutic level (ng/ml)	Half-life (hr)	Time to steady state (days)
Tricyclic antidepressants (tertiary amines)			
amitriptyline hydrochloride	110-250	31-46	4-10
clomipramine hydrochloride	80-100	19-37	7-14
doxepin hydrochloride	100-200	8-24	2-8
imipramine	200-350	11-25	2-5
trimipramine hydrochloride	180	7-30	2-6
Tricyclic antidepressants (secondary amines)			
amoxapine	200-500	8	2-7
desipramine hydrochloride	125-300	12-24	2-11
nortriptyline hydrochloride	50-150	18-44	4-19
protriptyline hydrochloride	100-200	67-89	14-19
Tetracyclic antidepressants			
maprotiline hydrochloride	200-300	21-25	6-10
mirtazapine	Not applicable	20-40	5
Triazolopryidine antidepressants			
trazadone hydrochloride	800-1,600	4-9	3-7
Aminoketine antidepressants			
bupropion hydrochloride	Not applicable	8-24	1.5-8
Phenethylamine antidepressants			
venlafaxine hydrochloride	Not applicable	5-11	3-4
Phenylpiperazine antidepressants			
nefazodone hydrochloride	Not applicable	2-4	4-5
Selective serotonin reuptake inhibitors			
citalopram hydrobromide	Not applicable	33	7
fluoxetine hydrochloride	Not applicable	24-384	14-28
fluvoxamine maleate	Not applicable	15.6	7
paroxetine hydrochloride	Not applicable	10-24	7-14
sertraline hydrochloride	Not applicable	1-4	7
MAO inhibitors			
phenelzine sulfate	Not applicable	Not applicable	Not applicable
tranylcypromine sulfate	Not applicable	2.4-2.8	Not applicable

0 = none   + = slight   ++ = moderate   +++ = high   ++++ = very high   +++++ = highest

Norepinephrine blocking activity	Serotonin blocking activity	Anticholinergic effects	Sedation	Orthostatic hypotension
++	++++	++++	++++	++
++	+++++	+++	+++	++
+	++	++	+++	++
++	++++	++	++	+++
+	+	++	+++	++
+++	++	+++	++	+
++++	++	+	+	+
++	+++	++	++	+
++++	++	+++	+	+
+++	0/+	++	++	+
+++	+++	++	+++	++
0	+++	+	++++	++
0/+	0/+	++	++	+
+++	+++	0	0	0
0/+	+++++	0/+	++	+
0/+	++++	0/+	0/+	0/+
0/+	+++++	0/+	0/+	0/+
0/+	+++++	0/+	0/+	0
0/+	+++++	0	0/+	0
0/+	+++++	0	0/+	0
Not applicable	Not applicable	+	+	+
Not applicable	Not applicable	+	+	0

tient's blood pH at 7.45 to 7.55. If hypotension is unresponsive to sodium bicarbonate, you may need to use fluid expansion and vasopressors (norepinephrine 0.1 to 0.2 mcg/kg/minute) or dopamine (10 to 20 mcg/kg/minute).

Cardiac arrthymias may respond to lidocaine, bretylium, or phenytoin. Isoproterenol may control bradycardia and torsades de pointes. For a life-threatening ventricular arrhythmia, give propranolol. For a child, give 0.01 to 0.1 mg/kg over 10 minutes to a maximum of 1 mg. For an adult, give 1 mg I.V. over 1 minute every 2 to 5 minutes to a maximum of 5 mg.

PATIENT TEACHING

For any patient who takes an antidepressant, make sure to offer the following teaching points.

■ Urge the patient to mention all co-exisiting medical conditions and all prescribed drugs, over-the-counter medications, and herbal remedies she takes.

■ Encourage the patient to take the antidepressant exactly as prescribed. Mention that the full effects of the therapy may take 4 to 6 weeks to develop.

■ Tell the patient not to crush or chew a sustained-release drug form. This form should be swallowed whole.

■ Caution the patient to avoid alcohol, barbiturates, and other CNS depressants. Besides increasing CNS depression, alcohol may interfere with selective serotonin reuptake inhibitors.

■ Caution the patient to avoid hazardous activities until the full effects of the drug are known.

Antidepressants may cause drowsiness, dizziness, or blurred vision.

■ Tell the patient to avoid prolonged exposure to sunlight or sunlamps because photosensitivity may occur.

■ If the patient takes a selective serotonin reuptake inhibitor, tell her to notify the prescriber if she develops a jittery feeling, insomnia, anxiety, nausea, or headache. She may need a dosage adjustment.

■ If the patient takes an MAO inhibitor, tell her to avoid foods that contain tyramine.

■ Warn the patient not to take the smoking cessation aid Zyban while taking bupropion because the two drugs contain the same active ingredient.

■ Caution the patient not to stop an antidepressant abruptly. Doing so may cause nausea, headache, dizziness, rebound irritability, a jarring "electric" sensation, and malaise.

■ Urge the patient to promptly notify the prescriber about planned, suspected, or known pregnancy. Also, urge the patient to notify the prescriber about planned breast-feeding.

■ Warn the patient about an increased risk of seizures, especially if she takes bupropion.

■ Warn the patient about an increased risk of tardive dyskinesia.

■ Tell the patient to stop the drug and immediately notify the prescriber if she develops seizures, difficult or rapid breathing, fever with sweating, a loss of bladder control, severe muscle stiffness, or unusual weakness or tiredness.

amitriptyline hydrochloride
Apo-Amitriptyline, Elavil, Endep, Levate◇, Novotriptyn◇

Pharmacologic classification: tricyclic antidepressant

Therapeutic classification: antidepressant

Pregnancy risk category D

How supplied
Available by prescription only
Injection: 10 mg/ml
Tablets: 10 mg, 25 mg, 50 mg, 75 mg, 100 mg, 150 mg

Indications and dosages
Depression
Anorexia or bulimia with depression*, neurogenic pain (adjunctive)*
Adults: Initial outpatient, 75 to 150 mg/day P.O. in divided doses or 50 to 150 mg h.s. For inpatient, 100 to 300 mg/day. I.M. dosage is 20 to 30 mg q.i.d. and should be changed to P.O. as soon as possible. Maintenance dosage is 50 to 100 mg/day.
▶ DOSAGE ADJUSTMENT. For elderly or adolescent patients, give 10 mg P.O. t.i.d. and 20 mg h.s.

Pharmacodynamics
Antidepressant action: Amitriptyline probably exerts an antidepressant effect by inhibiting reuptake of norepinephrine and serotonin in CNS nerve terminals (presynaptic neurons), resulting in increased levels and activity of these neurotransmitters in the synaptic cleft. Amitriptyline inhibits reuptake of serotonin more actively than it does norepinephrine. The drug commonly causes undesirable levels of sedation, but tolerance to this effect usually develops within a few weeks.

Pharmacokinetics
Absorption: Amitriptyline is absorbed rapidly from the GI tract after oral administration and from muscle tissue after I.M. administration.
Distribution: Drug is distributed widely into the body, including the CNS and breast milk. It's 96% protein-bound. Effects peak 2 to 12 hours after a dose is given, and steady state occurs in 4 to 10 days. Full therapeutic effect usually occurs in 2 to 4 weeks.
Metabolism: Drug is metabolized by the liver to the active metabolite nortriptyline. A significant first-pass effect may account for the variability of serum levels in different patients taking the same dosage.
Excretion: Drug is excreted mostly in urine.

Contraindications and precautions
Contraindicated during acute recovery phase after MI, in patients hypersensitive to drug, and within 14 days of taking an MAO inhibitor.

Use cautiously in patients with a recent history of MI and in those with unstable heart disease or renal or hepatic impairment.

Interactions
Drug-drug
Antiarrhythmics (quinidine, disopyramide, procainamide), pimozide, thyroid hormones: may increase risk of arrhythmias and conduction defects. Avoid concomitant use.

Atropine, other anticholinergic drugs: may cause oversedation, paralytic ileus, visual changes, and severe constipation. Monitor patient.

Barbiturates: increased amitriptyline metabolism, decreasing therapeutic efficacy. Monitor patient for loss of effect.

Beta blockers, cimetidine, oral contraceptives, methylphenidate, propoxyphene, selective serotonin reuptake inhibitors: may inhibit amitriptyline metabolism, increasing plasma levels and toxicity. Monitor patient and serum levels closely.

Central-acting antihypertensives (clonidine, guanabenz, guanadrel, guanethidine, methyldopa, reserpine): amitriptyline may decrease antihypertensive effects. Monitor patient's blood pressure.

CNS depressants (analgesics, anesthetics, barbiturates, narcotics, tranquilizers): additive effects and oversedation are likely to occur. Monitor patient closely.

Disulfiram, ethchlorvynol: may cause delirium and tachycardia. Avoid concomitant use.

Haloperidol, phenothiazines: decreased amitriptyline metabolism, increasing the risk of toxicity. Monitor patient and serum levels closely.

Metrizamide: increased risk of seizures. Use together with extreme caution.

Sympathomimetics (ephedrine, epinephrine, phenylephrine, phenylpropanolamine,) commonly found in nasal sprays: may increase blood pressure. Monitor patient closely.

Warfarin: may increase PT and INR and increase risk of bleeding. Monitor patient for loss of therapeutic warfarin levels.

Drug-lifestyle
Alcohol use: additive effects are likely. Discourage concomitant use.

Heavy smoking: increased amitriptyline metabolism and decreased efficacy. Discourage concomitant use, and urge smoking cessation.

Sun exposure: photosensitivity reactions may result. Recommend precautions.

Adverse reactions
CNS: anxiety, ataxia, ***coma,*** delusions, disorientation, dizziness, drowsiness, extrapyramidal symptoms, fatigue, hallucinations, headache, insomnia, peripheral neuropathy, restlessness, ***seizures,*** tremor, weakness.

CV: ***arrhythmias, CVA,*** *ECG changes,* edema, heart block, hypertension, ***MI,*** *orthostatic hypotension, tachycardia.*

EENT: *blurred vision,* increased intraocular pressure, mydriasis, tinnitus.

GI: anorexia, constipation, diarrhea, *dry mouth,* epigastric distress, nausea, paralytic ileus, vomiting.

GU: urine retention.

Hematologic: ***agranulocytosis,*** eosinophilia, ***leukopenia, thrombocytopenia.***

Hepatic: elevated liver function test results.

Reactions may be *common,* uncommon, ***life-threatening,*** or COMMON AND LIFE-THREATENING.

Metabolic: decreased or increased serum glucose levels.
Skin: diaphoresis, photosensitivity, rash, urticaria.
Other: *hypersensitivity reaction.*

Overdose and treatment

The first 12 hours after acute ingestion are a stimulatory phase characterized by excessive anticholinergic activity, which may include agitation, irritation, confusion, hallucinations, hyperthermia, parkinsonian symptoms, seizures, urine retention, dry mucous membranes, pupil dilation, constipation, and ileus. This phase is followed by CNS depression—including hypothermia, decreased or absent reflexes, sedation, hypotension, and cyanosis—and such cardiac irregularities as tachycardia, conduction disturbances, and quinidine-like effects on the ECG.

Widening of the QRS complex usually indicates a serum level above 1,000 mg/ml. Metabolic acidosis may follow hypotension, hypoventilation, and seizures. Delayed cardiac anomalies and death may occur.

Treatment is symptomatic and supportive, and includes managing the patient's airway, body temperature, and fluid and electrolyte balance. Induce emesis with ipecac if the gag reflex is intact; follow with gastric lavage and activated charcoal to prevent further absorption. Dialysis is of little use.

Physostigmine may be used cautiously to reverse the symptoms of tricyclic antidepressant poisoning in life-threatening situations. Give parenteral diazepam or phenytoin for seizures. Give parenteral phenytoin or lidocaine for arrhythmias. Give sodium bicarbonate for acidosis. Don't give barbiturates; they may increase CNS and respiratory depressant effects.

Special considerations

■ Depressed patients, particularly those with manic depressive illness, may shift toward mania or hypomania.
■ Avoid giving drug to patient who has a history of attempted suicide by overdose.
■ I.M. administration may produce a more rapid onset of action than oral administration.
■ Switch from parenteral to oral administration as soon as possible.
■ Therapeutic plasma levels range from 110 to 250 ng/ml.
■ Expect amitriptyline to cause sedation; tolerance to sedative effects may develop over several weeks.
■ Give the full dose at bedtime, as needed, to help offset daytime sedation.
■ Don't withdraw drug abruptly, especially after long-term therapy, because nausea, headache, and malaise may result.
■ Discontinue drug at least 48 hours before surgical procedures.
■ Besides standard indications, drug has been used to prevent migraine, cluster headaches, intractable hiccups, and postherpetic neuralgia.

Breast-feeding patients

■ Drug is excreted in breast milk at levels equal to or greater than those in maternal serum. About 1% of the ingested dose appears in the breast-fed infant's serum. Weigh the possible benefit of therapy for the mother against possible adverse effects of therapy on the infant.

Pediatric patients
■ Drug isn't recommended for children under age 12.

Geriatric patients
■ Expect elderly patients to have an increased risk of adverse cardiac effects.

Patient teaching
■ Tell patient to take drug exactly as prescribed and not to double up after missing a dose.
■ Inform patient that the full dose may be taken at bedtime to reduce daytime sedation. To avoid morning hangover, it may be taken in the early evening.
■ Advise patient to lie down for about 30 minutes after taking initial doses, and caution her to rise to slowly to an upright position to prevent dizziness or fainting.
■ Suggest taking drug with food or milk if it causes stomach upset.
■ Tell patient to avoid hazardous activities until drug's full effects are clear.
■ Explain that drug's full effects may not become apparent for up to 4 weeks after therapy starts.
■ Suggest using ice or sugarless chewing gum or hard candy to alleviate a dry mouth. Stress the importance of regular dental hygiene because a dry mouth can raise the risk of dental caries.
■ Warn patient not to drink alcoholic beverages during therapy.
■ Advise women to use a reliable form of contraception during therapy and to immediately notify prescriber about planned, suspected, or known pregnancy.
■ Warn patient not to abruptly stop taking drug.
■ Encourage patient to report troublesome or unusual effects, especially confusion, movement disorders, rapid heartbeat, dizziness, fainting, or difficulty urinating.

amoxapine
Asendin

Pharmacologic classification: **dibenzoxazepine, tricyclic antidepressant**

Therapeutic classification: **antidepressant**

Pregnancy risk category C

How supplied
Available by prescription only
Tablets: 25 mg, 50 mg, 100 mg, 150 mg

Indications and dosages
Depression
Adults: initially, 50 mg P.O. b.i.d. or t.i.d; may increase to 100 mg b.i.d. or t.i.d. by end of first week. Increase above 300 mg daily only if this dosage has been ineffective for at least 2 weeks. When effective dosage is established, entire daily dose (not exceeding 300 mg) may be given h.s. Maximum dosage in hospitalized patients is 600 mg in divided doses.
▶ **DOSAGE ADJUSTMENT.** In elderly patients, recommended starting dose is 25 mg P.O. b.i.d. to t.i.d. May increase to 50 mg P.O. b.i.d. to t.i.d. Maximum, 300 mg/day.

Pharmacodynamics

Antidepressant action: Drug is thought to exert antidepressant effects by inhibiting reuptake of norepinephrine and serotonin in CNS nerve terminals (presynaptic neurons), which results in increased levels and enhanced activity of these neurotransmitters in the synaptic cleft. Amoxapine has a greater inhibitory effect on norepinephrine reuptake than on serotonin reuptake. Drug also blocks CNS dopamine receptors, which may account for the higher likelihood of movement disorders during therapy.

Pharmacokinetics

Absorption: Amoxapine is absorbed rapidly and completely from the GI tract after oral administration.

Distribution: Drug is distributed widely into the body, including the CNS and breast milk. It is 92% protein-bound. Effects peak in 8 to 10 hours; steady state occurs in 2 to 7 days. Proposed therapeutic plasma levels (parent drug and metabolite) range from 200 to 500 ng/ml.

Metabolism: Drug is metabolized by the liver to the active metabolite 8-hydroxyamoxapine. A significant first-pass effect may explain the variability of serum levels in different patients taking the same dosage.

Excretion: Amoxapine is excreted in urine and feces (7% to 18%); about 60% of a given dose is excreted as the conjugated form within 6 days.

Contraindications and precautions

Contraindicated during acute recovery phase after MI, in patients hypersensitive to drug, and within 14 days of taking an MAO inhibitor.

Use with extreme caution if patient has a history of seizures. Also, use cautiously in patients with a history of urine retention, CV disease, angle-closure glaucoma, or increased intraocular pressure.

Interactions
Drug-drug

Antiarrhythmics (disopyramide, quinidine, procainamide), pimozide, thyroid hormones: may increase the risk of arrhythmias and conduction defects. Avoid concomitant use.

Atropine, other anticholinergic drugs: may cause oversedation, paralytic ileus, visual changes, and severe constipation. Use with extreme caution.

Barbiturates: induced amoxapine metabolism and decreased efficacy. Monitor patient closely.

Beta blockers, cimetidine, methylphenidate, oral contraceptives, propoxyphene: may inhibit amoxapine metabolism, increasing plasma levels and toxicity. Monitor patient and serum levels closely.

Central-acting antihypertensives, such as clonidine, guanabenz, guanadrel, guanethidine, methyldopa, reserpine: amoxapine may decrease antihypertensive effects. Monitor patient for loss of drug effect.

CNS depressants, such as analgesics, anesthetics, barbiturates, narcotics, tranquilizers: may cause oversedation. Monitor patient closely.

Disulfiram, ethchlorvynol: may cause delirium and tachycardia. Avoid concomitant use.
Haloperidol, phenothiazines: decreased amoxapine metabolism, increasing the risk of toxicity. Monitor patient's serum levels closely.
Metrizamide: additive effects are likely, along with increased risk of seizures. Monitor patient closely.
Sympathomimetics (including ephedrine, epinephrine, phenylephrine, phenylpropanolamine,) commonly found in nasal sprays: may increase blood pressure. Monitor patient's blood pressure.
Warfarin: may increase PT, INR, and risk of bleeding. Monitor patient for increased anticoagulant effect.

Drug-lifestyle
Alcohol use: additive effects are likely. Discourage concomitant use.
Heavy smoking: increased amoxapine metabolism and decreased efficacy. Discourage concomitant use, and urge smoking cessation.
Sun exposure: photosensitivity reactions may result. Recommend precautions.

Adverse reactions
CNS: anxiety, ataxia, *dizziness, drowsiness,* confusion, *EEG changes,* excitation, extrapyramidal symptoms, fatigue, headache, insomnia, nervousness, **neuroleptic malignant syndrome,** nightmares, restlessness, **seizures,** *tardive dyskinesia,* tremor, weakness.
CV: hypertension, *orthostatic hypotension,* palpitations, *tachycardia.*
EENT: *blurred vision.*

GI: *constipation, dry mouth,* excessive appetite, nausea.
GU: **acute renal failure** (with overdose), *urine retention.*
Skin: *diaphoresis,* edema, rash.

Overdose and treatment
The first 12 hours after acute ingestion are a stimulatory phase characterized by excessive anticholinergic activity, which may include agitation, irritation, confusion, hallucinations, hyperthermia, parkinsonian symptoms, seizures, urine retention, dry mucous membranes, pupil dilation, constipation, and ileus. This phase is followed by CNS depression— including hypothermia, decreased or absent reflexes, sedation, hypotension, and cyanosis—and such cardiac irregularities as tachycardia, conduction disturbances, and quinidine-like effects on the ECG.

Amoxapine overdose produces a much higher likelihood of CNS toxicity than other antidepressants. Acute deterioration of renal function (evidenced by myoglobin in urine) occurs in 5% of overdosed patients, especially those who have repeated seizures after the overdose. Seizures may progress to status epilepticus within 12 hours.

Widening of the QRS complex usually indicates a serum level above 1,000 mg/ml. (Serum levels aren't helpful.) Metabolic acidosis may follow hypotension, hypoventilation, and seizures.

Treatment is symptomatic and supportive, and includes managing the patient's airway, body temperature, and fluid and electrolyte balance. Closely monitor the patient's renal function because of the risk

---

Reactions may be *common,* uncommon, *life-threatening,* or COMMON AND LIFE-THREATENING.

of renal failure. Induce emesis with ipecac if the gag reflex is intact and the patient is conscious; follow with gastric lavage and activated charcoal to prevent further absorption. Dialysis is of little use.

Treat seizures with parenteral diazepam or phenytoin (the value of physostigmine is less certain). Give parenteral phenytoin or lidocaine for arrhythmias. Give sodium bicarbonate for acidosis. Don't give barbiturates; they may enhance CNS and respiratory depression.

Special considerations
- Drug produces a high risk of seizures.
- To help reduce daytime sedation, give the full dose at bedtime.
- Don't give more than 300 mg in a single dose.
- Expect tolerance to sedative effects to develop over the first few weeks of therapy.
- Tardive dyskinesia and other extrapyramidal effects may occur because of drug's dopamine-blocking activity.
- If patient has bipolar disorder, expect that drug may cause manic episodes during the depressed phase.
- Watch for evidence of neuroleptic malignant syndrome, such as a high fever, tachycardia, tachypnea, and profuse diaphoresis.
- Gynecomastia may occur in both male and female patients because amoxapine may increase cellular division in breast tissue.
- Amoxapine may prolong conduction time (elongation of QT and PR intervals, flattened T waves on ECG); it also may elevate liver function test results, decrease WBC counts, and decrease or increase serum glucose levels.
- Taper drug to discontinue it rather than stopping it abruptly. Abrupt withdrawal of long-term therapy can cause nausea, headache, and malaise (not a result of addiction).
- Discontinue drug at least 48 hours before surgical procedures.

Breast-feeding patients
- Amoxapine is excreted in breast milk as parent drug at about 20% the level of maternal serum and as metabolites at about 30% the level of maternal serum. The potential benefits to the mother should outweigh the possible adverse reactions in the infant.

Pediatric patients
- Drug isn't recommended for patients under age 16.

Geriatric patients
- Elderly patients are much more susceptible to tardive dyskinesia and extrapyramidal symptoms.

Patient teaching
- Tell patient to take drug exactly as prescribed and not to double up after missing a dose.
- Inform patient that the full dose may be taken at bedtime to reduce daytime sedation.
- Advise patient to lie down for about 30 minutes after taking initial doses, and caution her to rise to slowly to an upright position to prevent dizziness or fainting.
- Suggest taking drug with food or milk if it causes stomach upset.
- Tell patient to avoid hazardous activities until full effects are clear.

■ Explain that full effects may not occur for 2 weeks, possibly 4 to 6 weeks, after therapy starts.

■ Suggest using ice or sugarless chewing gum or hard candy to alleviate a dry mouth. Stress the importance of regular dental hygiene because a dry mouth can raise the risk of dental caries.

■ Warn patient not to drink alcoholic beverages during therapy.

■ Warn patient not to abruptly stop taking drug.

■ Caution patient that exposure to sunlight, sunlamps, or tanning beds may burn the skin or cause abnormal pigment changes.

■ Encourage patient to report troublesome or unusual effects, especially confusion, movement disorders, rapid heartbeat, dizziness, fainting, or difficulty urinating.

---

bupropion hydrochloride
Wellbutrin, Wellbutrin SR

Pharmacologic classification: aminoketone

Therapeutic classification: antidepressant

Pregnancy risk category B

How supplied
Available by prescription only
Tablets: 75 mg, 100 mg
Tablets (sustained-release): 100 mg, 150 mg

Indications and dosages
Depression
Adults: initially, 100 mg P.O. b.i.d. If necessary, increase after 3 days to usual dosage of 100 mg P.O. t.i.d. If no response occurs after several weeks of therapy, consider increasing to 150 mg t.i.d. For sustained-release tablets, start with 150 mg P.O. q morning; increase to target of 150 mg P.O. b.i.d. as tolerated as early as day 4 of dosing. Maximum, 450 mg/day.

Pharmacodynamics
Antidepressant action: Mechanism of action is unknown. Bupropion weakly inhibits norepinephrine, dopamine, and serotonin reuptake. It doesn't inhibit MAO.

Pharmacokinetics
Absorption: Animal studies indicate that only 5% to 20% of the drug is bioavailable. Plasma levels peak in 2 to 3 hours.
Distribution: At plasma levels up to 200 mcg/ml, drug appears to be about 80% bound to plasma proteins.
Metabolism: Metabolism is probably hepatic; several active metabolites have been identified. With prolonged use, active metabolites accumulate in the plasma and their level may exceed that of the parent compound. Bupropion appears to induce its own metabolism.
Excretion: Excretion is primarily renal; elimination half-life of parent compound in single-dose studies ranges from 8 to 24 hours.

Contraindications and precautions
Contraindicated in patients with hypersensitivity to drug, seizure disorders, or bulimia or anorexia nervosa because of the increased risk of seizures. Also contraindicated within 14 days of taking an

---

MAO inhibitor and in patients who take Zyban (bupropion packaged as a smoking cessation aid).

Use cautiously in patients with recent MI, unstable heart disease, or renal or hepatic impairment.

Interactions
Drug-drug
Benzodiazepines after recent and rapid withdrawal, levodopa, MAO inhibitors, phenothiazines, tricyclic antidepressants: increased risk of adverse effects, including seizures. Avoid concomitant use.

Adverse reactions
CNS: *agitation,* akathisia, akinesia, anxiety, *confusion,* delusions, *dizziness,* euphoria, fatigue, *headache,* hostility, impaired sleep quality, *insomnia, sedation,* **seizures,** *tremor.*
CV: *arrhythmias,* hypertension, hypotension, palpitations, syncope, *tachycardia.*
EENT: *auditory disturbances,* blurred vision.
GI: *anorexia, constipation,* diarrhea, *dry mouth,* dyspepsia, increased appetite, *nausea,* taste disturbance, *vomiting.*
GU: decreased libido, impotence, menstrual complaints, urinary frequency, urine retention.
Metabolic: *weight gain or loss.*
Musculoskeletal: arthritis.
Skin: cutaneous temperature disturbance, *excessive diaphoresis,* pruritus, rash.
Other: chills, fever.

Overdose and treatment
Overdose may cause labored breathing, salivation, an arched back, ptosis, ataxia, and seizures.

If the ingestion was recent, empty the patient's stomach by using gastric lavage or inducing emesis with ipecac, as appropriate; follow with activated charcoal. Treatment should be supportive. Control seizures with I.V. benzodiazepines. Stuporous, comatose, or convulsing patients may need intubation. No data are available regarding the benefits of dialysis, hemoperfusion, or diuresis.

Special considerations
■ Consider the patient to have some risk of suicide until depression improves significantly. Supervise high-risk patients closely early in therapy. To reduce the risk of intentional overdose, provide the smallest quantity of drug consistent with good management.
■ Many patients have a period of increased restlessness at the start of therapy. It may include agitation, insomnia, and anxiety. Some patients may need a sedative-hypnotic drug; about 2% may need to stop taking bupropion.
■ If patient has bipolar disorder, anticipate an increased risk of manic episodes during the depressed phase.
■ Make sure the patient isn't taking Zyban, which is bupropion packaged under a different trade name for smoking cessation.

Breast-feeding patients
■ Because of the potential for serious adverse reactions in the infant, breast-feeding during therapy isn't recommended.

Pediatric patients
- Safety in children under age 18 hasn't been established.

Patient teaching
- Tell patient to take daily dosage in three divided doses, preferably at 6-hour intervals, to minimize the risk of seizures.
- Urge patient not to chew, divide, or crush sustained-release tablets.
- Warn patient to avoid alcohol during therapy because it may raise the risk of seizures.
- Caution patient to avoid hazardous activities until drug's full effect is clear.
- Instruct patient not to take Zyban in combination with Wellbutrin. Also, caution against taking other drugs, including OTC medications, dietary supplements, and herbal remedies, without consulting the prescriber.

---

citalopram hydrobromide
Celexa

Pharmacologic classification: selective serotonin reuptake inhibitor

Therapeutic classification: antidepressant

Pregnancy risk category C

How supplied
Available by prescription only
Tablets: 20 mg, 40 mg

Indications and dosages
Depression
Adults: initially, 20 mg P.O. once daily, increasing to 40 mg/day after no less than 1 week. Maximum recommended is 40 mg/day.
▶ **Dosage adjustment.** For elderly patient or patient with hepatic impairment, give 20 mg/day P.O. and adjust to 40 mg/day if patient fails to respond.

Pharmacodynamics
Antidepressant action: Drug's action is presumed to be linked to potentiation of serotonergic activity in the CNS that results from inhibited neuronal reuptake of serotonin.

Pharmacokinetics
Absorption: Absolute bioavailability is 80% following oral administration. Serum levels peak in 4 hours.
Distribution: Drug is highly bound to plasma proteins (80%).
Metabolism: Drug is extensively metabolized to inactive metabolites, primarily by cytochrome P-450 3A4 and cytochrome P-450 2C19.
Excretion: About 20% of drug is excreted in urine. Elimination half-life is about 35 hours. In patients over age 60, half-life is increased by up to 30%.

Contraindications and precautions
Contraindicated in patients hypersensitive to drug or its inactive ingredients, and within 14 days of taking an MAO inhibitor.

Use cautiously in patients with a history of mania, seizures, suicidal ideation, or hepatic or renal impairment.

Interactions
Drug-drug
Carbamazepine: may increase citalopram clearance; monitor patient for lack of effect.

CNS drugs: additive effects. Use together cautiously.

Drugs that inhibit cytochrome P-450 isoenzymes 3A4 and 2C19: decreased clearance of citalopram and increased risk of toxicity. Monitor patient and serum levels.

Imipramine, other tricyclic antidepressants: imipramine metabolite desipramine increased by about 50%. Use together cautiously.

Lithium: may enhance serotonergic effect of citalopram. Use cautiously, and monitor lithium levels.

MAO inhibitors: serious, sometimes fatal, reactions may occur. Don't use drug within 14 days of MAO inhibitor use.

Warfarin: PT increases by 5%. Monitor PT and INR closely.

Drug-lifestyle
Alcohol use: may increase CNS effects. Discourage concomitant use.

Adverse reactions
CNS: agitation, amnesia, anxiety, apathy, confusion, depression, dizziness, fatigue, impaired concentration, *insomnia*, migraine, paresthesia, *somnolence,* **suicide risk,** tremor.

CV: hypotension, orthostatic hypotension, tachycardia.

EENT: abnormal accommodation, rhinitis, sinusitis.

GI: abdominal pain, anorexia, diarrhea, *dry mouth*, dyspepsia, flatulence, increased appetite, increased saliva, *nausea*, taste perversion, vomiting.

GU: amenorrhea, dysmenorrhea, ejaculation disorder, impotence, polyuria.

Metabolic: weight gain or loss.

Musculoskeletal: arthralgia, myalgia.

Respiratory: cough, upper respiratory infection.

Skin: *increased diaphoresis,* pruritus, rash.

Other: decreased libido, fever, yawning.

Overdose and treatment
Overdose may cause dizziness, diaphoresis, nausea, vomiting, tremor, somnolence, and tachycardia. Treatment is symptomatic and supportive. Establish and maintain a patent airway to ensure adequate oxygenation. Also, provide continuous ECG monitoring. Perform gastric lavage, and administer activated charcoal. Forced diuresis and dialysis probably won't be helpful.

Special considerations
■ Expect that drug could impair judgment, thinking, or motor skills.

■ Consider the patient to have some risk of suicide until depression improves significantly. Supervise high-risk patients closely early in therapy. To reduce the risk of intentional overdose, provide the smallest quantity of drug consistent with good management.

■ Don't give citalopram within 14 days of an MAO inhibitor.

Breast-feeding patients
■ Drug is excreted in breast milk and will affect a breast-feeding infant. Either discontinue drug dur-

ing breast-feeding or discontinue breast-feeding during therapy.

Geriatric patients
■ Use cautiously in elderly patients because they may have greater sensitivity to drug.

Patient teaching
■ Tell patient that drug may be taken in the morning or evening without regard to meals.
■ Instruct patient to continue therapy as prescribed, even though she may feel better in 1 to 4 weeks.
■ Warn patient to avoid alcohol.
■ Tell patient to avoid hazardous tasks until drug effects are clear.
■ Warn against stopping drug abruptly.
■ Urge patient to consult prescriber before taking other prescribed drugs, OTC medications, and herbal remedies.
■ Caution patient against taking an MAO inhibitor with citalopram.

---

clomipramine hydrochloride
Anafranil

Pharmacologic classification: **tricyclic antidepressant**

Therapeutic classification: **antiobsessional**

Pregnancy risk category C

How supplied
Available by prescription only
Capsules: 25 mg, 50 mg, 75 mg

Indications and dosages
Obsessive-compulsive disorder
Adults: initially, 25 mg P.O. daily, gradually increased over the first 2 weeks to 100 mg P.O. daily, given in divided doses with meals. Maximum, 250 mg/day. After dosage is stabilized, entire daily dose may be given h.s.
Children and adolescents: initially, 25 mg P.O. daily, gradually increased over the first 2 weeks to a maximum of 3 mg/kg or 100 mg P.O. daily, whichever is smaller, given in divided doses with meals. Maximum daily dose is 3 mg/kg or 200 mg, whichever is smaller. After dosage is stabilized, entire daily dose may be given h.s.

Pharmacodynamics
Antiobsessional action: Drug selectively inhibits reuptake of serotonin into neurons in the CNS, although its exact mechanism is unknown. It may also have some blocking activity at postsynaptic dopamine receptors.

Pharmacokinetics
Absorption: Clomipramine is well absorbed from GI tract, but extensive first-pass metabolism limits its bioavailablity to about 50%.
Distribution: Drug distributes well into lipophilic tissues. The volume of distribution is about 12 L/kg; 98% is bound to plasma proteins.
Metabolism: Drug's metabolism is primarily hepatic. Several metabolites have been identified; desmethylclomipramine is the primary active metabolite.
Excretion: About 66% of drug is excreted in urine and the remainder in feces. Mean elimination

---

half-life of the parent compound is about 36 hours. The elimination half-life of desmethylclomipramine has a mean of 69 hours. After multiple doses, the half-life may increase.

Contraindications and precautions
Contraindicated in patients with hypersensitivity to drug or other tricyclic antidepressants, in patients who have taken an MAO inhibitor within 14 days, and in patients in the acute recovery period after an MI.

Use cautiously in patients with urine retention, suicidal tendencies, glaucoma, increased intraocular pressure, brain damage, or seizure disorders. Also, use cautiously in patients with impaired renal or hepatic function, hyperthyroidism, or tumors of the adrenal medulla. And use cautiously in patients taking drugs that may lower the seizure threshold and in those undergoing elective surgery or receiving thyroid medication or electroconvulsive treatment.

Interactions
Drug-drug
Barbiturates: repeated doses increase the activity of hepatic microsomal enzymes and may decrease clomipramine levels. Monitor patient for decreased effectiveness and for possibly exaggerated depressant effect.
CNS depressants: may cause an exaggerated depressant effect. Monitor patient closely.
Epinephrine, norepinephrine: may produce an increased hypertensive effect. Use together cautiously.

MAO inhibitors: may cause hyperpyretic crisis, seizures, coma, and death. Avoid concomitant use.
Methylphenidate: may increase clomipramine levels. Monitor patient and serum levels closely.

Drug-lifestyle
Alcohol use: may cause an exaggerated depressant effect when used with tricyclic antidepressants. Discourage concomitant use.

Adverse reactions
CNS: *dizziness,* EEG changes, *fatigue, headache, insomnia, myoclonus, nervousness,* **seizures,** *somnolence, tremor.*
CV: orthostatic hypotension, palpitations, tachycardia.
EENT: *pharyngitis, rhinitis, visual changes.*
GI: *abdominal pain, anorexia, constipation,* diarrhea, *dry mouth, dyspepsia, increased appetite, nausea.*
GU: *dysmenorrhea, ejaculation failure, impotence, urinary hesitancy,* urinary tract infection.
Hematologic: anemia, purpura.
Metabolic: *weight gain.*
Musculoskeletal: *myalgia.*
Skin: *diaphoresis,* dry skin, rash, pruritus.
Other: *altered libido.*

Overdose and treatment
Overdose may cause changes similar to those of other tricyclic antidepressant overdoses, including sinus tachycardia, intraventricular block, hypotension, irritability, fixed and dilated pupils, drowsiness, delirium, stupor, hyperreflexia, and hyperpyrexia.

Treatment should include gastric lavage with large quantities of fluid. Lavage should be continued for 12 hours because the anticholinergic effects of the drug slow gastric emptying. Hemodialysis, peritoneal dialysis, and forced diuresis are ineffective because of the high degree of plasma protein binding. Support respirations and monitor patient's cardiac function. Treat shock with plasma expanders or corticosteroids; treat seizures with diazepam.

Special considerations
■ Therapeutic plasma levels range from 80 to 100 ng/ml.
■ Monitor patient for urine retention and constipation. Give a stool softener or high-fiber diet, as needed, and provide adequate fluids.
■ Clomipramine may activate mania or hypomania.
■ To minimize the risk of overdose, dispense drug in small quantities.
■ Discontinue drug before elective surgical procedures.
■ Don't stop drug abruptly.

Breast-feeding patients
■ No data exist to demonstrate whether drug appears in breast milk. Use cautiously in breast-feeding women.

Patient teaching
■ Tell patient that adverse GI effects can be minimized by taking drug with meals during the initial adjustment period. Later, the entire daily dose may be taken at bedtime to limit daytime drowsiness.
■ Instruct patient to avoid alcohol and other CNS depressants.
■ Caution patient to avoid hazardous activities until full effects of drug are clear, especially early in therapy, when daytime sedation and dizziness may occur.
■ Suggest using a saliva substitute or sugarless candy or gum to relieve a dry mouth.
■ Caution patient to avoid herbal remedies or OTC medications, particularly antihistamines and decongestants, unless recommended by the prescriber.
■ Encourage patient to continue therapy, even if adverse reactions are troublesome. Advise patient not to stop taking drug without consulting prescriber.
■ Advise women to use effective contraception during therapy and to immediately notify prescriber about planned, suspected, or known pregnancy.

desipramine hydrochloride
Norpramin

Pharmacologic classification: dibenzazepine tricyclic antidepressant

Therapeutic classification: antidepressant

Pregnancy risk category NR

How supplied
Available by prescription only
Tablets: 10 mg, 25 mg, 50 mg, 75 mg, 100 mg, 150 mg

Indications and dosages
Depression
Adults: 100 to 200 mg P.O. daily in divided doses, increasing to a maximum of 300 mg daily.

Alternatively, the entire dosage can be given once daily, usually h.s.

▶ DOSAGE ADJUSTMENT. For elderly or adolescent patients, give 25 to 100 mg P.O. daily, increasing gradually to a maximum of 100 mg daily (150 mg daily for severely ill patients in these age groups).

Pharmacodynamics
Antidepressant action: Drug is thought to exert its antidepressant effect by inhibiting reuptake of norepinephrine and serotonin in CNS nerve terminals (presynaptic neurons), which results in increased amounts and enhanced activity of these neurotransmitters in the synaptic cleft. Desipramine inhibits reuptake of norepinephrine more strongly than serotonin; it causes fewer sedative effects and has less anticholinergic and hypotensive activity than its parent compound, imipramine.

Pharmacokinetics
Absorption: Drug is absorbed rapidly from the GI tract after oral administration.
Distribution: Drug is distributed widely into the body, including the CNS and breast milk. Drug is 90% protein-bound. Effects peak in 4 to 6 hours, steady state occurs in 2 to 11 days, and full therapeutic effect takes place in 2 to 4 weeks. Proposed therapeutic plasma levels (parent drug and metabolite) range from 125 to 300 ng/ml.
Metabolism: Desipramine is metabolized by the liver. A significant first-pass effect may explain the variability of serum levels in different patients taking the same dosage.

Excretion: Drug is excreted primarily in urine.

Contraindications and precautions
Contraindicated in patients hypersensitive to drug, in patients who have taken an MAO inhibitor within 14 days, and in patients in the acute recovery period after an MI.

Use with extreme caution in patients who have history of seizure disorders, urine retention, CV disease, thyroid disease, or glaucoma, and in those taking thyroid medication.

Interactions
Drug-drug
Antiarrhythmics (disopyramide, procainamide, quinidine), pimozide, thyroid hormones: may increase risk of cardiac arrhythmias and conduction defects. Use with extreme caution.
Anticholinergic drugs, such as antihistamines, antiparkinsonian drugs, atropine, meperidine, phenothiazines: may cause oversedation, paralytic ileus, visual changes, and severe constipation. Monitor patient closely.
Barbiturates: may induce desipramine metabolism and decrease therapeutic efficacy. Monitor patient for lack of therapeutic effect.
Beta blockers, methylphenidate, oral contraceptives, propoxyphene: may inhibit desipramine metabolism, increasing plasma levels and toxicity. Monitor patient closely.
Central-acting antihypertensives, such as clonidine, guanabenz, guanadrel, guanethidine, methyldopa, reserpine: decreased antihyperten-

---

◊ Available in Canada only · *Unlabeled use

sive effects. Monitor patient and blood pressure closely.
Cimetidine, fluoxetine, fluvoxamine, paroxetine, sertraline: may increase serum desipramine levels.
CNS depressants, including analgesics, anesthetics, barbiturates, narcotics, tranquilizers: may cause oversedation. Use cautiously.
Disulfiram, ethchlorvynol: may cause delirium and tachycardia. Monitor patient closely.
Haloperidol, phenothiazines: decreased desipramine metabolism and increased risk of toxicity. Monitor serum levels closely.
MAO inhibitors: may cause severe excitation, hyperpyrexia, or seizures, usually with high dosage. Avoid concomitant use.
Metrizamide: additive effects likely, increasing the risk of seizures and other adverse effects. Monitor patient closely.
Selective serotonin reuptake inhibitors: possible toxic reaction to tricyclic antidepressant at much lower dosages. Monitor patient closely.
Sympathomimetics (including ephedrine, epinephrine, phenylephrine, phenylpropanolamine) commonly found in nasal sprays: may increase blood pressure.
Warfarin: may elevate PT and INR, increasing the risk of bleeding. Monitor patient closely.

Drug-lifestyle
Alcohol use: may enhance CNS depression. Discourage use together.
Heavy smoking: may lower plasma desipramine levels. Discourage concomitant use, and encourage smoking cessation.

Sun exposure: may increase risk of photosensitivity. Urge patient to take precautions.

Adverse reactions
CNS: agitation, anxiety, confusion, *dizziness, drowsiness,* EEG changes, excitation, extrapyramidal reactions, headache, nervousness, restlessness, *seizures,* tremor, weakness.
CV: *ECG changes,* hypertension, orthostatic hypotension, *tachycardia.*
EENT: *blurred vision,* mydriasis, tinnitus.
GI: anorexia, *constipation, dry mouth,* nausea, paralytic ileus, vomiting.
GU: *urine retention.*
Hematologic: decreased WBC counts.
Hepatic: elevated liver function test results.
Metabolic: hyperglycemia, hypoglycemia.
Skin: *diaphoresis,* photosensitivity, rash, urticaria.
Other: *hypersensitivity reaction, sudden death* (in children).

Overdose and treatment
The first 12 hours after acute ingestion are a stimulatory phase characterized by excessive anticholinergic activity, which may include agitation, irritation, confusion, hallucinations, hyperthermia, parkinsonian symptoms, seizures, urine retention, dry mucous membranes, pupil dilation, constipation, and ileus. This phase is followed by CNS depression—including hypothermia, decreased or absent reflexes, sedation, hypotension, and cyanosis—and such car-

---

Reactions may be *common,* uncommon, *life-threatening,* or COMMON AND LIFE-THREATENING.

diac irregularities as tachycardia, conduction disturbances, and quinidine-like effects on the ECG.

Widening of the QRS complex usually indicates a serum level above 1,000 mg/ml. Metabolic acidosis may follow hypotension, hypoventilation, and seizures.

Treatment is symptomatic and supportive, and includes managing the patient's airway, body temperature, and fluid and electrolyte balance. Induce emesis with ipecac if the patient is conscious; follow with gastric lavage and activated charcoal to prevent further absorption. Dialysis is of little use.

Physostigmine may be used cautiously to reverse CV abnormalities or coma; too rapid administration may cause seizures. Give parenteral diazepam or phenytoin for seizures. Give parenteral phenytoin or lidocaine for arrhythmias. Give sodium bicarbonate for acidosis. Don't give barbiturates; they may increase CNS and respiratory depressant effects.

Special considerations

■ Because drug has been used to commit suicide, dispense smallest prudent amount to depressed patient.
■ If patient has bipolar disorder, drug may induce a hypomanic state.
■ Tolerance to sedative effects usually develops during initial weeks of therapy.
■ Check patient's standing and sitting blood pressures to assess orthostasis before giving drug.
■ Drug causes fewer sedative, anticholinergic, and hypotensive effects than its parent compound, imipramine.
■ Discontinue drug at least 48 hours before surgical procedures.
■ To discontinue drug, taper gradually over 3 to 6 weeks rather than stopping abruptly. Abrupt withdrawal of long-term therapy may cause nausea, headache, and malaise (which doesn't indicate addiction).

Breast-feeding patients
■ Drug is excreted in breast milk at levels equal to those in maternal serum. Make sure possible benefits to mother outweigh possible risk to infant.

Pediatric patients
■ Drug isn't recommended for patients under age 12.

Geriatric patients
■ Elderly patients may be more susceptible to adverse CV and anticholinergic effects.

Patient teaching

■ Tell patient to take the drug exactly as prescribed and not to double up if she misses a dose.
■ Tell patient to take the full dose at bedtime to minimize daytime sedation.
■ To prevent dizziness, urge patient to lie down for about 30 minutes after each dose at the start of therapy and to avoid sudden postural changes, especially when rising to an upright position.
■ Explain that full effects of drug may not be apparent for 4 weeks or more after therapy starts.

- Suggest that patient use ice or sugarless gum or hard candy if a dry mouth develops.
- Stress the importance of regular dental hygiene because a dry mouth increases the risk of dental caries.
- Warn patient not to suddenly stop taking drug.
- Encourage patient to report unusual or troublesome effects, especially confusion, movement disorders, rapid heartbeat, dizziness, fainting, or difficulty urinating.
- Advise women to use effective contraception during therapy and to immediately notify presciber about planned, suspected, or known pregnancy.

doxepin hydrochloride
Adapin, Sinequan, Triadapin ◊

Pharmacologic classification: tricyclic antidepressant

Therapeutic classification: antidepressant

Pregnancy risk category C

How supplied
Available by prescription only
Capsules: 10 mg, 25 mg, 50 mg, 75 mg, 100 mg, 150 mg
Oral concentrate: 10 mg/ml

Indications and dosages
Depression, anxiety
Adults: initially, 25 to 75 mg P.O. daily in divided doses, to a maximum of 300 mg daily. Or give entire maintenance dosage once daily to a maximum of 150 mg P.O.

▶ **DOSAGE ADJUSTMENT.** Reduce dosage in elderly, debilitated, or adolescent patients and in those taking other drugs, especially anticholinergics.

Pharmacodynamics
Antidepressant action: Doxepin is thought to exert antidepressant effects by inhibiting reuptake of norepinephrine and serotonin in CNS nerve terminals (presynaptic neurons), which results in increased levels and enhanced activity of these neurotransmitters in the synaptic cleft. Doxepin inhibits serotonin reuptake more actively than norepinephrine reuptake. Doxepin also may be used as an anxiolytic; anxiolytic effects usually precede antidepressant effects. Drug has the greatest sedative effect of all tricyclic antidepressants; tolerance to this effect usually develops in a few weeks.

Pharmacokinetics
Absorption: Drug is absorbed rapidly from the GI tract after oral administration.
Distribution: Doxepin is distributed widely into the body, including the CNS and breast milk. Drug is 90% protein-bound. Effects peak in 2 to 4 hours; steady state occurs within 7 days. Therapeutic levels (parent drug and metabolite) are thought to range from 150 to 250 ng/ml.
Metabolism: Drug is metabolized by the liver to the active metabolite desmethyldoxepin. A significant first-pass effect may explain the variability of serum levels in different patients taking the same dosage.

Reactions may be *common,* uncommon, *life-threatening,* or COMMON AND LIFE-THREATENING.

Excretion: Drug is excreted mostly in urine.

Contraindications and precautions

Contraindicated in patients with hypersensitivity to drug, glaucoma, or tendency to retain urine.

Use with caution in patients who have CV disease because of possible conduction problems.

Interactions
Drug-drug

Antiarrhythmics (disopyramide, procainamide, quinidine), pimozide, thyroid hormones: may increase risk of cardiac arrhythmias and conduction defects. Use with extreme caution.

Anticholinergics, such as antihistamines, antiparkinsonian drugs, atropine, meperidine, phenothiazines: may cause oversedation, paralytic ileus, visual changes, and severe constipation. Monitor patient closely.

Barbiturates: may induce doxepin metabolism and decrease its efficacy. Dosage adjustment may be necessary.

Beta blockers, cimetidine, fluoxetine, methylphenidate, oral contraceptives, propoxyphene, sertraline: may inhibit doxepin metabolism, increasing plasma levels and toxicity. Monitor patient closely.

Central-acting antihypertensive drugs, such as clonidine, guanabenz, guanadrel, guanethidine, methyldopa, reserpine: doxepin may decrease antihypertensive effects. Monitor patient closely.

Clonidine: increases hypertensive effect. Monitor patient closely.

CNS depressants, including analgesics, anesthetics, barbiturates, narcotics, tranquilizers: may cause oversedation. Monitor patient.

Disulfiram, ethchlorvynol: may cause delirium and tachycardia. Avoid concomitant use.

Haloperidol, phenothiazines: decreased doxepin metabolism and increased risk of toxicity. Dosage adjustment may be necessary.

MAO inhibitors: may cause severe excitation, hyperpyrexia, or seizures, usually with high dose. Avoid concomitant use.

Metrizamide: additive effects are likely, increasing the risk of seizures or other adverse effects. Avoid use together.

Sympathomimetics (including ephedrine, epinephrine, phenylephrine, phenylpropanolamine) commonly found in nasal sprays: may increase blood pressure. Monitor patient's blood pressure.

Warfarin: may increase PT, INR, and risk of bleeding. Monitor patient, PT, and INR closely.

Drug-food

Carbonated beverages, grape juice: may affect drug metabolism. Don't give together.

Drug-lifestyle

Alcohol use: induces doxepin metabolism, decreases therapeutic efficacy, and enhances CNS depression. Discourage concomitant use.

Heavy smoking: induces doxepin metabolism and decreases therapeutic efficacy. Caution against concomitant use, and encourage smoking cessation.

Sun exposure: increases risk of photosensitivity reactions. Tell patient to take precautions.

Adverse reactions
CNS: ataxia, confusion, *dizziness, drowsiness,* extrapyramidal reactions, hallucinations, headache, numbness, paresthesia, **seizures,** weakness.
CV: *conduction disorder*, ECG changes, *orthostatic hypotension, tachycardia.*
EENT: *blurred vision,* tinnitus.
GI: anorexia, *constipation, dry mouth,* nausea, vomiting.
GU: urine retention.
Hematologic: *bone marrow depression,* eosinophilia.
Hepatic: elevated liver function test results.
Metabolic: hyperglycemia, hypoglycemia. *weight gain.*
Skin: *diaphoresis,* photosensitivity, rash, urticaria.
Other: *hypersensitivity reaction.*

Overdose and treatment
The first 12 hours after acute ingestion are a stimulatory phase characterized by excessive anticholinergic activity, which may include agitation, irritation, confusion, hallucinations, hyperthermia, parkinsonian symptoms, seizures, urine retention, dry mucous membranes, pupil dilation, constipation, and ileus. This phase is followed by CNS depression—including hypothermia, decreased or absent reflexes, sedation, hypotension, and cyanosis—and such cardiac irregularities as tachycardia, conduction disturbances, and quinidine-like effects on the ECG.

Widening of the QRS complex usually indicates a serum level above 1,000 mg/ml. Metabolic acidosis may follow hypotension, hypoventilation, and seizures.

Treatment is symptomatic and supportive, and includes managing the patient's airway, body temperature, and fluid and electrolyte balance. Induce emesis with ipecac if the patient is conscious; follow with gastric lavage and activated charcoal to prevent further absorption. Dialysis is of little use.

Physostigmine may be used cautiously to reverse central anticholinergic effects. Give parenteral diazepam or phenytoin for seizures. Give parenteral phenytoin or lidocaine for arrhythmias. Give sodium bicarbonate for acidosis. Don't give barbiturates; they may increase CNS and respiratory depressant effects.

Special considerations
■ Consider the patient to have some risk of suicide until depression improves significantly. Supervise high-risk patients closely early in therapy. To reduce the risk of intentional overdose, provide the smallest quantity of drug consistent with good management.
■ Full antidepressant effect may take up to three weeks.
■ Doxepin may prolong conduction time (elongation of QT and PR intervals, flattened T waves). It also may elevate liver function test results, decrease WBC counts, and decrease or increase serum glucose levels.
■ Watch for serotonin syndrome if drug is combined with other antidepressants, particularly selective

---

Reactions may be *common,* uncommon, **life-threatening,** or COMMON AND LIFE-THREATENING.

serotonin reuptake inhibitors. Symptoms include tremor, agitation, rigidity, delirium, hyperthermia, obtundation, and myoclonus.
■ Abrupt withdrawal of long-term therapy may cause nausea, headache, malaise (which doesn't indicate addiction).

Breast-feeding patients
■ Drug is excreted in breast milk. Avoid use of drug, especially at high doses, in breast-feeding patients.

Pediatric patients
■ Doxepin is rarely used for treating anxiety in children.

Geriatric patients
■ Elderly patients are more likely to develop orthostatic hypotension and adverse CNS, GI, and GU reactions.

Patient teaching
■ Teach patient to dilute oral concentrate with 120 ml of water, milk, or juice (orange, pineapple, prune, or tomato). Caution against mixing drug in carbonated beverages.
■ Instruct patient to take full dose at bedtime.
■ Suggest ice chips, sugarless gum or hard candy, or saliva substitutes to relieve a dry mouth.
■ Warn patient to avoid hazardous activities until full effects of drug are known.
■ Tell patient that drowsiness usually decreases with time.
■ Warn patient to avoid taking other prescribed drugs, OTC medications, or herbal remedies during therapy without consulting prescriber.
■ Advise women to use effective contraception and to immediately notify prescriber about planned, suspected, or known pregnancy.

---

fluoxetine hydrochloride
Prozac, Prozac Pulvules

Pharmacologic classification: **selective serotonin reuptake inhibitor**

Therapeutic classification: **antidepressant**

Pregnancy risk category B

How supplied
Available by prescription only
Capsules: 10 mg, 20 mg
Oral solution: 20 mg/5 ml

Indications and dosages
Depression
Panic disorder*, bipolar disorder*, alcohol dependence*, cataplexy*, narcolepsy*, myoclonus*
Adults: 20 mg P.O. daily in the morning. Increase to 40 mg daily p.r.n. after several weeks with doses morning and midday. Don't exceed 80 mg daily.

Obsessive-compulsive disorder, Trichotillomania*
Adults: initially, 20 mg P.O. daily. Gradually increase dosage as needed and tolerated to 60 to 80 mg daily.

Eating disorders*, kleptomania*
Adults: 60 to 80 mg P.O. daily.

Attention-deficit hyperactivity disorders*, schizophrenia*
Adults: 20 to 60 mg P.O. daily.

Borderline personality disorder*
Adults: 5 to 80 mg P.O. daily.

Social phobia*
Adults: 10 to 60 mg P.O. daily.

Tourette syndrome*
Adults: 20 to 40 mg P.O. daily.

Premenstrual syndrome*, recurrent syncope*
Adults: 20 mg P.O. daily.

Post-traumatic stress disorder*
Adults: 10 to 80 mg P.O. daily.

▶ DOSAGE ADJUSTMENT. Administer lower or less frequent doses to patients with renal or hepatic impairment. Also, consider lower or less frequent doses in elderly patients and patients with concurrent disease or multiple drug therapy.

Pharmacodynamics
Antidepressant action: Drug's antidepressant action is probably related to its inhibition of neuronal uptake of serotonin at the presynaptic neuronal membrane, which increases synaptic levels of serotonin in the CNS. Drug appears to have little or no effect on norepinephrine. In fact, animal studies suggest that it's a much more potent uptake inhibitor of serotonin than of norepinephrine.

Pharmacokinetics
Absorption: Drug is well absorbed after oral administration. Absorption isn't altered by food.

Distribution: Drug is apparently highly protein-bound (about 95%).
Metabolism: Drug is metabolized primarily in the liver to active metabolites.
Excretion: Drug is excreted by the kidneys. Elimination half-life is 2 to 3 days. Norfluoxetine (the primary active metabolite) has an elimination half-life of 7 to 9 days.

Contraindications and precautions
Contraindicated in patients hypersensitive to drug and in patients who take an MAO inhibitor within 14 days of fluoxetine.
    Use cautiously in patients at high risk of suicide and those with a history of seizures, diabetes mellitus, or renal, hepatic, or CV disease.

Interactions
Drug-drug
Antidepressants, including MAO inhibitors, selective serotonin reuptake inhibitors: increased risk of serotonin syndrome (tremor, agitation, rigidity, delirium, hyperthermia, obtundation, myoclonus). Avoid concomitant use. Don't give fluoxetine within 14 days of an MAO inhibitor.
Benzodiazepams, carbamazepine, flecainide, vinblastine: may increase serum levels of these drugs. Dosage adjustment may be required.
Cimetidine, other highly protein-bound drugs, warfarin: may increase plasma levels of fluoxetine or other highly protein-bound drugs. Dosage adjustment may be required.

Reactions may be *common*, uncommon, *life-threatening*, or COMMON AND LIFE-THREATENING.

Cisapride: may increase serum cisapride levels and cause lethal arrythmias. Don't administer together.
Insulin, oral antidiabetic drugs: may alter blood glucose levels. Dosage adjustment may be required.
Lithium, tricyclic antidepressants: may increase adverse CNS effects. Monitor patient closely.
Phenytoin: may increase plasma phenytoin levels and risk of toxicity. Dosage adjustment may be required.
Tryptophan: may increase adverse CNS effects (agitation, restlessness) and GI distress. Avoid concomitant use.

Drug-herb
St. John's wort: increased risk of serotonin syndrome (tremor, agitation, rigidity, delirium, hyperthermia, obtundation, myoclonus). Avoid concomitant use.

Drug-lifestyle
Alcohol use: may increase CNS depression. Discourage alcohol use.

Adverse reactions
CNS: *anxiety, asthenia, dizziness, drowsiness,* fatigue, *headache, insomnia, nervousness, tremor.*
CV: hot flashes, palpitations.
EENT: cough, nasal congestion, pharyngitis, sinusitis.
GI: abdominal pain, *anorexia,* constipation, *diarrhea, dry mouth, dyspepsia,* flatulence, increased appetite, *nausea,* vomiting.
GU: sexual dysfunction.
Metabolic: *weight loss.*
Musculoskeletal: muscle pain.
Respiratory: respiratory distress, upper respiratory infection.
Skin: diaphoresis, *pruritus, rash.*

Other: fever, flulike syndrome.

Overdose and treatment
Overdose may cause agitation, restlessness, hypomania, and other signs of CNS excitation. At higher doses, it may cause nausea and vomiting. Among about 38 reports of acute fluoxetine overdose, two fatalities involved plasma levels of 4.57 mg/L and 1.93 mg/L. One involved 1.8 g of fluoxetine with an undetermined amount of maprotiline; another death involved combined ingestion of fluoxetine, codeine, and temazepam. One other patient developed two tonic-clonic seizures after taking 3 g of fluoxetine; these seizures stopped spontaneously and didn't require anticonvulsant treatment.

To treat fluoxetine overdose, establish and maintain an airway; ensure adequate oxygenation and ventilation. Activated charcoal, possibly with sorbitol, may be as effective as emesis or lavage. Monitor patient's cardiac and vital signs, and provide supportive care. Fluoxetine-induced seizures that don't subside spontaneously may respond to diazepam. Forced diuresis, dialysis, hemoperfusion, and exchange transfusion are unlikely to help.

Special considerations
■ Consider the patient to have some risk of suicide until depression improves significantly. Supervise high-risk patients closely early in therapy. To reduce the risk of intentional overdose, provide the smallest quantity of drug consistent with good management.

■ Treatment of acute depression usually requires at least several months of continuous therapy; optimal duration hasn't been established.
■ Fluoxetine therapy may activate mania or hypomania.
■ Full antidepressant effects may take 4 weeks or longer to appear.
■ Because of its long elimination half-life, changes in fluoxetine dosage won't be reflected in plasma levels for several weeks, which may affect adjustment to final dosage and withdrawal from treatment.

Patient teaching
■ Tell patient to avoid hazardous activities until full effects of drug are clear.
■ Caution patient to avoid alcohol during therapy.
■ Urge patient to avoid other prescribed drugs, OTC medications, and herbal remedies without first consulting prescriber.
■ Tell patient to promptly report rash, hives, anxiety, nervousness, or anorexia (especially if underweight).
■ Urge patient to notify prescriber about planned, suspected, or known pregnancy.

fluvoxamine maleate
Luvox

Pharmacologic classification: **selective serotonin reuptake inhibitor**

Therapeutic classification: **anticompulsive**

Pregnancy risk category C

How supplied
Available by prescription only
Tablets: 50 mg, 100 mg

Indications and dosages
Obsessive-compulsive disorder
Adults: initially, 50 mg P.O. daily h.s. Increase in 50-mg increments q 4 to 7 days until maximum benefit is achieved. Maximum is 300 mg daily; daily amounts above 100 mg should be divided in half and given as two doses.
⟩ DOSAGE ADJUSTMENT. Because elderly patients and those with hepatic impairment may have decreased clearance of fluvoxamine maleate, gradual dosage adjustment may be appropriate.

Pharmacodynamics
Anticompulsive action: The exact mechanism of action is unknown. Fluvoxamine is a potent selective inhibitor of neuronal serotonin uptake, which is thought to reduce obsessive-compulsive behavior.

Pharmacokinetics
Absorption: Absolute bioavailability of drug is 53%.
Distribution: Mean apparent volume of distribution is about 25 L/kg. About 80% of drug is

bound to plasma protein (mostly albumin).

Metabolism: Drug is extensively metabolized in the liver, mostly by oxidative demethylation and deamination.

Excretion: Metabolites are excreted primarily in urine.

Contraindications and precautions

Contraindicated in patients with hypersensitivity to drug or to other phenylpiperazine antidepressants and within 14 days of taking an MAO inhibitor.

Use cautiously in patients with hepatic dysfunction, conditions that may affect hemodynamic responses or metabolism, or a history of mania or seizures.

Interactions
Drug-drug

Antidepressants, including selective serotonin reuptake inhibitors: Increased risk of serotonin syndrome (tremor, agitation, rigidity, delirium, hyperthermia, obtundation, myoclonus). Monitor patient.

Benzodiazepines, theophylline, warfarin: reduced clearance of these drugs. Use together cautiously.

Carbamazepine, clozapine, methadone, metoprolol, propranolol, tricyclic antidepressants: may elevate serum levels of these drugs. Use together cautiously, and monitor patient closely for adverse reactions. Dosage adjustments may be necessary.

Diltiazem: may cause bradycardia. Monitor patient's heart rate.

Lithium, tryptophan: may enhance effects of fluvoxamine. Use together cautiously.

MAO inhibitors: may cause severe excitation, hyperpyrexia, myoclonus, delirium, and coma. Avoid use together.

Drug-herb

St. John's wort: may increase risk of serotonin syndrome (tremor, agitation, rigidity, delirium, hyperthermia, obtundation, myoclonus). Avoid concurrent use.

Drug-lifestyle

Smoking: may decrease effectiveness of drug. Discourage concomitant use, and encourage smoking cessation.

Adverse reactions

CNS: agitation, anxiety, asthenia, CNS stimulation, depression, dizziness, headache, hypertonia, insomnia, nervousness, somnolence, tremor.

CV: palpitations, vasodilation.

EENT: amblyopia, taste perversion.

GI: anorexia, *constipation, diarrhea, dry mouth, dyspepsia,* dysphagia, flatulence, *nausea,* tooth disorder, *vomiting.*

GU: abnormal ejaculation, anorgasmia, decreased libido, impotence, urinary frequency, urine retention.

Respiratory: dyspnea, upper respiratory infection, yawning.

Skin: diaphoresis.

Other: chills, flulike syndrome.

Overdose and treatment

Overdose may cause drowsiness, vomiting, diarrhea, and dizziness. It also may cause coma, tachycardia, bradycardia, hypotension, ECG abnormalities, liver function abnormalities, and seizures. Loss of consciousness or vomiting may lead to aspiration pneumonitis, respiratory difficulties, or hypokalemia.

Treatment is supportive. Besides maintaining an open airway and monitoring the patient's vital signs and ECG, give activated charcoal, which may be as effective as emesis or lavage. Because absorption may be delayed in an overdose, measures to minimize absorption may be necessary for up to 24 hours after ingestion. Dialysis probably is not beneficial.

Special considerations
■ Record patient's mood changes during therapy. Monitor patient for suicidal tendencies, and provide a minimum supply of drug.
■ At least 14 days should elapse between therapy with an MAO inhibitor and use of fluvoxamine.
■ Besides standard indication, drug is being studied as a treatment for depression.

Breast-feeding patients
■ Drug is excreted in breast milk and should not be given to breast-feeding women. Either drug therapy should stop during breast-feeding or breast-feeding should stop during drug therapy.

Pediatric patients
■ Safety and effectiveness in children under age 18 haven't been established.

Geriatric patients
■ Drug clearance is decreased by about 50% in elderly patients compared with younger patients. Administer drug cautiously to pa-

tients in this age group, and adjust dosage during start of therapy.

Patient teaching
■ Inform patient that full antidepressant effect may take several weeks to develop.
■ Urge patient to continue taking drug as prescribed, even when she starts feeling better.
■ Caution patient to avoid hazardous activities until full effects of drug are clear.
■ Urge patient to avoid alcoholic beverages during therapy.
■ Inform patient that smoking may decrease effectiveness of drug.
■ Tell patient to report rash, hives, or a related allergic reaction.
■ Caution patient not to take other prescribed drugs, OTC medications, or herbal remedies without consulting prescriber.
■ Instruct women to immediately notify prescriber about planned, suspected, or known pregnancy.

---

imipramine hydrochloride
Apo-imipramine◇, Impril◇, Novopramine◇, Tofranil

imipramine pamoate
Tofranil-PM

Pharmacologic classification: **dibenzazepine tricyclic antidepressant**

Therapeutic classification: **antidepressant**

Pregnancy risk category B

How supplied
Available by prescription only
imipramine hydrochloride

Tablets: 10 mg, 25 mg, 50 mg
Injection: 12.5 mg/ ml
imipramine pamoate
Capsules: 75 mg, 100 mg, 125 mg, 150 mg

Indications and dosages
Depression
Adults: initially, 75 to 100 mg P.O. or I.M. daily in divided doses, increased by 25 to 50 mg up to 200 mg. Alternatively, some patients can start with lower doses (25 mg P.O.) and increase in 25-mg increments every other day. Maximum, 300 mg/day. Alternatively, entire dosage may be given h.s. Maximum dosage is 200 mg/day for outpatients, 300 mg/day for inpatients.
▶ DOSAGE ADJUSTMENT. Maximum dosage for elderly patients is 100 mg/day.

Childhood enuresis*
Children age 6 and over: 25 to 75 mg P.O. daily, 1 hour before bedtime. Usual dose 1.5 mg/kg/day in three divided doses. Maximum, 5 mg/kg/day.

Pharmacodynamics
Antidepressant action: Imipramine is thought to exert antidepressant effects by inhibiting reuptake of norepinephrine and serotonin in CNS nerve terminals (presynaptic neurons), which results in increased levels and enhanced activity of these neurotransmitters in the synaptic cleft. Drug also has anticholinergic activity and can be used to treat nocturnal enuresis in children.

Pharmacokinetics
Absorption: Drug is absorbed rapidly from the GI tract and muscle tissue after oral and I.M. administration.
Distribution: Imipramine is distributed widely into the body, including the CNS and breast milk. Drug is 90% protein-bound. Effects peak in 30 minutes to 2 hours; steady state occurs in 2 to 5 days. Therapeutic plasma levels (parent drug and metabolite) are thought to range from 150 to 300 ng/ml.
Metabolism: Drug is metabolized by the liver to the active metabolite desipramine. A significant first-pass effect may explain the variability of serum levels in different patients who take the same dosage.
Excretion: Drug is excreted mostly in urine.

Contraindications and precautions
Contraindicated during acute recovery phase after MI, in patients hypersensitive to drug, and within 14 days of taking an MAO inhibitor.
Use cautiously in patients at risk for suicide, in patients receiving thyroid hormones, and in those with impaired renal function, impaired hepatic function, a history of urine retention, angle-closure glaucoma, increased intraocular pressure, CV disease, hyperthyroidism, seizure disorders, or allergy to injectable sulfites.

Interactions
Drug-drug
Antiarrhythmics (disopyramide, procainamide, quinidine), pimozide, thyroid hormones: may increase risk

of arrhythmias and conduction defects. Monitor patient closely.
Anticholinergics, such as antihistamines, antiparkinsonians, atropine, meperidine, phenothiazines: may cause oversedation, paralytic ileus, visual changes, and severe constipation. Monitor patient closely.
Antidepressants, such as selective serotonin reuptake inhibitors: increased risk of serotonin syndrome (tremor, agitation, rigidity, delirium, hyperthermia, obtundation, myoclonus). Monitor patient closely.
Barbiturates: induced imipramine metabolism and decreased therapeutic efficacy. Monitor patient for loss of imipramine effect.
Beta blockers, cimetidine, methylphenidate, oral contraceptives, propoxyphene: may inhibit imipramine metabolism, increasing plasma levels and toxicity. Monitor patient closely.
Central-acting antihypertensives, such as clonidine, guanabenz, guanadrel, guanethidine, methyldopa, reserpine: decreased antihypertensive effects. Monitor patient's blood pressure closely.
CNS depressants, such as analgesics, anesthetics, barbiturates, narcotics, tranquilizers: may cause oversedation. Monitor patient closely.
Disulfiram, ethchlorvynol: may cause delirium and tachycardia. Monitor patient closely.
Haloperidol, phenothiazines: decreased imipramine metabolism and increased risk of toxicity. Use together with extreme caution.
MAO inhibitors: increased risk for hyperpyretic crisis or severe convulsions. Use of imipramine within 14 days of an MAO inhibitor is contraindicated.
Metrizamide: additive effects and increased risk of seizures are likely. Monitor patient closely.
Sympathomimetics (including ephedrine, epinephrine, phenylephrine, phenylpropanolamine) commonly found in nasal sprays: may increase blood pressure. Monitor patient's blood pressure closely.
Warfarin: may increase PT, INR, and risk of bleeding. Monitor serum levels.

Drug-lifestyle
Alcohol use: may cause additive effects. Discourage alcohol use during therapy.
Heavy smoking: induces imipramine metabolism and decreases therapeutic efficacy. Discourage concomitant use, and encourage smoking cessation.
Sun exposure: photosensitivity reaction may occur. Tell patient to take precautions.

Adverse reactions
CNS: anxiety, ataxia, confusion, *dizziness, drowsiness,* EEG changes, excitation, extrapyramidal reactions, hallucinations, nervousness, paresthesia, **seizures,** tremor.
CV: **arrhythmias, CVA,** *ECG changes,* **heart block, heart failure,** hypertension, **MI,** *orthostatic hypotension, tachycardia.*
EENT: blurred vision, mydriasis, tinnitus.
GI: abdominal cramps, anorexia, *constipation, dry mouth,* nausea, paralytic ileus, vomiting.
GU: altered libido, galactorrhea and breast enlargement (in females), gynecomastia (in males),

impotence, testicular swelling, *urine retention.*
Metabolic: increased or decreased blood glucose.
Skin: *diaphoresis,* photosensitivity, pruritus, rash, urticaria.
Other: *hypersensitivity reaction,* SIADH.

Overdose and treatment

Imipramine overdose is commonly life-threatening, particularly when combined with alcohol. The first 12 hours after acute ingestion are a stimulatory phase characterized by excessive anticholinergic activity, which may include agitation, irritation, confusion, hallucinations, hyperthermia, parkinsonian symptoms, seizures, urine retention, dry mucous membranes, pupil dilation, constipation, and ileus. This phase is followed by CNS depression—including hypothermia, decreased or absent reflexes, sedation, hypotension, and cyanosis—and such cardiac irregularities as tachycardia, conduction disturbances, and quinidine-like effects on the ECG.

Widening of the QRS complex usually indicates a serum level above 1,000 mg/ml. Metabolic acidosis may follow hypotension, hypoventilation, and seizures.

Treatment is symptomatic and supportive, and includes managing the patient's airway, body temperature, and fluid and electrolyte balance. Induce emesis with ipecac if the gag reflex is intact; follow with gastric lavage and activated charcoal to prevent further absorption. Dialysis is of little use.

Don't give quinidine, procainamide, or atropine during an imipramine overdose. Give parenteral diazepam or phenytoin for seizures. Give parenteral phenytoin or lidocaine for arrhythmias. Give sodium bicarbonate for acidosis. Don't give barbiturates; they may increase CNS and respiratory depressant effects.

Special considerations

■ Drug commonly causes orthostatic hypotension. Check patient's seated and standing blood pressures after giving first dose.
■ Tolerance to sedative effects usually develops over several weeks.
■ Don't stop drug abruptly; instead, taper it gradually.
■ Abrupt withdrawal of long-term therapy may cause nausea, headache, and malaise (which doesn't indicate addiction).
■ Discontinue drug at least 48 hours before surgical procedures.
■ I.M. route of administration is rarely used.

Breast-feeding patients

■ Low levels of imipramine are excreted in breast milk. Make sure possible benefits to mother outweigh possible risks to infant.

Pediatric patients

■ Drug may be used to treat nocturnal enuresis in children. Don't use pamoate salt for this purpose.
■ Drug isn't recommended for treating depression in patients under age 12.

Patient teaching

■ Tell patient to take drug exactly as prescribed.

◇ Available in Canada only　　　　　　　　　　　*Unlabeled use

- Explain that full effects of drug may not occur for 4 to 6 weeks after therapy starts.
- Tell patient to take drug with food or milk if it causes stomach upset.
- Suggest using ice chips or sugarless gum or hard candy to relieve a dry mouth. Encourage good dental hygiene because a dry mouth raises the risk of dental caries.
- Caution patient not to drink alcoholic beverages during therapy.
- Warn patient not to stop drug abruptly.
- Encourage patient to report unusual or troublesome effects immediately, including confusion, movement disorders, rapid heartbeat, dizziness, fainting, or difficulty urinating.

---

maprotiline hydrochloride
Ludiomil

Pharmacologic classification:
tetracyclic antidepressant

Therapeutic classification:
antidepressant

Pregnancy risk category B

How supplied
Available by prescription only
Tablets: 25 mg, 50 mg, 75 mg

Indications and dosages
Depression, anxiety with depression
Adults: initially, 75 mg/day P.O. for patients with mild to moderate depression. After 2 weeks, increase p.r.n. by 25-mg increments to 150 mg/day, usually given t.i.d., although it may be given as a single daily dose. Maximum, 225 mg in hospitalized patients.
▶ DOSAGE ADJUSTMENT. Start elderly patients with 25 mg/day; maintenance dosage is 25 to 75 mg/day.

Pharmacodynamics
Antidepressant action: Maprotiline is thought to exert antidepressant effects by inhibiting reuptake of norepinephrine and serotonin in CNS nerve terminals (presynaptic neurons), which results in increases concentration of and enhances activity of these neurotransmitters in the synaptic cleft. Maprotiline has minimal inhibitory effect on serotonin reuptake. Drug also has anxiolytic effects.

Pharmacokinetics
Absorption: Drug is absorbed slowly but completely from the GI tract after oral administration.
Distribution: Maprotiline is distributed widely into the body, including the CNS and breast milk. It is 88% protein-bound. Serum levels peak 8 to 24 hours after an oral dose; steady state plasma levels and peak therapeutic effect usually occur within 2 weeks. Proposed therapeutic serum levels are 200 to 300 ng/ml.
Metabolism: Drug is metabolized slowly by the liver to the active metabolite desmethylmaprotiline; a significant first-pass effect may account for variability of serum levels in different patients taking the same dosage. Drug half-life is 51 hours.
Excretion: Most of drug is excreted in urine as metabolites with 3

---

weeks. About 30% is excreted in feces via the bilary tract.

Contraindications and precautions

Contraindicated during acute recovery phase after MI, within 14 days of taking an MAO inhibitor, and in patients hypersensitive to drug or patients with seizure disorders.

Use cautiously in adolescents, in elderly or debilitated patients, and in patients with suicidal tendencies, increased intraocular pressure, or a history of MI, CV disease, urine retention, or angle-closure glaucoma.

Interactions
Drug-drug

Antiarrhythmics (such as disopyramide, procainamide, quinidine) pimozide, thyroid hormones: may increase the risk of arrhythmias and conduction defects. Monitor patient closely.

Anticholinergics, such as antihistamines, antiparkinsonian drugs, atropine, meperidine, phenothiazines: may cause oversedation, paralytic ileus, visual changes, and severe constipation. Monitor patient closely.

Barbiturates: induces maprotiline metabolism and decreases therapeutic efficacy. Monitor patient for loss of therapeutic effect.

Beta blockers, cimetidine, methylphenidate, oral contraceptives, propoxyphene: may inhibit maprotiline metabolism, increasing plasma levels and toxicity. Monitor patient closely.

Central-acting antihypertensives, such as clonidine, guanabenz, gua-

nadrel, guanethidine, methylopa, reserpine: decreased antihypertensive effects. Monitor patient's blood pressure closely.

CNS depressants, such as analgestics, anesthetics, barbiturates, narcotics, tranquilizers: may cause oversedation. Monitor patient closely.

Disulfiram, ethchlorvynol: increased risk of delirium, tachycardia.

Haloperidol, phenothiazines: decreased maprotiline metabolism and decreased therapeutic efficacy. Use together caustiously.

MAO inhibitors: increased risk of nonfatal hyperpyrexia, hypertension, tachycardia, confusion, and seizures. Use within 14 days of an MAO inhibitor is contraindicated.

Metrizamide: increased risk of seizures. Monitor patient closely.

Phenothiazines: increased risk of seizures. Monitor patient closely.

Sympathomimetics (including ephedrine, epinephrine, phenlephrine, phenlpropanolamine) commonly found in nasal sprays: may increase blood pressure. Monitor patient's blood pressure closely.

Warfarin: may increase PT and risk of bleeding. Monitor serum levels.

Drug-lifestyle

Alcohol use: may cause additive effects. Discourage alcohol use during therapy.

Heavy smoking: induces maprotiline metabolism and decreases therapeutic efficacy. Discourage concomitant use, and encourage smoking cessation.

Adverse reactions

CNS: agitation, anxiety, confusion, *dizziness, drowsiness,* extrapyrami-

dal symptoms, headache, insomnia, nervousness, numbness, *seizures*, tremor, weakness.
CV: *arrhythmias, ECG changes, heart block,* hypertension, *orthostatic hypotension,* syncope, *tachycardia.*
EENT: *blurred vision,* mydriasis, tinnitus.
GI: *constipation,* diarrhea, *dry mouth,* nausea, vomiting.
GU: urine retention.
Skin: *diaphoresis,* photosensitivity, rash, urticaria.
Other: *hypersensitivity reaction.*

Overdose and treatment
The first 12 hours after acute ingestion are a stimulatory phase characterized by excessive anticholinergic activity, which may include agitation, irritation, confusion, hallucinations, hyperthermia, parkinsonian symptoms, seizures, urine retention, dry mucous membranes, pupil dilation, constipation, and ileus. This phase is followed by CNS depression—including hypothermia, decreased or absent reflexes, sedation, hypotension, and cyanosis—and such cardiac irregularities as tachycardia, conduction disturbances, and quinidine-like effects on the ECG.

Widening of the QRS complex usually indicates a serum level above 1,000 mg/ml. Metabolic acidosis may follow hypotension, hypoventilation, and seizures.

Treatment is symptomatic and supportive, and includes managing the patient's airway, body temperature, and fluid and electrolyte balance. Induce emesis with ipecac if the patient is conscious; follow with gastric lavage and activated charcoal to prevent further absorption. Dialysis is of little use.

Give parenteral diazepam or phenytoin for seizures. Give parenteral phenytoin or lidocaine for arrhythmias. Give sodium bicarbonate for acidosis. Don't give barbiturates; they may increase CNS and respiratory depressant effects. Also, don't give group 1 antiarrhythmic drugs.

Special considerations
■ Maprotiline may produce a higher risk of seizures than other tricyclic antidepressants. If patient has an abnormal EEG, watch her closely.
■ To minimize the risk of seizures, keep daily dose below 200 mg.
■ Although rare, hypomania or manic episodes may develop in some patients with cyclic disorders who take maprotiline.
■ Maprotiline may prolong conduction time (elongation of QT and PR intervals, flattened T waves). It also may elevate liver function test results, decrease WBC counts, and decrease or increase serum glucose levels.
■ Abrupt withdrawal of long-term therapy may cause nausea, headache, and malaise (which don't indicate addiction).

Breast-feeding patients
■ Maprotiline appears in breast milk at levels equal to or greater than those in mother's serum. Make sure potential benefits to woman outweighs risks to infant.

Pediatric patients
■ Maprotiline isn't recommended for children under age 18.

Patient teaching
- Tell patient to take drug exactly as prescribed.
- Tell patient not to take the full daily dose at one time, unless directed by prescriber, and not to double up to compensate for a missed dose.
- Explain that full effects of the drug may not occur for up to 4 weeks.
- Warn patient not to stop drug abruptly.
- Caution patient to avoid alcohol during therapy.
- Urge patient to report unusual or troublesome effects immediately, such as confusion, movement disorders, a rapid heartbeat, dizziness, fainting, or difficulty urinating.

mirtazapine
Remeron

Pharmacologic classification:
piperazinoazepine

Therapeutic classification:
tetracyclic antidepressant

Pregnancy risk category C

How supplied
Available by prescription only
Tablets: 15 mg, 30 mg, 45 mg

Indications and dosages
Depression
Adults: initially, 15 mg P.O. h.s. Maintenance dosage ranges from 15 mg to 45 mg daily. Make dosage adjustments no more often than every 1 to 2 weeks.

Pharmacodynamics
Antidepressant action: Mirtazapine is a potent antagonist of 5-HT_2, 5-HT_3, and histamine. It moderately antagonizes muscarinic receptors and peripheral alpha receptors.

Pharmacokinetics
Absorption: Mirtazapine is rapidly and completely absorbed from the GI tract. Absolute bioavailability is about 50%. Plasma levels peak in about 2 hours.
Distribution: About 85% of drug is bound to plasma protein.
Metabolism: Drug is extensively metabolized in the liver.
Excretion: Drug is predominantly eliminated in urine (75%) with 15% excreted in feces. Half-life is between 20 and 40 hours.

Contraindications and precautions
Contraindicated in patients hypersensitive to drug and patients who have taken an MAO inhibitor within 14 days of mirtazapine.
  Use cautiously in patients with CV or cerebrovascular disease, seizure disorders, suicidal ideation, impaired hepatic or renal function, increased intraocular pressure, or a history of mania, hypomania, urine retention, or angle-closure glaucoma. Also, use cautiously in patients with conditions that predispose them to hypotension, such as dehydration, hypovolemia, or antihypertensive therapy.

Interactions
Drug-drug
Diazepam, other CNS depressants: may cause additive CNS effects. Avoid concomitant use.

MAO inhibitors: may cause life-threatening interaction. Don't administer mirtazapine within 14 days of an MAO inhibitor.

Drug-lifestyle
Alcohol use: may cause additive CNS effects. Discourage alcohol use.

Adverse reactions
CNS: abnormal dreams, abnormal thinking, asthenia, confusion, dizziness, *seizures, somnolence,* tremor.
CV: edema, peripheral edema.
GI: *constipation, dry mouth, increased appetite,* nausea.
GU: urinary frequency.
Hematologic: *agranulocytosis.*
Hepatic: increased cholesterol, triglyceride, and ALT serum levels.
Metabolic: *weight gain.*
Musculoskeletal: back pain, myalgia.
Respiratory: dyspnea.
Other: flulike syndrome.

Overdose and treatment
Overdose may cause disorientation, drowsiness, impaired memory, and tachycardia.

Treatment resembles that used for any antidepressant overdose. If patient is unconscious, establish an airway and provide adequate oxygenation. Perform gastric lavage, induce emesis, or use both procedures if needed. Consider activated charcoal as well. Monitor patient's cardiac and vital signs, and provide general symptomatic and supportive measures.

Special considerations
■ Monitor patient closely during therapy because no data are available to show whether drug causes physical or psychological dependence.
■ Monitor patient's liver function tests because drug may increase cholesterol, triglycerides, and ALT levels.
■ Although agranulocytosis is a rare adverse effect, watch for evidence of it (sore throat, fever, stomatitis, or other signs of infection together with a low WBC count) and discontinue drug as needed.

Breast-feeding patients
■ Use cautiously in breast-feeding women because no data are available to show whether it appears in breast milk.

Pediatric patients
■ Safety and effectiveness in children haven't been established.

Geriatric patients
■ Elderly patients have decreased drug clearance.

Patient teaching
■ Urge patient to take drug exactly as prescribed.
■ Caution patient to avoid hazardous activities if drug causes somnolence.
■ Urge patient to avoid alcohol and other CNS depressants during therapy because of their additive effects.
■ Caution patient not to take any other prescribed drugs, OTC medications, or herbal remedies without consulting prescriber.

Reactions may be *common,* uncommon, *life-threatening,* or COMMON AND LIFE-THREATENING.

- Tell patient to report signs and symptoms of infection, such as fever, chills, sore throat, flulike symptoms, mucous membrane ulceration, or other possible signs of infection.
- Tell women to immediately report planned, suspected, or known pregnancy.

nefazodone hydrochloride
Serzone

Pharmacologic classification:
phenylpiperazine

Therapeutic classification:
antidepressant

Pregnancy risk category C

How supplied
Available by prescription only
Tablets: 100 mg, 150 mg, 200 mg, 250 mg

Indications and dosages
Depression
Adults: initially, 200 mg/day P.O. divided into two doses. Increase in 100- to 200-mg/day increments at intervals of no less than 1 week, p.r.n. Usual range, 300 to 600 mg/day.
▶ DOSAGE ADJUSTMENT. For elderly patients, start with 100 mg/day P.O. divided into two doses and increase over the standard dosage range used for younger adults.

Pharmacodynamics
Antidepressant action: Drug action isn't precisely defined. It inhibits neuronal uptake of serotonin and norepinephrine. It also occupies central 5-HT (serotonin) and alpha-adrenergic receptors.

Pharmacokinetics
Absorption: Nefazodone is rapidly and completely absorbed but, because of extensive metabolism, its absolute bioavailability is only about 20%.
Distribution: Drug is widely distributed in body tissues, including the CNS. More than 99% of drug is bound to plasma proteins.
Metabolism: Drug is extensively metabolized by n-dealkylation and aliphatic and aromatic hydroxylation.
Excretion: Nefazodone and its metabolites are excreted in urine. Half-life of drug is 2 to 4 hours.

Contraindications and precautions
Contraindicated in patients with hypersensitivity to drug or other phenylpiperazine antidepressants. Don't use within 14 days of MAO inhibitor therapy or together with pimozide or cisapride.

Use cautiously in patients with CV or cerebrovascular disease that could be worsened by hypotension (such as MI, angina, or CVA) and conditions that predispose patients to hypotension (such as dehydration, hypovolemia, and antihypertensive drug therapy). Also, use cautiously in patients with a history of mania.

Interactions
Drug-drug
Alprazolam, triazolam: nefazodone potentiates the effects of these drugs. Avoid concurrent administration if possible. If not, dosage of

alprazolam or triazolam may need pronounced reduction.

Cisapride, pimozide: may cause decreased metabolism of these drugs, leading to increased levels and cardiotoxicity. Avoid giving together.

CNS-active drugs: may alter CNS activity. Use together cautiously.

Digoxin: may increase digoxin level. Use together cautiously, and monitor patient's digoxin levels.

MAO inhibitors: may cause severe excitation, hyperpyrexia, seizures, delirium, or coma. Avoid concomitant use.

Highly plasma-protein-bound drugs: may increase occurrence and severity of adverse reactions. Monitor patient closely.

Drug-food
Any food: decreases absorption. Give drug on empty stomach.

Adverse reactions
CNS: abnormal dreams, *asthenia,* ataxia, *confusion,* decreased concentration, *dizziness, headache,* hypertonia, incoordination, insomnia, *light-headedness,* memory impairment, paresthesia, psychomotor retardation, *somnolence,* tremor.
CV: hypotension, orthostatic hypotension, peripheral edema, vasodilation.
EENT: *abnormal vision, blurred vision,* pharyngitis, taste perversion, tinnitus, visual field defect.
GI: *constipation,* diarrhea, *dry mouth,* dyspepsia, increased appetite, *nausea,* thirst, vomiting.
GU: urinary frequency, urinary tract infection, urine retention, vaginitis.

Musculoskeletal: arthralgia, neck rigidity.
Respiratory: cough.
Skin: pruritus, rash.
Other: breast pain, chills, fever, flu-like syndrome, infection.

Overdose and treatment
Overdose may cause nausea, vomiting, and somnolence. Other drug-related adverse reactions may occur as well.

Provide symptomatic and supportive treatment if patient develops hypotension or excessive sedation. Perform gastric lavage if needed.

Special considerations
■ Record patient's mood changes during therapy. Monitor patient for suicidal tendencies, and provide a minimum supply of drug.
■ Monitor liver function test results if patient has evidence of possible hepatic dysfunction (nausea, vomiting, abdominal pain, dark urine).
■ Wait at least 1 week after stopping nefazodone before giving an MAO inhibitor. Wait at least 14 days after stopping an MAO inhibitor before giving nefazodone.

Breast-feeding patients
■ Use caution when giving drug to breast-feeding women because no data are available to document drug excretion into breast milk.

Pediatric patients
■ Safety and effectiveness in children under age 18 haven't been established.

Reactions may be *common,* uncommon, *life-threatening,* or COMMON AND LIFE-THREATENING.

Geriatric patients
■ Observe usual precautions in elderly patients who have ongoing medical illnesses or are receiving other drugs.

Patient teaching
■ Inform patient that full antidepressant effect may take several weeks to occur. Advise patient to keep taking drug, as prescribed, even after she feels better.
■ Instruct patient not to drink alcoholic beverages during therapy.
■ Warn patient to avoid hazardous activities until full effects of drug are clear.
■ Tell patient to report rash, hives, or any related allergic reaction.
■ Instruct male patient to stop drug immediately and to seek medical attention if he develops prolonged or inappropriate erections.
■ Instruct women to report planned, suspected, or known pregnancy.

nortriptyline hydrochloride
Aventyl, Pamelor

Pharmacologic classification: tricyclic antidepressant

Therapeutic classification: antidepressant

Pregnancy risk category D

How supplied
Available by prescription only
Capsules: 10 mg, 25 mg, 50 mg, 75 mg
Solution: 10 mg/5 ml (4% alcohol)

Indications and dosages
Depression, panic disorder*
Adults: 25 mg P.O. t.i.d. or q.i.d., gradually increasing to a maximum of 150 mg/day. Alternatively, entire dose may be given h.s.
▶ DOSAGE ADJUSTMENT. For elderly or adolescent patients, give 30 to 50 mg P.O., in divided doses as needed.

Analgesia (adjunct) for phantom limb pain and chronic pain caused by migraine, chronic tension headache, diabetic neuropathy, tic douloureux, cancer, peripheral neuropathy, postherpetic neuralgia, arthritis*
Adults: 50 to 150 mg P.O. daily.

Premenstrual syndrome*
Adults: 50 to 125 mg P.O. daily.

Dermatologic disorders (chronic urticaria and angioedema, nocturnal pruritus in atopic eczema)*
Adults: 20 to 75 mg P.O. daily.

Pharmacodynamics
Antidepressant action: Drug inhibits reuptake of norepinephrine and serotonin in CNS nerve terminals (presynaptic neurons), which yields increased levels and enhanced activity of these neurotransmitters in the synaptic cleft. Drug inhibits reuptake of serotonin more actively than norepinephrine; it is less likely than other tricyclic antidepressants to cause orthostatic hypotension.

Pharmacokinetics
Absorption: Drug is absorbed rapidly from the GI tract after oral administration.

Distribution: Drug is distributed widely into the body, including the CNS and breast milk. It is 95% protein-bound. Plasma levels peak within 8 hours after giving a dose; steady state serum levels occur in 2 to 4 weeks. Therapeutic serum level ranges from 50 to 150 ng/ml.

Metabolism: Drug is metabolized by the liver. A significant first-pass effect may account for the variability of serum levels in different patients who take the same dosage.

Excretion: Drug is mostly excreted in urine. Some is excreted in feces via the biliary tract.

Contraindications and precautions
Contraindicated in patients hypersensitive to drug, in patients who have taken an MAO inhibitor within 14 days, and in patients in the acute recovery period after an MI.

Use cautiously in patients with a history of urine retention, seizures, glaucoma, suicidal tendencies, CV disease, or hyperthyroidism and in those receiving thyroid hormones.

Interactions
Drug-drug
Antiarrhythmics (such as disopyramide, procainamide, quinidine), grepafloxacin, pimozide, quinolones, thyroid hormones: may increase risk of cardiac arrhythmias and conduction defects. Use together with extreme caution.

Anticholinergic drugs, such as antihistamines, antiparkinsonian drugs, atropine, meperidine, phenothiazines: may cause oversedation, paralytic ileus, visual changes, and severe constipation. Monitor patient closely.

Barbiturates: may induce nortriptyline metabolism and decrease therapeutic efficacy. Monitor patient for loss of therapeutic effect.

Beta blockers, bupropion, cimetidine, H_2 blockers, methylphenidate, oral contraceptives, propoxyphene, selective serotonin reuptake inhibitors, valproic acid: may inhibit nortriptyline metabolism, increasing plasma levels and toxicity. Monitor patient and serum levels closely.

Carbamazepine: nortriptyline levels may decrease and carbamazepine levels may increase. Monitor patient closely.

Central-acting antihypertensives, such as clonidine, guanabenz, guanadrel, guanethidine, methyldopa, reserpine: decreased antihypertensive effects. Monitor patient and blood pressure closely.

CNS depressants, including analgesics, anesthetics, barbiturates, narcotics, tranquilizers: may cause oversedation. Use together cautiously.

Disulfiram, ethchlorvynol: may cause delirium and tachycardia. Avoid concomitant use.

Haloperidol, phenothiazines: decreased nortriptyline metabolism and increased risk of toxicity. Monitor patient and serum levels closely.

Metrizamide: additive effects likely, increasing the risk of seizures and other adverse effects. Monitor patient closely.

Rifampicin: may decrease nortriptyline levels. Monitor patient for decreased effectiveness.
Sympathomimetics (including ephedrine, epinephrine, phenylephrine, phenylpropanolamine,) commonly found in nasal sprays: may increase blood pressure.
Warfarin: may increase PT, INR, and the risk of bleeding. Monitor patient closely.

Drug-lifestyle
Alcohol use: may enhance CNS depression. Discourage use together.
Heavy smoking: induces nortriptyline metabolism and decreases efficacy. Discourage concomitant use, and encourage smoking cessation.

Adverse reactions
CNS: agitation, ataxia, confusion, *dizziness, drowsiness,* EEG changes, extrapyramidal reactions, hallucinations, headache, insomnia, nervousness, nightmares, paresthesia, *seizures,* tremor, weakness.
CV: *CVA, heart block,* hypertension, hypotension, *MI,* prolonged conduction time causing elongation of QT and PR intervals or flattened T waves, *tachycardia.*
EENT: *blurred vision,* mydriasis, tinnitus.
GI: anorexia, *constipation,* dry mouth, nausea, paralytic ileus, vomiting.
GU: *urine retention.*
Hematologic: *agranulocytosis,* bone marrow depression, eosinophilia, *thrombocytopenia.*
Hepatic: elevated liver function test results.
Metabolic: increased serum glucose levels.

Skin: diaphoresis, photosensitivity, rash, urticaria.
Other: *hypersensitivity reaction.*

Overdose and treatment
The first 12 hours after acute ingestion are a stimulatory phase characterized by excessive anticholinergic activity, which may include agitation, irritation, confusion, hallucinations, hyperthermia, parkinsonian symptoms, seizures, urine retention, dry mucous membranes, pupil dilation, constipation, and ileus. This phase is followed by CNS depression—including hypothermia, decreased or absent reflexes, sedation, hypotension, and cyanosis—and such cardiac irregularities as tachycardia, conduction disturbances, and quinidine-like effects on the ECG.

Widening of the QRS complex usually indicates a serum level above 1,000 mg/ml. Metabolic acidosis may follow hypotension, hypoventilation, and seizures.

Treatment is symptomatic and supportive and includes managing the patient's airway, body temperature, and fluid and electrolyte balance. Induce emesis with ipecac if the patient is conscious; follow with gastric lavage and activated charcoal to prevent further absorption. Dialysis is usually ineffective.

Consider giving physostigmine or cardiac glycosides if patient has serious CV abnormalities or cardiac failure. Give parenteral diazepam or phenytoin for seizures. Give parenteral phenytoin or lidocaine for arrhythmias. Give sodium bicarbonate for acidosis. Don't give quinidine, procainamide, or disopyramide for arrhythmias because they may further depress myocardial conduction and contractility. Don't give barbiturates either; they may increase CNS and respiratory depressant effects.

Special considerations
- Drug is available in liquid form.
- To reduce daytime sedation, give drug at bedtime. Tolerance to sedative effects usually develops during first few weeks of therapy.
- Monitor plasma drug levels if patient receives more than 100 mg/day to ensure a level between 50 and 150 ng/ml.
- Check patient's WBC, CBC, and liver function test results periodically.
- Nortriptyline is less likely than other tricyclic antidepressants to cause hypotension.
- If patient has bipolar disorder, expect nortriptyline to raise the risk of manic symptoms.
- Stopping drug abruptly after long-term therapy may cause nausea, headache, and malaise (which don't indicate addiction). Withdraw drug gradually over a few weeks.
- Stop therapy at least 48 hours before surgical procedures.

Breast-feeding patients
- Low levels of nortriptyline are excreted into breast milk; make sure benefits to mother outweigh risks to infant.

Pediatric patients
- Drug is not recommended for children.

Geriatric patients
- Elderly patients have an increased risk of adverse cardiac effects and may benefit from reduced dosages.

Patient teaching
- Tell patient to take full daily dose at bedtime to minimize daytime sedation.
- Explain that drug's full antidepressant effect may take up to 4 weeks to occur.
- To minimize dizziness early in therapy, recommend that patient lie down for about 30 minutes and avoid sudden position changes after each dose.
- Suggest using sugarless gum or hard candy to relieve dry mouth.
- Caution patient to avoid hazardous activities until drug's full effects are clear.
- Tell patient to avoid alcohol during therapy.
- Caution against doubling up after missing a dose. Also, warn against stopping drug abruptly without consulting prescriber.
- Instruct patient to report development of a sore throat or fever, which may be evidence of neutrophil depression.
- Urge patient to report unusual reactions promptly, such as confusion, movement disorders, fainting, a rapid heartbeat, or difficulty urinating.
- Advise women to use effective contraception during therapy and to notify prescriber about planned, suspected, or known pregnancy.

Reactions may be *common,* uncommon, *life-threatening,* or COMMON AND LIFE-THREATENING.

paroxetine hydrochloride
Paxil, Paxil CR

Pharmacologic classification: selective serotonin reuptake inhibitor

Therapeutic classification: antidepressant

Pregnancy risk category C

How supplied
Available by prescription only
Suspension: 10 mg/5ml
Tablets: 10 mg, 20 mg, 30 mg, 40 mg
Tablets (controlled-release): 12.5 mg, 25 mg

Indications and dosages
Depression
Adults: initially, 20 mg P.O. daily, preferably in the morning. Increase by 10 mg/day at 1-week intervals to a maximum of 50 mg daily, if needed. For controlled-release form, 25 mg P.O. daily in the morning. If patient fails to respond, increase by 12.5 mg daily at 1-week intervals to a maximum of 62.5 mg daily.

Obsessive-compulsive disorder
Adults: initially, 20 mg P.O. daily, preferably in the morning. Increase by 10 mg/day at 1-week intervals to a target dose of 40 mg/day. Maximum, 60 mg/day.

Social anxiety disorder
Adults: initially, 20 mg P.O. daily in the morning. Usual range is 20 to 60 mg daily. Maintain the lowest effective dose.

Panic disorder
Adults: initially, 10 mg P.O. daily, preferably in the morning. Increase by 10 mg/day at 1-week intervals to a target dose of 40 mg/day. Maximum, 60 mg/day.

▶ **DOSAGE ADJUSTMENT.** For elderly or debilitated patients or patients with severe hepatic or renal disease, start with 10 mg P.O. daily, preferably in the morning. Increase by 10 mg/day at 1-week intervals, p.r.n., to a maximum of 40 mg/day.

Diabetic neuropathy*
Adults: 10 to 60 mg P.O. daily.

Headaches*
Adults: 10 to 50 mg P.O. daily.

Premature ejaculation*
Adults: 20 mg P.O. daily.

Pharmacodynamics
Antidepressant action: Drug inhibits neuronal uptake of serotonin, which potentiates serotonergic activity in the CNS.

Pharmacokinetics
Absorption: Paroxetine is completely absorbed after oral dosing.
Distribution: Drug is distributed throughout the body, including the CNS, with only 1% remaining in plasma. About 93% to 95% of paroxetine is bound to plasma protein.
Metabolism: About 36% of drug is metabolized in the liver. The principal metabolites are polar and conjugated products of oxidation and methylation, which are readily cleared.

◊ Available in Canada only   *Unlabeled use

Excretion: About 64% is excreted in urine (2% as parent compound and 62% as metabolite).

Contraindications and precautions

Contraindicated within 14 days of taking an MAO inhibitor.

Use cautiously in patients with a history of seizures or mania; in patients with severe, concurrent systemic illness; in patients at risk for volume depletion; and in patients hypersensitive to selective serotonin reuptake inhibitors.

Interactions
Drug-drug

Cimetidine: decreases hepatic metabolism of paroxetine, increasing risk of toxicity. Dosage adjustments may be needed.

Digoxin: may decrease digoxin levels. Monitor patient and serum digoxin levels closely.

MAO inhibitors: may increase the risk of serious, possibly fatal, adverse reactions. Concomitant use is contraindicated.

Phenobarbital: induces paroxetine metabolism, thereby reducing plasma drug levels. Monitor plasma levels closely.

Phenytoin: may alter phenytoin pharmacokinetics. Dosage adjustment may be needed.

Procyclidine: may increase procyclidine levels. Monitor patient for excessive anticholinergic effects.

Phenothiazine, theophylline: may increase levels of these drugs. Monitor patient closely.

Drug-herb
St. John's wort: may cause sedative-hypnotic intoxication. Avoid concomitant use.

Drug-food
Tryptophan: may increase the risk of adverse reactions, such as diaphoresis, headache, nausea, and dizziness. Avoid using together.
Warfarin: risk of bleeding may increase. Monitor patient's INR.

Drug-lifestyle
Alcohol use: may increase risk of CNS adverse effects. Discourage alcohol use during treatment.
Sunlight: photosensitivity may occur. Recommend precautions.

Adverse reactions
CNS: abnormal dreams, agitation, anxiety, confusion, *dizziness, headache, insomnia, nervousness,* paresthesia, *somnolence, tremor.*
CV: chest pain, orthostatic hypotension, palpitations, vasodilation.
EENT: double vision, dysgeusia, lump or tightness in throat, visual disturbances.
GI: abdominal pain, *constipation, diarrhea, dry mouth,* dyspepsia, flatulence, increased or decreased appetite, *nausea,* vomiting.
GU: decreased libido, ejaculatory disturbances, female genital disorders (including anorgasmia, difficulty with orgasm), male genital disorders (including anorgasmia, erectile difficulties, delayed ejaculation or orgasm, impotence, and sexual dysfunction), urinary frequency and other urinary disorders.

Reactions may be *common,* uncommon, *life-threatening,* or COMMON AND LIFE-THREATENING.

Musculoskeletal: *asthenia,* myalgia, myasthenia, myopathy.
Skin: *diaphoresis,* pruritus, rash.
Other: yawning.

Overdose and treatment
Overdose may cause nausea, vomiting, dizziness, sweating, facial flushing, drowsiness, sinus tachycardia, and dilated pupils.

Treatment includes induced emesis, gastric lavage, or both. Consider also giving 20 to 30 g of activated charcoal every 4 to 6 hours for the first 24 to 48 hours after ingestion. Also, provide supportive care, frequent monitoring of vital signs, and careful observation. Any evidence of abnormality warrants monitoring of patient's ECG and cardiac function.

Use special caution if patient's overdose involves paroxetine and an excessive amount of a tricyclic antidepressant. Accumulation of the parent tricyclic and its active metabolite may increase the risk of adverse effects and extend the time during which the patient needs close medical observation.

Special considerations
■ Hyponatremia may occur, especially in elderly patients, those who take diuretics, and those who are volume depleted. Monitor patient's serum sodium levels.
■ If signs of psychosis occur or increase, reduce dosage. Monitor patient for suicidal tendencies, and provide only a minimum supply of drug.
■ Drug may not be effective for treating social anxiety disorder or panic disorder for more than 12 weeks. If patient continues to respond, however, treatment may continue. Periodically reassess patient to reevaluate treatment.
■ Wait at least 14 days after giving an MAO inhibitor before giving paroxetine. Also, wait at least 14 days after giving paroxetine before giving an MAO inhibitor.

Breast-feeding patients
■ Paroxetine appears in breast milk. Either stop breast-feeding during therapy or stop therapy during breast-feeding.

Patient teaching
■ Explain that symptoms typically improve in 1 to 4 weeks, but that patient should continue taking drug as prescribed, even after she feels better.
■ Warn patient not to chew, crush, or cut controlled-release tablets.
■ Urge patient to avoid alcohol.
■ Tell patient to avoid hazardous tasks until drug effects are clear.
■ Tell patient not to take other prescribed drugs, OTC medications, or herbal remedies during therapy without consulting the prescriber.

phenelzine sulfate
Nardil

Pharmacologic classification: MAO inhibitor

Therapeutic classification: antidepressant

Pregnancy risk category C

How supplied
Available by prescription only
Tablets: 15 mg

Indications and dosages
Severe depression
Adults: 15 mg P.O. t.i.d. Increase rapidly to 60 mg/day. Maximum daily dose, 90 mg. Onset of maximum therapeutic effect, 2 to 6 weeks. Some clinicians reduce dosage after response occurs. Maintenance dosage may be as low as 15 mg daily or every other day.

Post-traumatic stress disorder*
Adults: 60 to 75 mg P.O. daily.

Pharmacodynamics
Antidepressant action: Phenelzine inhibits MAO, an enzyme that normally inactivates amine-containing substances, such as the neurotransmitters norepinephrine and serotonin. By inhibiting MAO, phenelzine increases neurotransmitter levels and activity, thus helping to relieve depression.

Pharmacokinetics
Absorption: Drug is absorbed rapidly and completely from the GI tract.
Distribution: Unknown.
Metabolism: Drug is metabolized in the liver.
Excretion: Drug is excreted primarily in urine within 24 hours; some drug is excreted in feces via the biliary tract. Half-life is relatively short, but enzyme inhibition is prolonged and unrelated to half-life.

Contraindications and precautions
Contraindicated in patients hypersensitive to drug and in patients with heart failure, pheochromocytoma, hypertension, liver disease, and CV disease. Also contraindicated within 10 days of therapy with other MAO inhibitors (such as isocarboxazid, tranylcypromine) or within 10 days of taking cocaine, receiving local anesthesia that contains sympathomimetic vasoconstrictors, or undergoing elective surgery that requires general anesthesia. Contraindicated within 2 weeks of taking a selective serotonin reuptake inhibitor or during therapy with bupropion. Contraindicated by some manufacturers in patients over age 60 because of the possibility of cerebrosclerosis with damaged vessels.

Use cautiously in patients at risk for diabetes, suicide, or seizures disorders and in those receiving thiazide diuretics or spinal anesthesics.

Interactions
Drug-drug
Barbiturates, beta blockers, dextromethorphan, narcotics, sedatives, tricyclic antidepressants: use cautiously and give reduced dosages.
Disulfiram: may cause tachycardia, flushing, or palpitations. Monitor patient closely.
General or spinal anesthetics normally metabolized by MAO: may cause severe hypotension and excessive CNS depression. Monitor patient closely.
Insulin, sulfonylureas: hypoglycemic effects may be increased. Dosage adjustments may be necessary.
Local anesthetics (lidocaine, procaine): phenelzine decreases effectiveness, resulting in poor nerve

block. Discontinue phenelzine for at least 1 week before giving these drugs.

OTC cold, hay fever, and weight-loss products that contain amphetamines, dextromethorphan, ephedrine, phenylephrine, phenylpropanolamine: phenelzine enhances pressor effects and may result in serious CV toxicity. Avoid concomitant use.

Serotonergic drugs (fluoxetine, fluvoxamine, paroxetine, sertraline): may cause serious adverse effects. Wait at least 2 weeks between drugs.

Drug-herb

Ginseng, St. John's wort: increased risk of adverse reactions, including headache, tremors, mania. Avoid concomitant use.

Cacao: may potentiate vasopressor effects. Avoid concomitant use.

Drug-food

Foods high in caffeine, tryptophan, tyramine: may precipitate hypertensive crisis. Avoid concomitant use.

Drug-lifestyle

Alcohol use: many forms contain tyramine (beer, red wine, distilled spirits) and may precipitate hypertensive crisis. Avoid concomitant use.

Adverse reactions

CNS: *dizziness,* drowsiness, fatigue, headache, hyperreflexia, *insomnia,* muscle twitching, vertigo, tremor, weakness.

CV: edema, orthostatic hypotension.

GI: *anorexia,* constipation, dry mouth, nausea.

GU: sexual disturbances.

Metabolic: weight gain.

Skin: diaphoresis.

Overdose and treatment

Overdose may exacerbate adverse reactions or cause exaggerated responses to normal pharmacologic activity. Symptoms become apparent slowly (over 24 to 48 hours) and may persist for up to 2 weeks. They may include agitation, flushing, tachycardia, hypotension, hypertension, palpitations, increased motor activity, twitching, increased deep tendon reflexes, seizures, hyperpyrexia, cardiorespiratory arrest, and coma. Doses of 375 mg to 1.5 g have been ingested with fatal and nonfatal results.

Induce vomiting or perform gastric lavage with charcoal slurry early in the overdose. Treat symptomatically and supportively. Give 5 to 10 mg phentolamine I.V. push for hypertensive crisis. Give I.V. diazepam to treat seizures, agitation, and tremors. Give beta blockers to treat tachycardia. Use cooling blankets for fever. Monitor patient's vital signs and fluid and electrolyte balance. Don't give sympathomimetics (such as norepinephrine or phenylephrine) in hypotension caused by MAO inhibitors.

Special considerations

■ Use caution when giving any drugs within 14 days of MAO inhibitor therapy.

■ Consider the patient to have some risk of suicide until depression improves significantly. Supervise high-risk patients closely

early in therapy. To reduce the risk of intentional overdose, provide the smallest quantity of drug consistent with good management.
■ To minimize dizziness from orthostatic hypotension, have patient lie down and avoid sudden position changes for 1 hour after taking phenelzine at the start of therapy.
■ Phenelzine therapy elevates liver function test results and urinary catecholamine levels, and it may elevate WBC count.
■ Drug is rarely used as first-line treatment, but it may be appropriate for treatment-resistant patients.
■ Unlike with other MAO inhibitors, combination therapy with phenelzine and tricyclic antidepressants is usually well tolerated.

Pediatric patients
■ Drug isn't recommended for use in patients under age 16.

Geriatric patients
■ Drug isn't recommended for use in patients over age 60.

Patient teaching
■ Instruct patient to take drug exactly as prescribed and not to double up to compensate for a missed dose.
■ Suggest taking drug at bedtime to minimize daytime sedation.
■ Warn patient about the possibility of dizziness and falls.
■ Tell patient to avoid alcohol, other CNS depressants, or self-prescribed medications (such as cold, hay fever, or diet preparations) or herbal remedies without consulting prescriber.
■ Explain that many foods and beverages (such as wine, beer,

cheeses, preserved fruits, meats, and vegetables) may interact with drug. If possible, obtain a list of foods to avoid from a hospital dietary department or pharmacy.
■ Tell patient to avoid hazardous tasks until drug's effects are clear.
■ Instruct patient to report problems or adverse effects because dosage may need to be reduced.
■ Caution patient not to discontinue drug abruptly.
■ Urge women to use effective contraception and to report planned, suspected, or known pregnancy.

---

protriptyline hydrochloride
Triptil, Vivactil

Pharmacologic classification:
tricyclic antidepressant

Therapeutic classification:
antidepressant

Pregnancy risk category C

How supplied
Available by prescription only
Tablets: 5 mg, 10 mg

Indications and dosages
Depression
Adults: 15 to 40 mg P.O. daily in divided doses, increasing gradually to a maximum of 60 mg/day.
▶ DOSAGE ADJUSTMENT. For elderly and adolescent patients, start with 5 mg P.O. t.i.d.

Pharmacodynamics
Antidepressant action: Protriptyline is thought to exert antidepressant effects by inhibiting reuptake of

norepinephrine and serotonin in CNS nerve terminals (presynaptic neurons), which increases concentrations of these neurotransmitters in the synaptic cleft. Protriptyline inhibits reuptake of serotonin and norepinephrine equally. It stimulates the CNS and may be most useful in treating withdrawn, depressed patients.

Pharmacokinetics

Absorption: Protriptyline is absorbed slowly from the GI tract after oral administration. Plasma levels peak in 24 to 30 hours. Steady state plasma levels and peak therapeutic effects occur within 2 weeks.

Distribution: Drug is distributed widely into the body and is 90% protein-bound. Proposed therapeutic levels range from 70 to 170 ng/ml.

Metabolism: Protriptyline is metabolized by the liver. A significant first-pass effect may account for variability of serum levels in different patients taking the same dosage.

Excretion: Most of drug is excreted slowly in urine; some is excreted in feces via the biliary tract. About 50% of dose is excreted as metabolites within 16 days.

Contraindications and precautions

Contraindicated during acute recovery phase after MI, within 14 days of taking an MAO inhibitor, and in patients hypersensitive to drug or patients with seizure disorders.

Use cautiously in adolescents, in elderly or debilitated patients, in patients who take thyroid medication, and in patients with suicidal tendencies, increased intraocular pressure, CV disorders, urine retention, or hyperthyroidism.

Interactions
Drug-drug

Antiarrhythmics (such as disopyramide, procainamide, quindine) pimozide, thyroid hormones: may increase risk of arrhythmias and conduction defects. Monitor patient closely.

Anticholinergics, such as antihistamines, antiparkinsonian drugs, atropine, meperidine, phenothiazines: may cause oversedation, paralytic ileus, visual changes, and severe constipation. Monitor patient closely.

Barbiturates: induces maprotiline metabolism and decreases therapeutic efficacy. Monitor patient for loss of therapeutic effect.

Beta blockers, cimetidine, methylphenidate, oral contraceptives, propoxyphene: may inhibit maprotiline metabolism, increasing plasma levels and toxicity. Monitor patient closely.

Central-acting antihypertensives, such as clonidine, guanabenz, guanadrel, guanethidine, methylopa, reserpine: decreased antihypertensive effects. Monitor patient's blood pressure closely.

CNS depressants, such as analgestics, anesthetics, barbiturates, narcotics, tranquilizers: may cause oversedation. Monitor patient closely.

Disulfiram, ethchlorvynol: increased risk of delirium.

Haloperidol, phenothiazines: decreased maprotiline metabolism

---

and decreased therapeutic efficacy. Use together caustiously.
Metrizamide: increased risk of seizures. Monitor patient closely.
Sympathomimetics (including ephedrine, epinephrine, phenlephrine, phenlpropanolamine) commonly found in nasal sprays: may increase blood pressure. Monitor patient's blood pressure closely
Warfarin: may increase PT and risk of bleeding. Monitor serum levels.

Drug-lifestyle
Alcohol use: may cause additive effects. Discourage alcohol use during therapy.
Heavy smoking: induces maprotiline metabolism and decreases therapeutic efficacy. Discourage concomitant use, and encourage smoking cessation.

Adverse reactions
CNS: anxiety, ataxia, confusion, disorientation, dizziness, EEG changes, extrapyramidal symptoms, hallucinations, headache, insomnia, nervousness, paresthesia, restlessness, *seizures,* tremor, weakness.
CV: *arrhythmias, CVA, heart block,* hypertension, *MI,* orthostatic hypotension, *tachycardia.*
EENT: *blurred vision,* mydriasis, tinnitus.
GI: anorexia, constipation, *dry mouth,* nausea, paralytic ileus, vomiting.
GU: *urine retention.*
Skin: *diaphoresis,* photosensitivity, rash, urticaria.
Other: *hypersensitivity reaction.*

Overdose and treatment
The first 12 hours after acute ingestion are a stimulatory phase characterized by excessive anticholinergic activity, which may include agitation, irritation, confusion, hallucinations, hyperthermia, parkinsonian symptoms, seizures, urine retention, dry mucous membranes, pupil dilation, constipation, and ileus. This phase is followed by CNS depression—including hypothermia, decreased or absent reflexes, sedation, hypotension, and cyanosis—and such cardiac irregularities as tachycardia, conduction disturbances, and quinidine-like effects on the ECG.

Widening of the QRS complex usually indicates a serum level above 1,000 mg/ml (serum levels aren't usually helpful). Metabolic acidosis may follow hypotension, hypoventilation, and seizures.

Treatment is symptomatic and supportive, and includes managing the patient's airway, body temperature, and fluid and electrolyte balance. Induce emesis with ipecac if the patient is conscious; follow with gastric lavage and activated charcoal to prevent further absorption. Dialysis is of little use.

Give parenteral diazepam or phenytoin for seizures. Give parenteral phenytoin or lidocaine for arrhythmias. Give sodium bicarbonate for acidosis. Don't give barbiturates; they may increase CNS and respiratory depressant effects.

Special considerations
■ Consider the patient to have some risk of suicide until depression improves significantly.

Supervise high-risk patients closely early in therapy. To reduce the risk of intentional overdose, provide the smallest quantity of drug consistent with good management.
■ Protriptyline stimulates the CNS and may be better suited for withdrawn patients. It also has a weaker sedative effect and a lower risk of orthostatic hypotension.
■ If patient has manic-depressive psychosis, anticipate that drug may promote a shift toward the manic phase.
■ Give ice chips or sugarless chewing gum or hard candy to ease a dry mouth.
■ Drug may prolong conduction time (elongated QT and PR intervals, flattened T waves). It also may elevate liver enzyme levels, decrease WBC counts, and decrease or increase serum glucose levels.
■ Don't withdraw drug abruptly; instead, withdraw it gradually over a few weeks.
■ Abrupt withdrawal of long-term therapy may cause nausea, headache, and malaise (which don't indicate addiction).
■ Discontinue drug at least 48 hours before surgical procedures.

Breast-feeding patients
■ Protriptyline may be excreted in breast milk. Make sure potential benefits to mother outweigh possible risk to the infant.

Pediatric patients
Protriptyline is not recommended for children under age 12.

Geriatric patients
■ Elderly patients are more sensitive to therapeutic effects and more prone to adverse cardiac effects.
■ Monitor CV status closely in elderly patients who take more than 20 mg/day.

Patient teaching
■ Tell patient to take drug exactly as prescribed. Caution against double dosing to compensate for a missed dose.
■ Suggest taking drug with food or milk if it causes stomach upset.
■ To prevent dizziness or fainting at the start of therapy, tell patient to lie down for about 30 minutes after taking each dose and to avoid sudden postural changes, especially when rising to an upright position.
■ Explain that full drug effects may take up to 4 weeks to occur, possibly longer.
■ Explain that drug may cause stimulation or dizziness. Caution against hazardous activities until full effects of drug are known.
■ Urge patient to avoid alcohol during therapy.
■ Suggest using ice chips or sugarless gum or hard candy to ease a dry mouth.
■ Urge patient not to stop taking drug suddenly.
■ If patient develops insomnia, advise taking drug as early in the day as possible.
■ Tell patient to promptly notify prescriber about confusion, movement disorders, a rapid heartbeat, dizziness, fainting, or difficulty urinating.

---

sertraline hydrochloride
Zoloft

Pharmacologic classification: selective serotonin reuptake inhibitor

Therapeutic classification: antidepressant

Pregnancy risk category C

How supplied
Available by prescription only
Tablets: 25 mg, 50 mg, 100 mg

Indications and dosages
Depression, obsessive-compulsive disorder
Adults: 50 mg P.O. daily. Adjust dosage as needed and tolerated; clinical trials involved 50 to 200 mg daily. Adjust dosage at intervals of no less than 1 week.

Panic disorder
Adults: 25 mg P.O. daily. Adjust dose as needed and tolerated at intervals of no less than 1 week.; clinical trials involved 50 to 200 mg daily.
▶ **DOSAGE ADJUSTMENT.** If patient has hepatic impairment, give a smaller amount or use a less frequent dosing schedule.

Pharmacodynamics
Antidepressant action: Sertraline probably acts by blocking serotonin reuptake into presynaptic neurons in the CNS, thus prolonging its action.

Pharmacokinetics
Absorption: Drug is well absorbed after oral administration; absorption rate and extent increase when drug is taken with food. Serum level peaks 4.5 to 8.5 hours after a dose.
Distribution: In vitro studies indicate that drug is highly protein-bound (more than 98%).
Metabolism: Metabolism is probably hepatic; drug undergoes significant first-pass metabolism. N-desmethylsertraline is substantially less active than the parent compound.
Excretion: Drug is excreted mostly as metabolites in urine and feces. Mean elimination half-life is 26 hours. Steady state levels occur within 1 week of daily use in young, healthy patients.

Contraindications and precautions
Contraindicated in patients receiving MAO inhibitors.
Use cautiously in patients at risk for suicide and in those with seizure disorders, bipolar affective disorder, or conditions that affect metabolism or hemodynamic responses.

Interactions
Drug-drug
Desipramine, imipramine: decreased clearance. Dosage adjustments may be needed.
Diazepam, tolbutamide: clearance is decreased by sertraline. Monitor patient for increased drug effects.
MAO inhibitors: may cause serious mental status changes, hyperthermia, autonomic instability, rapid fluctuations of vital signs, delirium, coma, and death. Avoid concomitant use.

Reactions may be *common,* uncommon, *life-threatening,* or COMMON AND LIFE-THREATENING.

Warfarin and other highly protein-bound drugs: may cause interactions, increasing plasma levels of sertraline or other highly bound drug. Small (8%) increases in PT have occurred with warfarin. Monitor patient closely.

Adverse reactions
CNS: agitation, anxiety, confusion, *dizziness, fatigue, headache,* hypertonia, hypoesthesia, *insomnia,* nervousness, paresthesia, *somnolence, tremor,* twitching.
CV: chest pain, hot flashes, palpitations.
GI: abdominal pain, anorexia, constipation, *diarrhea, dry mouth, dyspepsia,* flatulence, increased appetite, *loose stools, nausea,* thirst, vomiting.
GU: dysuria, nocturia, polyuria, *sexual dysfunction.*
Hepatic: elevated liver enzymes.
Metabolic: decreased uric acid, minor increases in serum cholesterol and triglycerides, weight gain.
Musculoskeletal: myalgia.
Skin: *diaphoresis,* pruritus, rash.

Overdose and treatment
Overdose may cause somnolence, nausea, vomiting, tachycardia, ECG changes, anxiety, and pupil dilation.

Experience with sertraline overdose is limited, and treatment is supportive. Establish an airway, and maintain adequate ventilation. Because recent studies question the value of induced emesis or gastric lavage, consider activated charcoal in sorbitol to bind the drug in the GI tract.

No specific antidote exists for sertraline overdose. Monitor patient's vital signs closely. Because drug has a large volume of distribution, hemodialysis, peritoneal dialysis, or forced diuresis probably aren't useful.

Special considerations
■ Patients who respond to therapy during the first 8 weeks usually continue to respond, although limited data are available regarding therapy lasting longer than 16 weeks. If patient receives prolonged therapy, monitor effectiveness periodically. It is unknown if periodic dose adjustments can help to maintain effectiveness.
■ Drug may activate mania or hypomania in patients with cyclic disorders.
■ Don't give sertraline within 14 days of stopping an MAO inhibitor. Don't give an MAO inhibitor within 14 days of stopping sertraline.

Breast-feeding patients
■ Sertraline is excreted in breast milk. Use cautiously in breast-feeding women.

Pediatric patients
■ Safety and efficacy in children haven't been established.

Geriatric patients
■ Plasma clearance is slower in elderly patients, and it may take 2 to 3 weeks of daily dosing to reach steady state levels. Monitor patient closely for dose-related adverse effects.

Patient teaching
- Instruct patient to take drug once daily, either in the morning or evening, with or without food.
- Tell patient to avoid hazardous activities until drug's full effects are clear.
- Advise patient to avoid alcohol during therapy.
- Tell patient not to take other prescribed drugs, OTC medications, or herbal remedies without consulting prescriber.
- Explain the risks of orthostatic hypotension and falls, especially to elderly patients.
- Advise women to use effective contraception and to notify prescriber about planned, suspected, or known pregnancy.

tranylcypromine sulfate
Parnate

Pharmacologic classification:
MAO inhibitor

Therapeutic classification:
antidepressant

Pregnancy risk category C

How supplied
Available by prescription only
Tablets: 10 mg

Indications and dosages
Severe depression
Panic disorder*
Adults: 30 mg P.O. daily in divided doses. If no improvement occurs after 2 weeks, increase by 10 mg/day q 1 to 3 weeks. Maximum, 60 mg daily.

Pharmacodynamics
Antidepressant action: Tranylcypromine inhibits MAO, an enzyme that normally inactivates amine-containing substances, such as the neurotransmitters norepinephrine and serotonin. By inhibiting MAO, phenelzine increases neurotransmitter levels and activity, thus helping to relieve depression.

Pharmacokinetics
Absorption: Drug is rapidly and completely absorbed from the GI tract. Serum levels peak at 1 to 3 hours. Therapeutic activity may not begin for 3 to 4 weeks.
Distribution: Not fully understood. Dosage adjustments are determined by therapeutic response and adverse reaction profile.
Metabolism: Drug is metabolized in the liver.
Excretion: Drug is excreted primarily in urine within 24 hours; some is excreted in feces via the biliary tract. Half-life is 2½ hours. Enzyme inhibition is prolonged and unrelated to half-life.

Contraindications and precautions
Contraindicated in patients receiving anesthetics, antihistaminics, antihypertensives, bupropion, buspirone, dextromethorphan, dibenzazepine derivatives, diuretics, MAO inhibitors, meperidine, sedatives, selective serotonin reuptake inhibitors, some CNS depressants (including narcotics and alcohol), or sympathomimetics (including amphetamines). Also contraindicated with cheese, other foods high in tyramine or tryptophan, or excessive quantities of caffeine.

Reactions may be *common,* uncommon, ***life-threatening,*** or COMMON AND LIFE-THREATENING.

Contraindicated in patients with suspected or confirmed cerebrovascular defect, pheochromocytoma, a history of liver disease, severely impaired renal function, CV disease, hypertension, a history of headache, or upcoming elective surgery. Also contraindicated in patients hypersensitive to drug or its components.

Use cautiously in patients with renal disease, diabetes, seizure disorders, Parkinson's disease, or hyperthyroidism; in patients at risk for suicide; and in patients with a history of mania or undergoing current therapy with antiparkinsonians or spinal anesthetics.

Interactions
Drug-drug
Barbiturates, dextromethorphan, narcotics, sedatives: Use cautiously and in reduced doses.
Cocaine, local anesthetics that contain vasoconstrictors: avoid concomitant use.
Disulfiram: may cause tachycardia, flushing, or palpitations. Avoid concomitant use.
General or spinal anesthetics (normally metabolized by MAO inhibitors): may cause severe hypotension and excessive CNS depression. Discontinue tranylcypromine for at least 1 week before giving these drugs.
Insulin, sulfonylureas: may potentiate a hypoglycemic response. Dosage adjustment may be needed.
Local anesthetics that don't contain vasoconstrictors (such as lidocaine, procaine): Tranylcypromine decreases effectiveness, resulting in poor nerve block.

Meperidine: increased risk of circulatory collapse and death. Avoid concomitant use.
OTC cold, hay fever, and weight-loss products that contain amphetamines, ephedrine, phenylephrine, phenylpropanolamine, methylphenidate or related drugs: may result in serious CV toxicity. Avoid concomitant use.
Sulfonamides: may cause toxicity from either drug. Dosage adjustment may be needed.

Drug-herb
Ginseng: may produce adverse reactions, such as headache, tremors, mania. Avoid concomitant use.

Drug-food
Foods high in tryptophan, tyramine, or caffeine: may cause hypertensive crisis. Avoid concomitant use.

Drug-lifestyle
Alcohol use: may potentiate CNS effects. Advise against alcohol consumption during therapy.

Adverse reactions
CNS: agitation, anxiety, confusion, *dizziness,* drowsiness, headache, jitters, lethargy, numbness, paresthesia, sedation, syncope, tremor, weakness.
CV: edema, *orthostatic hypotension,* palpitations, paradoxical hypertension, *tachycardia.*
EENT: blurred vision, tinnitus.
GI: abdominal pain, *anorexia,* constipation, diarrhea, dry mouth, nausea.
GU: elevated urine catecholamine levels, impaired ejaculation, impotence, SIADH, urine retention.

Hematologic: *agranulocytosis,* anemia, *leukopenia, thrombocytopenia.*
Hepatic: elevated liver function test results, *hepatitis.*
Musculoskeletal: muscle spasm, myoclonic jerks.
Skin: diaphoresis, rash.
Other: chills.

Overdose and treatment
Overdose may worsen adverse reactions or cause an exaggerated response to normal pharmacologic activity. Signs and symptoms arise slowly (over 24 to 48 hours) and may persist for up to 2 weeks. They may include agitation, respiratory failure, vascular collapse, flushing, tachycardia, hypotension, hypertension, palpitations, increased motor activity, twitching, increased deep tendon reflexes, seizures, hyperpyrexia, respiratory failure, vascular collapse, cardiopulmonary arrest, and coma. Doses of 350 mg have been fatal.

Treat symptomatically and supportively. Give 5 to 10 mg of phentolamine I.V. push for hypertensive crisis. Give I.V. diazepam for seizures, agitation, or tremors. Give beta blockers for tachycardia. Give I.V. fluids for hypotension and vascular collapse. Use cooling blankets for fever. Monitor the patient's vital signs and fluid and electrolyte balance. Don't give sympathomimetics (such as norepinephrine and phenylephrine) for hypotension caused by MAO inhibitors.

Special considerations
■ Consider the patient to have some risk of suicide until depression improves significantly. Supervise high-risk patients closely early in therapy. To reduce the risk of intentional overdose, provide the smallest quantity of drug consistent with good management.
■ Tranylcypromine may have a more rapid onset of antidepressant effect (7 to 10 days) than other MAO inhibitors (21 to 30 days). MAO activity also returns rapidly to pretreatment values.

Breast-feeding patients
■ Drug is excreted in breast milk; avoid administering it when patient is breast-feeding.

Pediatric patients
■ Drug is not recommended for children under age 16.

Geriatric patients
■ Avoid giving drug to patients over age 60 because elderly patients have less compensatory reserve to cope with serious adverse effects.

Patient teaching
■ Tell patient to take drug exactly as prescribed and not to double up if she misses a dose.
■ To minimize daytime sedation, tell patient to take drug at bedtime.
■ To minimize the effects of orthostatic hypotension, instruct patient to lie down after taking drug and to avoid abrupt postural changes, especially from a sitting or lying position to a standing one.
■ Explain that many foods and beverages that contain tyramine or tryptophan (such as wines, beer, cheeses, preserved fruits, meats, and vegetables) may interact with drug. If possible, obtain a list of

---

these foods from a hospital dietary department or pharmacy.
- Tell patient to avoid hazardous activities until full effects of drug are clear.
- Warn patient not to drink alcohol or take other prescribed drugs, OTC medications, or herbal remedies without consulting prescriber.
- Tell patient to notify prescriber about adverse reactions, including severe headache, palpitations, tachycardia, sweating, tightness in throat and chest, dizziness, stiff neck, nausea, vomiting, or other unusual symptoms.
- Caution patient not to abruptly stop taking drug.
- Tell patient to inform dentist and other health care providers that she takes an MAO inhibitor.

trazodone hydrochloride
Desyrel

Pharmacologic classification: triazolopyridine derivative

Therapeutic classification: antidepressant

Pregnancy risk category C

How supplied
Available by prescription only
Tablets: 50 mg, 100 mg
Tablets (film-coated): 50 mg, 100 mg
Dividose tablets: 150 mg, 300 mg

Indications and dosages
Depression
Adults: initially, 150 mg daily in divided doses. May increase by 50 mg/day q 3 to 4 days. Average

dosage ranges from 150 mg to 400 mg/day. Maximum, 400 mg/day in outpatients, 600 mg/day in inpatients.

Aggressive behavior*
Adults: 50 mg P.O. b.i.d.

Panic disorder*, agoraphobia with panic attacks*
Adults: 300 mg P.O. daily.

Insomnia*
Adults: 25 to 75 mg P.O. h.s., commonly with a selective serotonin reuptake inhibitor.

Alcohol cravings*, anxiety and depression with alcoholism*
Adults: 50 to 100 mg P.O. daily.
▶ **DOSAGE ADJUSTMENT.** Elderly patients usually require lower initial doses.

Pharmacodynamics
Antidepressant action: Trazodone probably relieves depression by inhibiting reuptake of norepinephrine and serotonin in CNS nerve terminals (presynaptic neurons), which increases the level and enhances the activity of these neurotransmitters in the synaptic cleft. Trazodone shares some properties with tricyclic antidepressants: It has antihistaminic, alpha-blocking, analgesic, and sedative effects as well as relaxant effects on skeletal muscle. Unlike tricyclic antidepressants, however, trazodone counteracts the pressor effects of norepinephrine, has limited effects on the CV system and, in particular, has no direct quinidine-like effects on cardiac tissue. It also has fewer anticholinergic effects. Trazodone has

been used in alcohol-dependent patients to decrease tremors, anxiety, and depression. Adverse reactions are somewhat dose-related.

Pharmacokinetics
Absorption: Drug is well absorbed from the GI tract after oral administration. Effects peak in 1 hour. Taking drug with food delays absorption, extends peak effect to 2 hours, and increases the amount of drug absorbed by 20%.
Distribution: Drug is widely distributed in the body. It doesn't concentrate in any particular tissue, but small amounts may appear in breast milk. About 90% is protein-bound. Proposed therapeutic drug levels haven't been established. Steady state plasma levels occur in 3 to 7 days, and therapeutic activity starts in 7 days.
Metabolism: Trazodone is metabolized by the liver. More than 75% of metabolites are excreted within 3 days.
Excretion: Drug is mostly excreted in feces via the biliary tract; the rest is excreted in urine.

Contraindications and precautions
Contraindicated in patients hypersensitive to the drug and in patients in the initial recovery phase after an MI.

Use cautiously in patients with cardiac disease and in those at risk for suicide.

Interactions
Drug-drug
*Antihypertensives, such as clonidine, guanabenz, guanadrel, guanethi-*dine, methyldopa, reserpine:* increased risk of hypotension. Monitor patient closely.
CNS depressants, such as analgesics, anesthetics, barbiturates, narcotics, tranquilizers: increased risk of oversedation. Monitor patient closely.
Digoxin, phenytoin: serum levels of these drugs may increase. Monitor serum levels closely.

Drug-herb
St. John's wort: increased risk of serotonin syndrome. Avoid concomitant use.

Drug-lifestyle
Alcohol use: may worsen CNS depression. Discourage alcohol use during therapy.

Adverse reactions
CNS: anger, confusion, *dizziness, drowsiness,* fatigue, ***generalized tonic-clonic seizures,*** headache, hostility, insomnia, nervousness, nightmares, tremor, vivid dreams, weakness.
CV: hypertension, orthostatic hypotension, prolonged conduction time on ECG, shortness of breath, syncope, tachycardia.
EENT: blurred vision, nasal congestion, tinnitus.
GI: anorexia, constipation, dry mouth, dysgeusia, nausea, vomiting.
GU: decreased libido, hematuria, priapism (possibly leading to impotence), urine retention.
Hematologic: anemia, decreased WBC counts.
Hepatic: elevated liver function test results.

Reactions may be *common,* uncommon, *life-threatening,* or COMMON AND LIFE-THREATENING.

Metabolic: altered serum glucose levels.
Skin: diaphoresis, rash, urticaria.

Overdose and treatment

Overdose may cause drowsiness, vomiting, orthostatic hypotension, tachycardia, headache, shortness of breath, dry mouth, seizures, ECG changes, and incontinence. Coma may occur as well.

Treatment is symptomatic and supportive and includes maintaining the patient's airway and stabilizing vital signs and fluid and electrolyte balance. Induce emesis if the gag reflex is intact. Follow with gastric lavage (start with lavage if gag reflex is absent) and activated charcoal to prevent further absorption. Forced diuresis may aid elimination. Dialysis is usually ineffective.

Special considerations

■ Consider the patient to have some risk of suicide until depression improves significantly. Supervise high-risk patients closely early in therapy. To reduce the risk of intentional overdose, provide the smallest quantity of drug consistent with good management.
■ Give trazodone with food to help prevent GI upset and increase absorption.
■ As needed, break a scored 150-mg tablet to obtain doses of 50 mg, 75 mg, or 100 mg.
■ To minimize drowsiness, give a major portion of the daily dose at bedtime. Alternatively, reduce the dosage.
■ Give ice, sugarless gum, or sugarless hard candy to help relieve a dry mouth.

■ Monitor patient's blood pressure because hypotension may occur.
■ Drug competes with vitamin B_6 (pyridoxine) for the carrier protein. Give vitamin B_6 supplement daily to prevent cognitive impairment.
■ Tolerance to adverse effects (especially sedative effects) usually develops after 1 to 2 weeks of treatment.
■ Drug has fewer adverse cardiac and anticholinergic effects than tricyclic antidepressants. Adverse effects are more common at doses above 300 mg/day.
■ Use caution when giving drug to male patients, especially sexually active ones, because drug can cause prolonged, painful erections that may require surgical correction.
■ Don't withdraw drug abruptly. Do discontinue it at least 48 hours before surgical procedures.

Breast-feeding patients
■ Drug is excreted in breast milk. Give cautiously to breast-feeding women.

Pediatric patients
■ Drug is not recommended for children under age 18.

Geriatric patients
■ Elderly patients have an increased risk of adverse reactions. However, drug may be preferred over other tricyclic antidepressants in elderly patients because it has fewer adverse cardiac effects.

Patient teaching
■ Instruct patient to take drug exactly as prescribed and not to double up if she misses a dose.

- Tell patient that full effects of drug may take up to 2 weeks to occur.
- Suggest taking drug with food or milk if it causes stomach upset.
- To minimize dizziness, tell patient to lie down for about 30 minutes after each dose and to avoid sudden position changes, especially rising from sitting or lying to standing.
- Suggest sugarless gum or hard candy to relieve a dry mouth.
- Warn patient to avoid hazardous activities until full effects of drug are clear.
- Tell patient to avoid alcohol.
- Advise patient to report unusual effects immediately, including dizziness, fainting, rapid heartbeat, sexual dysfunction, or a prolonged, painful erection. Tell male patient to consider an involuntary erection lasting more than 1 hour a medical emergency.
- Caution patient not to stop drug abruptly.

---

trimipramine maleate
Surmontil

Pharmacologic classification:
tricyclic antidepressant

Therapeutic classification:
antidepressant

Pregnancy risk category C

How supplied
Available by prescription only
Capsules: 25 mg, 50 mg, 100 mg

Indications and dosages
Depression
Adults: For outpatients, give 75 mg/day P.O. in divided doses, and increase to 200 mg/day. Maintenance, 50 to 150 mg/day. May be given as a single bedtime dose. For inpatients, give 100 mg/day in divided doses, and increase p.r.n. Maximum, 300 mg/day.
▶ DOSAGE ADJUSTMENT. For elderly or adolescent patients, give 50 to 100 mg/day P.O.

Pharmacodynamics
Antidepressant action: Trimipramine is thought to exert antidepressant effects by equally inhibiting reuptake of norepinephrine and serotonin in CNS nerve terminals (presynaptic neurons), which results in increased levels and enhanced activities of these neurotransmitters in the synaptic cleft. Trimipramine also has anxiolytic effects and inhibits gastric acid secretion.

Pharmacokinetics
Absorption: Drug is absorbed rapidly from the GI tract after oral administration.
Distribution: Drug is distributed widely in the body and is 90% protein-bound. Effects peak in 2 hours; steady state occurs within 7 days.
Metabolism: Drug is metabolized by the liver. A significant first-pass effect may explain the variability of serum levels in different patients taking the same dosage.
Excretion: Drug is mostly excreted in urine; some is excreted in feces via the biliary tract.

Contraindications and precautions

Contraindicated during the acute recovery phase of MI, in patients hypersensitive to drug, and in those who received an MAO inhibitor within 14 days.

Use cautiously in adolescents, in elderly or debilitated patients, in patients receiving thyroid medications, and in those with CV disease, increased intraocular pressure, hyperthyroidism, impaired hepatic function, or a history of seizures, urine retention, or angle-closure glaucoma.

Interactions
Drug-drug

Antiarrhythmics (quinidine, disopyramide, procainamide), pimozide, thyroid hormones: may increase risk of cardiac arrhythmias and conduction defects. Use with extreme caution.

Anticholinergic drugs, such as antihistamines, antiparkinsonian drugs, atropine, meperidine, phenothiazines: may cause oversedation, paralytic ileus, visual changes, and severe constipation. Monitor patient closely.

Barbiturates, carbamazepine: may induce trimipramine metabolism and decrease efficacy. Dosage adjustment may be needed.

Beta blockers, cimetidine, methylphenidate, oral contraceptives, propoxyphene: may inhibit trimipramine metabolism, increasing plasma levels and toxicity. Monitor patient closely and adjust dosage as needed.

Central-acting antihypertensives, such as clonidine, guanabenz, guanadrel, guanethidine, methyldopa,

reserpine: decreased antihypertensive effects. Monitor patient and blood pressure closely.

CNS depressants, including analgesics, anesthetics, barbiturates, narcotics, tranquilizers: may cause oversedation. Use cautiously.

Disulfiram, ethchlorvynol: may cause delirium and tachycardia. Avoid concomitant use.

Haloperidol, phenothiazines: decreased trimipramine metabolism and increased risk of toxicity. Monitor serum levels closely.

Metrizamide: additive effects likely, increasing the risk of seizures and other adverse effects. Monitor patient closely.

Selective serotonin reuptake inhibitors (fluoxetine, paroxetine, sertraline): increased pharmacologic and toxic effects of trimipramine. Dose adjustment may be needed.

Sympathomimetics (including ephedrine, epinephrine, phenylephrine, phenylpropanolamine) commonly found in nasal sprays: may increase blood pressure.

Warfarin: may increase PT, INR, and the risk of bleeding. Monitor patient closely.

Drug-lifestyle

Alcohol use: additive effects are likely. Discourage alcohol use during therapy.

Heavy smoking: induces trimipramine metabolism and decreases efficacy. Discourage concomitant use, and encourage smoking cessation.

Sun exposure: increased risk of photosensitivity reactions. Recommend precautions.

Adverse reactions

CNS: agitation, anxiety, ataxia, confusion, delusions, *dizziness, drowsiness,* EEG changes, extrapyramidal symptoms, hallucinations, headache, insomnia, paresthesia, *seizures,* tremor, weakness,
CV: *arrhythmias, CVA, heart block,* hypertension, *MI, orthostatic hypotension,* prolonged conduction time on ECG, tachycardia.
EENT: *blurred vision,* mydriasis, tinnitus.
GI: anorexia, *constipation, dry mouth,* nausea, paralytic ileus, vomiting.
GU: *urine retention.*
Hematologic: *agranulocytosis,* altered PT and INR, decreased WBC counts, *esinophilia, purpura, thrombocytopenia.*
Hepatic: elevated liver function test results.
Metabolic: altered serum glucose levels, weight loss or weight gain.
Skin: *diaphoresis,* photosensitivity, rash, urticaria.
Other: *hypersensitivity reaction.*

Overdose and treatment

The first 12 hours after acute ingestion are a stimulatory phase characterized by excessive anticholinergic activity, which may include agitation, irritation, confusion, hallucinations, hyperthermia, parkinsonian symptoms, seizures, urine retention, dry mucous membranes, pupil dilation, constipation, and ileus. This phase is followed by CNS depression—including hypothermia, decreased or absent reflexes, sedation, hypotension, and cyanosis—and such cardiac irregularities as tachycardia, conduction disturbances, and quinidine-like effects on the ECG.

Widening of the QRS complex usually indicates a serum level above 1,000 mg/ml. (Serum levels aren't helpful.) Metabolic acidosis may follow hypotension, hypoventilation, and seizures.

Treatment is symptomatic and supportive, and includes managing the patient's airway, body temperature, and fluid and electrolyte balance. Induce emesis with ipecac if the gag reflex is intact and the patient is conscious; follow with gastric lavage and activated charcoal to prevent further absorption. Dialysis is of little use.

Physostigmine given slowly by the I.V. route may help to reverse most CV and CNS effects when other treatments fail. Treat seizures with parenteral diazepam or phenytoin. Give parenteral phenytoin or lidocaine for arrhythmias. Give sodium bicarbonate for acidosis. Don't give barbiturates; they may enhance CNS and respiratory depressant effects.

Special considerations

■ To reduce daytime sedation, give the full dose at bedtime.
■ Consider the patient to have some risk of suicide until depression improves significantly. Supervise high-risk patients closely early in therapy. To reduce the risk of intentional overdose, provide the smallest quantity of drug consistent with good management.
■ Tolerance usually develops to sedative effects of drug.
■ Manic or hypomanic episodes may occur in some patients, especially those with cyclic disorders.

- Watch for bleeding because drug may alter PT and INR.
- Don't withdraw drug abruptly because doing so may result in nausea, headache, and malaise (which don't indicate addiction).
- Discontinue drug at least 48 hours before surgical procedures.

Breast-feeding patients
- Drug is excreted in breast milk. Use caution when treating breast-feeding patients.

Pediatric patients
- Safety and effectiveness in children hasn't been established.

Patient teaching
- Tell patient to take drug exactly as prescribed and not to double up if she misses a dose.
- Explain that full effects of drug may not become apparent for 4 to 6 weeks after therapy begins.
- To minimize daytime sedation, tell patient to take full dose at bedtime.
- Suggest taking drug with food or milk if it causes stomach upset.
- Warn patient that drug may cause drowsiness or dizziness. Tell her to avoid hazardous activities until full effects of drug are clear.
- Caution patient not to drink alcohol during therapy.
- Suggest ice, sugarless gum, or sugarless hard candy to relieve a dry mouth.
- To prevent dizziness, instruct patient to lie down for about 30 minutes after each dose and to avoid abrupt postural changes, especially from lying or sitting to standing.
- Caution patient not to stop drug abruptly.

- Tell patient to report adverse reactions promptly, especially confusion, movement disorders, a rapid heartbeat, dizziness, fainting, or difficulty urinating.
- Elderly patients may be more vulnerable to adverse cardiac effects.
- Tell women to use contraception during therapy and to promptly notify prescriber about planned, suspected, or known pregnancy.

venlafaxine hydrochloride
Effexor, Effexor XR

Pharmacologic classification: neuronal serotonin, norepinephrine, and dopamine reuptake inhibitor

Therapeutic classification: antidepressant

Pregnancy risk category C

How supplied
Available by prescription only
Capsules (extended-release): 37.5 mg, 75 mg, 150 mg
Tablets: 25 mg, 37.5 mg, 50 mg, 75 mg, 100 mg

Indications and dosages
Depression
Adults: initially, 75 mg P.O. daily in two or three divided doses with food. Increase dosage by 75 mg/day as needed and tolerated at intervals no shorter than q 4 days. For moderately depressed outpatients, usual maximum dosage is 225 mg/day; in severely depressed patients, dosage may be as high as 375 mg/day divided into 3 doses. For ex-

tended-release capsules, give 75 mg P.O. daily in a single dose. For some patients (especially those who should avoid overstimulation), it may be better to start at 37.5 mg P.O. daily for 4 to 7 days before increasing to 75 mg daily. Dosage may be increased by 75 mg/day q 4 days to a maximum of 225 mg/day.

Generalized anxiety disorder

Adults: For extended-release capsules, 75 mg P.O. daily in a single dose. For some patients (especially those who should avoid overstimulation), it may be better to start at 37.5 mg P.O. daily for 4 to 7 days before increasing to 75 mg daily. Dosage may be increased by 75 mg/day q 4 days to a maximum of 225 mg/day.

▷ **Dosage adjustment.** Reduce dosage by 50% in patients with impaired hepatic function. In patients with moderate renal impairment (glomerular filtration rate of 10 to 70 ml/minute), reduce daily dose by 25%. In hemodialysis patients, reduce dosage by 50% and hold drug until after dialysis treatment.

Pharmacodynamics

Antidepressant action: Venlafaxine and its active metabolite, O-desmethylvenlafaxine (ODV) probably potentiate neurotransmitter activity in the CNS by strongly inhibiting neuronal serotonin and norepinephrine reuptake and weakly inhibiting dopamine reuptake.

Pharmacokinetics

Absorption: About 92% of drug is absorbed after oral administration.

Distribution: Drug is 25% to 29% protein-bound in plasma.
Metabolism: Drug is extensively metabolized in the liver, with ODV being the only major active metabolite.
Excretion: About 87% of dose is recovered in urine within 48 hours (5% as unchanged venlafaxine, 29% as unconjugated ODV, 26% as conjugated ODV, and 27% as minor inactive metabolites).

Contraindications and precautions

Contraindicated in patients hypersensitive to drug and within 14 days of MAO inhibitor therapy.

Use cautiously in patients with impaired renal or hepatic function, conditions that could affect hemodynamic responses or metabolism, or a history of seizures or mania.

Interactions
Drug-drug

Cimetidine, CNS-active drugs: possible increase in venlafaxine level, especially in elderly patients or patients with hepatic dysfunction or hypertension. Use together cautiously.
MAO inhibitors: increased risk of a condition similar to neuroleptic malignant syndrome. Don't give venlafaxine within 14 days after patient takes an MAO inhibitor. Don't give an MAO inhibitor within 7 days after patient takes venlafaxine.

Drug-herb

Yohimbe: may cause additive stimulation. Use together cautiously.

Reactions may be *common,* uncommon, *life-threatening,* or COMMON AND LIFE-THREATENING.

Drug-lifestyle
Alcohol use: additive effects are likely. Discourage alcohol use during therapy.

Adverse reactions
CNS: abnormal dreams, agitation, anxiety, *asthenia, dizziness, headache, insomnia, nervousness,* paresthesia, *somnolence,* tremor.
CV: hypertension, tachycardia, vasodilation.
EENT: blurred vision, mydrias, tinnitus.
GI: *anorexia, constipation,* diarrhea, *dry mouth,* dyspepsia, flatulence, *nausea,* vomiting.
GU: *abnormal ejaculation,* impaired urination, impotence, urinary frequency.
Metabolic: weight loss.
Skin: *diaphoresis,* rash.
Other: chills, infection, yawning.

Overdose and treatment
Overdose may cause no symptoms, or it may cause somnolence, generalized seizures, and prolongation of the QT interval.

Treatment involves ensuring an adequate airway, providing oxygenation and ventilation, and monitoring the patient's cardiac rhythm and vital signs. Also, provide supportive, symptomatic treatment. Consider inducing emesis, performing gastric lavage, or administering activated charcoal. Forced diuresis, dialysis, hemoperfusion, and exchange transfusion probably won't help. No specific antidotes are known for venlafaxine overdose.

Special considerations
■ Monitor patient's blood pressure regularly because drug may cause sustained increases. If patient develops a sustained increase in blood pressure during therapy, she may need a dosage reduction or discontinuation of the drug.
■ Closely monitor a patient with a major affective disorder because venlafaxine may activate mania or hypomania.
■ When discontinuing therapy after more than 1 week, taper the dose. If therapy has lasted 6 weeks or more, taper the dose over 2 weeks.
■ If patient develops seizures, discontinue the drug.

Breast-feeding patients
■ Drug is excreted in breast milk. Use it cautiously in breast-feeding women.

Pediatric patients
■ Safety and effectiveness haven't been established in children under age 18.

Patient teaching
■ Tell patient to avoid alcohol.
■ Warn patient to avoid hazardous tasks until drug effects are clear.
■ Instruct patient not to take other prescribed drugs, OTC medications, or herbal remedies without consulting prescriber.
■ Instruct patient to report a rash, hives, or other allergic reaction.
■ Urge women to notify prescriber about planned, suspected, or known pregnancy.

◊ Available in Canada only   *Unlabeled use

CHAPTER 7

Mood stabilizing drugs

219 ■ **Introduction**

222 ■ **Generic drugs**

■ **carbamazepine** (See Chapter 5, ANTICONVULSANTS)

■ **lithium carbonate, lithium citrate**

■ **valproic acid, divalproex sodium, valproate sodium** (See Chapter 5, ANTICONVULSANTS)

Mood stabilizing drugs are used mainly to treat bipolar disorder, in which the patient has alternating or occasionally simultaneous periods of mania (or hypomania) and depression.

UNDERSTANDING BIPOLAR DISORDER

Bipolar disorder affects about 1.5% of Americans and occurs equally often among men and women. The symptoms typically begin in a person's early 20s.

Bipolar disorder probably results fully or partly from alterations in the levels of certain neurotransmitters in the brain, such as norepinephrine, serotonin, dopamine, gamma-aminobutyric acid, and glutamate. Some evidence also suggests that electrolyte or second messenger systems—such as the phosphoinositide system, sodium-potassium pumps, or calcium channels—may be responsible. The disorder also may stem in part from an increased sensitization to stressors. This sensitization may take the form of a "kindling response," which involves the kind of repeated, subthreshold stimulation that can lead to seizures.

A person's genetic makeup may influence his risk for bipolar disorder as well. In fact, this disorder occurs in about 67% of monozygotic twins. About half of patients with bipolar disorder have a parent who also has a mood disorder.

Mood swings

A patient with bipolar disorder typically complains of mood swings. The patient shifts from mania (or hypomania) to depres-

---

Characteristics of bipolar disorder

In bipolar disorder, patients experience both manic and depressive phases of the illness.

Manic phase
In the manic phase of bipolar disorder, patients usually have one or more of the following symptoms:
- decreased need for sleep
- distractibility
- elevated mood
- increased drive for pleasurable, high-risk behaviors
- increased goal-oriented activity
- inflated self-esteem
- racing thoughts
- rapid speech.

Depressive phase
In the depressive phase of bipolar disorder, patients usually have some or all of the following symptoms:
- altered appetite
- depressed mood
- disturbed sleep
- feelings of guilt
- loss of interest in pleasurable activities
- problems concentrating.

---

sion and back. (See *Characteristics of bipolar disorder*.) Manic symptoms typically develop rapidly and may intensify over several weeks. Untreated, a manic episode can last 3 months, sometimes longer. The frequency of these episodes increases as the disorder progresses.

A patient may have one of two subtypes of bipolar disorder based on the severity and duration of his symptoms. In type I bipolar disorder, the patient has mania and major depressive symptoms. In type II bipolar disorder, the patient has hypomania and major depressive symptoms. The difference between mania and hypomania is one of degree; symptoms of hypomania are similar to those of mania, but are less severe.

Patients with type I bipolar disorder have a 40% to 50% chance of experiencing a second manic episode within 2 years of the first. They also may have what's known as a mixed episode, in which the patient experiences both manic and major depressive symptoms at the same time for at least one week. A patient who has four or more separate mood disturbances during a single year is known as a "rapid cycler."

TREATING BIPOLAR DISORDER

Treatment for bipolar disorder focuses on controlling both mania and depression. Mood stabilizers form the mainstay of treatment. They include lithium salts, valproic acid derivatives, and carbamazepine. Other mood stabilizers are under investigation, notably gabapentin and lamotrigine. Antidepressants may be given with mood stabilizers to treat depressive symptoms.

Initial treatment

Once a diagnosis of bipolar disorder has been made, a patient should be started on a mood stabilizer or lithium, with the goal of treatment being a return to euthymia. For a patient in a manic episode, the treatment of choice is either lithium or valproic acid. For a patient undergoing a mixed episode or rapid cycling, valproic acid is considered the treatment of choice. Lithium and carbamazepine provide alternative treatments for mixed episodes; carbamazepine provides an alternative treatment for rapid cycling.

For a patient in the depressive phase of bipolar disorder, treatment usually includes both a mood stabilizer and an antidepressant. Keep in mind that antidepressant therapy alone can raise the risk of shifting into mania; that's why therapy should include both a mood stabilizer and an antidepressant.

Bupropion and selective serotonin reuptake inhibitors form the first line of therapy for the depressive phase of bipolar disorder. Bupropion seems to cause the smallest risk of mania and usually forms the first choice. This is particularly true in patients who have a history of switching from depression to mania and in patients who are rapid cyclers. Lithium can also effectively treat depressive symptoms in bipolar patients and may be used as monotherapy in patients with mild symptoms. Tricyclic antidepressants typically aren't used for patients with bipolar disorder.

Once the patient starts taking a mood stabilizer, expect the effect to begin within the first 2 weeks. Monitor serum levels of the drug to help adjust the dosage and maintain a therapeutic level. Based on the kinetic properties of these drugs, a steady state typically occurs in 5 to 7 days; that's the best time to check the level of drug in the patient's blood.

Depending on the patient's response and any adverse effects he's experiencing, dosage adjustments can be made at that point. Because carbamazepine has a unique metabolism, more frequent monitoring may be needed at the start of therapy and any time the dosage changes.

If the patient doesn't respond to first-line treatment, you may need to increase the dosage, if possible. If not, or if an increase doesn't improve the patient's response, then the patient may need to switch to a different mood stabilizer or a second mood stabilizer given along with the first.

Besides an antidepressant and a mood stabilizer, the patient also may need short-term adjunctive treatment to help reduce agitation, psychotic symptoms, or insomnia. Treatment for these problems typically involves an antipsychotic or a benzodiazepine, and it typically lasts only a short time.

Ongoing treatment

After the acute phase of treatment, the patient should continue taking a mood stabilizer for at least 6 months while adjunctive drugs are tapered and discontinued. If the patient has type I bipolar disorder and has experienced either two manic episodes or a severe first episode with a positive family history, he should expect to take a mood stabilizer for the rest of his life.

Certain adverse effects are common to all mood stabilizers and include nausea, vomiting, and drowsiness. Adverse gastrointestinal effects can be minimized by giving low doses at the start of treatment, by giving smaller doses more frequently, by giving doses with food, or by switching to an extended-release product if available.

PATIENT TEACHING

Many teaching points are specific only to certain drugs used to treat bipolar disorder. However, some teaching points can be applied to all mood stabilizers:

■ Caution the patient to swallow a sustained-release product whole and not to break, chew, or crush it.

■ Suggest that the patient take the drug with food to minimize stomach upset. If that change isn't helpful, consider switching to a sustained-release product.

■ Tell the patient to expect a response to the treatment about 1 to 2 weeks after it begins.

■ Stress that the patient will need to take the drug exactly as prescribed, on a regular basis rather than an as-needed basis.

■ Explain that additional drugs may be prescribed together with a mood stabilizer to help control the patient's symptoms.

■ Advise the patient that the duration of treatment depends on the severity of his symptoms, his family history, and the recurrence of symptoms. Some patients may need permanent drug therapy.

■ Explain that periodic laboratory tests to determine the level of drug in the patient's blood are a requirement of continued treatment.

■ Caution the patient to avoid alcohol during therapy.

■ Tell the patient that mood stabilizing drugs can harm a developing fetus. Urge women to notify the prescriber about suspected, planned, or known pregnancy.

lithium carbonate
Carbolith◇, Duralith◇, Eskalith,
Eskalith CR, Lithane, Lithizine◇,
Lithobid, Lithonate, Lithotabs

lithium citrate
Cibalith-S

Pharmacologic classification:
alkali metal

Therapeutic classification:
antimanic, antipsychotic

Pregnancy risk category D

How supplied
Available by prescription only
lithium carbonate
Capsules: 150 mg, 300 mg, 600 mg
Tablets: 300 mg
Tablets (sustained-release): 300 mg,
450 mg
lithium citrate
Syrup (sugarless): 300 mg/5 ml
(with 0.3% alcohol)

Indications and dosages
Mania, depression in patients
with bipolar disorder
Adults: 900 mg (sustained-release
tablet) P.O. morning and h.s., or
600 mg (tablet or capsule) morning, noon, and h.s.

Major depression*,
schizoaffective disorder*,
schizophrenic disorder*, alcohol
dependence*
Adults: 300 mg lithium carbonate
P.O. t.i.d. or q.i.d.

Apparent mixed bipolar
disorder in children*
Children: initially, 15 to 60 mg/kg
or 0.5 to 1.5 g/m^2 of lithium car-

bonate P.O. daily in three divided
doses. Don't exceed usual adult
dosage. Adjust dosage based on patient response and serum lithium
levels; usual range is 150 to 300 mg
daily in divided doses.

Pharmacodynamics
Antimanic and antipsychotic ac-
tions: Lithium probably competes
with other cations for exchange at
the sodium-potassium ion pump,
thus altering cation exchange at the
tissue level. It also inhibits adeny-
late cyclase, reducing intracellular
levels of cAMP and, to a lesser extent, cyclic guanosine monophos-
phate.

Pharmacokinetics
Absorption: The rate and extent of
absorption vary with dosage form;
absorption is complete within 6
hours after oral administration of
standard tablets and capsules.
Distribution: Drug is distributed
widely into the body, including
breast milk. Levels in thyroid
gland, bone, and brain tissue exceed serum levels. Levels peak in 30
minutes to 3 hours; with liquid
form, they peak in 15 minutes to 1
hour. Serum level reaches steady
state in 12 hours. Therapeutic effects start in 5 to 10 days and peak
within 3 weeks. Therapeutic and
toxic serum levels and therapeutic
effects correlate well. Therapeutic
range is 0.6 to 1.2 mEq/L. Adverse
reactions increase as level reaches
1.5 to 2 mEq/L, but such levels may
be needed in acute mania. Toxicity
usually occurs at levels above
2 mEq/L.
Metabolism: Lithium isn't metabolized.

Excretion: Drug is excreted 95% unchanged in urine; about 50% to 80% of a dose is excreted within 24 hours. The level of renal function determines the elimination rate.

Contraindications and precautions

Contraindicated during pregnancy and for patients who can't be closely monitored.

Use cautiously in elderly patients and patients with thyroid disease, seizure disorders, renal disease, CV disease, severe dehydration, debilitation, or sodium depletion. Also, use cautiously in patients who take neuroleptics, neuromuscular blockers, or diuretics.

Interactions
Drug-drug
Antacids and drugs that contain aminophylline, caffeine, calcium, sodium, or theophylline: may increase lithium excretion by renal competition for elimination, thus decreasing lithium's therapeutic effect. Dosage adjustment may be needed.
Carbamazepine, mazindol, methyldopa, phenytoin, tetracyclines: may increase lithium toxicity. Monitor patient carefully.
Chlorpromazine: may decrease chlorpromazine effects. Dosage adjustment may be needed.
Fluoxetine: increases serum lithium levels. Dosage adjustment may be needed.
Haloperidol: may cause severe encephalopathy with confusion, tremors, extrapyramidal effects, and weakness. Use together cautiously.

Neuromuscular blockers, such as atracurium, pancuronium, and succinylcholine: potentiated neuromuscular blocking effects.
NSAIDs, such as indomethacin, phenylbutazone, piroxicam: decrease renal excretion of lithium and may require a 30% reduction in lithium dosage.
Sympathomimetics: lithium may interfere with sympathomimetic pressor effects. Dosage adjustment may be needed.
Thiazide diuretics: may decrease renal excretion and enhance lithium toxicity. Diuretic dosage may need a 30% reduction.

Drug-herb
Parsley: may promote or produce serotonin syndrome. Avoid concurrent use.
Psyllium seed: may inhibit GI absorption of lithium. Avoid concurrent use.

Drug-food
Caffeine: may increase lithium excretion by renal competition for elimination, thus decreasing lithium's therapeutic effect. Dosage adjustment may be needed.
Dietary sodium: increased sodium intake may increase renal elimination of lithium; decreased intake may decrease elimination. Dosage adjustment may be needed.

Adverse reactions
CNS: ataxia, blackouts, ***coma,*** confusion, dizziness, drowsiness, EEG changes, ***epileptiform seizures,*** headache, impaired speech, incoordination, lethargy, muscle weakness, psychomotor retardation,

restlessness, tremors, worsened organic mental syndrome.

CV: *arrhythmias, bradycardia,* hypotension, peripheral edema, *peripheral vascular collapse* (rare), *reversible ECG changes.*

EENT: blurred vision, tinnitus.

GI: abdominal pain, anorexia, diarrhea, dry mouth, flatulence, indigestion, metallic taste, nausea, *thirst,* vomiting.

GU: albuminuria, decreased creatinine clearance, glycosuria, *polyuria, renal toxicity* with long-term use.

Hematologic: *leukocytosis with WBC count of 14,000 to 18,000/mm* (reversible).

Metabolic: goiter, hyponatremia, hypothyroidism (decreased T_3, T_4, and protein-bound iodine, but increased ^{131}I uptake), transient hyperglycemia.

Skin: acne, alopecia, diminished or absent sensation, drying and thinning of hair, pruritus, psoriasis, rash.

Overdose and treatment

Acute overdose may cause vomiting and diarrhea, typically within 1 hour after ingestion. Patients have ingested up to 6 g of lithium with minimal toxic effects; however, patients who ingested 10 to 60 g of lithium have died. Serum lithium levels above 3.4 mEq/L may be fatal.

Long-term ingestion of lithium may lead to overdose as well, typically after an alteration in pharmacokinetics, a drug interaction, or volume or sodium depletion. The patient may develop ataxia, confusion, hand tremors, increased deep tendon reflexes, joint pain, muscle stiffness, nystagmus, sedation, and visual changes. The condition may progress to include movement abnormalities, tremors, seizures, coma, and CV collapse.

Treatment is symptomatic and supportive; monitor the patient's vital signs closely. Induce emesis after acute overdose if the patient isn't comatose and isn't already vomiting. If induced emesis isn't feasible, perform gastric lavage. Monitor the patient's fluid and electrolyte balance, and correct sodium depletion with normal saline solution.

The patient may undergo hemodialysis if his serum level is above 3 mEq/L, he's severely symptomatic and unresponsive to fluid and electrolyte correction, or if his urine output decreases significantly. Serum rebound of tissue lithium stores commonly occurs after dialysis and may demand prolonged or repeated hemodialysis. Peritoneal dialysis may help but is less effective.

Special considerations

■ Check patient's baseline ECG, thyroid function, renal studies, and electrolyte levels.

■ Give drug with food or milk to reduce GI upset.

■ Shake syrup form before giving it.

■ Because lithium toxicity may occur at close to therapeutic serum levels, make sure that patient undergoes repeated testing of serum drug levels. The usual testing schedule is 8 to 12 hours after the first dose (usually before morning dose), two or three times weekly for the first month, and then weekly to monthly during maintenance therapy.

Reactions may be *common,* uncommon, *life-threatening,* or COMMON AND LIFE-THREATENING.

- Don't give drug if patient or family members can't commit to compliance with follow-up testing schedule.
- Make sure patient consumes 2,500 to 3,000 ml of fluid daily and a balanced diet that includes adequate salt. Adjust fluid and salt levels to compensate if protracted sweating or diarrhea causes excessive fluid loss. Likewise, watch for signs of edema or sudden weight gain.
- Expect beneficial effects of drug to start in 1 to 3 weeks. Give other psychotropic drugs (such as chlorpromazine) in the interim, as needed.
- Monitor lithium doses carefully when patient's manic symptoms begin to subside because the ability to tolerate high serum lithium levels decreases as symptoms resolve.
- Arrange for outpatient follow-up of thyroid and renal functions every 6 to 12 months. Thyroid should be palpated to check for enlargement.
- Reduce lithium dosage or withdraw drug before patient undergoes electroconvulsive therapy because the combination raises the risk of acute neurotoxicity with delirium.
- Expect EEG changes during therapy, including diffuse slowing, widening of frequency spectrum, potentiation, and disorganization of background rhythm.
- Drug causes false-positive test results on thyroid function tests; it also elevates neutrophil count.
- When lithium blood levels are below 1.5 mEq/L, adverse reactions usually remain mild.

- Check patient's urine to rule out a specific gravity level below 1.015, because it may indicate diabetes insipidus.
- Because drug may alter glucose tolerance in diabetic patients, monitor their blood glucose levels closely.
- Lithane tablets contain tartrazine, a dye that may cause an allergic reaction in certain people, particularly people with asthma who are sensitive to aspirin.
- Lithium is used investigationally to increase the WBC count in patients receiving chemotherapy and to treat cluster headaches, aggression, organic brain syndrome, tardive dyskinesia, and SIADH.

Breast-feeding patients
- Lithium level in breast milk is 33% to 50% that of maternal serum level. Patients shouldn't breast-feed during lithium therapy.

Pediatric patients
- Drug isn't recommended for children under age 12.

Geriatric patients
- Elderly patients are more susceptible to overdose and toxic effects, especially dyskinesias. These patients usually respond to a lower dosage.

Patient teaching
- Instruct patient to take drug with food or milk.
- Tell patient to expect transient nausea, polyuria, thirst, and discomfort for the first few days of therapy.
- Explain that lithium has a narrow therapeutic margin of safety. A

serum drug level that's even slightly high can be dangerous.

■ Warn ambulatory patient to avoid hazardous activities until full CNS effects of drug are known.

■ Advise patient to maintain adequate water intake and adequate—but not excessive—salt in the diet.

■ Tell patient to avoid large amounts of caffeine because they interfere with drug's effectiveness.

■ Explain the importance of regular follow-up visits to measure serum lithium levels.

■ Tell patient not to switch brands of lithium or take other prescribe drugs, OTC medications, or herbal remedies without consulting the prescriber. Different brands may not provide the same effects.

■ Advise patient to consult prescriber before starting a weight-loss program.

■ Warn patient and family members to watch for signs of toxicity, such as diarrhea, vomiting, dehydration, drowsiness, muscle weakness, tremor, fever, and ataxia. If symptoms of toxicity occur, tell patient to withhold one dose and promptly call the prescriber.

■ Tell patient to make sure his close friends and family members can recognize the signs of lithium overdose in case he needs emergency care.

■ Warn patient not to stop drug abruptly.

■ Instruct patient to carry or wear medical identification that describes his lithium regimen and provides emergency information.

CHAPTER 8

Antiparkinsonians

229 ■ **Introduction**

233 ■ **Generic drugs**

■ amantadine hydrochloride

■ benztropine mesylate

■ biperiden hydrochloride, biperiden lactate

■ bromocriptine mesylate

■ diphenhydramine hydrochloride

■ entacapone

■ levodopa

■ levodopa-carbidopa

■ pergolide mesylate

■ pramipexole dihydrochloride

■ ropinirole hydrochloride

■ selegiline hydrochloride

■ tolcapone

■ trihexyphenidyl hydrochloride

Parkinson's disease is a degenerative neurologic disorder that causes progressive motor impairments. It usually occurs late in life and produces characteristic hand tremors, weakness, and changes in posture and gait. Although several drugs are available to treat it, Parkinson's disease eventually overcomes their effects.

UNDERSTANDING PARKINSON'S DISEASE

No one knows exactly what causes Parkinson's disease, but we understand some of its characteristics. Its major traits include a loss of neurons in the substantia nigra of the central nervous system (CNS) and the presence of Lewy bodies. These round, concentrically laminated structures appear in vacuoles in the cytoplasm of some neurons in the midbrain.

Normally, brain cells in the substantia nigra communicate with the striatum by using the neurotransmitter dopamine. As Parkinson's disease progresses, a loss of nigral cells causes levels of striatal dopamine to decline. The development of Lewy bodies and related gliosis seem to result from the degenerating neurons in this dopaminergic area.

Several internal and environmental factors may be linked to Parkinson's disease. For example, the disease may result in part from inadequate oxygen or neurotropic proteins important to the normal functioning of nerve cells. A deficiency of these substances could hamper the survival of dopaminergic neurons. Environmental toxins, infectious agents, and ischemia also can damage neurons, a process that theoretically could hasten the path to Parkinson's disease.

Identifying symptoms

Patients may lose nearly 80% of their dopaminergic neurons before the symptoms of Parkinson's disease begin to appear. When they do, they typically start with akinesia. This state of decreased spontaneous motor activity causes such symptoms as a decreased length of stride, joint pains, a shuffling gait, decreased arm swing, lack of facial expression, and decreased blinking. Later, other symptoms may include paresthesias, numbness, and coldness.

As the disease progresses, the patient develops a resting tremor, rigidity, bradykinesia, impaired reflexes, and changes in posture: The neck becomes bent and the shoulders become stooped. Micrographia and dysarthria may also accompany the disease.

Between 20% and 60% of people with Parkinson's disease also develop dementia. This condition arises most commonly in older people and people with advanced disease. Parkinson's dementia is a subcortical dementia characterized by poor concentration, a slowing of cognitive and motor function, difficulties with memory retrieval, cumulative memory loss, and disturbances in executive functioning.

TREATING PARKINSON'S DISEASE

Most attention for the treatment of Parkinson's disease has been focused on the loss of dopaminergic neurons that project into the CNS.

Parkinson's disease: Choosing a drug regimen

Use this table to help choose a drug regimen based on the underlying mechanism of your patient's Parkinson's disease and on whether she's already taking levodopa.

DRUG	Postencephalic parkinsonism	Arteriosclerotic parkinsonism	Idiopathic parkinsonism	Drug-induced parkinsonism	Disease that needs adjunct to levodopa
Anticholinergics					
benztropine	■	■	■	■	
biperiden	■	■	■	■	
diphenhydramine	■	■	■	■	
trihexyphenidyl	■	■	■	■	■
Dopaminergics					
amantadine	■	■	■	■	
bromocriptine	■		■	■	
levodopa	■	■	■	■	
levodopa-carbidopa	■		■	■	
pergolide			■		■
selegiline					■
Catechol-O-methyltransferase inhibitors					
entacapone					■
tolcapone					■
Dopamine receptor agonists (Non-ergot)					
pramipexole			■		■
ropinirole			■		■

Five human dopamine receptors (D_1 through D_5) have been identified. Most of the drugs currently available to treat Parkinson's disease interact with one or more of the receptors in varying degrees.

Many drugs can be used to help reduce the symptoms of Parkinson's disease. (See *Parkinson's disease: Choosing a drug regimen.*) The drugs with the longest history as a treatment for Parkinson's disease are the anticholinergics. These drugs competitively antagonize the actions of acetylcholine and other cholinergic agonists in the parasympathetic nervous system. However, they lack a specific site of action, which raises the risk of adverse effects.

Belladonna alkaloids are active as anticholinergics and have a higher selectivity for CNS receptors. Antihistamines have central anticholinergic effects and may be used early in Parkinson's disease because they produce fewer peripheral adverse effects than belladonna alkaloids, including the synthetic derivatives.

Levodopa, a dopamine precursor, has proven to be the most effective treatment for Parkinson's disease because it's converted into dopamine in the brain. (See *How levodopa works*.) Dopamine agonists, such as bromocriptine and pergolide, stimulate dopamine receptors D_1 and D_2 to help alleviate symptoms of the disease.

Newer treatments for Parkinson's disease include the non-ergot dopamine agonists, pramipexole and ropinirole. These drugs have a higher affinity for D_3 receptors than for D_2 or D_4 receptors, which means that they can provide more benefits with fewer adverse reactions.

The antiviral drug amantadine can help ease the symptoms of Parkinson's disease as well, possibly by somehow potentiating dopaminergic neurotransmission in the CNS. It also may block the reuptake of dopamine into presynaptic neurons, causing dopamine to accumulate.

How levodopa works

No one knows exactly how levodopa raises levels of dopamine in the brain. But it probably works something like this: A certain amount of each dose that crosses the blood-brain barrier is decarboxylated. The dopamine that results from that decarboxylation then stimulates dopaminergic receptors in the basal ganglia. This stimulation enhances the balance between cholinergic and dopaminergic activity. The result? Improved modulation of voluntary nerve impulses transmitted to the motor cortex.

Selegiline is a relatively selective inhibitor of MAO-B, a mitochondrial enzyme that metabolizes dopamine; thus, the drug enhances dopaminergic activity in the substantia nigra and acts to prolong the effects of levodopa. At higher doses, selegiline also affects MAO-A. It may also directly increase dopamine levels by decreasing the reuptake of dopamine into nerve cells. Inhibition of MAO-B may stop or at least delay nigrostriatal degeneration, which means that it could act as a neuroprotective substance.

Cathechol-0-methyltransferase (COMT), is the major metabolizing enzyme for levodopa in the brain and periphery. Tolcapone is a potent, selective reversible inhibitor of COMT in the periphery and, to a lesser extent, in central areas. Entacapone reversibly inhibits COMT in the peripheral tissues. When these drugs are given with levodopa or levodopa-carbidopa, plasma levodopa levels are higher and more sustained than when they're given without these drugs. Thus, these drugs help to maintain dopaminergic stimulation in the brain, yielding a greater reduction in Parkinson's disease symptoms.

Another group of substances—antioxidants—may prove useful in slowing Parkinson's disease as well. That's because the free radical known as methyl-4-phenyl-1,2,3,6 tetrahydropyridine (MPTP) is highly toxic to dopamine-producing nerve cells in the substantia nigra. Its toxicity stems from its interference with mitochondrial function in those cells. Some scientists believe that such antioxidants as beta-carotene, vitamin C, vitamin E, and coenzyme Q10 may help to protect against the development of Parkinson's disease by working against MPTP.

PATIENT TEACHING

If your patient receives drug treatment for Parkinson's disease, make sure to review the following teaching topics.
- Tell her to take the drug with a small amount of food if it causes GI upset.
- If she'll be taking an anticholinergic, explain that the drug may make her drowsy. Urge her to avoid hazardous activities until she understands how the drug affects her.
- Mention that anticholinergic drugs may cause a dry mouth, difficult urination, or constipation. Recommend that she maintain an adequate fluid intake, use stool softeners if needed, and try sugarless gum, sugarless hard candy, or ice chips to help relieve the symptoms.
- Warn her not to consume alcohol or other CNS depressants during therapy.
- If the patient takes levodopa, tell her to avoid vitamin products that contain pyridoxine (vitamin B_6) or iron salts.
- Tell her to notify the prescriber if she feels light-headed or dizzy.
- Inform her that levodopa may discolor her urine, saliva, or sweat.
- If the patient is diabetic, caution her that levodopa may interfere with urine glucose tests.
- Tell the patient to immediately notify the prescriber about uncontrollable movements of the face, eyelids, mouth, tongue, neck, arms, hands, or legs.
- If the patient takes selegiline, stress that she should avoid foods that contain tyramine because they raise the risk of a hypertensive reaction, especially if she takes a larger-than-normal amount of the drug.
- If the patient takes tolcapone, review the signs and symptoms of hepatic failure (persistent nausea, fatigue, lethargy, anorexia, jaundice, dark urine, pruritus, right upper quadrant tenderness) and tell her to report them to the prescriber immediately if they develop.
- No matter which drug or drugs the patient takes to treat Parkinson's disease, remind her to take it exactly as prescribed.

amantadine hydrochloride
Symmetrel

Pharmacologic classification:
synthetic cyclic primary amine

Therapeutic classification:
antiparkinsonian, antiviral

Pregnancy risk category C

How supplied
Available by prescription only
Capsules: 100 mg
Syrup: 50 mg/5 ml
Tablets: 100 mg

Indications and dosages
Drug-induced extrapyramidal reactions
Adults: 100 to 300 mg/day P.O. in divided doses.

Idiopathic parkinsonism, parkinsonian syndrome
Adults: 100 mg P.O. b.i.d. In patients who are seriously ill or receiving other antiparkinsonians, 100 mg/day for at least 1 week, then 100 mg b.i.d., p.r.n. Patient may need up to 400 mg/day, but doses over 200 mg require close supervision.

▶ **DOSAGE ADJUSTMENT.** If creatinine clearance is 30 to 50 ml/minute/1.73m², give 200 mg of syrup or capsule form on day 1 followed by 100 mg daily. If creatinine clearance is 15 to 29 ml/minute/1.73m², give 200 mg on day 1 followed by 100 mg on alternating days. If creatinine clearance is below 15 ml/minute/1.73m², give 200 mg q 7 days. If patient receives chronic hemodialysis, give 200 mg q 7 days.

Pharmacodynamics
Antiparkinsonian action: Amantadine probably causes the release of dopamine in the substantia nigra and other central sites.
Antiviral action: Amantadine interferes with viral uncoating of RNA in lysosomes of influenza type A virus. Drug may protect against influenza type A virus in 70% to 90% of patients, and it reduces the duration of fever and other symptoms when given within 48 hours (preferably 24) of onset of illness.

Pharmacokinetics
Absorption: With oral administration, drug is well absorbed from the GI tract. Serum levels peak in 1 to 8 hours; usual serum level is 0.2 to 0.9 mcg/ml. Neurotoxicity may occur at levels exceeding 1.5 mcg/ml.
Distribution: Drug is distributed widely throughout body and crosses the blood-brain barrier.
Metabolism: About 10% of dose is metabolized.
Excretion: About 90% of dose is excreted unchanged in urine, primarily by tubular secretion. Excretion rate depends on urine pH (acidic pH enhances excretion). Elimination half-life in patients with normal renal function is about 24 hours; in those with renal dysfunction, it may extend to 10 days. Some drug may be excreted in breast milk.

Contraindications and precautions
Contraindicated in patients hypersensitive to drug.
  Use cautiously in elderly patients and those with seizure disorders,

heart failure, peripheral edema, hepatic disease, mental illness, eczematoid rash, renal impairment, orthostatic hypotension, or CV disease.

Interactions
Drug-drug
Benztropine and trihexyphenidyl in high doses: possible confusion and hallucinations. Monitor patient closely.
CNS stimulants: may cause additive stimulation. Use together cautiously.
Hydrochlorothiazide, triamterene: may decrease urinary amantadine excretion, causing increased serum levels and possible toxicity. Monitor patient and serum amantadine levels closely.

Drug-herb
Jimson weed: may adversely affect CV function. Avoid use together.

Drug-lifestyle
Alcohol use: may cause light-headedness, confusion, fainting, and hypotension. Discourage use together.

Adverse reactions
CNS: anxiety, ataxia, confusion, depression, *dizziness,* fatigue, hallucinations, headache, *insomnia, irritability, light-headedness.*
CV: **heart failure,** orthostatic hypotension, peripheral edema.
GI: anorexia, constipation, dry mouth, *nausea,* vomiting.
Skin: *livedo reticularis* with prolonged use.

Overdose and treatment
Overdose may cause nausea, vomiting, anorexia, hyperexcitability, tremors, slurred speech, blurred vision, lethargy, anticholinergic effects, seizures, and possible ventricular arrhythmias, including torsades de pointes and ventricular fibrillation. CNS effects result from increased levels of dopamine in the brain.

Treatment includes immediate gastric lavage or induced emesis, along with supportive measures, forced fluids and, if necessary, I.V. administration of fluids. Urine acidification may be used to increase drug excretion. Physostigmine may be given (1 to 2 mg by slow I.V. infusion at 1- to 2-hour intervals) to counteract CNS toxicity. Seizures or arrhythmias may be treated with conventional therapy. Monitor patient closely.

Special considerations
■ If patient complains of insomnia, give drug several hours before bedtime.
■ Patients who initially benefit from amantadine commonly experience decreased effectiveness after a few months. To restore benefits, increase to 300 mg/day or discontinue drug for several weeks. Other antiparkinsonians may be needed during that time.
■ Besides standard indications, drug has been used to prevent influenza type A virus and other respiratory tract illnesses in elderly or debilitated patients.

Breast-feeding patients
■ Drug is excreted in breast milk. Avoid breast-feeding during amantadine therapy.

Pediatric patients
- Safety and effectiveness in children under age 1 haven't been established.

Geriatric patients
- Elderly patients are more susceptible to adverse neurologic effects; dividing daily amount into two doses may reduce this risk.

Patient teaching
- Tell patient to take drug after meals to ensure best absorption.
- To prevent effects of orthostatic hypotension, tell patient to change positions slowly, especially when rising to a sitting or standing position.
- Warn patient that drug may impair mental alertness.
- Caution patient to avoid alcohol during therapy.
- If patient takes drug for parkinsonism, warn against stopping abruptly. A parkinsonian crisis could ensue.
- Urge patient to report adverse effects promptly, especially dizziness, depression, anxiety, nausea, and urine retention.
- Tell women to use effective contraception and to promptly report planned, suspected, or known pregnancy.

benztropine mesylate
Cogentin

Pharmacologic classification:
anticholinergic

Therapeutic classification:
antiparkinsonian

Pregnancy risk category C

How supplied
Available by prescription only
Injection: 1 mg/ml in 2-ml ampule
Tablets: 0.5 mg, 1 mg, 2 mg

Indications and dosages
Acute dystonic reaction
Adults: 1 to 2 mg I.M. or I.V. followed by 1 to 2 mg P.O. b.i.d. to prevent recurrence.

Parkinsonism
Adults: initially, 0.5 to 1 mg, increased 0.5 mg q 5 to 6 days. Range, 0.5 to 6 mg P.O. daily, adjusted to meet individual requirements. Maximum, 6 mg/day.

Drug-induced extrapyramidal reactions
Adults: 1 to 4 mg P.O. or I.V. daily or b.i.d., adjusted to meet individual requirements. Maximum, 6 mg/day.

Pharmacodynamics
Antiparkinsonian action: Benztropine blocks central cholinergic receptors, helping to balance cholinergic activity in the basal ganglia. It may also prolong the effects of dopamine by blocking dopamine reuptake and storage at central receptor sites.

Pharmacokinetics
Absorption: Drug is absorbed from the GI tract.
Distribution: Largely unknown; however, drug crosses the blood-brain barrier and may cross the placenta.
Metabolism: Unknown.
Excretion: Like other muscarinics, benztropine is excreted in the urine as unchanged drug and metabolites. After oral therapy, small amounts are probably also excreted in feces as unabsorbed drug.

Contraindications and precautions
Contraindicated in patients hypersensitive to drug or its components, in patients with acute angle-closure glaucoma, and in children under age 3.

Use cautiously in hot weather, in patients with mental disorders, and in children over age 3.

Interactions
Drug-drug
Amantadine: may amplify such adverse anticholinergic effects as confusion and hallucinations. Decrease benztropine dosage before giving amantadine.
Antacids, antidiarrheals: may decrease benztropine absorption. Give benztropine at least 1 hour before these drugs.
CNS depressants: increased sedative effects of benztropine. Monitor patient closely.
Haloperidol: may decrease effects of haloperidol, possibly reflecting direct CNS antagonism. Monitor patient closely.

Phenothiazines: may decrease the effects of these drugs, possibly reflecting direct CNS antagonism. Also increases the risk of adverse anticholinergic effects. Monitor patient closely.

Drug-lifestyle
Alcohol use: increases the sedative effects of benztropine. Discourage concomitant use.

Adverse reactions
CNS: confusion, depression, disorientation, hallucinations, memory impairment, nervousness, toxic psychosis.
CV: tachycardia.
EENT: dilated pupils, blurred vision.
GI: dry mouth, *constipation,* nausea, vomiting, paralytic ileus.
GU: urine retention, dysuria.

Overdose and treatment
Overdose may cause central stimulation followed by depression and psychotic symptoms, such as disorientation, confusion, hallucinations, delusions, anxiety, agitation, and restlessness. Peripheral effects may include dilated, nonreactive pupils; blurred vision; hot, flushed, dry skin; dry mucous membranes; dysphagia; decreased or absent bowel sounds; urine retention; hyperthermia; tachycardia; hypertension; and increased respiration.

Treatment is primarily symptomatic and supportive. Maintain a patent airway. If patient is alert, induce emesis or perform gastric lavage. Follow with a sodium chloride cathartic and activated charcoal to prevent further absorption. In severe cases, you may give physostigmine to block the anti-muscarinic effects of benztropine. Give fluids as needed for shock, diazepam for psychotic symptoms, and pilocarpine (ophthalmic) to relieve mydriasis. If urine retention occurs, catheterization may be needed.

Special considerations
- To help prevent gastric irritation, give drug after meals.
- Never discontinue drug abruptly.
- Monitor patient for intermittent constipation and abdominal distention and pain, which may indicate paralytic ileus.
- Some adverse reactions may result from atropine-like toxicity and are dose related.
- Give I.M. form of drug for rapid relief of acute dystonic reaction.

Breast-feeding patients
- Drug may be excreted in breast milk, possibly causing toxicity in infant. Benztropine also may decrease milk production. Avoid using drug in breast-feeding women.

Pediatric patients
- Drug is not recommended for children under age 3.

Patient teaching
- Explain that drug's full effect may not occur for 2 to 3 days after therapy begins.
- Caution patient not to discontinue drug suddenly; instead, dosage should be reduced gradually.
- Tell patient that drug may increase sensitivity of eyes to light.

biperiden hydrochloride, biperiden lactate
Akineton

Pharmacologic classification: anticholinergic

Therapeutic classification: antiparkinsonian

Pregnancy risk category C

How supplied
Available by prescription only
biperiden hydrochloride
Tablets: 2 mg biperiden lactate
Injection: 5 mg/ml in 1-ml ampule

Indications and dosages
Extrapyramidal disorders
Adults: 2 mg P.O. daily, b.i.d., or t.i.d., depending on severity. Usual dose is 2 mg daily. To treat drug-induced extrapyramidal symptoms, give 2 mg I.M. or slow I.V. q 30 minutes, not to exceed 8 mg in a 24-hour period.

Parkinsonism
Adults: 2 mg P.O., t.i.d., or q.i.d. For prolonged therapy, adjust to no more than 16 mg daily.

Pharmacodynamics
Antiparkinsonian action: Drug blocks central cholinergic receptors, helping to balance cholinergic activity in the basal ganglia. It may also prolong the effects of dopamine by blocking dopamine reuptake and storage at central receptor sites.

Pharmacokinetics
Absorption: Drug is well absorbed from the GI tract.

Distribution: Poorly understood based on limited studies in humans.
Metabolism: Exact metabolic fate is unknown.
Excretion: Drug is excreted in urine as unchanged drug and metabolites. After oral therapy, small amounts are probably excreted as unabsorbed drug.

Contraindications and precautions

Contraindicated in patients with hypersensitivity to drug, angle-closure glaucoma, bowel obstruction, or megacolon.

Use cautiously in patients with prostatic hyperplasia, arrhythmias, or seizure disorders.

Interactions
Drug-drug

Amantadine: may amplify the anticholinergic adverse effects of biperiden, such as confusion and hallucinations. Decrease biperiden dosage before giving amantadine.
Antacids, antidiarrheals: may decrease biperiden absorption. Give biperiden at least 1 hour before these drugs.
CNS depressants: increased sedative effects of biperiden. Monitor patient closely.
Digoxin: plasma digoxin levels may rise. Dose adjustment may be needed.
Haloperidol: may decrease the antipsychotic effectiveness of these drugs, possibly by direct CNS antagonism.
Phenothiazines: may decrease the antipsychotic effectiveness of these drugs, possibly by direct CNS antagonism. Also increases the risk

of anticholinergic adverse effects. Monitor patient closely.

Drug-lifestyle
Alcohol use: increases sedative effects of biperiden. Discourage concomitant use.

Adverse reactions
CNS: agitation, disorientation, drowsiness, euphoria.
CV: transient orthostatic hypotension (with parenteral use).
EENT: blurred vision.
GI: *constipation,* dry mouth.
GU: urine retention.

Overdose and treatment
Overdose may cause central stimulation followed by depression and psychotic symptoms, such as disorientation, confusion, hallucinations, delusions, anxiety, agitation, and restlessness. Peripheral effects may include dilated, nonreactive pupils; blurred vision; hot, dry, flushed skin; dry mucous membranes; dysphagia; decreased or absent bowel sounds; urine retention; hyperthermia; headache; tachycardia; hypertension; and increased respirations.

Treatment is primarily symptomatic and supportive. Maintain a patent airway. If the patient is alert, induce emesis or perform gastric lavage. Follow with a sodium chloride cathartic and activated charcoal to prevent further absorption of orally administered drug. In severe cases, physostigmine may be administered to block the antimuscarinic effects of biperiden. Give fluids, as needed, for shock, diazepam for psychotic symptoms, and pilocarpine (ophthalmic) for

---

Reactions may be *common,* uncommon, *life-threatening,* or COMMON AND LIFE-THREATENING.

mydriasis. If urine retention occurs, catheterization may be needed.

Special considerations
■ When giving biperiden I.V., inject drug slowly.
■ Keep patient supine during parenteral administration to minimize transient orthostatic hypotension and disturbed coordination.
■ Because biperiden may cause dizziness, assist patient during ambulation.
■ In patients with severe parkinsonism, tremors may increase when drug is given to relieve spasticity.
■ Adverse reactions are dose-related and may resemble atropine toxicity.

Breast-feeding patients
■ Drug may be excreted in breast milk, possibly causing toxicity in infants. It may also decrease milk production. Avoid use of drug in breast-feeding women.

Pediatric patients
■ Drug isn't recommended for children.

Geriatric patients
■ Use cautiously in elderly patients, and give reduced doses.

Patient teaching
■ Instruct patient to take drug with food to avoid GI upset.
■ Tell patient that drug may increase sensitivity of the eyes to light.
■ Tell patient that tolerance to therapeutic and adverse effects can occur with long-term use.

bromocriptine mesylate
Parlodel

Pharmacologic classification: dopamine receptor agonist

Therapeutic classification: semisynthetic ergot alkaloid, dopaminergic agonist, antiparkinsonian, inhibitor of prolactin release, inhibitor of growth hormone release

Pregnancy risk category B

How supplied
Available by prescription only
Capsules: 5 mg
Tablets: 2.5 mg

Indications and dosages
Parkinson's disease
Adults: initially, 1.25 to 2.5 mg P.O. b.i.d. with meals. Dosage may be increased by 2.5 mg daily q 14 to 28 days, up to 100 mg daily or until maximum therapeutic response occurs. Usual range is 10 to 40 mg daily. Safety in dosages over 100 mg daily has not been established.

Pharmacodynamics
Antiparkinsonian action: Drug activates dopaminergic receptors in the neostriatum of the CNS, which may produce antiparkinsonian action. Dysregulation of brain serotonin activity also may occur. The precise role of bromocriptine in long-term treatment of parkinsonism syndrome needs further study.
Prolactin-inhibiting action: Drug reduces prolactin levels by acting directly on the anterior pituitary gland to inhibit prolactin release. It may also stimulate the release of

prolactin-inhibitory factor from postsynaptic dopamine receptors in the hypothalamus via a complicated catecholamine pathway. Drug reduces high serum prolactin levels and restores ovulation and ovarian function in amenorrheic women and suppresses puerperal or non-puerperal lactation in women with adequate gonadotropin levels and ovarian function. Average time to reverse amenorrhea is 6 to 8 weeks, but it may take up to 24 weeks.

Pharmacokinetics

Absorption: Drug is 28% absorbed when given orally and peaks in about 1 to 3 hours. After an oral dose, serum prolactin decreases within 2 hours, reaches maximum decrease at 8 hours, and remains decreased at 24 hours.

Distribution: About 90% to 96% is bound to serum albumin.

Metabolism: First-pass metabolism occurs with more than 90% of absorbed dose. Drug is metabolized completely in the liver, mainly by hydrolysis, before excretion. The metabolites are not active or toxic.

Excretion: Drug is primarily excreted through bile. Almost all (85%) of dose appears in feces within 5 days. Only 2.5% to 5.5% of dose is excreted in urine.

Contraindications and precautions

Contraindicated in patients with hypersensitivity to ergot derivatives, uncontrolled hypertension, or toxemia of pregnancy.

Use cautiously in patients with renal impairment, hepatic impairment, or a history of MI with residual arrhythmias.

Interactions

Drug-drug

Antihypertensives: bromocriptine may potentiate antihypertensive action. Reduced antihypertensive dosage may be needed to prevent hypotension.

Drugs that increase prolactin levels, such as amitriptyline, butyrophenones, imipramine, methyldopa, phenothiazines, reserpine: may decrease the efficacy of bromocriptine and create a need for increased bromocriptine dosage.

Erythromycin: Bromocriptine levels may be increased resulting in toxicity. Monitor patient and serum levels closely.

Sympathomimetics, such as isometheptene, phenylpropanolamine: Increased risk of adverse effects, including ventricular tachycardia and cardiac dysfunction. Avoid concomitant use.

Drug-lifestyle

Alcohol use: intolerance to alcohol may result from high doses of bromocriptine. Tell patient to limit concomitant use.

Adverse reactions

CNS: delusions, depression, *dizziness,* drowsiness, fatigue, *headache,* insomnia, light-headedness, mania, nervousness, **seizures.**

CV: *acute MI, CVA,* hypotension.

EENT: blurred vision, nasal congestion.

GI: *abdominal cramps,* anorexia, *constipation,* diarrhea, *nausea,* vomiting.

GU: urinary frequency, urine retention.

Skin: coolness, pallor of fingers and toes.

Overdose and treatment

Overdose may cause nausea, vomiting, and severe hypotension.

Treatment includes emptying the stomach by aspiration and lavage, and administering I.V. fluids to treat hypotension.

Special considerations

- For antiparkinsonism, drug is usually given with levodopa or levodopa-carbidopa.
- Give drug with meals, milk, or snacks to minimize GI distress.
- Give drug cautiously, especially if patient receives long-term, high-dose therapy. Perform regular physical assessments, noting changes in pulmonary function.
- First-dose phenomenon occurs in 1% of patients. Sensitive patients may experience syncope for 15 to 60 minutes, but can usually tolerate continued treatment. Patient should begin therapy with lowest dosage, taken at bedtime.
- Examine patient carefully for pituitary tumor (Forbes-Albright syndrome). Bromocriptine doesn't affect tumor size, but it may alleviate amenorrhea or galactorrhea.
- Adverse reactions are more common at high doses.
- Drug is also given for female infertility, acromegaly, and amenorrhea and galactorrhea caused by hyperprolactinemia.

Breast-feeding patients

- Because drug inhibits lactation, it shouldn't be given to women who intend to breast-feed.

Pediatric patients

- Drug isn't recommended for children under age 15.

Geriatric patients

- Safety hasn't been established for long-term use in elderly patients at doses needed to treat Parkinson's disease.

Patient teaching

- Tell patient to take drug with meals to avoid GI upset.
- Tell patient that drowsiness is commonly at start of therapy. Urge her to lie down after first dose.
- Warn patient that drug may impair alertness and coordination.
- Instruct patient to report visual problems, severe nausea and vomiting, or acute headaches.
- Tell patient to limit alcohol during therapy because alcohol intolerance may occur, especially at high bromocriptine doses.

---

diphenhydramine hydrochloride
Benadryl, Benylin, Compoz, Diphen AF, Diphenadryl, Hydramine, Nervine Nighttime Sleep-Aid, Nytol, Sleep-Eze 3, Sominex, Tusstat, Twilite

Pharmacologic classification: ethanolamine-derivative antihistamine

Therapeutic classification: sedative-hypnotic, antidyskinetic (anticholinergic), antiemetic, antivertigo, antihistamine (H_2-receptor antagonist), antitussive

Pregnancy risk category B

How supplied
Available with or without a prescription

Capsules: 25 mg, 50 mg
Capsules (chewable): 12.5 mg
Elixir: 12.5 mg/5 ml (14% alcohol)
Injection: 50 mg/ml
Syrup: 12.5 mg/5 ml (5% alcohol)
Tablets: 25 mg, 50 mg

Indications and dosages
Parkinson's disease, motion sickness
Adults and children age 12 and older: 25 to 50 mg P.O. t.i.d. or q.i.d.; or 10 to 50 mg I.V. or deep I.M. Maximum I.M. or I.V. dose is 400 mg daily.
Children under age 12: 5 mg/kg daily P.O., deep I.M., or I.V. in divided doses q.i.d. Maximum, 300 mg daily.

Insomnia
Adults: 50 mg P.O. h.s.

Sedation induction
Adults: 25 to 50 mg P.O., or deep I.M., p.r.n.

Pharmacodynamics
Anesthetic action: Drug is structurally related to local anesthetics, which prevent initiation and transmission of nerve impulses; this is the probable source of its topical and local anesthetic effects.
Antihistamine action: Antihistamines compete for H_2-receptor sites on the smooth muscles of the bronchi, GI tract, uterus, and large blood vessels. By binding to cellular receptors, they prevent histamine from binding and thus suppress histamine-induced allergic symptoms. They don't prevent histamine release.

Antitussive action: Drug suppresses the cough reflex by directly affecting the cough center.
Antivertigo, antiemetic, antidyskinetic actions: Central antimuscarinic actions of antihistamines probably produce these effects.
Sedative action: Mechanism of CNS depression is unknown.

Pharmacokinetics
Absorption: Drug is well absorbed from the GI tract. Action begins in 15 to 30 minutes and peaks in 1 to 4 hours.
Distribution: Drug is distributed widely throughout the body, including the CNS; drug crosses the placenta and is excreted in breast milk. Drug is about 82% protein-bound.
Metabolism: About 50% to 60% of an oral dose is metabolized by the liver before reaching the systemic circulation (first-pass effect); virtually all available drug is metabolized by the liver in 24 to 48 hours.
Excretion: Plasma elimination half-life is about 2½ to 9 hours; drug and metabolites are excreted mainly in urine.

Contraindications and precautions
Contraindicated in patients hypersensitive to drug; in newborns, premature neonates, or breast-feeding patients; and during acute asthma attacks.

Use with extreme caution in patients with angle-closure glaucoma, prostatic hyperplasia, pyloroduodenal or bladder neck obstruction, asthma, COPD, increased intraocular pressure, hyperthyroidism, CV disease, hypertension, or stenosing peptic ulcer.

Interactions

Drug-drug

CNS depressants, such as antianxiety drugs, barbiturates, sleeping aids, tranquilizers: additive CNS depression may occur. Monitor patient closely.

Epinephrine: enhanced effects. Don't use together.

Heparin: partially counteracted anticoagulant effects. Monitor patient's PT and INR as indicated.

MAO inhibitors: interference with detoxification of diphenhydramine, thus prolonging central depressant and anticholinergic effects. Monitor patient closely.

Sulfonylureas: diphenhydramine may diminish their effects. Monitor patient closely.

Drug-lifestyle

Alcohol use: may cause additive CNS depression. Discourage use.

Sun exposure: may cause photosensitivity reactions. Urge precautions.

Adverse reactions

CNS: confusion, *dizziness, drowsiness,* fatigue, headache, *incoordination,* insomnia, nervousness, restlessness, *sedation,* **seizures,** *sleepiness,* tremor, vertigo.

CV: hypotension, palpitations, tachycardia.

EENT: blurred vision, diplopia, tinnitus.

GI: anorexia, constipation, diarrhea, *dry mouth, epigastric distress, nausea,* vomiting.

GU: dysuria, urinary frequency, urine retention.

Hematologic: *agranulocytosis, hemolytic anemia, thrombocytopenia.*

Respiratory: nasal congestion, *thickening of bronchial secretions.*

Skin: photosensitivity, rash, urticaria.

Other: *anaphylactic shock.*

Overdose and treatment

Overdose usually causes drowsiness. Profound overdose may cause respiratory depression, seizures, and coma. Anticholinergic symptoms, such as dry mouth, flushed skin, fixed and dilated pupils, and GI symptoms, are common, especially in children.

Treat overdose by inducing emesis with ipecac syrup if patient is conscious. Perform gastric lavage if patient is unconscious or ipecac fails. Follow with activated charcoal to reduce further drug absorption. Treat hypotension with vasopressors. Control seizures with diazepam or phenytoin. Don't give stimulants.

Special considerations

■ Injectable and elixir solutions are light-sensitive; protect them from light.

■ Diphenhydramine injection is compatible with most I.V. solutions but is incompatible with some drugs; check compatibility before mixing in the same I.V. line.

■ Alternate injection sites to prevent irritation. Administer deep I.M. into a large muscle.

■ Drowsiness is the most common adverse effect during initial therapy; it usually resolves with continued therapy.

■ Discontinue drug 4 days before diagnostic skin tests; antihistamines can prevent, reduce, or mask positive skin test response.
■ Besides standard indications, drug has been used to treat rhinitis, allergy symptoms, and nonproductive cough.

Breast-feeding patients
■ Avoid giving antihistamines during breast-feeding. Many antihistamines are secreted in breast milk and may cause unusual excitability in the infant; premature infants are at particular risk for seizures.

Geriatric patients
■ Elderly patients are usually more sensitive to adverse antihistamine effects than younger patients and are especially likely to experience dizziness, sedation, hyperexcitability, dry mouth, and urine retention. Symptoms usually respond to decreased dosage.

Patient teaching
■ Explain that drowsiness is very common initially but usually declines with continued therapy.
■ Urge patient to avoid alcohol during therapy.
■ Tell patient to notify physician about use of diphenhydramine before undergoing skin tests for allergies.
■ Tell patient to avoid prolonged use of diphenhydramine for insomnia because rebound insomnia may occur when therapy stops. Advise patient to see primary care provider if insomnia persists for longer than 2 weeks because it may indicate a need for medical attention.

entacapone
Comtan

Pharmacologic classification: **catechol-O-methyltransferase (COMT) inhibitor**

Therapeutic classification: **antiparkinsonian**

Pregnancy risk category C

How supplied
Available by prescription only
Tablets: 200 mg

Indications and dosages
Adjunct to levodopa-carbidopa for patients with idiopathic Parkinson's disease who experience end-of-dose wearing off of levodopa-carbidopa
Adults: 200 mg P.O. with each dose of levodopa-carbidopa to a maximum of eight times daily (1,600 mg/day). Reducing daily levodopa dose or extending the interval between doses may be needed to optimize patient's response.

Pharmacodynamics
Antiparkinsonian action: Entacapone is a reversible inhibitor of peripheral COMT, which is responsible for eliminating various catecholamines, including dopamine. Blocking this pathway when administering levodopa-carbidopa yields higher serum levodopa levels, thereby allowing greater dopaminergic stimulation in the CNS and a greater clinical effect in treating parkinsonian symptoms.

Pharmacokinetics
Absorption: Absorption is rapid, with serum levels peaking in about 1 hour. Food doesn't affect absorption.
Distribution: Drug is about 98% protein-bound, mainly to albumin, and doesn't distribute widely into tissues.
Metabolism: Drug is almost completely metabolized by glucuronidation before elimination. No active metabolites have been identified.
Excretion: About 10% of drug is excreted in urine; the rest is excreted in bile and feces. The half-life of entacapone is biphasic: 0.4 to 0.7 hours for first phase and 2.4 hours for second phase.

Adverse reactions
CNS: agitation, anxiety, asthenia, dizziness, *dyskinesia,* fatigue, hallucinations, *hyperkinesia,* hypokinesia, somnolence.
GI: abdominal pain, constipation, *diarrhea,* dry mouth, dyspepsia, gastritis, *nausea,* taste perversion, vomiting, flatulence.
GU: *urine discoloration.*
Hematologic: purpura.
Musculoskeletal: back pain, *rhabdomyolysis* (rare).
Respiratory: dyspnea.
Skin: sweating.
Other: bacterial infection.

Interactions
Drug-drug
Ampicillin, chloramphenicol, cholestyramine, erythromycin, probenecid: may block biliary excretion, raising serum entacapone levels. Use cautiously.

CNS depressants: additive effect. Use cautiously.
Drugs metabolized by COMT, such as bitolterol, dobutamine, dopamine, epinephrine, isoetharine, isoproterenol, norepinephrine: may raise serum levels of these drugs, causing increased heart rate, altered blood pressure, or possible arrhythmias. Use cautiously.
Nonselective MAO inhibitors, such as phenelzine, tranylcypromine: may inhibit normal catecholamine metabolism. Avoid concomitant use.

Drug-lifestyle
Alcohol use: may cause additive CNS effects. Avoid concomitant use.

Overdose and treatment
There are no reported cases of overdose. Management would be symptomatic. Expect that hemodialysis wouldn't be effective because of drug's high protein-binding time. In acute stages, gastric lavage or activated charcoal may be helpful to limit absorption in GI tract.

Contraindications and precautions
Contraindicated in patients hypersensitive to drug.
    Use cautiously in patients with hepatic impairment, biliary obstruction, or orthostatic hypotension.

Special considerations
■ Give drug with immediate- or sustained-release levodopa-carbidopa, with or without food. Entacapone monotherapy produces no antiparkinsonian effects.

- To minimize adverse effects, levodopa-carbidopa dosage should be lowered or dosing interval lengthened when given with entacapone.
- Hallucinations may develop or worsen when taking this drug.
- Monitor patient's blood pressure closely. Observe for orthostatic hypotension.
- Diarrhea most commonly begins 4 to 12 weeks after therapy starts, but it may begin during the first week or not until after many months of therapy.
- Drug may discolor urine.
- Rapid withdrawal of drug or abrupt reduction in dose could cause signs and symptoms of Parkinson's disease, hyperpyrexia, confusion, or a condition that resembles neuroleptic malignant syndrome. Discontinue drug slowly, and monitor patient closely. Adjust other dopaminergic treatments as needed.
- Entacapone may cause or worsen existing dyskinesia despite reduction of levodopa-carbidopa dosage.

Patient teaching
- Instruct patient not to crush or break tablet and to take it at same time as levodopa-carbidopa.
- Warn patient to avoid hazardous activities until full CNS effects of drug are known.
- Advise patient to avoid alcohol during treatment.
- Instruct patient to use caution when rising to a sitting or standing position after a prolonged period of sitting or lying down because dizziness may occur. This effect is more common early in therapy.

- Warn patient that hallucinations, increased dyskinesia, nausea, and diarrhea could occur.
- Inform patient that drug may turn urine brownish orange.
- Advise patient never to stop or decrease dose of drug without consulting with physician first.
- Tell patient to notify prescriber about planned, suspected, or known pregnancy, and about planned or current breast-feeding.

---

levodopa
Dopar, Larodopa

Pharmacologic classification: dopamine precursor

Therapeutic classification: antiparkinsonian

Pregnancy risk category C

How supplied
Available by prescription only
Capsules: 100 mg, 250 mg, 500 mg
Tablets: 100 mg, 250 mg, 500 mg

Indications and dosages
Idiopathic, postencephalitic, arteriosclerotic parkinsonism; symptomatic parkinsonism caused by injury to the nervous system from carbon monoxide or manganese intoxication
Adults: initially, 0.5 to 1 g P.O. daily, given b.i.d., t.i.d., or q.i.d. Increase by no more than 0.75 g daily q 3 to 7 days, as tolerated. Usually, optimal dose is 3 to 6 g daily divided into three doses. Don't exceed 8 g daily for most patients. Larger dose requires close supervision. Significant therapeu-

tic response may not occur for 6 months.

Pharmacodynamics
Antiparkinsonian action: Precise mechanism is unknown. A small percentage of each dose crossing the blood-brain barrier is decarboxylated. The dopamine then stimulates dopaminergic receptors in the basal ganglia to enhance the balance between cholinergic and dopaminergic activity, yielding improved modulation of voluntary nerve impulses transmitted to the motor cortex.

Pharmacokinetics
Absorption: Drug is absorbed rapidly from the small intestine by an active amino acid transport system, with 30% to 50% reaching general circulation.
Distribution: Drug is distributed widely to most body tissues, but not to the CNS, which receives less than 1% of dose because of extensive metabolism in the periphery.
Metabolism: 95% of levodopa is converted to dopamine by l-aromatic amino acid decarboxylase enzyme in the lumen of the stomach and intestines and on the first pass through the liver.
Excretion: Drug is excreted primarily in urine; 80% of dose is excreted within 24 hours as dopamine metabolites. Half-life is 1 to 3 hours.

Contraindications and precautions
Contraindicated within 14 days of taking an MAO inhibitor, in patients hypersensitive to drug, and in patients with acute angle-closure glaucoma, melanoma, or undiagnosed pigmented skin lesions.

Use cautiously in patients with peptic ulcer, psychiatric illness, MI with residual arrhythmias, bronchial asthma, emphysema, endocrine disorders, or severe renal, CV, hepatic, or pulmonary disorders.

Interactions
Drug-drug
Amantadine, benztropine, procyclidine, or *trihexyphenidyl:* may increase the efficacy of levodopa. Monitor patient.
Bromocriptine: may produce additive effects, allowing reduced levodopa dosage. Monitor patient.
Anesthetics or *hydrocarbon inhalation:* may cause arrhythmias because of increased endogenous dopamine concentration. Levodopa should be discontinued 6 to 8 hours before administration of anesthetics such as halothane.
Antacids that contain calcium, magnesium, or sodium bicarbonate: may increase levodopa absorption. Monitor patient closely.
Anticholinergics: may produce a mild synergy and increased efficacy. Gradually reduce anticholinergic dosage.
Anticonvulsants (such as hydantoins, phenytoin), benzodiazepines, haloperidol, papaverine, phenothiazines, rauwolfia alkaloids, thioxanthenes: may decrease therapeutic effects of levodopa. Monitor patient closely.
Antihypertensives: concurrent use may increase hypotensive effects. Monitor patient closely.
MAO inhibitors: may cause hypertensive crisis. Discontinue MAO

inhibitors for 2 to 4 weeks before starting levodopa.

Methyldopa: may alter antiparkinsonian effects of levodopa and produce additive toxic CNS effects. Use with extreme caution.

Pyridoxine: in a small dose (10 mg), reverses the antiparkinsonian effects of levodopa. Avoid use together.

Sympathomimetics: may increase the risk of arrhythmias. Reduce sympathomimetic dosage. Giving levodopa-carbidopa reduces the tendency of sympathomimetics to cause dopamine-induced arrhythmias; however, levodopa dose should be reduced.

Tricyclic antidepressants: may increase sympathetic activity, with sinus tachycardia and hypertension. Use with caution.

Drug-herb
Jimson weed: may adversely affect CV function. Avoid use together.
Kava: may increase parkinsonian symptoms. Avoid use together.
Rauwolfia: may decrease levodopa effectiveness. Monitor patient closely.

Adverse reactions
CNS: *aggressive behavior,* anxiety, ataxia, bradykinetic episodes, *choreiform movements,* delirium, dementia, disturbing dreams, *dyskinetic movements, dystonic movements,* euphoria, fatigue, hallucinations (may require reduction or withdrawal of drug), *head movements, involuntary grimacing,* malaise, mood changes, muscle twitching, *myoclonic body jerks,* nervousness, psychiatric disturbances, *seizures,* severe depression, tremor, *suicidal tendencies.*

CV: cardiac irregularities, *orthostatic hypotension,* phlebitis.
EENT: activation of latent Horner's syndrome, blepharospasm, blurred vision, diplopia, excessive salivation, miosis, mydriasis, oculogyric crisis.
GI: abdominal pain, *anorexia,* bitter taste, constipation, diarrhea, dry mouth, flatulence, *nausea, vomiting.*
GU: darkened urine, incontinence, priapism, urinary frequency, urine retention.
Hematologic: *agranulocytosis, hemolytic anemia, leukopenia.*
Hepatic: elevated liver enzymes, *hepatotoxicity.*
Metabolic: weight loss at start of therapy.
Respiratory: hiccups, hyperventilation.
Other: dark perspiration.

Overdose and treatment
Overdose may cause spasm or closing of eyelids, irregular heartbeat, or palpitations.

Treatment includes immediate gastric lavage, maintenance of an adequate airway, and judicious administration of I.V. fluids. It may include antiarrhythmic drugs as well. Pyridoxine 10 to 25 mg P.O. may reverse toxic and therapeutic effects of levodopa, although its usefulness hasn't been established in acute overdose.

Special considerations
■ Treat psychotic patients cautiously, and watch all patients for depression and suicidal tendencies.
■ Protect drug from heat, light, and moisture. If preparation dark-

ens, it has lost potency and should be discarded.

■ Give drug between meals with a low-protein snack to maximize absorption and minimize GI upset. High-protein foods seems to interfere with drug transport.

■ If patient has trouble swallowing pills, crush drug and mix with applesauce or fruit baby food.

■ Maximum drug effectiveness may not occur for several weeks or months after therapy starts.

■ Monitor patient's vital signs carefully, especially while adjusting dosage.

■ Although controversial, a medically supervised period of drug discontinuance (called a drug holiday) may reestablish the effectiveness of a lower-dose regimen.

■ Coombs' test occasionally becomes positive during extended drug use. Expect uric acid elevation with colorimetric method but not with uricase method.

■ Combining levodopa and carbidopa usually reduces the amount of levodopa needed, thus reducing adverse reactions.

■ Assess patient for muscle twitching and blepharospasm (twitching of eyelids); they may be an early sign of drug overdose.

■ Observe patient closely when reducing or abruptly stopping levodopa because of the risk of a condition similar to neuroleptic malignant syndrome.

■ If patient receives long-term therapy, test regularly for diabetes and acromegaly. Also, check blood tests and liver and kidney function studies periodically for adverse effects. Leukopenia may require end of therapy.

■ Watch suspicious moles because drug can activate malignant melanoma.

■ If patient will be undergoing surgery, continue giving levodopa as long as oral intake is permitted, usually 6 to 24 hours before surgery. Resume drug as soon as patient can take drug orally.

■ If restarting therapy after a long interruption, adjust dosage gradually to previous level.

■ Besides standard indications, levodopa has also been used for restless leg syndrome and to relieve the pain of herpes zoster.

Breast-feeding patients
■ Drug may inhibit lactation and shouldn't be used by breast-feeding women.

Pediatric patients
■ Safe use of levodopa in children under age 12 hasn't been established.

Geriatric patients
■ Elderly patients have a higher risk of psychic adverse effects, such as anxiety, confusion, or nervousness. Those with heart disease have a higher risk of cardiac effects.

■ Elderly patients, especially those with osteoporosis, should resume normal activities gradually, because increased mobility may increase the risk of fractures.

Patient teaching
■ Explain that therapeutic response may not occur for up to 6 months.

■ Tell patient not to take drug with food, but mention that eating something about 15 minutes afterward may help reduce GI upset.

■ Teach patient to recognize therapeutic effects and adverse reactions. Stress the need to report changes to prescriber.

■ Warn patient of possible dizziness and orthostatic hypotension, especially at the start of therapy. Tell patient to change positions slowly and to dangle her legs before getting out of bed. Teach patient how to use elastic stockings to reduce the effects of orthostatic hypotension if appropriate.

■ Inform patient that urine, sweat, and other body fluids may darken during therapy.

■ Warn patient and family not to increase dosage without consulting prescriber; they may be tempted to do so as Parkinson's disease progresses.

■ Advise patient and family that multivitamin preparations, fortified cereals, and certain OTC products may contain pyridoxine (vitamin B_6), which can reverse the effects of levodopa.

■ Tell patient to take a missed dose as soon as possible unless the next scheduled dose is within 2 hours. Warn against doubling the dose.

■ Advise women to use contraception during therapy and to report planned, suspected, or known pregnancy.

levodopa-carbidopa
Sinemet, Sinemet CR

Pharmacologic classification: decarboxylase inhibitor–dopamine precursor combination

Therapeutic classification: antiparkinsonian

Pregnancy risk category C

How supplied
Available by prescription only
Tablets: 10 mg carbidopa with 100 mg levodopa (Sinemet 10-100), 25 mg carbidopa with 100 mg levodopa (Sinemet 25-100), 25 mg carbidopa with 250 mg levodopa (Sinemet 25-250)
Tablets (sustained-release): 50 mg carbidopa with 200 mg levodopa (Sinemet CR 50-200), 25 mg carbidopa with 100 mg levodopa (Sinemet CR 25-100)

Indications and dosages
Parkinsonism
Adults: Most patients respond to a 25 mg/100 mg combination (1 tablet t.i.d.). Dosage may be increased q 1 or 2 days.

Give 1 to 2 tablets of 10 mg/100-mg strength t.i.d. or q.i.d. or 1 sustained-release tablet b.i.d. at intervals of 6 hours or more. Intervals may be adjusted based on patient response. Usual dose is 2 to 8 tablets daily in divided doses q 4 to 8 hours while awake. Maintenance therapy must be carefully adjusted based on patient tolerance and desired therapeutic response.

Usual daily dosage is 3 to 6 tablets of 25 mg/250 mg strength daily in divided doses. Don't exceed 8 tablets daily. Optimum daily dose must be adjusted carefully for each patient. Daily dose of carbidopa should be 70 mg or above to suppress peripheral metabolism of levodopa, but it shouldn't exceed 200 mg.

Pharmacodynamics
Decarboxylase-inhibiting action: Carbidopa inhibits the peripheral decarboxylation of levodopa, thus slowing its conversion to dopamine in extracerebral tissues. This results in an increased availability of levodopa for transport to the brain, where it undergoes decarboxylation to dopamine.

Pharmacokinetics
Absorption: 40% to 70% of dose is absorbed after oral administration. Plasma levodopa levels rise when carbidopa and levodopa are given together because carbidopa inhibits peripheral metabolism of levodopa.
Distribution: Carbidopa is distributed widely in body tissues except the CNS. Levodopa is also distributed into breast milk.
Metabolism: Carbidopa is not metabolized extensively. It inhibits metabolism of levodopa in the GI tract, thus increasing levodopa absorption from the GI tract and its level in plasma.
Excretion: 30% of dose is excreted unchanged in urine within 24 hours. When given with carbidopa, the amount of levodopa excreted unchanged in urine is increased by about 6%. Half-life is 1 to 2 hours.

Contraindications and precautions
Contraindicated in patients hypersensitive to drug, patients who took an MAO inhibitor within 14 days, and patients with acute angle-closure glaucoma, melanoma, or undiagnosed skin lesions.

Use cautiously in patients with peptic ulcer, psychiatric illness, MI with residual arrhythmias, bronchial asthma, emphysema, well-controlled chronic open-angle glaucoma, or severe CV, endocrine, pulmonary, renal, or hepatic disorders.

Interactions
Drug-drug
Amantadine, benztropine, procyclidine, trihexyphenidyl: may increase the efficacy of levodopa. Monitor patient for drug effects.
Halogenated general anesthetics: may cause arrhythmias by increasing endogenous dopamine level. Use other anesthetics if possible. Levodopa-carbidopa should be stopped 6 to 8 hours before giving anesthetics.
Antacids that contain calcium, magnesium, or sodium bicarbonate: may increase levodopa absorption. Monitor patient closely.
Anticonvulsants (hydantoin), benzodiazepines, droperidol, haloperidol, loxapine, metyrosine, papaverine, phenothiazines, rauwolfia alkaloids, thioxanthenes: may decrease therapeutic effects of levodopa. Monitor patient and serum levels closely.
Antihypertensives: may increase hypotensive effects. Use with caution.

Bromocriptine: may produce additive effects. Reduce levodopa dosage as needed.

MAO inhibitors: may cause hypertensive crisis. Stop MAO inhibitor for 2 to 4 weeks before starting levodopa-carbidopa.

Methyldopa: may alter antiparkinsonian effects of levodopa and may produce additive toxic CNS effects. Monitor patient closely.

Molindone: may inhibit antiparkinsonian effects of levodopa by blocking dopamine receptors in the brain. Monitor patient closely.

Sympathomimetics: may increase risk of arrhythmia, although giving carbidopa with levodopa reduces the risk of dopamine-induced arrhythmias. Reduce sympathomimetic dosage.

Adverse reactions

CNS: agitation, anxiety, *ataxia,* bradykinetic episodes, *choreiform movements,* confusion, delirium, dementia, disturbing dreams, *dystonic movements, dyskinetic movements,* euphoria, fatigue, hallucinations, *head movements,* insomnia, *involuntary grimacing,* malaise, muscle twitching, *myoclonic body jerks,* psychiatric disturbances, severe depression, **suicidal tendencies,** tremor.

CV: **cardiac irregularities,** *orthostatic hypotension,* phlebitis.

EENT: blepharospasm, blurred vision, diplopia, excessive salivation, miosis, mydriasis, oculogyric crises.

GI: abdominal pain, *anorexia,* bitter taste, constipation, diarrhea, *dry mouth,* flatulence, *nausea, vomiting.*

GU: darkened urine, priapism, urinary frequency, urinary incontinence, urine retention.

Hematologic: **agranulocytosis, hemolytic anemia, leukopenia, thrombocytopenia.**

Hepatic: *hepatotoxicity.*

Metabolic: weight loss at start of therapy.

Respiratory: hiccups, hyperventilation.

Other: dark perspiration.

Overdose and treatment

There have been no reports of overdose with carbidopa. Levodopa overdose may cause irregular heartbeat, palpitations, continuous severe nausea and vomiting, and spasm or closing of eyelids.

Treatment of overdose includes immediate gastric lavage and antiarrhythmic drugs, if needed. Pyridoxine doesn't reverse the actions of levodopa-carbidopa combinations.

Special considerations

■ Treat psychotic patients cautiously, and watch all patients for depression and suicidal tendencies.

■ If patient is receiving levodopa, discontinue it at least 8 hours before starting levodopa-carbidopa.

■ Sustained-release tablets may be split but not crushed or chewed.

■ Adjust dosage based on patient's response and tolerance to drug. Monitor patient's vital signs, especially while adjusting dosage.

■ Maximum drug effectiveness may not occur for several weeks or months after therapy starts.

■ Pryidoxine (vitamin B_6) doesn't reverse beneficial effects of levodopa-carbidopa. Multivitamins

---

can be taken without fear of losing control of symptoms.

■ Coombs' test is occasionally positive after long-term use. In thyroid function tests, the response of thyroid-stimulating hormone to protirelin may be inhibited.

■ Levodopa-carbidopa therapy may elevate serum gonadotropin levels. Serum and urine uric acid levels may show false elevations.

■ Urine glucose tests using the copper reduction method may show false-positive results; tests using the glucose oxidase method may show false-negative results. Urine ketone tests using the dipstick method, urine norepinephrine tests, and urine protein tests using the Lowery test may show false-positive results.

■ Systemic drug effects may elevate BUN, ALT, AST, alkaline phosphatase, serum bilirubin, LD, and serum protein-bound iodine levels.

■ Hallucinations may require reduction or withdrawal of drug.

■ Assess patient for muscle twitching and blepharospasm (twitching of eyelids); they may be an early sign of drug overdose.

■ Watch suspicious moles because drug can activate malignant melanoma.

■ If patient receives long-term therapy, test regularly for diabetes and acromegaly. Also, check blood tests and liver and kidney function studies periodically for adverse effects. Leukopenia may require discontinuation of therapy.

■ If patient will be undergoing surgery, continue giving levodopa as long as oral intake is permitted, usually 6 to 24 hours before surgery. Resume drug as soon as patient can take drug orally.

Breast-feeding patients

■ Because levodopa may inhibit lactation, breast-feeding women shouldn't use it.

Pediatric patients

■ Safe use of drug in children under age 18 hasn't been established.

Geriatric patients

■ Elderly patients have a higher risk of psychic adverse effects, such as anxiety, confusion, or nervousness. Those with heart disease have a higher risk of cardiac effects. Elderly patients, especially those with osteoporosis, should resume normal activities gradually, because increased mobility may increase the risk of fractures.

Patient teaching

■ Tell patient not to take drug with food, but mention that eating something about 15 minutes afterward may help reduce GI upset.

■ Teach patient to recognize therapeutic effects and adverse reactions. Stress the need to report changes to prescriber.

■ Warn patient of possible dizziness and orthostatic hypotension, especially at the start of therapy. Tell patient to change positions slowly and to dangle her legs before getting out of bed. Teach patient how to use elastic stockings to reduce the effects of orthostatic hypotension if appropriate.

■ Inform patient that urine, sweat, and other body fluids may darken during therapy.

■ Caution against stopping drug abruptly without consulting prescriber.

■ Tell patient to take a missed dose as soon as possible unless the next scheduled dose is within 2 hours. Warn against doubling the dose.

■ Teach patient and family how to recognize condition that resembles neuroleptic malignant syndrome. Symptoms include muscle rigidity, fever, tachycardia, mental status changes, and tachypnea.

---

pergolide mesylate
Permax

Pharmacologic classification: dopaminergic agonist

Therapeutic classification: antiparkinsonian

Pregnancy risk category B

How supplied
Available by prescription only
Tablets: 0.05 mg, 0.25 mg, 1 mg

Indications and dosages
Parkinson's disease (adjunct to levodopa-carbidopa)
Adults: 0.05 mg P.O. daily for first 2 days, increased by 0.1 to 0.15 mg q third day for next 12 days. May continue to increase by 0.25 mg q third day until optimum response occurs. Gradual reduction in levodopa-carbidopa dosage may occur during pergolide adjustment. Usual dosage is 3 mg/day, usually given t.i.d. in divided doses. Maximum, 5 mg/day.

Pharmacodynamics
Antiparkinsonian action: Pergolide stimulates dopamine receptors at D_2 and D_3 sites. It acts by directly stimulating postsynaptic receptors in the nigrostriatal system.

Pharmacokinetics
Absorption: Drug is well absorbed after oral administration. Half-life is about 24 hours.
Distribution: Pergolide is about 90% bound to plasma proteins.
Metabolism: Drug is metabolized to at least 10 different compounds, some of which retain some pharmacologic activity.
Excretion: Drug is excreted primarily by the kidneys.

Contraindications and precautions
Contraindicated in patients hypersensitive to drug or to ergot alkaloids.
   Use cautiously in patients prone to arrhythmias and in patients with underlying psychiatric disorders.

Interactions
Drug-drug
Dopamine antagonists, including butyrophenones, metoclopramide, phenothiazines, thioxanthines: may antagonize the effects of pergolide. Monitor patient closely.
Drugs known to affect protein binding: altered protein binding of pergolide or other protein-bound drugs. Give together cautiously.

Adverse reactions
CNS: abnormal dreams, abnormal gait, akathisia, akinesia, anxiety, asthenia, *confusion,* depression, *dizziness, dyskinesia, dystonia,*

Reactions may be *common,* uncommon, *life-threatening,* or COMMON AND LIFE-THREATENING.

extrapyramidal symptoms, *hallucinations,* headache, hypertonia, incoordination, insomnia, neuralgia, paresthesia, personality disorder, psychosis, *somnolence,* speech disorder, tremor, twitching.
CV: *arrhythmias,* hypertension, hypotension, *MI, orthostatic hypotension,* palpitations, syncope, vasodilation.
EENT: abnormal vision, diplopia, epistaxis, eye disorder, *rhinitis,* taste perversion.
GI: abdominal pain, anorexia, *constipation,* diarrhea, dry mouth, dyspepsia, *nausea,* vomiting.
GU: hematuria, urinary frequency, UTI.
Hematologic: anemia.
Musculoskeletal: arthralgia, bursitis, myalgia, pain in chest, neck, and back.
Respiratory: dyspnea.
Skin: diaphoresis, rash.
Other: chills, facial edema, flulike syndrome, infection, peripheral or generalized edema, weight gain.

Overdose and treatment
Overdose caused hypotension and vomiting in one patient who intentionally ingested 60 mg of drug. Overdose also may cause hallucinations, involuntary movements, palpitations, and arrhythmias.

Provide supportive treatment. Monitor patient's cardiac function, and maintain patient's airway. Give antiarrhythmics and sympathomimetics as needed to support CV function. Give dopaminergic antagonists (such as phenothiazines) for adverse CNS effects. If indicated, empty stomach by gastric lavage or induced emesis. Follow with oral dose of activated charcoal to help reduce absorption if needed.

Special considerations
■ Gradual dosage adjustment, especially early in therapy, may help patient tolerate orthostatic hypotension.
■ Rapid dosage reduction may cause a condition that resembles neuroleptic malignant syndrome, with muscle rigidity, mental status changes, fever, and autonomic instability.
■ In early clinical trials, 27% of patients who started pergolide therapy stopped because of adverse effects, mainly hallucinations and confusion.

Breast-feeding patients
■ Safety in breast-feeding women hasn't been established.

Pediatric patients
■ Safety in children hasn't been established.

Patient teaching
■ Explain the likelihood of adverse effects and what to report.
■ Warn patient to avoid activities that could raise the risk of injury from orthostatic hypotension or syncope.
■ Caution patient to rise slowly to minimize the effects of orthostatic hypotension, particularly at the start of therapy.
■ Tell women to notify prescriber about planned, suspected, or known pregnancy.

pramipexole dihydrochloride
Mirapex

Pharmacologic classification:
nonergot dopamine agonist

Therapeutic classification:
antiparkinsonian

Pregnancy risk category C

How supplied
Available by prescription only
Tablets: 0.125 mg, 0.25 mg, 0.5 mg,
1 mg, 1.5 mg

Indications and dosages
Idiopathic Parkinson's disease
Adults: initially, 0.375 mg P.O. daily, given in three divided doses. Increase by 0.75 mg in divided doses no more often than q 5 to 7 days until you reach of 1.5 mg t.i.d. after 7 weeks of therapy. Maintenance, 1.5 to 4.5 mg daily in three divided doses.

▶ DOSAGE ADJUSTMENT. If patient's creatinine clearance is 35 to 59 ml/minute, start with 0.125 mg P.O. b.i.d.; maximum maintenance dose is 1.5 mg b.i.d. If patient's creatinine clearance is 15 to 34 ml/minute, start with 0.125 mg P.O. daily; maximum maintenance dose is 1.5 mg daily.

Pharmacodynamics
Antiparkinsonian action: Drug probably stimulates D_2 and D_3 dopamine receptors in striatum. In animal studies, it influences striatal neuron firing rates by activating dopamine receptors in the striatum and substantia nigra, where neurons send projections to the striatum.

Pharmacokinetics
Absorption: Drug is rapidly absorbed, peaking in about 2 hours. Absolute bioavailability of drug is above 90%, suggesting that it is well absorbed and undergoes little presystemic metabolism. Food doesn't affect extent of absorption but does increase time to maximum plasma level by about 1 hour.
Distribution: Drug is extensively distributed, with a volume of distribution of about 500 L. About 15% is bound to plasma proteins. Drug also is distributed into RBCs. Terminal half-life is 8 to 12 hours; steady state occurs within 2 days.
Metabolism: 90% of dose is excreted unchanged in urine.
Excretion: Drug is excreted mainly in urine. A small amount may be eliminated by nonrenal routes, although no metabolites have been identified in plasma or urine. Drug is secreted by the renal tubules, probably by the organic transport system.

Contraindications and precautions
Contraindicated in patients hypersensitive to drug or its components.

Use cautiously in patients with renal impairment, including elderly patients; dosage may need adjustment.

Interactions
Drug-drug
Cimetidine: increases pramipexole's bioavailability and half-life. Dosage adjustments may be needed.

Reactions may be *common,* uncommon, *life-threatening,* or COMMON AND LIFE-THREATENING.

Dopamine antagonists, such as butyrophenones, metoclopramide, phenothiazines, thiothixenes: may reduce pramipexole effectiveness. Dosage adjustments may be needed.
Drugs eliminated by renal secretion, such as diltiazem, quinidine, quinine, ranitidine, triamterene, verapamil: decreased clearance of oral pramipexole by about 20%. Dosage adjustments may be needed.
Levodopa: increases levodopa's maximum plasma levels. Dosage adjustments may be needed.

Adverse reactions

CNS: *abnormal dreams*, abnormal gait, akathisia, amnesia, *asthenia*, *confusion*, delusions, *dizziness*, *dyskinesia*, dystonia, *extrapyramidal symptoms*, *insomnia*, hallucinations, hypertonia, hypesthesia, malaise, myoclonus, paranoid reaction, sleep disorders, somnolence, thought abnormalities.
CV: chest pain, *orthostatic hypotension*, peripheral edema.
EENT: abnormal accommodation, diplopia, dry mouth, rhinitis, vision changes.
GI: anorexia, *constipation*, dysphagia, nausea.
GU: decreased libido, impotence, urinary frequency, urinary incontinence, UTI.
Musculoskeletal: arthritis, bursitis, myasthenia, twitching.
Respiratory: dyspnea, pneumonia.
Skin: skin disorders.
Other: *accidental injury*, fever, general edema, unevaluable reaction.

Overdose and treatment

Overdose may cause CNS overstimulation.

No known antidote exists; if signs of CNS stimulation occur, give a phenothiazine or other butyrophenone neuroleptic drug. Also, provide supportive measures, such as gastric lavage, I.V. fluids, and ECG monitoring.

Special considerations

- Adjust dosage gradually, increasing it to attain maximum therapeutic effect while minimizing the main adverse effects: dyskinesia, hallucinations, somnolence, and dry mouth.
- Drug may cause orthostatic hypotension, especially when increasing dosage. Monitor patient carefully.
- Avoid abrupt withdrawal of drug, rapid dose reduction, and large changes in therapy because these actions may raise the patient's risk of neuroleptic malignant syndrome, which causes fever, muscle rigidity, altered consciousness, and autonomic instability.
- If drug must be discontinued, withdraw it over a 1-week period.

Breast-feeding patients

- Give drug cautiously to breast-feeding women; no data exist to demonstrate whether drug appears in breast milk.

Pediatric patients

- Safety and efficacy in children haven't been established.

Geriatric patients

- In elderly patients, drug clearance decreases because half-life is about 40% longer and clearance is about 30% lower.

◊ Available in Canada only   *Unlabeled use

Patient teaching

- Tell patient to take drug only as prescribed.
- Suggest that patient take drug with food if nausea develops.
- Instruct patient to rise slowly from lying or sitting positions to minimize the effects of orthostatic hypotension.
- Caution patient to avoid hazardous activities until full effects of drug are known.
- Tell patient to use caution when taking drug with other CNS depressants.
- Warn patient not to stop drug abruptly.
- Tell women to notify prescriber about planned, suspected, or known pregnancy.

ropinirole hydrochloride
Requip

Pharmacologic classification:
nonergoline dopamine agonist

Therapeutic classification:
antiparkinsonian

Pregnancy risk category C

How supplied
Available by prescription only
Tablets: 0.25 mg, 0.5 mg, 1 mg, 2 mg, 5 mg

Indications and dosages
Idiopathic Parkinson's disease
Adults: initially, 0.25 mg P.O. t.i.d. Based on patient response, adjust dosage q week: 0.5 mg t.i.d. after first week, 0.75 mg t.i.d. after second week, and 1 mg t.i.d. after third week. After fourth week, dosage may be increased q week by 1.5 mg/day up to 9 mg/day and then q week by up to 3 mg/day to maximum dose of 24 mg/day.
▷ **DOSAGE ADJUSTMENT.** If patient has severe renal or hepatic impairment, reduce dosage cautiously. If patient has mild to moderate renal impairment, adjustment isn't needed.

Pharmacodynamics
Antiparkinsonian action: Exact mechanism of action is unknown. Ropinirole is a nonergoline dopamine agonist thought to stimulate postsynaptic dopamine D_2 receptors in the caudate-putamen in the brain.

Pharmacokinetics
Absorption: Drug is rapidly absorbed, peaking in 1 to 2 hours. Absolute bioavailability is 55%.
Distribution: Drug is widely distributed throughout the body, with an apparent volume of distribution of 7.5 L/kg. Up to 40% is bound to plasma proteins.
Metabolism: Drug is extensively metabolized by cytochrome P-450 isoenzyme CYP1A2 to inactive metabolites.
Excretion: Less than 10% of an administered dose is excreted unchanged in the urine. Elimination half-life is 6 hours.

Contraindications and precautions
Contraindicated in patients hypersensitive to drug or its components.
Use cautiously in patients with severe renal or hepatic impairment.

Reactions may be *common*, uncommon, *life-threatening*, or COMMON AND LIFE-THREATENING.

Interactions
Drug-drug
Ciprofloxacin: increased ropinirole level. Ropinirole dosage may need adjustment during concomitant use.

CNS depressants, such as antidepressants, antipsychotics, benzodiazepines: increased CNS effects. Use together cautiously.

Dopamine antagonists, such as butyrophenones, metoclopramide, phenothiazines, thioxanthenes: may decrease ropinirole effectiveness when administered together. Monitor patient carefully.

Estrogens: reduced ropinirole clearance. Adjust ropinirole dosage if estrogen therapy begins or ends during ropinirole treatment.

Inhibitors or substrates of cytochrome P-450 CYP1A2 isoenzyme, such as ciprofloxacin, fluvoxamine, mexiletine, norfloxacin: altered clearance of ropinirole. Ropinirole dosage may need adjustment.

Drug-lifestyle
Alcohol use: increases CNS effects. Discourage concomitant use.
Smoking: may increase ropinirole clearance. Encourage smoking cessation; discourage concomitant use.

Adverse reactions
Early Parkinson's disease (without levodopa)
CNS: aggravated Parkinson's disease, amnesia, asthenia, confusion, *dizziness, fatigue,* hallucinations, headache, hyperkinesia, hypesthesia, impaired concentration, malaise, *somnolence,* vertigo.
CV: atrial fibrillation, chest pain, edema, hypertension, extrasystoles, orthostatic hypotension, palpitations, *syncope,* tachycardia.
EENT: abnormal vision, dry mouth, eye abnormality, pharyngitis, rhinitis, sinusitis, xerophthalmia.
GI: abdominal pain, anorexia, *dyspepsia,* flatulence, *nausea, vomiting.*
GU: impotence, UTI.
Respiratory: bronchitis, dyspnea.
Skin: flushing, increased sweating.
Other: pain, peripheral ischemia, *viral infection,* yawning.

Advanced Parkinson's disease (with levodopa)
CNS: abnormal dreams, aggravated parkinsonism, amnesia, anxiety, confusion, *dizziness, dyskinesia, hallucinations, headache,* hypokinesia, insomnia, nervousness, paresis, paresthesia, *somnolence,* tremor.
CV: hypotension, syncope.
EENT: diplopia, dry mouth.
GI: abdominal pain, constipation, diarrhea, dysphagia, flatulence, increased salivation, *nausea,* vomiting.
GU: pyuria, urinary incontinence, UTI.
Hematologic: anemia.
Metabolic: weight loss.
Musculoskeletal: arthralgia, arthritis.
Respiratory: dyspnea, upper respiratory infection.
Skin: increased sweating.
Other: *falls,* injuries, pain, viral infection.

Overdose and treatment
Overdose may cause mild or facial dyskinesia, agitation, increased dyskinesia, grogginess, sedation, orthostatic hypotension, chest pain, confusion, vomiting, and nausea.

Treatment includes supportive measures and removal of unabsorbed drug.

Special considerations
- Drug may increase alkaline phosphatase and BUN levels.
- Monitor patient carefully for orthostatic hypotension, especially during dosage increases. Symptomatic hypotension may occur because dopamine agonists impair systemic regulation of blood pressure.
- Watch for syncope with or without bradycardia, especially about 4 weeks after therapy starts and when dosage increases.
- Assess patient for other adverse events caused by dopaminergic therapy, such as withdrawal, emergent hyperpyrexia, confusion, and fibrotic complications.
- Ropinirole can potentiate the dopaminergic adverse effects of levodopa and may cause or worsen dyskinesia. If so, levodopa dosage may need to be decreased.
- Avoid abrupt withdrawal of drug, rapid dose reduction, and large changes in therapy because these actions may raise the patient's risk of neuroleptic malignant syndrome, which causes fever, muscle rigidity, altered consciousness, and autonomic instability. This syndrome hasn't been reported among patients taking ropinirole; if it occurs, stop drug gradually over 7 days by reducing frequency of administration to twice daily for 4 days and then once daily for the remaining 3 days.

Breast-feeding patients
- Drug inhibits prolactin secretion and could, in theory, inhibit lactation. It isn't known whether drug appears in breast milk. Consider whether to stop the drug or breast-feeding based on importance of drug to mother.

Pediatric patients
- Safety and effectiveness in children haven't been established.

Patient teaching
- Tell patient to take drug with food to reduce nausea.
- Inform patient that hallucinations may occur. Elderly patients face a greater risk than younger patients with Parkinson's disease.
- Instruct patient to rise slowly from sitting or lying position to minimize the effects of orthostatic hypotension, which may occur during initial therapy or after a dosage increase.
- Tell patient to avoid hazardous activities until full CNS effects of drug are known.
- Advise patient to avoid alcohol and other CNS depressants.
- Tell women to notify prescriber about planned, suspected, or known pregnancy and about planned or current breast-feeding.

---

selegiline hydrochloride (L-deprenyl hydrochloride)
Atapryl, Carbex, Eldepryl, Selpak

Pharmacologic classification:
MAO inhibitor

Therapeutic classification:
antiparkinsonian

Pregnancy risk category C

How supplied
Available by prescription only
Capsules: 5 mg
Tablets: 5 mg

Indications and dosages
Parkinson's disease (adjunct to levodopa-carbidopa)
Adults: 10 mg P.O. daily, 5 mg at breakfast and 5 mg at lunch. After 2 to 3 days, begin gradually decreasing levodopa-carbidopa dosage.

Pharmacodynamics
Antiparkinsonian action: Probably acts by selectively inhibiting MAO-B, found mostly in the brain. At higher-than-recommended doses, it is a nonselective inhibitor of MAO, including MAO-A in the GI tract. It may also directly increase dopaminergic activity by decreasing reuptake of dopamine into nerve cells. Its pharmacologically active metabolites (amphetamine and methamphetamine) may contribute to this effect.

Pharmacokinetics
Absorption: Drug is rapidly absorbed; about 73% of dose is absorbed. Bioavailability is increased if taken with food.

Distribution: Drug and metabolites are up to 94% protein-bound.
Metabolism: Three metabolites have been detected in serum and urine: N-desmethylselegiline, L-amphetamine, and L-methamphetamine.
Excretion: 45% of drug appears as a metabolite in the urine after 48 hours.

Contraindications and precautions
Contraindicated in patients hypersensitive to drug, patients receiving meperidine or other opioids, and patients who took an antidepressant within 14 days (5 weeks for fluoxetine) because of the increased risk of serotonin syndrome.

Interactions
Drug-drug
Adrenergics: may increase the pressor response, particularly if patient has taken an overdose of selegiline. Use with caution.
Mereperidine: fatal interaction may occur. Don't use together.

Drug-herb
Cacao: may cause vasopressor effects. Discourage concomitant use.
Ginseng: may cause adverse reactions, such as headache, tremors, mania. Discourage concomitant use.

Drug-food
Food: increases bioavailability. Tell patient to take drug with food.
Foods high in tyramine: may cause hypertensive crisis. Tell patient which foods to avoid.

Drug-lifestyle
Alcohol use: May cause excessive depressant effect. Discourage concomitant use.

Adverse reactions
CNS: anxiety, behavior changes, chorea, confusion, *dizziness,* dyskinesia, fatigue, grimacing, hallucinations, headache, increased apraxia, increased bradykinesia, increased tremor, insomnia, involuntary movements, lethargy, loss of balance, malaise, restlessness, stiff neck, twitching, vivid dreams.
CV: *arrhythmias,* hypertension, hypotension, new or increased angina, orthostatic hypotension, palpitations, peripheral edema, syncope, tachycardia.
EENT: blepharospasm.
GI: abdominal pain, anorexia, constipation, diarrhea, dry mouth, dysphagia, GI bleeding, heartburn, *nausea,* peptic ulcer, vomiting, weight loss.
GU: prostatic hyperplasia, sexual dysfunction, slow urination, transient nocturia, urinary frequency, urinary hesitancy, urine retention.
Skin: diaphoresis, hair loss, rash.

Overdose and treatment
Overdose may cause hypotension and psychomotor agitation. Because selegiline becomes a nonselective MAO inhibitor at high doses, it also may cause symptoms of MAO inhibitor poisoning: drowsiness, dizziness, hyperactivity, respiratory depression and collapse, agitation, seizures, coma, hypertension, hypotension, cardiac conduction disturbances, and CV collapse. These symptoms may not develop immediately after ingestion; in fact, delays of 12 hours or more are possible.

Provide supportive treatment and closely monitor the patient for worsening of symptoms. Induced emesis or gastric lavage may be helpful in the early stages of treatment. Give I.V. fluids and pressor drugs to combat hypotension and vascular collapse, if necessary. Avoid phenothiazine derivatives and CNS stimulants; adrenergics may provoke an exaggerated pressor response. Diazepam may be useful in treating seizures.

Special considerations
■ Selegiline is usually administered with levodopa-carbidopa.
■ If patient develops increased adverse reactions (including dyskinesias) with levodopa, reduce levodopa-carbidopa dosage. Most such patients need a reduction of 10% to 30%.

Breast-feeding patients
■ It isn't known whether drug appears in breast milk. Give cautiously to breast-feeding women.

Patient teaching
■ Instruct patient to take second dose with lunch to avoid nighttime sedation.
■ Tell patient not to take more than 10 mg daily. No evidence exists to suggest that higher doses improve efficacy, and they may increase adverse reactions.
■ Tell patient to avoid hazardous activities until full sedative effects of drug are known.
■ Caution patient to change positions slowly, especially early in

therapy, to minimize dizziness and the risk of falls.

■ Emphasize the danger of combining drug with alcohol. Excessive depressant effects are possible even if drug is taken the evening before alcohol consumption.

■ Explain the possibility of interactions with foods that contain tyramine, such as cheese, red wine, and herring. Mention that this interaction typically occurs only at higher-than-recommended doses and that dietary restrictions probably aren't necessary as long as patient doesn't exceed recommended dosage. Nonetheless, urge patient to immediately report signs or symptoms of hypertension, including a severe headache.

tolcapone
Tasmar

Pharmacologic classification: catechol-O-methyltransferase (COMT) inhibitor

Therapeutic classification: antiparkinsonian

Pregnancy risk category C

How supplied
Available by prescription only
Tablets: 100 mg, 200 mg

Indications and dosages
Idiopathic Parkinson's disease (adjunct to levodopa-carbidopa)
Adults: Recommended dosage is 100 mg P.O. t.i.d. Give 200 mg P.O. t.i.d. only if anticipated benefits outweigh the risk for fulminant liver failure. Maximum, 600 mg

daily. Always give drug with levodopa-carbidopa. The first daily dose of tolcapone should always be taken with the first daily dose of levodopa-carbidopa.

▶ DOSAGE ADJUSTMENT. If patient has severe hepatic or renal dysfunction, adjust dosage cautiously, and don't give more than 100 mg t.i.d. If patient has mild to moderate renal dysfunction, dosage adjustment isn't needed.

Pharmacodynamics
Antiparkinsonian action: Exact mechanism of action isn't known. Drug probably reversibly inhibits human erythrocyte COMT when given with levodopa-carbidopa. As a result, levodopa clearance declines and bioavailability rises twofold. Decreased clearance lengthens elimination half-life of levodopa from 2 to 3½ hours.

Pharmacokinetics
Absorption: Drug is rapidly absorbed; plasma levels peak within 2 hours. After oral administration, absolute bioavailability is 65%. Effects begin after administration of first dose. Drug can be administered without regard to meals, but absorption decreases when tolcapone is given within 2 hours before or 1 hour after food.
Distribution: Drug is highly bound (over 99.9%) to plasma proteins, primarily albumin. The steady state volume of distribution is small.
Metabolism: Drug is almost completely metabolized before excretion. The main mechanism of metabolism is glucuronidation.

Excretion: Only 0.5% of dose appears unchanged in urine. Tolcapone is a low-extraction-ratio drug with a systemic clearance of 7 L/hour. Elimination half-life is 2 to 3 hours. Dialysis probably doesn't affect clearance because of the high protein binding.

Contraindications and precautions

Contraindicated in patients hypersensitive to drug or its components, in patients with liver disease or ALT or AST values beyond the upper limit of normal, in patients withdrawn from therapy because of drug-induced hepatocellular injury, and in patients with a history of nontraumatic rhabdomyolysis or hyperpyrexia and confusion that may be drug-related.

Use cautiously in patients with Parkinson's disease because syncope and orthostatic hypotension may worsen.

Interactions
Drug-drug

Desipramine: increased risk of adverse effects. Use together cautiously, and monitor patient closely.
Nonselective MAO inhibitors, such as phenelzine, tranylcypromine: avoid concurrent use because of an increased risk of hypertensive crisis. Risk doesn't appear to exist with selective MAO-B inhibitors, such as selegiline.

Adverse reactions
CNS: *confusion,* depression, *dizziness, dyskinesia, dystonia, excessive dreaming,* falling, fatigue, *hallucinations, headache,* hyperkinesia, loss of balance, paresthesia, *sleep disorder, somnolence,* speech disorder, tremor.
CV: chest discomfort, chest pain, hypotension, *orthostatic complaints,* palpitations, syncope.
EENT: pharyngitis, tinnitus.
GI: abdominal pain, *anorexia,* constipation, *diarrhea,* dry mouth, dyspepsia, flatulence, *nausea, vomiting.*
GU: hematuria, impotence, urine discoloration, urinary incontinence, UTI.
Hepatic: *fulminant liver failure.*
Musculoskeletal: arthritis, neck pain, stiffness, *muscle cramps,* myalgia.
Respiratory: bronchitis, dyspnea, upper respiratory infection.
Skin: increased sweating, rash.

Overdose and treatment
Overdose at 800 mg t.i.d. has caused nausea, vomiting, and dizziness.

If overdose occurs, provide supportive care. Hospitalization is recommended. Hemodialysis probably won't be helpful.

Special considerations
■ Because drug raises the risk of life-threatening fulminant liver failure, give it only to patients who take levodopa-carbidopa and either haven't responded or aren't suitable for other adjunctive therapy.
■ Don't give drug until patient has been fully informed of its risks and has given written informed consent.
■ If patient shows no improvement after 3 weeks of tolcapone treatment, discontinue drug.
■ Diarrhea commonly results from tolcapone therapy. It typically occurs either 2 weeks after therapy

---

begins or after 6 to 12 weeks. Although it usually resolves with discontinuation of drug, hospitalization may be required in rare cases.

■ Monitor patient's liver enzymes every 2 weeks for the first year of therapy and every 8 weeks thereafter. Stop drug if hepatic transaminases exceed the upper limit of normal or if patient appears jaundiced.

■ Don't use drug with a nonselective MAO inhibitor.

Breast-feeding patients
■ Because of the risk that drug may appear in breast milk, use caution when giving drug to breast-feeding woman.

Pediatric patients
■ No potential use has been identified for children.

Patient teaching
■ Tell patient to take drug exactly as prescribed.

■ To minimize the effects of orthostatic hypotension, caution patient to change positions slowly and to rise slowly from lying or sitting positions.

■ Warn patient to avoid hazardous activities until the full CNS effects of drug are known.

■ Tell patient that drug poses the risk of liver injury; stress the need to immediately report nausea, right upper quadrant pain, yellowing of the skin and eyes, and dark urine.

■ Advise patient that drug increases the risk of worsened dyskinesia or dystonia.

■ Inform patient that hallucinations may occur.

■ Tell patient to notify prescriber about planned, suspected, or known pregnancy.

trihexyphenidyl hydrochloride
Apo-Trihex◊, Artane, Artane Sequels, Trihexane, Trihexy-2, Trihexy-5

Pharmacologic classification: anticholinergic

Therapeutic classification: antiparkinsonian

Pregnancy risk category C

How supplied
Available by prescription only
Capsules (sustained-release): 5 mg
Elixir: 2 mg/5 ml
Tablets: 2 mg, 5 mg

Indications and dosages
Idiopathic parkinsonism
Adults: 1 mg P.O. on first day, 2 mg on second day, and then increase 2 mg q 3 to 5 days until patient receives 6 to 10 mg daily. Usually given t.i.d. with meals or q.i.d. if needed (last dose before bed). Postencephalitic parkinsonism may require 12 to 15 mg daily. Patients receiving levodopa may need 3 to 6 mg daily. Give sustained-release capsules after patient has been stabilized on conventional drug forms, not as initial therapy. They can be given mg-per-mg to match total daily dose, given as a single dose after breakfast or in 2 divided doses 12 hours apart.

Drug-induced extrapyramidal symptoms

Adults: initially, 1 mg P.O. If no benefit occurs after a few hours, progressively increase subsequent doses until control is achieved. Usual dosage is 5 to 15 mg daily.

Pharmacodynamics

Antiparkinsonian action: Trihexyphenidyl blocks central cholinergic receptors, helping to balance cholinergic activity in the basal ganglia. It may also prolong the effects of dopamine by blocking dopamine reuptake and storage at central receptor sites.

Pharmacokinetics

Absorption: Drug is rapidly absorbed after oral administration. Action begins within 1 hour. Oral availability is 100%.
Distribution: Drug crosses the blood-brain barrier; little else is known about its distribution.
Metabolism: Exact metabolic fate is unknown. Duration of effect is 6 to 12 hours.
Excretion: Drug is excreted in the urine as unchanged drug and metabolites.

Contraindications and precautions

Contraindicated in patients hypersensitive to drug.

Use cautiously in patients with glaucoma, obstructive disease of the GI or GU tract, prostatic hyperplasia, or impaired renal, cardiac, or hepatic function.

Interactions
Drug-drug

Amantadine: may increase adverse anticholinergic effects of trihexyphenidyl, causing confusion and hallucinations. Monitor patient closely.
Antacids, antidiarrheals: may decrease trihexyphenidyl absorption. Dosage adjustment may be needed.
CNS depressants, such as tranquilizers, sedative-hypnotics: increases sedative effects of trihexyphenidyl. Monitor patient closely.
Haloperidol, phenothiazines: may decrease antipsychotic effectiveness of these drugs, possibly from direct CNS antagonism. Also may increase the risk of adverse anticholinergic effects. Monitor patient closely.
Levodopa: synergistic anticholinergic effects and possible enhanced GI metabolism of levodopa from reduced gastric motility and delayed gastric emptying. Monitor patient closely. Dosage adjustment may be needed for both drugs.

Drug-lifestyle

Alcohol use: may increase sedative effects. Discourage concurrent use.

Adverse reactions

CNS: confusion, delirium, dizziness, drowsiness, headache, hallucinations, memory loss, nervousness, weakness.
CV: orthostatic hypotension, tachycardia.
EENT: blurred vision, increased intraocular pressure, mydriasis.
GI: constipation, *dry mouth, nausea,* vomiting.
GU: urinary hesitancy, urine retention.

Skin: decreased sweating.
Other: heat stroke.

Overdose and treatment
Overdose may cause central stimulation followed by depression, with such psychotic symptoms as disorientation, confusion, hallucinations, delusions, anxiety, agitation, and restlessness. Peripheral effects may include dilated, nonreactive pupils; blurred vision; flushed, dry, hot skin; dry mucous membranes; dysphagia; decreased or absent bowel sounds; urine retention; circulatory collapse; cardiac arrest; respiratory depression or arrest; seizures; shock; coma; hyperthermia; headache; tachycardia; hypertension; and increased respirations.

Treatment is primarily symptomatic and supportive. Maintain a patent airway. If the patient is alert, induce emesis or perform gastric lavage. Follow with a sodium chloride cathartic and activated charcoal to prevent further drug absorption. In severe cases, physostigmine may be administered to block the antimuscarinic effects of trihexyphenidyl. Give fluids, as needed, for shock. Give diazepam for psychotic symptoms and seizures. Give pilocarpine (ophthalmic) for mydriasis. If urine retention occurs, catheterization may be needed.

Special considerations
■ Store drug in a tight container.
■ Arrange for gonioscopic evaluation and close monitoring of intraocular pressure, especially if patient is over age 40.
■ Assess patient for urinary hesitancy.

■ Give drug cautiously in hot weather because of the increased risk of heat prostration.
■ To control drug-induced extrapyramidal symptoms more rapidly, decrease the dosage of the responsible drug, and then adjust the dosages of both drugs to achieve the desired therapeutic effect.
■ Tolerance may develop to drug, necessitating higher doses.

Breast-feeding patients
■ Avoid giving drug to breast-feeding women because it may be excreted in breast milk, possibly causing toxicity in infant. Drug also may decrease milk production.

Geriatric patients
■ Use caution and reduced dosages when giving drug to elderly patients.

Patient teaching
■ Tell patient to take drug with food if GI upset occurs.
■ Warn patient to avoid hazardous activities until full CNS effects of drug are known.
■ If patient develops dry mouth, suggest relieving it with cool drinks, ice chips, sugarless gum, or sugarless hard candy.
■ Urge patient to notify prescriber about urinary hesitation or urine retention.

CHAPTER 9

Antipsychotics

271 ■ Introduction

281 ■ Generic drugs

■ chlorpromazine hydrochloride

■ clozapine

■ fluphenazine decanoate, fluphenazine enanthate, fluphenazine hydrochloride

■ haloperidol, haloperidol decanoate, haloperidol lactate

■ loxapine hydrochloride, loxapine succinate

■ mesoridazine besylate

■ molindone hydrochloride

■ olanzapine

■ perphenazine

■ pimozide

■ prochlorperazine, prochlorperazine edisylate, prochlorperazine maleate

■ quetiapine fumarate

■ risperidone

■ thioridazine, thioridazine hydrochloride

■ thiothixene, thiothixene hydrochloride

■ trifluoperazine hydrochloride

Antipsychotic drugs are typically used to treat a heterogeneous group of related disorders collectively known as schizophrenia. Schizophrenia is characterized by disorganized and often bizarre thinking, withdrawn or bizarre behavior, a blunted or inappropriate affect (emotional tone), delusions, hallucinations, and poor interpersonal skills.

The theory that best explains the biochemical basis of schizophrenia focuses mainly on the neurotransmitter dopamine. In short, the theory states that excessive amounts of dopamine may play a profound and unique role in inducing psychotic illness. This theory is supported by the observation that drugs known to increase dopamine in the central nervous system (CNS)—such as levodopa, amphetamines, and apomorphine—can worsen psychotic symptoms. Fortunately, a number of drugs are available to help reduce the symptoms of schizophrenia and to help patients achieve an improved level of functioning.

TREATING SCHIZOPHRENIA

Antipsychotic drugs can be used to treat a wide range of problems, from migraine headaches to tetanus. (See *Antipsychotics: Comparing indications*, pages 272 and 273.) Usually, however, you'll be giving these drugs to patients who have schizophrenia. Depending on the drug, the therapeutic effects, pharmacokinetics, adverse effects, and overdose scenarios vary somewhat.

Drug effects

Antipsychotic drugs work by blocking postsynaptic receptors in dopamine-mediated pathways from the midbrain to the limbic system and to the temporal and frontal lobes of the cerebral cortex. They also block dopamine receptors in the substantia nigra, in the midbrain to the caudate nucleus, and in the basal ganglia.

Several types of dopamine receptors have been identified. Most antipsychotics block dopamine 1 (D_1) and dopamine 2 (D_2) receptors. However, the effectiveness of these drugs is correlated with the extent to which they block D_2 receptors. Therefore, a drug is considered a low-potency or a high-potency antipsychotic based on its affinity for D_2 receptors. Low-potency antipsychotics are more likely to cause sedation and other anticholinergic effects. High potency antipsychotics are more likely to produce extrapyramidal symptoms (EPS).

Conventional (also called *typical*) antipsychotics have a higher affinity for D_2 receptors than for D_1 receptors. They also bind with varying affinity to nondopaminergic sites (such as cholinergic, alpha-adrenergic, and histaminergic sites), which probably explains why antipsychotic drugs have differing adverse effect profiles.

Newer (also called *novel*) antipsychotics have a higher affinity for serotonin (5-HT_2) receptors than for D_2 receptors. They may interact with several dopaminergic receptors (D_1, D_2, D_4, and D_5) and may antagonize one or more serotonin receptors (5-HT_2, 5-HT_6, and 5-HT_7), alpha-adrenergic re-

Antipsychotics: Comparing indications

DRUG	Psychotic disorders	Behavioral disorders in children	Phencyclidine psychosis	Migraine	Schizophrenia	Alcoholism (acute and chronic)	
chlorpromazine hydrochloride	■	■	*	*			
clozapine	■						
fluphenazine	■						
haloperidol	■	■	*				
loxapine	■						
mesoridazine besylate		■			■	■	
molindone hydrochloride	■						
olanzapine	■						
perphenazine	■						
pimozide							
prochlorperazine	■			*			
quetiapine fumarate	■						
risperidone	■						
thioridazine	■	■					
thiothixene	■						
trifluoperazine hydrochloride	■						

* = unlabeled use

Psychoneurotic manifestations	Anxiety	Tourette syndrome	Hyperactivity	Surgery	Tetanus	Acute intermittent porphyria	Emesis
				■	■	■	■
		■	■				*
■							
							■
		■					
							■
■							
	■						

ceptors, muscarinic receptors, histaminergic receptors, or nicotinic receptors.

Not long ago, novel antipsychotics were known as *atypical* antipsychotics. Because these drugs have become much more typical in antipsychotic regimens, however, the term atypical has fallen out of favor. The main reason why novel antipsychotics are growing in popularity is their reduced likelihood of causing EPS and other adverse effects.

Keep in mind that shifting a patient from one antipsychotic class to another may reduce the adverse effects the patient experiences. However, giving two or more antipsychotics not only doesn't improve the therapeutic response, but it raises the risk of adverse effects.

Pharmacokinetics

Because absorption of oral antipsychotic drugs may vary, intramuscular injection usually offers the most reliable method for delivering an antipsychotic dose. This route also yields higher blood levels (by 4 to 10 times) in a shorter time than oral forms. Oral liquid forms are absorbed more predictably than tablets or capsules. They're highly protein-bound and extremely lipophilic. After oral administration, plasma levels peak in about 2 to 4 hours.

One exception to this general rule is the long-acting decanoate form (see fluphenazine and haloperidol). With this drug form, onset of action may take days; however, esterification of the drug slows its release from fatty tissues, thus prolonging the duration of action to a few weeks.

Distribution into the CNS exceeds that into plasma. Metabolism occurs via microsomal oxidation and by conjugation in the liver. Metabolites are excreted primarily in the urine with small amounts in the bile. Half-lives vary from 10 to 20 hours. With long-term administration, lipid tissue becomes saturated. As a result, drug effects may persist for months after therapy stops. Checking plasma levels as a way to monitor therapeutic response is controversial and not routinely done.

Adverse effects

As a group, antipsychotic drugs can cause many different adverse effects. Some of the adverse effects of greatest concern are agranulocytosis, anticholinergic effects, and EPS. (See *Antipsychotics: Comparing adverse effects*, pages 276 and 277.) Certain adverse effects may be linked to certain types of drugs or to certain levels of potency; they include seizures, cardiovascular (CV) effects, and some types of ocular, hepatic, genitourinary, skin, and endocrine problems. These drugs also may lead to neuroleptic malignant syndrome. Patients with brain damage or seizures may even face an increased risk of sudden death from high doses.

Agranulocytosis

By definition, agranulocytosis is a white blood cell (WBC) count below 500/mm³. Although this adverse effect is of highest concern with the novel antipsychotic clozapine, it may happen with any antipsychotic. It tends to occur most often between weeks 4 and 10 of therapy. Assess your patient for a sore throat, sore gums, or other signs of infection. During clozapine therapy, make sure your patient receives weekly laboratory tests to monitor his WBC count. This testing should continue for several weeks after therapy stops.

Anticholinergic effects

Antipsychotic drugs commonly cause anticholinergic effects, such as sedation, a dry mouth, constipation, dry nasal passages, dry skin, urinary hesitancy, urine retention, tachycardia, blurred vision, and inhibited ejaculation. These effects are more likely with low-potency antipsychotics than with high-potency drugs. Also, elderly patients may be more sensitive than younger patients to anticholinergic effects.

Extrapyramidal symptoms

The blockade of dopamine receptors in the nigrostriatal system can produce one of several variations of EPS. They include acute dystonia, akathisia, and tardive dyskinesia.

Acute dystonia

This type of EPS typically occurs during the first several days of antipsychotic therapy. It's more common among patients who take high-potency drugs. Symptoms usually involve the head and neck and may include oculogyric crisis (where the eyes roll back in the head), trismus (where the face twists to one side), a fixed and protruding tongue, and opisthotonus (where neck may arch and draw the patient's head backward).

Akathisia

This type of EPS causes an internal motor restlessness. Patients describe it as feeling "wound up like a top." They may appear restless and have trouble sitting or lying still. Their legs and arms may move constantly. Akathisia may appear early in antipsychotic therapy or after several months; it's most common in patients ages 30 to 60, but it may occur in patients as young as age 15. It also may appear as drug-induced Parkinsonism, in which the patient develops a characteristic triad that includes akinesia, rigidity, and tremors.

Tardive dyskinesia

This syndrome of abnormal involuntary muscle movements may appear after many years of antipsychotic therapy or after just 3 to 6 months. It's characterized by gross hyperactivity of the oro-bucco-lingual region, which leads to smacking, puckering, sucking lip movements; jaw movements; protrusion of the tongue; and difficulty swallowing. It also commonly causes choreoathetoid movements of the arms, hands, feet, and legs. Chronic EPS may appear months or years after drug therapy starts and may continue even after therapy stops.

Seizures

Although conventional antipsychotics decrease the seizure threshold, they usually don't lead to seizures at normal dosage levels. Rather, seizures are more likely to occur after an abrupt change in dosage or a sudden discontinuation of the drug. Clozapine may be most closely linked to an increased seizure risk; because it can increase

Antipsychotics: Comparing adverse effects

DRUG	ADVERSE EFFECTS	
	Sedation	Extrapyramidal symptoms
Aliphatic phenothiazines		
chlorpromazine	+++	++
Piperazine phenothiazines		
fluphenazine	+	+++
perphenazine	++	++
prochlorperazine	++	+++
trifluoperazine	+	+++
Piperidines		
mesoridazine	+++	+
thioridazine	+++	+
Thioxanthenes		
thiothixene	++	+++
Phenylbutylpiperadines		
haloperidol	+	+++
pimozide	++	+++
Dihydroindolones		
molindone	++	++
Dibenzepines		
loxapine	+	++
Dibenzodiazepines		
clozapine	+++	+
Thienbenzodiazepines		
olanzapine	+++	+
Dibenzothiazepines		
quetiapine	++	+
Benzisoxazoles		
risperidone	+	+

Key: + = low incidence; ++ = moderate incidence; +++ = high incidence

Anticholinergic effects	Orthostatic hypotension	Weight gain
++	+++	N/A
+	+	N/A
+	+	N/A
+	+	N/A
+	+	N/A
+++	++	N/A
+++	+++	N/A
+	++	N/A
+	+	N/A
++	+	N/A
+	+	N/A
+	+	N/A
+++	++	++
+++	++	++
N/A	++	+
N/A	+	+

the risk of seizures by about 5% to 14% at 600 to 900 mg daily, its maximum daily dose is 900 mg.

Cardiovascular effects

Keep in mind that antipsychotics have both antiarrhythmic and arrhythmogenic effects (similar to quinidine) on the myocardium and conduction system. Such effects typically include tachycardia and orthostatic hypotension. Electrocardiogram (ECG) changes may include prolonged QT and PR intervals, depressed T waves, and a depressed ST segment. These changes usually aren't clinically significant unless the patient already has cardiac problems. Low-potency antipsychotics are more likely to produce CV effects than high-potency drugs. These effects are usually attributed to piperazine and aliphatic phenothiazines.

Ocular problems

Many patients report blurred vision at the start of antipsychotic therapy; it typically dissipates after a few weeks. Patients also may complain of light sensitivity. And you may note the development of miosis, mydriasis, ptosis, star-shaped lenticular opacities, epithelial keratopathy, and pigmentary retinopathy. If your patient has glaucoma, administer antipsychotic therapy only in conjunction with an ophthalmologist because antipsychotics may increase intraocular pressure.

Certain ocular problems are more likely during therapy with novel rather than conventional antipsychotics; they include xerophthalmia, eye pain, blepharitis, cataracts, ocular muscle abnormality, and eye inflammation. Also, keep in mind that thioridazine given at more than 800 mg daily may cause pigmentary retinopathy from melanin deposits in the cornea. That's why the thioridazine daily dose shouldn't exceed 800 mg.

Hepatic problems

Although all antipsychotics are metabolized in the liver, hepatic abnormalities stem most commonly from therapy with chlorpromazine. Patents who develop jaundice while taking this drug typically do so between the second and fourth weeks of therapy; the condition is considered a hypersensitivity reaction. However, because antipsychotic drugs lead to jaundice infrequently, make sure to rule out other causes of jaundice before attributing the condition to antipsychotic therapy.

Genitourinary problems

Genitourinary problems are more likely to occur during therapy with a low-potency antipsychotic because these drugs are more likely to slow the smooth muscles and cause paralysis of the detrusor muscle of the bladder.

Skin reactions

Allergic skin reactions typically occur between weeks 2 and 10 of therapy and appear as maculopapular, erythematous, itchy rashes of the face, neck, limbs, and truck. Contact dermatitis can occur in any patient hypersensitive to an antipsychotic. Photosensitivity tends to occur more often during therapy with low-potency antipsychotics, especially chlorpromazine. High doses of low-potency antipsychotics given over prolonged periods may cause a blue-gray discoloration of the skin commonly known as "purple person syndrome" or "thorazine blue syndrome."

Endocrine problems

Antipsychotic drugs may cause several endocrine changes. For example, they may increase glucose levels by affecting glucose metabolism. Aliphatic and piperazine phenothiazines may affect the hypothalamus and the ability of the body to regulate its temperature.

Low-potency antipsychotics, particularly the novel drugs, commonly cause weight gain. Antipsychotics also may cause lactation and moderate breast engorgement in women, galactorrhea, syndrome of inappropriate antidiuretic hormone, mastalgia, amenorrhea, menstrual irregularities, gynecomastia in males who take large doses, libido changes, hyponatremia, glycosuria, increased plasma cholesterol levels, and pituitary tumor linked to hyperprolactinemia.

Neuroleptic malignant syndrome

Patients may face an increased risk of neuroleptic malignant syndrome while receiving antipsychotic therapy. The syndrome results from disrupted central thermoregulatory mechanisms and excess heat production caused either by muscle contraction that stems from dopamine blockade or by muscle contraction that results directly from the action of the antipsychotic. The syndrome is characterized by hyperpyrexia, altered consciousness, dyskinesia, increased muscle tone, dysarthria, autonomic changes of tachycardia, tachypnea, labile blood pressure, diaphoresis, and incontinence. Laboratory tests show the presence of urinary myoglobin along with increased WBCs, creatinine phosphokinase, and liver function test results.

Overdose and treatment

Antipsychotics have a wide therapeutic window, which makes overdose uncommon. When it does occur, however, symptoms typically include somnolence, a deep sleep from which the patient can be aroused, or coma. Hypotension and EPS may occur as well.

To treat an antipsychotic overdose, perform gastric lavage and give activated charcoal as needed to absorb remaining drug from the patient's stomach. Keep in mind that the anticholinergic properties of the drug may delay gastric emptying. Induced emesis usually isn't beneficial, however, because most antipsychotics have potent antiemetic properties that block the chemoreceptor trigger zone.

Hypotension after an overdose may require the use of an alpha-stimulating drug, such as norepinephrine or phenylephrine. Don't give epinephrine, dopamine, or other sympathomimetics that have beta-agonist activity because beta stimulation may worsen hypotension caused by drug-induced alpha blockade. If the patient develops a ventricular arrhythmia, give phenytoin 1 mg/kg intravenously and monitor the patient's ECG; repeat the phenytoin every 5 minutes up to 10 mg/kg. Hyperactivity or seizures may be controlled with pentobarbital or diazepam.

PATIENT TEACHING

Naturally, you'll need to convey particular information about each antipsychotic drug to the patient who takes it. In general, however, make sure your patient teaching includes these ideas.

- At the start of therapy, caution the patient about possible orthostatic hypotension.
- Because antipsychotics cause drowsiness, warn the patient to avoid hazardous activities, especially early in therapy.
- To minimize photosensitivity, tell the patient to avoid exposure to ultraviolet light or sunlight.
- If the patient takes a phenothiazine, warn him that it may discolor his urine.
- Warn the patient to avoid exertion during hot weather because some antipsychotics may increase the risk of heat stroke.
- Tell the patient to notify the prescriber about a sore throat, bleeding gums, or any other sign of infection.
- Tell women to notify the prescriber about planned, suspected, or known pregnancy during antipsychotic therapy.
- Urge the patient to consult the prescriber before taking any other prescribed drugs, over-the-counter medications, or herbal remedies during antipsychotic therapy.

chlorpromazine hydrochloride

Chlorpromanyl-5 ◊,
Chlorpromanyl-20 ◊, Largactil ◊,
Novo-Chlorpromazine ◊,
Ormazine, Thorazine, Thor-Prom

Pharmacologic classification:
aliphatic phenothiazine

Therapeutic classification:
antipsychotic, antiemetic

Pregnancy risk category C

How supplied

Available by prescription only
Capsules (sustained-release): 30 mg,
75 mg, 150 mg, 200 mg
Injection: 25 mg/ml
Oral concentrate: 30 mg/ml,
100 mg/ml
Suppositories: 25 mg, 100 mg
Syrup: 10 mg/5 ml
Tablets: 10 mg, 25 mg, 50 mg,
100 mg, 200 mg

Indications and dosages
Psychosis

Adults: 30 to 75 mg P.O. daily in
two to four divided doses. May increase twice weekly by 20 to 50 mg
until symptoms are controlled.
Most patients respond to 200 mg
daily, but some need up to 800 mg
daily.
Children age 6 months or over:
0.55 mg/kg P.O. q 4 to 6 hours or
I.M. q 6 to 8 hours; or 1.1 mg/kg
P.R. q 6 to 8 hours. Maximum I.M.
dosage in children uder age 5 or
weighing less than 22.7 kg (50 lb) is
40 mg. Maximum I.M. dosage in
children ages 5 to 12 years or weighing 22.7 to 45.5 kg (50 to 100 lb) is
75 mg.

Acute psychosis in severely agitated patients

Adults: initially, 25 mg I.M.
Additional 25- to 50-mg dose may
be given I.M. in 1 hour. Increase
dosage gradually over several days
to a maximum of 400 mg q 4 to 6
hours.

Mild alcohol withdrawal, acute intermittent porphyria

Adults: 25 to 50 mg I.M. t.i.d.
or q.i.d.

Pharmacodynamics

Antipsychotic action: Antipsychotic
action probably results from postsynaptic blockade of CNS dopamine receptors, which inhibits dopamine-mediated effects.
Antiemetic action: Probably results
from dopamine receptor blockade
in the medullary chemoreceptor
trigger zone.
Other actions: Drug also has many
other central and peripheral effects; it produces both alpha and
ganglionic blockade and counteracts histamine- and serotonin-mediated activity.

Pharmacokinetics

Absorption: Rate and extent of absorption vary with route of administration. Absorption of oral tablets
is erratic and variable, with onset
ranging from 30 minutes to 1 hour.
Effects peak at 2 to 4 hours; duration of action is 4 to 6 hours. Sustained-release forms have similar
absorption, but action lasts 10 to
12 hours. Suppositories act in 60
minutes and last 3 to 4 hours. Oral
concentrates and syrups are much
more predictable; I.M. drug is absorbed rapidly.

Distribution: Drug is distributed widely into the body, including breast milk. CNS levels usually exceed plasma levels. Serum level reaches steady state in 4 to 7 days. Drug is 91% to 99% protein-bound.

Metabolism: Drug is metabolized extensively by the liver and forms 10 to 12 metabolites; some are pharmacologically active.

Excretion: Drug is mostly excreted as metabolites in urine; some is excreted in feces via the biliary tract. It may undergo enterohepatic circulation.

Contraindications and precautions

Contraindicated in patients hypersensitive to drug and in patients with CNS depression, bone marrow suppression, subcortical damage, or coma.

Use cautiously in acutely ill or dehydrated children, in elderly or debilitated patients, and in patients with impaired renal or hepatic function, severe CV disease, glaucoma, prostatic hyperplasia, respiratory disorders, seizure disorders, hypocalcemia, reaction to insulin therapy, reaction to electroconvulsive therapy, or exposure to heat, cold, or organophosphate insecticides.

Interactions
Drug-drug

Antacids that contain aluminum or magnesium, antidiarrheals: decreased chlorpromazine absorption. Dosage adjustment may be needed.

Antiarrhythmics, such as quinidine, disopyramide, procainamide: increased risk of arrhythmias and conduction defects. Avoid concurrent use.

Anticholinergics (such as atropine), antidepressants, MAO inhibitors: increased risk of seizures. Avoid concurrent use in patients with seizure disorders.

Appetite suppressants, sympathomimetics (including ephedrine, phenylephrine, phenylpropanolamine): may decrease stimulatory and pressor effects when given with chlorpromazine. Dosage adjustment may be needed.

Beta blockers: may inhibit chlorpromazine metabolism, increasing plasma levels and the risk of toxicity from both drugs. Monitor blood levels carefully.

Bromocriptine: may antagonize the therapeutic effect of bromocriptine on prolactin secretion. Avoid concurrent use.

Central-acting antihypertensives, such as clonidine, guanabenz, guanadrel, guanethidine, methyldopa, and reserpine: blood pressure response may be inhibited. Adjust dose according to blood pressure.

CNS depressants (including analgesics, barbiturates, narcotics, tranquilizers, and general, spinal, or epidural anesthetics): additive effects likely. Use cautiously and adjust dosages as needed.

Dopamine: vasoconstricting effects at high dosages are decreased by chlorpromazine. Adjust dosages as needed.

Epinephrine: beta-adrenergic agonist effects of epinephrine continue, but alpha effects are blocked, leading to decreased diastolic and increased systolic pressures and

---

tachycardia. Avoid concomitant use.

Levodopa: decreased effectiveness and increased toxicity caused by chlorpromazine dopamine blockade. Adjust dosages as needed.

Lithium: may cause severe neurologic toxicity with an encephalitis-like syndrome and a decreased therapeutic response to chlorpromazine. Avoid concomitant use.

Phenobarbital: enhanced renal excretion and decreased therapeutic response to chlorpromazine. Dosage adjustment may be needed.

Phenytoin: chlorpromazine inhibits phenytoin metabolism, and risk of toxicity may increase. Monitor phenytoin levels and adjust dosage as needed.

Propylthiouracil: increased risk of agranulocytosis. Monitor patient's CBC with differential regularly.

Drug-food
Caffeine: may alter pharmacokinetics and decrease therapeutic response to chlorpromazine. Discourage caffeinated foods and beverages.

Drug-lifestyle
Alcohol use: increased risk of additive effects. Discourage use.

Heavy smoking: reduced therapeutic response to chlorpromazine. Discourage smoking.

Sun exposure: increased risk of photosensitivity reactions. Urge precautions.

Adverse reactions
CNS: dizziness, drowsiness, *extrapyramidal symptoms,* **neuroleptic malignant syndrome,** pseudoparkinsonism, *sedation,* **seizures,** *tardive dyskinesia.*

CV: ECG changes, *orthostatic hypotension,* tachycardia.

EENT: blurred vision, nasal congestion, ocular changes.

GI: *constipation, dry mouth,* nausea.

GU: gynecomastia, inhibited ejaculation, menstrual irregularities, priapism, *urine retention.*

Hematologic: *agranulocytosis,* **aplastic anemia,** eosinophilia, **hemolytic anemia, leukopenia, thrombocytopenia.**

Hepatic: abnormal liver function test results, jaundice.

Skin: allergic reactions, *mild photosensitivity, pain at I.M. injection site,* pigmentation, sterile abscess.

Overdose and treatment
Overdose may cause CNS depression characterized by deep, unarousable sleep and possible coma, hypotension or hypertension, extrapyramidal symptoms, involuntary muscle movements, agitation, seizures, arrhythmias, ECG changes, hypothermia or hyperthermia, and autonomic nervous system dysfunction.

Treatment is symptomatic and supportive. Maintain the patient's vital signs, airway, body temperature, and fluid and electrolyte balance. Don't induce vomiting because drug inhibits cough reflex, and aspiration may occur. Perform gastric lavage; then give activated charcoal and sodium chloride cathartics. Dialysis doesn't help to remove drug.

Regulate patient's body temperature as needed. Treat hypotension with I.V. fluids, but don't give epinephrine. Give parenteral diazepam or barbiturates for seizures, parenteral phenytoin (1 mg/kg adjusted to blood pressure) for arrhythmias, and benztropine (1 to 2 mg) or parenteral diphenhydramine (10 to 50 mg) for extrapyramidal symptoms.

Special considerations
■ Check patient's blood pressure before and after parenteral administration.
■ Solution for injection may be slightly discolored. Discard if drug is excessively discolored or a precipitate appears.
■ Use I.V. form only during surgery or for severe hiccups. Dilute injection to 1 mg/ml with normal saline solution and administer at 1 mg/2 minutes to a child or 1 mg/minute to an adult.
■ Give I.M. injection deep into upper, outer quadrant of buttocks. Injection is usually painful; massaging the area after administration may prevent abscess formation.
■ If tissue irritation occurs, dilute chlorpromazine injection with normal saline solution or 2% procaine.
■ Oral forms may cause stomach upset and may be given with food or fluid.
■ Don't crush or open sustained-release form; instead, have patient swallow drug whole.
■ Use caution when handling liquid or injectable forms; skin contact may cause a rash.
■ Dilute concentrate in 2 to 4 oz (60 to 120 ml) of liquid, preferably water, a carbonated drink, fruit juice, tomato juice, milk, pudding, or applesauce.

■ Urine may turn pink-brown during therapy.
■ The most prominent adverse effects of chlorpromazine are antimuscarinic and sedative. Drug commonly causes sedation, orthostatic hypotension, and photosensitivity reactions (3%).
■ Drug causes false-positive results on tests for urinary porphyrins, urobilinogen, amylase, and 5-hydroxyindoleacetic acid because metabolites darken urine. Drug also causes false-positive results on urine pregnancy tests that use human chorionic gonadotropin.
■ After abrupt withdrawal of long-term therapy, patient may develop gastritis, nausea, vomiting, dizziness, and tremor.
■ Store suppository form in a cool place.
■ Drug is also used to treat tetanus, nausea, vomiting, and intractable hiccups.

Breast-feeding patients
■ Because drug appears in breast milk, weigh potential benefits to mother against potential risk to infant when breast-feeding.

Pediatric patients
■ Drug isn't recommended for patients under age 6 months because therapy may raise the risk of sudden infant death syndrome in children under age 1.
■ Extrapyramidal effects may be more common in children than adults.

Geriatric patients
■ Older patients tend to require lower doses and are more likely to develop adverse effects, especially

tardive dyskinesia and other extrapyramidal effects. Dosages require individual adjustment.

Patient teaching
■ Teach patient how to use the prescribed drug form. For example, show him how to use a dropper to measure a liquid dose or how to prepare and insert the suppository form. Explain which fluids are appropriate for diluting liquid concentrate.
■ Instruct patient to take drug exactly as prescribed and not to double the dose to compensate for a missed dose.
■ Explain the risk of dystonic reactions and tardive dyskinesia, and tell patient to immediately report involuntary body movements or painful muscle contractions.
■ To prevent photosensitivity reactions, tell patient to minimize sun exposure, to wear sunscreen when going outdoors, and to avoid sunlamps and tanning beds.
■ Because drug may alter thermoregulation, warn patient to avoid exposure to temperature extremes, including very hot or cold baths.
■ Advise patient to avoid hazardous activities until full effects of drug are known. Mention that excessive sedative effects tend to subside after several weeks of therapy.
■ Tell patient to avoid skin contact with liquid form because a rash and irritation could result.
■ Tell patient to avoid alcohol and sedation-causing drugs.
■ Warn patient to change positions slowly and to rise slowly from lying or sitting positions to help minimize the effects of orthostatic hy-

potension and reduce the risk of falls and injuries.
■ If patient develops a dry mouth, suggest using sugarless chewing gum, sugarless hard candy, ice chips, or artificial saliva to ease the symptoms.
■ Caution patient that heavy smoking decreases the effectiveness of the drug.
■ Tell patient to notify prescriber about difficulty urinating, sore throat, dizziness, fever, or fainting.
■ Tell patient not to stop taking drug suddenly.
■ Urge patient to consult prescriber before taking any other prescribed, OTC, or herbal product because of the risk of drug interactions.

---

clozapine
Clozaril

Pharmacologic classification:
tricyclic dibenzodiazepine derivative

Therapeutic classification:
antipsychotic

Pregnancy risk category B

How supplied
Available by prescription only
Tablets: 25 mg, 100 mg

Indications and dosages
Schizophrenia in severely ill patients unresponsive to other therapies
Adults: initially, 25 mg P.O. once or twice daily, increased by 25 to 50 mg daily (if tolerated) to 300 to 450 mg daily by the end of 2 weeks.

Individual dosage is based on clinical response, patient tolerance, and adverse reactions. Subsequent dosage increases should occur no more than once or twice weekly and should not exceed 100 mg. Many patients respond to 300 to 600 mg daily, but some patients need as much as 900 mg daily. Don't exceed 900 mg/day.

Pharmacodynamics

Antipsychotic action: Clozapine binds to dopamine receptors (D_{1-5}) in the limbic system of the CNS. It also may interfere with adrenergic, cholinergic, histaminergic, and serotoninergic receptors.

Pharmacokinetics

Absorption: Levels peak about 2½ hours after oral administration. Food doesn't seem to interfere with bioavailability. Only 27% to 50% of a dose reaches systemic circulation.

Distribution: Drug is about 95% bound to serum proteins.

Metabolism: Metabolism is nearly complete; very little unchanged drug appears in the urine.

Excretion: About 50% of drug appears in urine and 30% in feces, mostly as metabolites. Elimination half-life appears proportional to dose and may range from 4 to 66 hours.

Contraindications and precautions

Contraindicated in patients with uncontrolled epilepsy, a history of clozapine-induced agranulocytosis, a WBC count below 3,500/mm, or severe CNS depression or coma. Drug is also contraindicated in patients taking other drugs that suppress bone marrow function and in those with myelosuppressive disorders.

Use cautiously in patients receiving general anesthesia and in those with prostatic hyperplasia, angle-closure glaucoma, or renal, hepatic, or cardiac disease.

Interactions
Drug-drug

Anticholinergics: may potentiate the anticholinergic effects of clozapine. Avoid concurrent use.

Antihypertensives: hypotensive effects are potentiated by clozapine. Monitor patient's blood pressure and adjust dose accordingly.

Benzodiazepine: may increase risk of respiratory arrest and severe hypotension if given to a patient taking clozapine. Avoid concurrent use.

CNS-active drugs: may cause additive effects. Use cautiously together.

Digoxin, warfarin, and other highly protein-bound drugs: increased serum levels when combined with clozapine. Monitor patient closely for adverse reactions, and check therapeutic levels frequently. Adjust dosage according to blood levels.

Drugs metabolized by cytochrome P-450 2D6, including antidepressants, carbamazepine, phenothiazines, and type IC antiarrhythmics (encainide, flecainide, propafenone) or drugs that inhibit this enzyme, such as quinidine: may have CV effects. Use cautiously or avoid concurrent use.

Drugs that suppress bone marrow function: may increase bone mar-

---

row toxicity. Avoid concurrent use.
Phenytoin: decreased phenytoin
levels and possible lowering of seizure threshold. Avoid use together.
If both must be given, monitor
phenytoin levels and adjust dosage
as needed.

Drug-herb
Nutmeg: may cause a loss of symptom control or interfere with psychiatric drug therapy. Urge avoidance of nutmeg.

Drug-food
Caffeine: may inhibit antipsychotic
effects of drug. Monitor patient
closely.

Drug-lifestyle
Alcohol use: increased CNS depression. Avoid concurrent use.

Adverse reactions
CNS: agitation, akathisia, anxiety,
ataxia, confusion, depression, disturbed sleep or nightmares, dizziness, *drowsiness,* fatigue, headache,
hyperkinesia, hypokinesia or akinesia, insomnia, lethargy, myoclonus, ***neuroleptic malignant syndrome,*** restlessness, rigidity, *sedation,* **seizures,** slurred speech,
syncope, tremor, vertigo, weakness.
CV: chest pain, ECG changes, hypertension, *hypotension, tachycardia,* orthostatic hypotension.
EENT: visual disturbances.
GI: *constipation,* diarrhea, *dry
mouth, excessive salivation,* heartburn, nausea, vomiting.
GU: abnormal ejaculation, incontinence, urinary frequency, urinary
urgency, urine retention.

Hematologic: *agranulocytosis,
leukopenia.*
Metabolic: weight gain.
Musculoskeletal: muscle pain or
spasm, muscle weakness.
Skin: diaphoresis, rash.
Other: fever.

Overdose and treatment
Overdose may cause drowsiness,
delirium, hypotension, hypersali-
vation, tachycardia, respiratory depression, coma and, rarely, seizures. Overdose may be fatal if it
involves more than 2.5 g of drug.

Treat symptomatically. Establish
an airway and ensure adequate ventilation. Monitor patient's vital
signs. Gastric lavage with activated
charcoal and sorbitol may be effective. Avoid epinephrine (and derivatives), quinidine, and procainamide when treating hypotension
and arrhythmias.

Special considerations
■ Because of the high rigk risk of
agranulocytosis and seizures, especially with long-term use, avoid
prolonged treatment periods for
patients who don't respond to
drug.
■ To prevent drug interactions,
make sure you know which other
prescribed drugs, OTC medications, and herbals remedies the patient takes or begins taking during
clozapine therapy.
■ For the first 6 months of clozapine therapy, patient should receive
no more than a 1-week supply of
drug and must participate in a
monitoring program with weekly
blood tests that include WBC
counts. After 6 months, blood tests
can be done every other week.

■ Some patients experience transient fevers (above 100.4° F [38° C]), especially in the first 3 weeks of therapy. Monitor patient closely.

■ Assess patient periodically for abnormal body movements.

■ To discontinue clozapine therapy, withdraw drug gradually over 1 to 2 weeks. If changes in the patient's clinical status (such as the development of leukopenia) require abrupt discontinuation of the drug, monitor patient closely for recurrence of psychotic symptoms and for seizures.

■ To reinstate therapy in patients withdrawn from drug, follow usual guidelines for dosage buildup. Keep in mind, however, that reexposure to drug may increase the risk and severity of adverse reactions. If therapy was terminated because WBC counts were below 2,000/mm³ or granulocyte counts were below 1,000/mm³, drug shouldn't be reinstated.

■ Instruct women to take an oral contraceptive during therapy.

Breast-feeding patients

■ Because drug may appear in breast milk, women who take clozapine shouldn't breast-feed.

Pediatric patients

■ Safe use in children hasn't been established.

Geriatric patients

■ Elderly patients may require reduced dosages because they may have a higher risk of adverse reactions, especially orthostatic hypotension, dry mouth, and constipation. Monitor elderly patients closely.

Patient teaching

■ Warn patient about the risk of developing agranulocytosis. Make sure he knows the importance of weekly blood tests for the first 6 months of therapy, biweekly thereafter, to monitor for agranulocytosis. Urge patient to promptly report flulike symptoms, fever, sore throat, lethargy, malaise, or other signs of infection.

■ Warn patient to rise slowly from lying or sitting positions to minimize the effects of orthostatic hypotension.

■ If patient develops a dry mouth, suggest using ice chips, sugarless candy, or sugarless gum to help relieve symptoms.

■ Tell patient to consult prescriber before taking any prescribed drugs, OTC medications, herbal remedies, or alcohol.

---

fluphenazine decanoate
Modecate◇, Prolixin Decanoate

fluphenazine enanthate
Moditen Enanthate◇, Prolixin Enanthate

fluphenazine hydrochloride
Permitil, Prolixin

Pharmacologic classification: phenothiazine (piperazine derivative)

Therapeutic classification: antipsychotic

Pregnancy risk category C

How supplied
Available by prescription only

---

fluphenazine decanoate
Depot injection: 25 mg/ml
fluphenazine enanthate
Depot injection: 25 mg/ml
fluphenazine hydrochloride
Elixir: 2.5 mg/5 ml (with 14% alcohol)
I.M. injection: 2.5 mg/ml
Oral concentrate: 5 mg/ml (Prolixin contains 14% alcohol; Permitil contains 1% alcohol)
Tablets: 1 mg, 2.5 mg, 5 mg, 10 mg

Indications and dosages
Psychotic disorders
Adults: initially, 0.5 to 10 mg fluphenazine hydrochloride P.O. daily in divided doses q 6 to 8 hours; may increase cautiously to 20 mg. Maintenance dosage is 1 to 5 mg P.O. daily. Usually, I.M. doses are one-third to one-half of oral doses (starting dose is 1.25 mg I.M.). Give decanoate form monthly starting with 12.5 to 25 mg I.M. or S.C. and increase gradually to desired response. Don't exceed 100 mg.

▶ **Dosage adjustment.** For elderly patients, initial dosing range is 1 to 2.5 mg P.O. daily.

Pharmacodynamics
Antipsychotic action: Fluphenazine is thought to exert antipsychotic effects by causing postsynaptic blockade of CNS dopamine receptors, which inhibits dopamine-mediated effects.
Other actions: The drug has many other central and peripheral effects as well; it produces both alpha and ganglionic blockade and counteracts histamine- and serotonin-mediated activity.

Pharmacokinetics
Absorption: Rate and extent of absorption vary with route of administration. Absorption of oral tablets is erratic and variable. Onset of oral and I.M. dosages is within 1 hour. Long-acting decanoate and enanthate salts begin acting in 24 to 72 hours.
Distribution: Drug is distributed widely into the body, including breast milk. CNS levels are usually higher than plasma levels. Drug is 91% to 99% protein-bound. Effects of oral dose usually peak at 2 hours; steady state serum levels occur in 4 to 7 days.
Metabolism: Fluphenazine is metabolized extensively by the liver, but no active metabolites are formed; duration of action is about 6 to 8 hours after oral administration and 1 to 6 weeks (average, 2 weeks) after I.M. depot administration.
Excretion: Drug is mostly excreted in urine via the kidneys; some is excreted in feces via the biliary tract.

Contraindications and precautions
Contraindicated in patients hypersensitive to drug and in patients experiencing coma, CNS depression, bone marrow suppression or other blood dyscrasia, subcortical damage, or liver damage.
Use cautiously in elderly or debilitated patients and in those with pheochromocytoma, severe CV disease, peptic ulcer disease, mitral insufficiency, glaucoma, prostatic hyperplasia, respiratory disorders, seizure disorders, hypocalcemia, a severe reaction to insulin, a severe

reaction to electroconvulsive therapy, or exposure to extreme heat or cold (including antipyretic therapy). Use parenteral form cautiously in patients with asthma and in patients allergic to sulfites.

Interactions
Drug-drug
Antacids that contain aluminum or magnesium, antidiarrheals, phenobarbital: decreased therapeutic response to fluphenazine. Separate administration times by several hours.

Antiarrhythmics (disopyramide, procainamide, quinidine): increased risk of arrhythmias and conduction defects. Avoid concurrent administration.

Anticholinergics (such as atropine), antidepressants, antihistamines, antiparkinsonians, MAO inhibitors, meperidine, phenothiazines: may cause oversedation, paralytic ileus, visual changes, and severe constipation. Monitor patient for adverse reactions and adjust dosage as needed.

Appetite suppressants, sympathomimetics (including ephedrine, epinephrine, phenylephrine, phenylpropanolamine): may decrease stimulatory and pressor effects. Dosage adjustment may be needed.

Beta blockers: may inhibit fluphenazine metabolism, increasing plasma levels and the risk of toxicity. Avoid concurrent use.

Bromocriptine: may antagonize the therapeutic effect of bromocriptine on prolactin secretion. Avoid concurrent use.

Central-acting antihypertensives, such as clonidine, guanabenz, guanadrel, guanethidine, methyldopa, *reserpine:* may inhibit blood pressure response. Adjust dosage according to blood pressure response.

CNS depressants, such as analgesics, barbiturates, narcotics, parenteral magnesium sulfate, tranquilizers, and general, spinal, or epidural anesthetics: may have added effects. Monitor patient for oversedation, respiratory depression, and hypotension, and adjust dosage as needed.

Dopamine: vasoconstricting effects at higher doses are decreased by fluphenazine. Avoid concurrent use.

Levodopa: possible decreased effectiveness of levodopa and loss of therapeutic effect caused by dopamine blockade. Avoid concurrent use.

Lithium: may result in severe neurologic toxicity, an encephalitis-like syndrome, and decreased therapeutic response to fluphenazine. Avoid concurrent use.

Metrizamide: increases the risk of seizures. Use cautiously in patients with seizure disorders.

Nitrates: may cause hypotension. Monitor patient's blood pressure and adjust dosage as needed.

Phenytoin, tricyclic antidepressants: inhibited metabolism of these drugs, which increases the risk of toxicity. Monitor patient's blood levels and adjust dosage as needed.

Propylthiouracil: increases the risk of agranulocytosis. Monitor patient's CBC with differential regularly.

Drug-food
Caffeine: may increase fluphenazine metabolism, decreasing its therapeutic effects. Discourage concurrent use of these substances.

Reactions may be *common,* uncommon, *life-threatening,* or COMMON AND LIFE-THREATENING.

Drug-lifestyle

Alcohol use: may increase CNS depression. Discourage alcohol consumption.

Smoking: may increase fluphenazine metabolism, decreasing its therapeutic effects. Recommend smoking cessation.

Sun exposure: may increase risk of photosensitivity. Avoid prolonged exposure to direct sunlight and wear sunscreen and protective clothing.

Adverse reactions

CNS: confusion, dizziness, *drowsiness, EEG changes, extrapyramidal symptoms,* **neuroleptic malignant syndrome,** *pseudoparkinsonism, sedation, tardive dyskinesia,* **seizures.**
CV: ECG changes, *orthostatic hypotension,* tachycardia.
EENT: *blurred vision,* nasal congestion, ocular changes.
GI: *constipation, dry mouth.*
GU: dark urine, gynecomastia, inhibited ejaculation, menstrual irregularities, *urine retention.*
Hematologic: *agranulocytosis, aplastic anemia,* eosinophilia, *hemolytic anemia, leukopenia, thrombocytopenia.*
Hepatic: abnormal liver function test results, cholestatic jaundice.
Metabolic: elevated protein-bound iodine, increased appetite, weight gain.
Skin: *allergic reactions, mild photosensitivity.*

Overdose and treatment

Overdose causes CNS depression characterized by deep, unarousable sleep, possible coma, hypotension, hypertension, extrapyramidal symptoms, dystonia, abnormal involuntary muscle movements, agitation, seizures, arrhythmias, ECG changes, hypothermia or hyperthermia, and autonomic nervous system dysfunction.

Treatment is symptomatic and supportive. Maintain the patient's vital signs, airway, body temperature, and fluid and electrolyte balance. Don't induce vomiting because drug inhibits cough reflex, and aspiration may occur. Perform gastric lavage, and then give activated charcoal and saline cathartics. Dialysis doesn't help.

Regulate patient's body temperature as needed. Treat hypotension with I.V. fluids; don't give epinephrine. Give parenteral diazepam or barbiturates for seizures, parenteral phenytoin (1 mg/kg adjusted to blood pressure) for arrhythmias, and benztropine (1 to 2 mg) or parenteral diphenhydramine (10 to 50 mg) for extrapyramidal symptoms.

Special considerations

■ Depot injection (25 mg/ml) and I.M. injection (2.5 mg/ml) aren't interchangeable.
■ Avoid depot injection in patients who aren't stabilized on a phenothiazine. This form has prolonged elimination, and its action couldn't be terminated if adverse reactions developed.
■ I.M. administration causes significantly more leakage than S.C. administration, a problem that should be considered if a patient receiving I.M. therapy fails to respond as expected.
■ Fluphenazine causes false-positive results on tests for urinary porphyrins, urobilinogen, amylase,

and 5-hydroxyindoleacetic acid because metabolites darken patient's urine. Drug also causes false-positive results on urine pregnancy tests that use human chorionic gonadotropin.
■ Fluphenazine causes elevated results on tests of liver enzymes and causes quinidine-like effects on an ECG.
■ The most prominent adverse effects of fluphenazine are extrapyramidal.
■ Abrupt withdrawal of long-term therapy may cause gastritis, nausea, vomiting, dizziness, tremor, a feeling of warmth or cold, diaphoresis, tachycardia, headache, and insomnia.

Breast-feeding patients
■ Because drug appears in breast milk, make sure benefits to mother outweigh possible risk to infant.

Pediatric patients
■ Safety and efficacy in children under age 12 haven't been established.

Patient teaching
■ Explain that drug may cause dizziness or drowsiness.
■ Tell patient to avoid hazardous activities until full CNS effects of drug are known.
■ Urge patient to avoid alcohol and to consult prescriber before taking other prescribed drugs, OTC medications, or herbal remedies.
■ Instruct patient to promptly notify prescriber about rash or hives, anxiety, nervousness, or anorexia (especially in underweight patients).

■ Tell patient to promptly notify prescriber about planned, suspected, or known pregnancy.

haloperidol
Apo-Haloperidol◊, Haldol, Novo-Peridol◊, Peridol◊

haloperidol decanoate
Haldol Decanoate, Haldol Decanoate 100, Haldol LA◊

haloperidol lactate
Haldol, Haldol Concentrate, Haloperidol Intensol

Pharmacologic classification: butyrophenone

Therapeutic classification: antipsychotic

Pregnancy risk category C

How supplied
Available by prescription only
haloperidol
Tablets: 0.5 mg, 1 mg, 2 mg, 5 mg, 10 mg, 20 mg
haloperidol decanoate
Injection: 50 mg/ml, 100 mg/ml
haloperidol lactate
Injection: 5 mg/ml
Oral concentrate: 2 mg/ml

Indications and dosages
Psychotic disorders, alcohol dependence*
Adults: Dosage varies based on patient's symptoms. Initial range is 0.5 to 5 mg P.O. b.i.d. or t.i.d.; or 2 to 5 mg I.M. q 4 to 8 hours, increased rapidly if necessary for prompt control. Maximum, 100 mg P.O. daily. Dosage above 100 mg

---

has been used for patients with severely resistant conditions.

Acute psychiatric situations*
Adults: 2 to 30 mg I.M. or I.V. q 1 hour at 5 mg/minute.

Chronic psychosis in patients who require prolonged therapy.
Adults: 100 mg I.M. of haloperidol decanoate q 4 weeks. Experience with dosages over 450 mg monthly is limited.

Control of tics, vocal utterances in Tourette syndrome.
Adults: 0.5 to 5 mg P.O. b.i.d. or t.i.d., increased p.r.n.
Children ages 3 to 12: 0.05 to 0.075 mg/kg/day given b.i.d. or t.i.d.

Agitation and hyperkinesia*
Children ages 3 to 6: 0.01 to 0.03 mg/ kg P.O. daily.

Pharmacodynamics
Antipsychotic action: Haloperidol probably exerts antipsychotic effects by creating a strong postsynaptic blockade of CNS dopamine receptors, which inhibits dopamine-mediated effects. Its pharmacologic effects are most similar to those of piperazine antipsychotics. Its mechanism of action in Tourette syndrome is unknown.
Other actions: Haloperidol has many other central and peripheral effects; it has weak peripheral anticholinergic effects and antiemetic effects, produces both alpha and ganglionic blockade, and counteracts histamine- and serotonin-mediated activity.

Pharmacokinetics
Absorption: Rate and extent of absorption vary with route of administration. Oral tablets yield 60% to 70% bioavailability. I.M. dose is 70% absorbed within 30 minutes. Plasma levels peak 2 to 6 hours after oral administration, 30 to 45 minutes after I.M. administration, and 6 to 7 days after I.M. administration of long-acting (decanoate) form.
Distribution: Haloperidol is distributed widely into the body, with high levels in adipose tissue. Drug is 90% to 92% protein-bound.
Metabolism: Haloperidol is metabolized extensively by the liver; there may be only one active metabolite that is less active than parent drug.
Excretion: About 40% of dose is excreted in urine within 5 days; about 15% is excreted in feces via the biliary tract.

Contraindications and precautions
Contraindicated in patients hypersensitive to drug and in those with parkinsonism, coma, or CNS depression.

Use cautiously in elderly or debilitated patients; patients with a history of seizures, EEG abnormalities, CV disorders, allergies, angle-closure glaucoma, or urine retention; and patients receiving lithium or anticoagulant, anticonvulsant, or antiparkinsonians.

Interactions
Drug-drug
Antacids that contain aluminum or magnesium, antidiarrheals: decreased therapeutic response to

fluphenazine. Separate administration times by several hours.

Antiarrhythmics (disopyramide, procainamide, quinidine): increased risk of arrhythmias and conduction defects. Avoid concurrent administration.

Anticholinergics (such as atropine), antidepressants, antihistamines, antiparkinsonians, MAO inhibitors, meperidine, phenothiazines: may cause oversedation, paralytic ileus, visual changes, and severe constipation. Monitor patient for adverse reactions and adjust dosage as needed.

Appetite suppressants, sympathomimetics (including ephedrine, epinephrine, phenylephrine, phenylpropanolamine): may decrease stimulatory and pressor effects. Dosage adjustment may be needed.

Beta blockers: may inhibit haloperidol metabolism, increasing plasma levels and the risk of toxicity. Monitor blood levels closely.

Bromocriptine: may antagonize the therapeutic effect of bromocriptine on prolactin secretion. Avoid concurrent use.

Central-acting antihypertensives, such as clonidine, guanabenz, guanadrel, guanethidine, methyldopa, reserpine: may inhibit blood pressure response. Adjust dosage according to blood pressure response.

CNS depressants, such as analgesics, barbiturates, narcotics, parenteral magnesium sulfate, tranquilizers, and general, spinal, or epidural anesthetics: may have added effects. Monitor patient for oversedation, respiratory depression, and hypotension, and adjust dosage as needed.

Dopamine: vasoconstricting effects at higher doses are decreased by haloperidol. Avoid concurrent use.

Levodopa: possible decreased effectiveness of levodopa and loss of therapeutic effect caused by dopamine blockade. Adjust dosage as needed.

Lithium: may result in severe neurologic toxicity, an encephalitis-like syndrome, and decreased therapeutic response to haloperidol. Avoid concurrent use.

Metrizamide: increases the risk of seizures. Avoid use in patients with seizure disorders.

Nitrates: may cause hypotension. Monitor patient's blood pressure and adjust dosage as needed.

Phenobarbital: increased renal excretion of phenobarbital causes decreased therapeutic response. Monitor blood levels and adjust the dose as needed.

Phenytoin: altered haloperidol metabolism of, which increases the risk of toxicity or underdosing. Monitor patient's blood levels and adjust dosage as needed.

Propylthiouracil: increases the risk of agranulocytosis. Monitor patient's CBC with differential regularly.

Drug-herb
Nutmeg: may cause a loss of symptom control or interfere with psychiatric drug therapy. Urge avoidance of nutmeg.

Drug-lifestyle
Alcohol use: increased CNS depression. Avoid concurrent use.

Reactions may be *common,* uncommon, ***life-threatening,*** or COMMON AND LIFE-THREATENING.

Adverse reactions

CNS: confusion, drowsiness, headache, insomnia, lethargy, ***neuroleptic malignant syndrome,*** sedation, ***seizures,*** *severe extrapyramidal reactions, tardive dyskinesia,* vertigo.
CV: ECG changes, hypertension, hypotension, tachycardia.
EENT: *blurred vision.*
GI: anorexia, constipation, diarrhea, dry mouth, dyspepsia, nausea, vomiting.
GU: gynecomastia, priapism, menstrual irregularities, urine retention.
Hematologic: leukocytosis, ***leukopenia.***
Hepatic: altered liver function tests, jaundice.
Skin: diaphoresis, rash, other skin reactions.

Overdose and treatment

Overdose causes CNS depression characterized by deep, unarousable sleep, possible coma, hypotension, hypertension, extrapyramidal symptoms, dystonia, abnormal involuntary muscle movements, agitation, seizures, arrhythmias, ECG changes (possible QT prolongation and torsades de pointes), hypothermia or hyperthermia, and autonomic nervous system dysfunction. Overdose with long-acting decanoate prolongs recovery time.

Treatment is symptomatic and supportive. Maintain the patient's vital signs, airway, body temperature, and fluid and electrolyte balance. Consider using ipecac to induce vomiting, but keep in mind the antiemetic properties of haloperidol and the increased risk of aspiration. Also, consider performing gastric lavage followed by activated charcoal and saline cathartics. Dialysis doesn't help.

Regulate patient's body temperature as needed. Treat hypotension with I.V. fluids; don't give epinephrine. Give parenteral diazepam or barbiturates for seizures. For arrhythmias, give parenteral phenytoin 1 mg/kg adjusted in response to patient's blood pressure. Monitor patient's ECG, and don't give more than 50 mg/minute. May repeat every 5 minutes up to 10 mg/kg. For extrapyramidal symptoms, give benztropine (1 to 2 mg) or parenteral diphenhydramine (10 to 50 mg). Watch for evidence of neurologic malignant syndrome, which may be life-threatening.

Special considerations

■ Drug has few CV adverse effects and may be preferred for patients with cardiac disease.
■ Drug is especially useful for agitation associated with senile dementia.
■ Give drug by deep I.M. injection. Don't give decanoate form by I.V. route.
■ A 2-mg dose is the therapeutic equivalent of 100 mg of chlorpromazine.
■ When changing from tablets to decanoate injection, patient should initially receive 10 to 20 times the oral dose once monthly (maximum, 100 mg).
■ Assess patient periodically for abnormal body movements and evidence of neuroleptic malignant syndrome.
■ Tardive dyskinesia may occur after prolonged use. It may not appear until months or years later,

and it may disappear spontaneously or persist for life.
- Don't withdraw drug abruptly except when required by a severe adverse reaction.
- The most prominent adverse reactions to haloperidol are extrapyramidal, such as neuroleptic malignant syndrome.
- Protect drug from light. Slight yellowing of injection or concentrate is common and doesn't affect potency. Discard markedly discolored solutions.
- Besides standard indications, drug is also used for phencyclidine psychosis (commonly called PCP psychosis), intractable hiccups, and prevention or control of severe nausea and vomiting such as that caused by chemotherapy.

Pediatric patients
- Drug isn't recommended for children under age 3. Children are especially prone to extrapyramidal effects.

Geriatric patients
- Elderly patients usually require lower initial doses and a more gradual dosage adjustment.

Patient teaching
- Before patient begins long-term therapy, explain the risk of potentially irreversible tardive dyskinesia.
- Warn patient to avoid hazardous activities until full CNS effects of drug are known.
- Tell patient that dizziness and drowsiness are common but usually subside after a few weeks.
- Warn patient to avoid alcohol and other CNS depressants during therapy.
- Tell patient to notify prescriber about adverse effects, such as extrapyramidal reactions.

---

loxapine hydrochloride
Loxitane C, Loxitane IM

loxapine succinate
Loxapac ◇, Loxitane

Pharmacologic classification:
dibenzoxazepine

Therapeutic classification:
antipsychotic

Pregnancy risk category C

How supplied
Available by prescription only
Capsules: 5 mg, 10 mg, 25 mg, 50 mg
Injection: 50 mg/ml
Oral concentrate: 25 mg/ml

Indications and dosages
Psychotic disorders
Adults: 10 mg P.O. b.i.d. to q.i.d., rapidly increased to 60 to 100 mg P.O. daily for most patients (dose varies with individual) or 12.5 to 50 mg I.M. q 4 to 6 hours. Maximum, 250 mg daily.

Pharmacodynamics
Antipsychotic action: Loxapine is the only tricyclic antipsychotic; it is structurally similar to amoxapine. Loxapine is thought to exert its antipsychotic effects by postsynaptic blockade of CNS dopamine receptors, which inhibits dopamine-mediated effects.
Other actions: Loxapine has many other central and peripheral effects.

Reactions may be *common,* uncommon, *life-threatening,* or COMMON AND LIFE-THREATENING.

Pharmacokinetics
Absorption: Drug is absorbed rapidly and completely from the GI tract. Levels peak later after I.M. dose (5 hours) than after oral dose (1 hour). First-pass metabolism results in lower systemic availability.
Distribution: Drug is distributed widely into the body, including breast milk. Peak effect occurs in 1½ to 3 hours; steady state serum level occurs in 3 to 4 days. Drug is 91% to 99% protein-bound.
Metabolism: Drug is metabolized extensively by the liver, forming a few active metabolites; duration of action is 12 hours.
Excretion: Drug is mostly excreted as metabolites in urine; some is excreted in feces via the biliary tract. About 50% of drug is excreted in urine and feces within 24 hours.

Contraindications and precautions
Contraindicated in patients hypersensitive to dibenzoxazepines and in patients experiencing drug-induced depressed states, severe CNS depression, or coma.

Use cautiously in patients with seizure or CV disorders, glaucoma, or history of urine retention.

Interactions
Drug-drug
Antacids that contain aluminum or magnesium, antidiarrheals: decreased loxapine absorption. Separate administration times by several hours.
Antiarrhythmics (disopyramide, procainamide, quinidine): increased risk of arrhythmias and conduction defects. Avoid concurrent administration.

Anticholinergics (such as atropine), antidepressants, antihistamines, antiparkinsonians, MAO inhibitors, meperidine, phenothiazines: may cause oversedation, paralytic ileus, visual changes, and severe constipation. Monitor patient for adverse reactions and adjust dosage as needed.
Appetite suppressants, sympathomimetics (including ephedrine, epinephrine, phenylephrine, phenylpropanolamine): may decrease stimulatory and pressor effects. Dosage adjustment may be needed.
Beta blockers: may inhibit loxapine metabolism, increasing plasma levels and the risk of toxicity. Monitor blood levels closely and adjust dosage as needed.
Bromocriptine: may antagonize the therapeutic effect of bromocriptine on prolactin secretion. Avoid concurrent use.
Central-acting antihypertensives, such as clonidine, guanabenz, guanadrel, guanethidine, methyldopa, reserpine: may inhibit blood pressure response. Adjust dosage according to blood pressure response.
CNS depressants, such as analgesics, barbiturates, narcotics, parenteral magnesium sulfate, tranquilizers, and general, spinal, or epidural anesthetics: may have added effects. Monitor patient for oversedation, respiratory depression, and hypotension, and adjust dosage as needed.
Dopamine: vasoconstricting effects at higher doses are decreased by loxapine. Avoid concurrent use.
Levodopa: possible decreased effectiveness of levodopa and loss of therapeutic effect caused by dopa-

---

mine blockade. Adjust dosage as needed.
Lithium: may result in severe neurologic toxicity, an encephalitis-like syndrome, and decreased therapeutic response to loxapine. Avoid concurrent use.
Nitrates: may cause hypotension. Monitor patient's blood pressure and adjust dosage as needed.

Drug-lifestyle
Alcohol use: may cause additive effects. Discourage alcohol consumption.

Adverse reactions
CNS: confusion, dizziness, *drowsiness,* EEG changes, *extrapyramidal symptoms,* **neuroleptic malignant syndrome,** numbness, pseudoparkinsonism, *sedation,* **seizures,** syncope, *tardive dyskinesia.*
CV: ECG changes, hypertension, *orthostatic hypotension, tachycardia.*
EENT: *blurred vision,* nasal congestion.
GI: *constipation, dry mouth,* nausea, paralytic ileus, vomiting.
GU: gynecomastia, menstrual irregularities, *urine retention.*
Hematologic: **agranulocytosis, leukopenia, thrombocytopenia.**
Hepatic: jaundice.
Metabolic: weight gain.
Skin: allergic reactions, *mild photosensitivity,* pruritus, rash.

Overdose and treatment
Overdose causes CNS depression characterized by deep, unarousable sleep, possible coma, hypotension, hypertension, extrapyramidal symptoms, dystonia, abnormal involuntary muscle movements, agitation, seizures, arrhythmias, ECG changes, hypothermia or hyperthermia, and autonomic nervous system dysfunction.

Treatment is symptomatic and supportive. Maintain the patient's vital signs, airway, body temperature, and fluid and electrolyte balance. Don't induce vomiting because drug inhibits cough reflex, and aspiration may occur. Perform gastric lavage, and then give activated charcoal and saline cathartics. Dialysis may be helpful.

Regulate patient's body temperature as needed. Treat hypotension with I.V. fluids; don't give epinephrine. Give parenteral diazepam or barbiturates for seizures, parenteral phenytoin (1 mg/kg adjusted to blood pressure) for arrhythmias, and benztropine (1 to 2 mg) or parenteral diphenhydramine (10 to 50 mg) for extrapyramidal symptoms.

Special considerations
- Obtain baseline blood pressure measurements before starting therapy, and monitor patient's blood pressure regularly.
- Don't give drug by I.V. route.
- Dilute liquid concentrate with orange juice or grapefruit juice just before administration.
- Assess patient periodically for abnormal body movements.
- Watch for tardive dyskinesia, especially after prolonged use. It may not appear until months or years after treatment, and it may disappear spontaneously or persist for life.
- Periodic ophthalmic tests are recommended.

- A 10-mg dose is the therapeutic equivalent of 100 mg of chlorpromazine.
- Avoid combining drug with alcohol or other depressants.
- Drug causes false-positive results on tests of urinary porphyrins, urobilinogen, amylase, and 5-hydroxyindoleacetic acid because metabolites darken patient's urine. Drug also causes false-positive results on urine pregnancy test that use human chorionic gonadotropin.
- The most prominent adverse reactions of loxapine are extrapyramidal.

Pediatric patients
- Drug isn't recommended for children under age 16.

Geriatric patients
- Elderly patients are highly sensitive to the antimuscarinic, hypotensive, and sedative effects of loxapine and have a higher risk of developing adverse extrapyramidal reactions, such as parkinsonism and tardive dyskinesia. These patients develop higher plasma levels and therefore require a lower initial dosage and more gradual increases.

Patient teaching
- Before patient begins long-term therapy, explain the risk of potentially irreversible tardive dyskinesia.
- Warn patient to avoid hazardous activities until full CNS effects of drug are known.
- Tell patient that dizziness and drowsiness are common but usually subside after a few weeks.
- If patient develops a dry mouth, recommend sugarless gum or candy, mouthwash, ice chips, or artificial saliva to help relieve symptoms.
- Tell patient to rise slowly from lying or sitting positions to minimize the effects of orthostatic hypotension.

---

mesoridazine besylate
Serentil

Pharmacologic classification: **phenothiazine (piperidine derivative)**

Therapeutic classification: **antipsychotic**

Pregnancy risk category C

How supplied
Available by prescription only
Injection: 25 mg/ml
Oral concentrate: 25 mg/ml (0.6% alcohol)
Tablets: 10 mg, 25 mg, 50 mg, 100 mg

Indications and dosages
Psychoneurotic manifestations (anxiety)
Adults and children over age 12: 10 mg P.O. t.i.d. to maximum of 150 mg/day.

Schizophrenia
Adults and children over age 12: initially, 50 mg P.O. t.i.d. to maximum of 400 mg/day; or 25 mg I.M. repeated in 30 to 60 minutes, p.r.n., not to exceed 200 mg I.M. daily.

Alcoholism
Adults and children over age 12: 25 mg P.O. b.i.d. to maximum of 200 mg/day.

Behavioral problems caused by chronic brain syndrome
Adults and children over age 12:
25 mg P.O. t.i.d. to maximum of 300 mg/day.
▶ DOSAGE ADJUSTMENT. Because elderly people commonly have decreased renal function, administer drug cautiously and adjust dosage as needed.

Pharmacodynamics
Antipsychotic action: Mesoridazine, a metabolite of thioridazine, is thought to exert antipsychotic effects by postsynaptic blockade of CNS dopamine receptors, which inhibits dopamine-mediated effects.
Other actions: The drug has many other central and peripheral effects as well; it produces both alpha and ganglionic blockade and counteracts histamine- and serotonin-mediated activity.

Pharmacokinetics
Absorption: Drug appears to be well absorbed from the GI tract following oral administration. I.M. dosage form is absorbed rapidly.
Distribution: Drug is distributed widely into the body, including breast milk. Effects peak at 2 to 4 hours; steady state serum level occurs in 4 to 7 days. Drug is 91% to 99% protein-bound.
Metabolism: Drug is metabolized extensively by the liver; no active metabolites are formed. Duration of action is 4 to 6 hours.
Excretion: Drug is mostly excreted as metabolites in urine; some is excreted in feces via the biliary tract.

Contraindications and precautions
Contraindicated in patients hypersensitive to drug and in those experiencing severe CNS depression or coma.

Interactions
Drug-drug
Antacids that contain aluminum or magnesium, antidiarrheals: decreased mesoridazine absorption. Separate administration times.
Antiarrhythmics (disopyramide, procainamide, quinidine): increased risk of arrhythmias and conduction defects. Avoid concurrent administration.
Anticholinergics (such as atropine), antidepressants, antihistamines, antiparkinsonians, MAO inhibitors, meperidine, phenothiazines: may cause oversedation, paralytic ileus, visual changes, and severe constipation. Monitor patient for adverse reactions and adjust dosage as needed.
Appetite suppressants, sympathomimetics (including ephedrine, epinephrine, phenylephrine, phenylpropanolamine): may decrease stimulatory and pressor effects. Dosage adjustment may be needed
Beta blockers: may inhibit mesoridazine metabolism, increasing plasma levels and the risk of toxicity. Monitor blood levels closely.
Bromocriptine: may antagonize the therapeutic effect of bromocriptine on prolactin secretion. Avoid concurrent use.
Central-acting antihypertensives, such as clonidine, guanabenz, guanadrel, guanethidine, methyldopa, reserpine: may inhibit blood pres-

sure response. Adjust dosage according to blood pressure response.

CNS depressants, such as analgesics, barbiturates, narcotics, parenteral magnesium sulfate, tranquilizers, and general, spinal, or epidural anesthetics: may have added effects. Monitor patient for oversedation, respiratory depression, and hypotension, and adjust dosage as needed.

Dopamine: decreased vasoconstricting effects of dopamine. Avoid concurrent use.

Epinephrine: mesoridazine may cause epinephrine reversal. Avoid concurrent use.

Levodopa: possible decreased effectiveness of levodopa and loss of therapeutic effect caused by dopamine blockade. Adjust dosage as needed.

Lithium: may result in severe neurologic toxicity, an encephalitis-like syndrome, and decreased therapeutic response to mesoridazine. Avoid concurrent use.

Metrizamide: increases the risk of seizures. Avoid use in patients with seizure disorders.

Nitrates: may cause hypotension. Monitor patient's blood pressure and adjust dosage as needed.

Phenobarbital: increased renal excretion of phenobarbital causes decreased therapeutic response to mesoridazine. Monitor blood levels and adjust the dose as needed.

Phenytoin: altered phenytoin metabolism, which increases the risk of toxicity or underdosing. Monitor patient's blood phenytoin levels and adjust dosage as needed.

Propylthiouracil: increases the risk of agranulocytosis. Monitor patient's CBC with differential regularly.

Drug-food
Caffeine: increased metabolism may cause decreased response to mesoridazine and may require dosage adjustment. Discourage foods and beverages that contain caffeine.

Drug-lifestyle
Alcohol use: may cause additive effects. Discourage concomitant use.

Heavy smoking: increased metabolism may cause decreased response to mesoridazine and may require dosage adjustment. Recommend smoking cessation.

Sun exposure: increased risk of photosensitivity reactions. Discourage prolonged or unprotected sun exposure.

Adverse reactions
CNS: confusion, dizziness, *drowsiness,* EEG changes, extrapyramidal symptoms, **neuroleptic malignant syndrome,** rigidity, sedation, tardive dyskinesia, tremor, weakness.
CV: ECG changes, *hypotension,* tachycardia.
EENT: blurred vision, nasal congestion, ocular changes, retinitis pigmentosa.
GI: constipation, dry mouth, nausea, vomiting.
GU: gynecomastia, inhibited ejaculation, menstrual irregularities, urine retention.
Hematologic: *agranulocytosis, aplastic anemia,* eosinophilia, *leukopenia, thrombocytopenia.*
Hepatic: abnormal liver function test results, jaundice.
Metabolic: weight gain.

Skin: allergic reactions, mild photosensitivity, pain at I.M. injection site, rash, sterile abscess.

Overdose and treatment
Overdose causes CNS depression characterized by deep, unarousable sleep, possible coma, hypotension, hypertension, extrapyramidal symptoms, dystonia, abnormal involuntary muscle movements, agitation, seizures, arrhythmias, ECG changes, hypothermia or hyperthermia, and autonomic nervous system dysfunction.

Treatment is symptomatic and supportive. Maintain the patient's vital signs, airway, body temperature, and fluid and electrolyte balance. Don't induce vomiting because drug inhibits cough reflex, and aspiration may occur. Perform gastric lavage, and then give activated charcoal and saline cathartics. Dialysis doesn't help.

Regulate patient's body temperature as needed. Treat hypotension with I.V. fluids; don't give epinephrine. Give parenteral diazepam or barbiturates for seizures. Give parenteral phenytoin for arrhythmias. Give and benztropine (1 to 2 mg) or parenteral diphenhydramine (10 to 50 mg) for extrapyramidal symptoms. Watch for evidence of potentially fatal neuroleptic malignant syndrome. Symptoms include hyperexia, muscle rigidity, altered mental status, and irregular pulse or blood pressure.

Special considerations
■ Mesoridazine causes fewer adverse reactions than other phenothiazine compounds.

■ The I.M. form of mesoridazine is irritating.
■ Mesoridazine causes false-positive results on tests of urinary porphyrins, urobilinogen, amylase, and 5-hydroxyindoleacetic acid because metabolites darken patient's urine. Drug also causes false-positive results on urine pregnancy tests that use human chorionic gonadotropin.
■ Mesoridazine causes elevated results on tests of liver function, prolactin and creatine phosphokinase levels, and protein-bound iodine. It causes quinidine-like effects on the patient's ECG.
■ After abrupt withdrawal of long-term therapy, patient may experience gastritis, nausea, vomiting, dizziness, tremor, a feeling of warmth or cold, diaphoresis, tachycardia, headache, and insomnia.
■ The most prominent adverse reactions of mesoridazine are antimuscarinic and sedative; it causes fewer extrapyramidal effects than other antipsychotics.

Pediatric patients
■ Drug isn't recommended for children under age 12.

Patient teaching
■ Before starting long-term therapy, explain the risk of developing possible permanent tardive dyskinesia.
■ Tell patient that drug commonly causes drowsiness and hypotension, both of which typically subside with prolonged use.
■ Warn patient not to consume excessive amounts of alcohol while taking mesoridazine.

■ Caution patient not to take other prescribed drugs, OTC medications, or herbal remedies without consulting prescriber.

---

molindone hydrochloride
Moban

Pharmacologic classification: dihydroindolone

Therapeutic classification: antipsychotic

Pregnancy risk category C

How supplied
Available by prescription only
Oral concentrate: 20 mg/ml
Tablets: 5 mg, 10 mg, 25 mg, 50 mg, 100 mg

Indications and dosages
Psychotic disorders
Adults: 50 to 75 mg P.O. daily, increased by 100 mg daily in 3 to 4 days to a maximum of 225 mg daily. Maintenance dose for mild disease is 5 to 15 mg t.i.d. or q.i.d., for moderate disease is 10 to 25 mg t.i.d. or q.i.d., and for severe disease is 225 mg daily.
▶ DOSAGE ADJUSTMENT. For elderly patients, lower doses are recommended; 30% to 50% of usual dose may be effective.

Pharmacodynamics
Antipsychotic action: Molindone is unrelated to all other antipsychotic drugs; it is thought to exert antipsychotic effects by postsynaptic blockade of CNS dopamine receptors, which inhibits dopamine-mediated effects.

Other actions: Molindone has many other central and peripheral effects; it also produces alpha and ganglionic blockade.

Pharmacokinetics
Absorption: Data are limited, but absorption appears rapid; effects peak within 1½ hours.
Distribution: Molindone is distributed widely into the body.
Metabolism: Drug is metabolized extensively; effects persist for 24 to 36 hours.
Excretion: Most of drug is excreted as metabolites in urine; some is excreted in feces via the biliary tract. Overall, 90% of a given dose is excreted within 24 hours.

Contraindications and precautions
Contraindicated in patients hypersensitive to drug and in those experiencing severe CNS depression or coma.

Use cautiously in patients at risk for seizures or when increased physical activity could harm patient.

Interactions
Drug-drug
Antacids that contain aluminum or magnesium, antidiarrheals: decreased molindone absorption. Separate administration times.
Antiarrhythmics (disopyramide, procainamide, quinidine): increased risk of arrhythmias and conduction defects. Avoid concurrent administration.
Anticholinergics (such as atropine), antidepressants, antihistamines, antiparkinsonians, MAO inhibitors, meperidine, phenothiazines: may

---

cause oversedation, paralytic ileus, visual changes, and severe constipation. Monitor patient for adverse reactions and adjust dosage as needed.

Appetite suppressants, sympathomimetics (including ephedrine, epinephrine, phenylephrine, phenylpropanolamine): may decrease stimulatory and pressor effects. Dosage adjustment may be needed.

Beta blockers: may inhibit molindone metabolism, increasing plasma levels and the risk of toxicity. Monitor blood levels closely.

Bromocriptine: may antagonize the therapeutic effect of bromocriptine on prolactin secretion. Avoid concurrent use.

Central-acting antihypertensives, such as clonidine, guanabenz, guanadrel, guanethidine, methyldopa, reserpine: may inhibit blood pressure response. Adjust dosage according to blood pressure response.

CNS depressants, such as analgesics, barbiturates, narcotics, parenteral magnesium sulfate, tranquilizers, and general, spinal, or epidural anesthetics: may have added effects. Monitor patient for oversedation, respiratory depression, and hypotension, and adjust dosage as needed.

Dopamine: decreased vasoconstricting effects of dopamine. Monitor patient for lack of therapeutic effect.

Epinephrine: molindone may cause epinephrine reversal. Avoid concurrent use.

Levodopa: possible decreased effectiveness of levodopa and loss of therapeutic effect caused by dopamine blockade. Adjust dosage as needed.

Lithium: may result in severe neurologic toxicity, an encephalitis-like syndrome, and decreased therapeutic response to molindone. Avoid concurrent use.

Metrizamide: increases the risk of seizures. Use cautiously in patients with seizure disorders.

Nitrates: may cause hypotension. Monitor patient's blood pressure and adjust dosage as needed.

Phenobarbital: increased renal excretion of phenobarbital causes decreased therapeutic response to molindone. Monitor blood levels and adjust the dose as needed.

Phenytoin: altered phenytoin metabolism of, which increases the risk of toxicity or underdosing. Monitor patient's blood phenytoin levels and adjust dosage as needed.

Propylthiouracil: increases the risk of agranulocytosis. Monitor patient's CBC with differential regularly.

Drug-food

Caffeine: increased metabolism may decrease effect of molindone and require a dosage adjustment. Discourage caffeine-containing foods and beverages.

Drug-lifestyle

Alcohol: may cause additive effects. Discourage concomitant use.

Heavy smoking: increased metabolism may decrease effect of molindone and require a dosage adjustment. Recommend smoking cessation.

Sun exposure: increased risk of photosensitivity reactions. Discourage prolonged or unprotected sun exposure.

Reactions may be *common,* uncommon, *life-threatening,* or COMMON AND LIFE-THREATENING.

Adverse reactions
CNS: depression, dizziness, *drowsiness,* EEG changes, euphoria, *extrapyramidal symptoms,* **neuroleptic malignant syndrome,** pseudoparkinsonism, *sedation, tardive dyskinesia.*
CV: ECG changes, *orthostatic hypotension,* tachycardia.
EENT: blurred vision.
GI: constipation, dry mouth, nausea.
GU: gynecomastia, inhibited ejaculation, menstrual irregularities, urine retention.
Hematologic: leukocytosis, *leukopenia.*
Hepatic: abnormal liver function test results, jaundice.
Skin: allergic reactions, mild photosensitivity.

Overdose and treatment
Overdose causes CNS depression characterized by deep, unarousable sleep, possible coma, hypotension, hypertension, extrapyramidal symptoms, dystonia, abnormal involuntary muscle movements, agitation, seizures, arrhythmias, ECG changes, hypothermia or hyperthermia, and autonomic nervous system dysfunction.

Treatment is symptomatic and supportive. Maintain the patient's vital signs, airway, body temperature, and fluid and electrolyte balance. Don't induce vomiting because drug inhibits cough reflex, and aspiration may occur. Perform gastric lavage, and then give activated charcoal and saline cathartics. Dialysis doesn't help.

Regulate patient's body temperature as needed. Treat hypotension with I.V. fluids; don't give epinephrine. Give parenteral diazepam or barbiturates for seizures, parenteral phenytoin for arrhythmias, and benztropine (1 to 2 mg) or parenteral diphenhydramine (10 to 50 mg) for extrapyramidal symptoms.

Special considerations
- Drug may cause GI distress and should be given with food or fluids.
- Protect liquid form from light.
- Dilute concentrate in 2 to 4 ounces of liquid, preferably soup, water, juice, carbonated (but non-caffeinated) drinks, milk, or puddings.
- Patient's urine may turn pink to brown.
- Expect an additive risk of seizures with metrizamide myelography.
- Drug's most prominent adverse reactions are extrapyramidal.

Pregnant patients
- Drug causes false-positive results in urine pregnancy tests that use human chorionic gonadotropin.

Pediatric patients
- Drug isn't recommended for children under age 12.

Geriatric patients
- Elderly patients have an increased risk of tardive dyskinesia and other extrapyramidal effects.

Patient teaching
- Explain the risk of dystonic reactions and possible permanent tardive dyskinesia, and urge the patient to notify prescriber about abnormal body movements.

■ Urge patient to take drug exactly as prescribed and not to change the dosage or double the dose after missing one.

■ Warn patient not to get liquid form on his skin because rash and irritation may result.

■ Tell patient to avoid temperature extremes (such as hot or cold baths, sunlamps, or tanning beds) because drug may alter thermoregulation.

■ If patient develops a dry mouth, suggest sugarless gum, sugarless candy, ice chips, or artificial saliva to help relieve the symptoms.

■ Caution patient not to take drug with antacids or antidiarrheals and not to drink alcohol or take sedating medications.

■ Tell patient to rise slowly from a lying or sitting position to minimize the effects of orthostatic hypotension, particularly light-headedness.

■ Tell patient not to stop therapy without consulting prescriber.

■ Warn patient about drug's sedative effect.

■ Tell patient to notify prescriber about difficult urination, sore throat, dizziness, or fainting.

■ Inform patient that drug may contain sodium metabisulfite, which can cause an allergic reaction in people allergic to sulfites.

---

olanzapine
Zyprexa

Pharmacologic classification:
thienobenzodiazepine derivative

Therapeutic classification:
antipsychotic

Pregnancy risk category C

How supplied
Available by prescription only
Tablets: 2.5 mg, 5 mg, 7.5 mg, 10 mg

Indications and dosages
Psychotic disorders
Adults: initially, 5 to 10 mg P.O. once daily. Adjust dosage by 5 mg daily at intervals of not less than 1 week. Most patients respond to 10 mg/day; don't exceed 20 mg/day.
▶ DOSAGE ADJUSTMENT. Begin therapy at 5 mg if patient is sensitive to drug, debilitated, predisposed to hypotension, or has an altered metabolism from smoking, gender, or age. Initial dosage may be lower in elderly patients because they tend to have decreased clearance.

Pharmacodynamics
Unknown. Acts as an antagonist at dopamine (D_{1-4}) and serotonin (5-$HT_{2A/2C}$) receptors; it may also exhibit antagonist-binding at adrenergic, cholinergic, and histaminergic receptors.

Pharmacokinetics
Absorption: Drug levels peak about 6 hours after an oral dose. Food doesn't affect the rate or extent of absorption. About 40% of

---

dose is eliminated by first-pass metabolism.

Distribution: Drug distributes extensively throughout the body, with a volume of distribution of about 1,000 L. Drug is 93% protein-bound, mainly to albumin and alpha-acid glycoprotein.

Metabolism: Drug is metabolized by direct glucuronidation and cytochrome P-450-mediated oxidation.

Excretion: About 57% of drug appears in urine and 30% in feces as metabolites. Only 7% of dose appears in urine unchanged. Elimination half-life ranges from 21 to 54 hours.

Contraindications and precautions

Contraindicated in patients hypersensitive to drug.

Use cautiously in elderly patients and patients with heart disease, cerebrovascular disease, conditions that predispose to hypotension (gradual dosage adjustment minimizes the risk), and hepatic impairment. Also, use cautiously in patients with a history of seizures, a condition that lowers the seizure threshold, paralytic ileus, significant prostatic hypertrophy, or angle-clososure glaucoma. Finally, use cautiously in patients at risk for aspiration pneumonia.

Interactions
Drug-drug

Antihypertensives, diazepam: may potentiate hypotensive effects. Monitor patient's blood pressure closely.

Carbamazepine, omeprazole, rifampin: may cause increased olanzapine clearance. Monitor patient, and adjust dosage as needed.

Dopamine agonists, levodopa: effects of these drugs may be antagonized. Adjust dosage as necessary.

Fluvoxamine: may inhibit olanzapine elimination. Dosage adjustment may be needed.

Drug-herb

Nutmeg: may interfere with symptom control or the effects of psychiatric therapy. Discourage consumption of food and beverages that contain nutmeg, and monitor patient closely.

Drug-lifestyle

Alcohol use: may potentiate hypotensive effects. Monitor patient's blood pressure closely, and discourage consumption of alcohol.

Adverse reactions

CNS: *agitation, akathisia,* amnesia, anxiety, articulation impairment, *dizziness,* dystonic/dyskinetic events, euphoria, *headache, hostility,* hypertonia, *insomnia, nervousness,* **neuroleptic malignant syndrome,** *parkinsonism,* personality disorder, *somnolence,* stuttering, tardive dyskinesia, tremor.

CV: chest pain, edema, hypotension, orthostatic hypotension, tachycardia.

EENT: amblyopia, blepharitis, corneal lesion, *rhinitis,* pharyngitis.

GI: abdominal pain, constipation, dry mouth, increased appetite, increased salivation, nausea, thirst, vomiting.

GU: hematuria, metrorrhagia, premenstrual syndrome, urinary incontinence, UTI.

Hepatic: increased ALT, AST, and GGT.
Metabolic: weight gain or loss.
Musculoskeletal: back pain, joint pain, limb pain, neck rigidity, twitching.
Respiratory: dyspnea, increased cough.
Skin: vesiculobullous rash.
Other: fever; flulike syndrome; increased serum prolactin, eosinophil count, and creatine kinase; intentional injury; suicide attempt.

Overdose and treatment
Overdose may cause drowsiness and slurred speech.

There is no specific antidote to olanzapine, and treatment should be symptomatic. Monitor patient for hypotension, circulatory collapse, obtundation, seizures, or dystonic reactions. Gastric lavage with activated charcoal and sorbitol may be effective. Dialysis isn't helpful. Avoid epinephrine, dopamine, or other sympathomimetics with beta-agonist activity.

Special considerations
■ Obtain baseline and periodic liver function tests.
■ Give drug cautiously if patient has a seizure disorder.
■ Efficacy for long-term use (more than 6 weeks) hasn't been established.
■ Watch for evidence of neuroleptic malignant syndrome (hyperpyrexia, muscle rigidity, altered mental status, autonomic instability), a rare but frequently fatal adverse reaction that may arise with antipsychotic therapy. If evidence appears, stop drug immediately and begin intensive monitoring and treatment.

Breast-feeding patients
■ Because drug probably appears in breast milk, a patient who takes olanzapine should avoid breast-feeding.

Pediatric patients
■ Safety and efficacy in children under age 18 haven't been established.

Geriatric patients
■ Drug half-life in elderly patients is 1½ times greater than in younger patients.

Patient teaching
■ Warn patient to avoid hazardous activities until full CNS effects of drug are known.
■ Caution patient against exposure to extreme heat; drug may impair body's ability to reduce core temperature.
■ Instruct patient to avoid alcohol during therapy.
■ Tell patient to rise slowly from lying or sitting positions to minimize the effects of orthostatic hypotension.
■ If patient develops a dry mouth, suggest using ice chips, sugarless candy, or sugarless gum to relieve the symptoms.
■ Tell patient not to take other prescribed drugs, OTC medications, or herbal remedies without consulting prescriber.

---

perphenazine
Apo-Perphenazine◊, Trilafon

Pharmacologic classification:
**phenothiazine (piperazine
derivative)**

Therapeutic classification:
antipsychotic, antiemetic

Pregnancy risk category C

How supplied
Available by prescription only
Injection: 5 mg/ml
Oral concentrate: 16 mg/5 ml
Tablets: 2 mg, 4 mg, 8 mg, 16 mg

Indications and dosages
Psychosis in hospitalized patients
Adults and children over age 12: initially, 8 to 16 mg P.O. b.i.d., t.i.d., or q.i.d. Don't exceed 64 mg P.O. daily in adults. Alternatively, give 5 mg I.M. q 6 hours, p.r.n. Severely agitated patients may need 10 mg I.M. for the first dose. Don't exceed 30 mg I.M. daily in a hospitalized patient. Change to P.O. as soon as possible (in 1-2 days).

Psychotic disorders in moderately disturbed outpatients
Adults and children over age 12: initially, 4 to 8 mg P.O. t.i.d. Reduce later doses to lowest effective level.
▶ DOSAGE ADJUSTMENT. If patient has hepatic dysfunction, adjustment may be needed. Also, elderly patients may need reduced initial dosages and gradual adjustment; 30% to 50% of the usual dose may be effective.

Pharmacodynamics
Antipsychotic action: Perphenazine is thought to exert antipsychotic effects by postsynaptic blockade of CNS dopamine receptors, which inhibits dopamine-mediated effects.
Antiemetic action: Its antiemetic effects are attributed to dopamine receptor blockade in the medullary chemoreceptor trigger zone.
Other actions: Perphenazine has many other central and peripheral effects as well: it produces both alpha and ganglionic blockade, and it counteracts histamine- and serotonin-mediated activity.

Pharmacokinetics
Absorption: Rate and extent of absorption vary with administration route: absorption of oral tablet is erratic and variable, with onset of action ranging from 30 minutes to 1 hour. Absorption of oral concentrate is much more predictable. Dose given by I.M. route is absorbed rapidly and peaks in about 8 days.
Distribution: Drug is distributed widely into the body, including breast milk. Drug is 91% to 99% protein-bound. After administration of oral tablet, effects peak in 2 to 4 hours; steady state serum levels occur in 4 to 7 days.
Metabolism: Drug is metabolized extensively by the liver, but no active metabolites are formed.
Excretion: Drug is mostly excreted in urine via the kidneys; some appears in feces via the biliary tract.

Contraindications and precautions
Contraindicated in patients hypersensitive to drug, in comatose pa-

tients, in patients receiving large doses of CNS depressants, and in patients with CNS depression, blood dyscrasia, bone marrow depression, liver damage, or subcortical damage.

Use cautiously in elderly or debilitated patients, in patients receiving other CNS depressants or anticholinergics, and in patients with alcohol withdrawal, psychic depression, suicidal tendencies, adverse reactions to other phenothiazines, impaired renal function, or respiratory disorders.

Interactions
Drug-drug
Antacids that contain aluminum or magnesium, antidiarrheals: decreased therapeutic response to fluphenazine. Separate administration times by several hours.

Antiarrhythmics (disopyramide, procainamide, quinidine): increased risk of arrhythmias and conduction defects. Avoid concurrent administration.

Anticholinergics (such as atropine), antidepressants, antihistamines, antiparkinsonians, MAO inhibitors, meperidine, phenothiazines: may cause oversedation, paralytic ileus, visual changes, and severe constipation. Monitor patient for adverse reactions and adjust dosage as needed.

Appetite suppressants, sympathomimetics (including ephedrine, epinephrine, phenylephrine, phenylpropanolamine): may decrease stimulatory and pressor effects. Dosage adjustment may be needed.

Beta blockers: may inhibit perphenazine metabolism, increasing plasma levels and the risk of toxicity. Monitor blood levels closely.

Bromocriptine: perphenazine may antagonize the therapeutic effect of bromocriptine on prolactin secretion. Avoid concurrent use.

Central-acting antihypertensives, such as clonidine, guanabenz, guanadrel, guanethidine, methyldopa, reserpine: may inhibit blood pressure response. Adjust dosage according to blood pressure response.

Cisapride, grepafloxacin, ibutilide, pimozide, sparfloxacin: increased risk of serious arrhythmias. Avoid concurrent use.

CNS depressants, such as analgesics, barbiturates, narcotics, parenteral magnesium sulfate, tranquilizers, and general, spinal, or epidural anesthetics: may have added effects. Monitor patient for oversedation, respiratory depression, and hypotension, and adjust dosage as needed.

Dopamine: decreased vasoconstricting effects of dopamine. Assess patient for lack of therapeutic response.

Epinephrine: may be reversed by perphenazine. Avoid concurrent use.

Levodopa: possible decreased effectiveness of levodopa and loss of therapeutic effect caused by dopamine blockade. Adjust dosage as needed.

Lithium: may result in severe neurologic toxicity, an encephalitis-like syndrome, and decreased therapeutic response to perphenazine. Avoid concurrent use.

Metrizamide: increases the risk of seizures. Use cautiously in patients with seizure disorders.

Reactions may be *common,* uncommon, ***life-threatening,*** or COMMON AND LIFE-THREATENING.

Nitrates: may cause hypotension. Monitor patient's blood pressure and adjust dosage as needed.

Phenobarbital: increased renal excretion of perphenazine causes decreased therapeutic response. Monitor blood levels and adjust the dosage as needed.

Phenytoin: altered phenytoin metabolism of, which increases the risk of toxicity or underdosing. Monitor patient's blood levels and adjust dosage as needed.

Propylthiouracil: increases the risk of agranulocytosis. Monitor patient's CBC with differential regularly.

Ritonavir: increases the effects of perphenazine. Monitor patient and adjust dosage as necessary.

Tramadol: increased risk of seizures. Avoid concurrent use.

Drug-food
Caffeine: may decrease therapeutic response to perphenazine. Avoid foods and beverages that contain caffeine.

Drug-lifestyle
Alcohol use: may cause additive effects. Discourage alcohol consumption.

Heavy smoking: may decrease therapeutic response to perphenazine. Recommend smoking cessation.

Adverse reactions
CNS: adverse behavioral effects, dizziness, drowsiness, EEG changes, *extrapyramidal symptoms,* **neuroleptic malignant syndrome,** pseudoparkinsonism, sedation, **seizures,** *tardive dyskinesia.*

CV: *cardiac arrest,* ECG changes, *orthostatic hypotension,* tachycardia.

EENT: *blurred vision,* nasal congestion, ocular changes.

GI: *constipation,* diarrhea, *dry mouth,* ileus, nausea, vomiting.

GU: dark urine, gynecomastia, inhibited ejaculation, menstrual irregularities, priapism, *urine retention.*

Hematologic: *agranulocytosis,* eosinophilia, galactorrhea, **hemolytic anemia, leukopenia, thrombocytopenia.**

Hepatic: abnormal liver function test results, jaundice.

Metabolic: hyperglycemia, hypoglycemia, SIADH, weight gain.

Skin: allergic reactions, *mild photosensitivity,* pain at I.M. injection site, sterile abscess.

Overdose and treatment
Overdose causes CNS depression characterized by deep, unarousable sleep, possible coma, hypotension, hypertension, extrapyramidal symptoms, dystonia, abnormal involuntary muscle movements, agitation, seizures, arrhythmias, ECG changes, hypothermia or hyperthermia, and autonomic nervous system dysfunction.

Treatment is symptomatic and supportive. Maintain the patient's vital signs, airway, body temperature, and fluid and electrolyte balance. Use ipecac syrup to induce vomiting if the patient is awake, even if the patient has already vomited. Don't induce vomiting if the patient has impaired consciousness. Perform gastric lavage, and then give activated charcoal and saline cathartics. Dialysis usually doesn't help.

Regulate patient's body temperature as needed. Treat hypotension with I.V. fluids; don't give epinephrine. Give parenteral diazepam or barbiturates for seizures, parenteral phenytoin (1 mg/kg adjusted to blood pressure) for arrhythmias, and benztropine (1 to 2 mg) or parenteral diphenhydramine (10 to 50 mg) for extrapyramidal symptoms.

Special considerations
■ Monitor patient's blood pressure before and after parenteral administration.
■ Discard injection form if it's excessively discolored or contains precipitate.
■ Administer I.M. injection deep into upper outer quadrant of buttocks. Massage the site to help prevent abscesses from forming.
■ Avoid extravasation when giving drug by I.M. route; it may cause skin necrosis.
■ Oral forms may cause stomach upset; give them with food or fluid.
■ Dilute every 5 ml of oral concentrate in 2 ounces (60 ml) of liquid, such as water, caffeine-free carbonated drinks, fruit juice, tomato juice, milk, or pudding. Shake oral concentrate before giving it.
■ Keep liquid form from contacting skin because rash or irritation may develop.
■ If patient receives doses of more than 24 mg, he should also receive trihexyphenidyl hydrochloride or benztropine mesylate to treat potential EPS.
■ The most serious adverse reactions caused by this drug are extrapyramidal.
■ Expect that abrupt withdrawal of long-term therapy may cause gastritis, nausea, vomiting, dizziness,

tremor, a feeling of warmth or cold, diaphoresis, tachycardia, headache, or insomnia.
■ Perphenazine causes false-positive results on tests of urinary porphyrins, urobilinogen, amylase, and 5-hydroxyindoleacetic acid because metabolites darken the patient's urine. Drug also causes false-positive results on urine pregnancy tests that use human chorionic gonadotropin.

Breast-feeding patients
■ Drug is widely distributed in breast milk. Use with caution, making sure that potential benefits to mother outweigh potential harm to infant.

Pediatric patients
■ Drug isn't recommended for children under age 12.

Geriatic patients
■ Elderly patients have an increased risk of adverse effects, especially tardive dyskinesia and other extrapyramidal effects.

Patient teaching
■ Explain the risks of dystonic reactions and tardive dyskinesia, and tell the patient to report abnormal body movements.
■ Urge the patient to take drug exactly as prescribed and not to double the next dose if he misses one.
■ Tell patient not to crush or chew sustained-release drug form.
■ Explain the dropper technique used to accurately measure a dose, and explain which fluids are appropriate for diluting the concentrate (not apple juice or caffeine-containing drinks).

■ Tell patient not to get liquid form on his skin; rash and irritation could result.

■ Inform patient that drug may interact with many other drugs. Urge him not to take other prescribed drugs, OTC medications, or herbal remedies without consulting prescriber.

■ Tell patient to avoid hazardous activities until the full CNS effects of the drug are known. Reassure patient that sedative effects should become tolerable in several weeks.

■ To prevent photosensitivity reactions, instruct patient to minimize sun exposure, and to wear sunscreen outdoors, and to avoid sun lamps and tanning beds.

■ Warn patient not to take extremely hot or cold baths and to avoid exposure to temperature extremes; drug may alter thermoregulation.

■ Tell patient not to drink alcohol or take other medications that may add to sedation.

■ If patient develops a dry mouth, suggest using sugarless hard candy, sugarless chewing gum, ice chips, or artificial saliva to relieve symptoms.

■ Warn patient not to abruptly stop taking drug.

■ Tell patient to promptly notify prescriber about difficulty urinating, sore throat, dizziness, or fainting.

pimozide
Orap

Pharmacologic classification:
diphenylbutylpiperidine

Therapeutic classification:
antipsychotic

Pregnancy risk category C

How supplied
Available by prescription only
Tablets: 2 mg

Indications and dosages
Severe motor and phonic tics in patients with Tourette syndrome
Adults: initially, 1 to 2 mg P.O. daily in divided doses. Increase dosage every other day, p.r.n. Most patients are adequately controlled on a maintenance dosage below 0.2 mg/kg (or 10 mg) daily.
Children over age 12: 0.05 mg/kg h.s. Increase at 3-day intervals to maximum of 0.2 mg/kg (or 10 mg) daily.

Pharmacodynamics
Antipsychotic action: Mechanism of action in Tourette syndrome is unknown. Drug is thought to exert its effects by postsynaptic blockade, presynaptic blockade, or both of CNS dopamine receptors, thus inhibiting dopamine-mediated effects. Pimozide also has anticholinergic, antiemetic, and anxiolytic effects and produces mild alpha blockade.

Pharmacokinetics
Absorption: Drug is absorbed slowly and incompletely from the

GI tract; bioavailability is about 50%. Plasma levels peak in 4 to 12 hours (usually 6 to 8 hours).
Distribution: Drug is distributed widely into the body.
Metabolism: Drug is metabolized by the liver and undergoes a significant first-pass effect.
Excretion: About 40% of a dose is excreted in urine as parent drug and metabolites in 3 to 4 days; about 15% is excreted in feces via the biliary tract within 3 to 6 days.

Contraindications and precautions

Contraindicated in patients hypersensitive to drug, in patients with simple tics or tics not caused by Tourette syndrome, in patients taking a drug known to cause motor and phonic tics, and in patients with congenital long QT syndrome, severe toxic CNS depression, coma, or a history of arrhythmias.

Use cautiously in patients with impaired renal or hepatic function, glaucoma, prostatic hyperplasia, seizure disorders, or EEG abnormalities.

Interactions
Drug-drug

Amphetamines, methylphenidate, pemoline: may induce Tourette-like tic and may exacerbate existing tics. Monitor patient and adjust dosage as needed.
Antiarrhythmics (disopyramide, procainamide, quinidine), antidepressants, antipsychotics, phenothiazines: may further depress cardiac conduction and prolong QT interval, resulting in serious arrhythmias. Avoid concurrent administration.

Anticonvulsants (carbamazepine, phenobarbital, phenytoin): may induce seizures, even in patients previously stabilized on an anticonvulsant. Anticonvulsant dosage may need to be increased.
Clarithromycin, dirithromycin, erythromycin: may inhibit pimozide metabolism, causing CV effects. Avoid concurrent use.
CNS depressants, such as analgesics, barbiturates, narcotics, parenteral magnesium sulfate, tranquilizers, and general, spinal, or epidural anesthetics: may have added effects. Monitor patient for oversedation, respiratory depression, and hypotension, and adjust dosage as needed.
Lithium, other antipsychotics: may cause encephalopathic symptoms. Avoid concurrent use.

Drug-lifestyle

Alcohol use: may cause oversedation and respiratory depression from additive CNS depression. Discourage concurrent use.

Adverse reactions

CNS: *adverse behavioral effects,* akathisia, drowsiness, dystonia, headache, hyperreflexia, insomnia, **neuroleptic malignant syndrome,** oculogyric crisis, opisthotonos, *parkinsonian-like symptoms, sedation, tardive dyskinesia.*
CV: *ECG changes (prolonged QT interval),* hypertension, hypotension, tachycardia.
EENT: visual disturbances.
GI: *anorexia, constipation, diarrhea, dry mouth, nausea.*
GU: impotence, urinary frequency.
Musculoskeletal: muscle rigidity.
Skin: diaphoresis, rash.

Reactions may be *common,* uncommon, *life-threatening,* or COMMON AND LIFE-THREATENING.

Overdose and treatment

Overdose may cause severe extrapyramidal symptoms, hypotension, respiratory depression, coma, and ECG abnormalities, including a prolonged QT interval, inverted or flattened T waves, and new U waves.

Perform gastric lavage to remove unabsorbed drug. Maintain patient's blood pressure with I.V. fluids, plasma expanders, or norepinephrine. Don't use epinephrine, and don't induce vomiting because of the potential for aspiration.

Treat extrapyramidal symptoms with parenteral diphenhydramine. Watch for adverse effects for at least 4 days because of prolonged half-life (55 hours) of drug.

Special considerations

■ Obtain a baseline ECG before therapy and periodically during therapy to monitor CV effects of the drug. Assess patient's QT interval for prolongation.

■ Keep patient's serum potassium level within the normal range; a decreased potassium level increases the risk of arrhythmias. Take special care to check potassium levels in patients with diarrhea and in those who take diuretics.

■ Extrapyramidal symptoms develop in about 10% to 15% of patients at normal dosage levels. They're especially likely during the early part of therapy.

■ Assess patient periodically for abnormal body movements.

■ If patient develops excessive restlessness and agitation, therapy with a beta blocker (such as propranolol or metoprolol) may be helpful.

Pediatric patients

■ Use and efficacy in children under age 12 are limited. Use of drug in children for any disorder other than Tourette syndrome isn't recommended.

Geriatric patients

■ Elderly patients have an increased risk of cardiac toxicity and tardive dyskinesia, even at normal dosage levels.

Patient teaching

■ Explain the risk of dystonic reactions and tardive dyskinesia, and teach the patient how to recognize their signs and symptoms.

■ Stress that drug's therapeutic effect may not be apparent for several weeks.

■ Caution patient to take drug exactly as prescribed and not to double a dose to make up for a missed one.

■ Urge the patient to lie down for 30 minutes after taking each dose and to rise slowly from a lying or sitting position to minimize the effects of orthostatic hypotension.

■ Tell patient to avoid alcohol, sleeping aids, and other drugs that may cause drowsiness during therapy.

■ If patient develops a dry mouth, suggest using sugarless hard candy, sugarless chewing gum, ice chips, or artificial saliva to ease the symptoms.

■ Caution patient to avoid hazardous activities until full CNS effects of drug are known.

■ To minimize daytime sedation, suggest taking the full daily dose at bedtime.

- Urge patient to report unusual effects promptly.
- Warn patient not to abruptly stop taking drug.

---

prochlorperazine
Compazine, Stemetil◇

prochlorperazine edisylate
Compazine

prochlorperazine maleate
Compazine, Compazine Spansule, Stemetil◇

Pharmacologic classification: phenothiazine (piperazine derivative)

Therapeutic classification: antianxiety drug, antiemetic, antipsychotic

Pregnancy risk category C

How supplied
Available by prescription only
prochlorperazine
Suppositories: 2.5 mg, 5 mg, 25 mg
prochlorperazine edisylate
Injection: 5 mg/ml
Syrup: 1 mg/ml
prochlorperazine maleate
Spansules (sustained-release): 10 mg, 15 mg, 30 mg
Tablets: 5 mg, 10 mg, 25 mg

Indications and dosages
Nonpsychotic anxiety
Adults: 5 mg P.O. t.i.d. or q.i.d., 15 mg sustained-release P.O. daily upon awakening, or 10 mg sustained-release P.O. q 12 hours. Maximum, 20 mg daily. Therapy should not exceed 3 months.

Psychotic disorders
Adults: 5 to 10 mg P.O. t.i.d or q.i.d. Increase gradually every 2 to 3 days until symptoms are controlled. Usual maintenance dose is 50 to 75 mg daily, although some severely disturbed patients have needed up to 150 mg daily. For rapid control of severe psychotic symptoms, give 10 to 20 mg I.M. Repeat as needed every 1 to 4 hours. Usually, symptoms will be controlled after 3 to 4 doses. Rarely, if patient needs prolonged parenteral administration, give 10 to 20 mg I.M. q 4 to 6 hours.
Children ages 2 to 12: 2.5 mg P.O. or P.R. b.i.d. or t.i.d. Maximum, 10 mg on the first day. May increase to 20 mg daily for children ages 2 to 5 and 25 mg daily for children ages 6 to 12. For prompt control of severe psychotic symptoms in children under age 12, give a single dose of 0.13 mg/kg I.M.
▷ **DOSAGE ADJUSTMENT.** Elderly patients tend to need lower doses, adjusted to achieve individual effects.

Pharmacodynamics
Antipsychotic action: Prochlorperazine is thought to exert antipsychotic effects by postsynaptic blockade of CNS dopamine receptors, which inhibits dopamine-mediated effects.
Antiemetic action: Antiemetic effects are attributed to dopamine receptor blockade in the medullary chemoreceptor trigger zone.
Other actions: Prochlorperazine has many other central and peripheral effects: It produces alpha and ganglionic blockade and counteracts histamine- and serotonin-mediated activity. It is used pri-

---

marily as an antiemetic; it is ineffective against motion sickness. This drug has weak anticholinergic and moderate sedative effects.

Pharmacokinetics
Absorption: Rate and extent of absorption vary with administration route. Absorption of oral tablet is erratic and variable, with onset of action ranging from 30 minutes to 1 hour. Absorption of oral concentrate is more predictable. Drug given by I.M. route is absorbed rapidly.
Distribution: Drug is distributed widely into the body, including breast milk. Drug is 91% to 99% protein-bound. Effects peak in 2 to 4 hours; serum levels reach steady state in 4 to 7 days.
Metabolism: Drug is metabolized extensively by the liver, but no active metabolites are formed; duration of action is about 3 to 4 hours, 10 to 12 hours for the sustained-release form.
Excretion: Drug is mostly excreted in urine via the kidneys; some is excreted in feces via the biliary tract.

Contraindications and precautions
Contraindicated in infants under age 2, in patients hypersensitive to phenothiazines, and in patients with CNS depression. Drug is also contraindicated during coma, pediatric surgery, spinal or epidural anesthesia, or use of adrenergic blockers or alcohol.

Use cautiously in acutely ill children, in patients who have been exposed to extreme heat or cold, and in patients with impaired CV function, glaucoma, prostatic hypertrophy, or seizure disorders.

Interactions
Drug-drug
Antacids that contain aluminum or magnesium, antidiarrheals: decreased prochlorperazine absorption. Avoid concurrent use.
Antiarrhythmics (disopyramide, procainamide, quinidine): increased risk of arrhythmias and conduction defects. Avoid concurrent use.
Anticholinergics (such as atropine), antidepressants, antihistamines, antiparkinsonians, MAO inhibitors, meperidine, phenothiazines: may cause oversedation, paralytic ileus, visual changes, and severe constipation. Monitor patient for adverse reactions and adjust dosage as needed.
Appetite suppressants, sympathomimetics (including ephedrine, epinephrine, phenylephrine, phenylpropanolamine): may decrease stimulatory and pressor effects. Dosage adjustment may be needed.
Beta blockers: may inhibit prochlorperazine metabolism, increasing plasma levels and the risk of toxicity. Monitor blood levels closely.
Bromocriptine: may antagonize the therapeutic effect of bromocriptine on prolactin secretion. Avoid concurrent use.
Central-acting antihypertensives, such as clonidine, guanabenz, guanadrel, guanethidine, methyldopa, reserpine: may inhibit blood pressure response. Adjust dosage according to blood pressure response.
CNS depressants, such as analgesics, barbiturates, narcotics, parenteral

---

◇ Available in Canada only   *Unlabeled use

magnesium sulfate, tranquilizers, and general, spinal, or epidural anesthetics: may have added effects. Monitor patient for oversedation, respiratory depression, and hypotension, and adjust dosage as needed.

Dopamine: decreased vasoconstricting effects of dopamine. Monitor patient for lack of therapeutic effect.

Epinephrine: prochlorperazine may cause epinephrine reversal. Avoid concurrent use.

Levodopa: possible decreased effectiveness of levodopa and loss of therapeutic effect caused by dopamine blockade. Adjust dosage as needed.

Lithium: may result in severe neurologic toxicity, an encephalitis-like syndrome, and decreased therapeutic response to prochlorperazine. Avoid concurrent use.

Metrizamide: increases the risk of seizures. Use cautiously in patients with seizure disorders.

Nitrates: may cause hypotension. Monitor patient's blood pressure and adjust dosage as needed.

Phenobarbital: increased renal excretion of prochlorperazine and causes decreased therapeutic response. Monitor patient's blood levels and adjust the dose as needed.

Phenytoin: altered phenytoin metabolism, which increases the risk of toxicity or underdosing. Monitor patient's blood phenytoin levels and adjust dosage as needed.

Propylthiouracil: increases the risk of agranulocytosis. Monitor patient's CBC with differential regularly.

Drug-food

Caffeine: increased metabolism may reduce drug effects and increase dosage requirement. Discourage consumption of caffeinated foods and beverages.

Drug-lifestyle

Alcohol use: may cause additive effects. Discourage concomitant use.

Heavy smoking: increased metabolism may reduce drug effects and increase dosage requirement. Recommend smoking cessation.

Sun exposure: increased risk of photosensitivity reactions. Discourage prolonged or unprotected sun exposure.

Adverse reactions

CNS: dizziness, EEG changes, *extrapyramidal symptoms,* **neuroleptic malignant syndrome,** pseudoparkinsonism, sedation.

CV: ECG changes, *orthostatic hypotension,* **seizures,** tachycardia.

EENT: *blurred vision, ocular changes.*

GI: *constipation, dry mouth,* ileus.

GU: dark urine, gynecomastia, hyperprolactinemia, inhibited ejaculation, menstrual irregularities, *urine retention.*

Hematologic: *agranulocytosis, aplastic anemia with pancytopenia, hemolytic anemia, thrombocytopenia, transient leukopenia.*

Hepatic: *cholestatic jaundice.*

Metabolic: decreased body temperature regulation, hyperglycemia, hypoglycemia, increased appetite, weight gain.

Skin: allergic reactions, *exfoliative dermatitis, mild photosensitivity.*

Other: hypersensitivity reactions.

Reactions may be *common,* uncommon, *life-threatening,* or COMMON AND LIFE-THREATENING.

Overdose and treatment

Overdose causes CNS depression characterized by deep, unarousable sleep, possible coma, hypotension, hypertension, extrapyramidal symptoms, dystonia, abnormal involuntary muscle movements, agitation, seizures, arrhythmias, ECG changes, hypothermia or hyperthermia, and autonomic nervous system dysfunction (tachycardia, miosis, ileus, cyanosis, respiratory collapse, or vasomotor collapse).

Treatment is symptomatic and supportive. Maintain the patient's vital signs, airway, body temperature, and fluid and electrolyte balance. Don't induce vomiting because drug inhibits cough reflex, and aspiration may occur. Perform gastric lavage, and then give activated charcoal and saline cathartics. Dialysis doesn't help.

Regulate patient's body temperature as needed. Treat hypotension with I.V. fluids; don't give epinephrine. Give parenteral diazepam or barbiturates for seizures, parenteral phenytoin (1 mg/kg adjusted to blood pressure) for arrhythmias, and benztropine or parenteral diphenhydramine for extrapyramidal symptoms.

Special considerations

- Check patient's blood pressure before and after parenteral administration.
- Solution for injection may be slightly discolored. Don't use if excessively discolored or contains a precipitate.
- Don't mix drug with other drugs in the same syringe.
- Give I.V. dose slowly (5 mg/minute).
- Administer I.M. injection deep into upper outer quadrant of buttock. Massage the area afterward to help prevent abscesses.
- Take special care to avoid extravasation when giving drug by I.M. route; it may cause skin necrosis.
- Don't give drug by the S.C. route.
- Liquid and injectable forms may cause a rash if they contact skin.
- Oral forms may cause stomach upset. Administer with food or fluid.
- Dilute the concentrate in 60 to 120 ml (2 to 4 oz) of water.
- Store the suppository form in a cool place.
- Protect the liquid formulation from light.
- Drug may cause urine to turn pink to brown.
- Prochlorperazine causes false-positive results on tests for urinary porphyrins, urobilinogen, amylase, and 5-hydroxyindoleacetic acid because metabolites darken patient's urine. It also causes false-positive results on urine pregnancy tests that use human chorionic gonadotropin. And it produces false-positive results on tests for phenylketonuria.
- Drug commonly causes extrapyramidal symptoms and photosensitivity reactions in hospitalized psychiatric patients. Protect patient from exposure to sunlight and heat lamps.

Breast-feeding patients

- Drug may enter breast milk and should be used with caution during breast-feeding. Potential benefits to mother should outweigh potential harm to infant.

Pediatric patients
- Prochlorperazine isn't recommended for patients who are under age 2 or who weigh less than 20 lb (9 kg).
- Don't give sustained-release form to children.

Geriatric patients
- Elderly patients have an increased risk for adverse reactions, especially tardive dyskinesia, other extrapyramidal effects, hypotension, and falls.

Patient teaching
- Explain the risks of dystonic reactions and tardive dyskinesia, and tell the patient to report abnormal body movements.
- Urge the patient to take drug exactly as prescribed and not to double the next dose if he misses one.
- Explain the dropper technique used to accurately measure a dose, and explain which fluids are appropriate for diluting the concentrate (not apple juice or caffeine-containing drinks).
- Teach patient how to administer the suppository form.
- Tell patient not to get liquid form on his skin; rash and irritation could result.
- Inform patient that drug may interact with many other drugs. Urge him not to take other prescribed drugs, OTC medications, or herbal remedies without consulting prescriber.
- Tell patient to avoid hazardous activities until the full CNS effects of the drug are known. Reassure patient that sedative effects should become tolerable in several weeks.

- To prevent photosensitivity reactions, instruct patient to minimize sun exposure, and to wear sunscreen outdoors, and to avoid sun lamps and tanning beds.
- Warn patient not to take extremely hot or cold baths and to avoid exposure to temperature extremes; drug may alter thermoregulation.
- Tell patient not to drink alcohol or take other medications that may add to sedation.
- If patient develops a dry mouth, suggest using sugarless hard candy, sugarless chewing gum, ice chips, or artificial saliva to relieve symptoms.
- Warn patient not to abruptly stop taking drug.

quetiapine fumarate
Seroquel

Pharmacologic classification:
dibenzothiazepine derivative

Therapeutic classification:
antipsychotic

Pregnancy risk category C

How supplied
Available by prescription only
Tablets: 25 mg, 100 mg, 200 mg

Indications and dosages
Psychotic disorders
Adults: initially, 25 mg P.O. b.i.d., increased by 25 to 50 mg b.i.d. or t.i.d. on days 2 and 3, as tolerated, to a target range of 300 to 400 mg daily by day 4, divided into two or three doses. Further dosage adjustments, if indicated, typically occur at no less than 2-day intervals.

Dosages can be increased or decreased by 25 to 50 mg b.i.d. Antipsychotic efficacy usually occurs at 150 to 750 mg/day. The safety of dosages above 800 mg/day hasn't been evaluated.

▶ **DOSAGE ADJUSTMENT.** For elderly patients, debilitated patients, and patients with hepatic impairment or a predisposition to hypotensive reactions, consider lower dosages, slower adjustments, and careful monitoring early in therapy.

Pharmacodynamics

Antipsychotic action: Exact mechanism of action is unknown. Quetiapine is a dibenzothiazepine derivative that is thought to exert antipsychotic activity through antagonism of dopamine type 2 (commonly known as D_2) and serotonin type 2 (commonly known as $5\text{-}HT_2$) receptors. Antagonism at serotonin $5\text{-}HT_{1A}$, D_1, H_1, and alpha$_1$- and alpha$_2$-adrenergic receptors may explain the drug's other effects.

Pharmacokinetics

Absorption: Drug is rapidly absorbed after oral administration. Plasma levels peak in about 1½ hours. Absorption is affected by food, with maximum level increasing 25% and bioavailability increasing 15%.

Distribution: Apparent volume of distribution is 10±4 L/kg. Drug is 83% plasma-protein bound. Steady state levels are reached within 2 days.

Metabolism: Drug is extensively metabolized by the liver via sulfoxidation and oxidation. Cytochrome P-450 3A4 is the major isoenzyme involved.

Excretion: Less than 1% of dose is excreted as unchanged drug. About 73% is recovered in the urine and 20% in the feces. Mean terminal half-life is about 6 hours.

Contraindications and precautions

Contraindicated in patients hypersensitive to drug or its ingredients.

Use cautiously in patients with CV disease, cerebrovascular disease, conditions that predispose the patient to hypotension, conditions that may lower the seizure threshold, conditions that raise the core body temperature, or a history of seizures. Also, use cautiously in patients at risk for aspiration pneumonia because of esophageal dysmotility and aspiration.

Interactions

Drug-drug

Antihypertensives: may potentiate hypotensive effect of both drugs. Monitor patient's blood pressure, and adjust dose as required.

Central-acting antihypertensives: may inhibit blood pressure response. Use cautiously together, and monitor patient's blood pressure.

Cimetidine: decreases clearance of oral quetiapine by 20%. Adjust dosage as needed.

Cytochrome P-450 3A inhibitors, such as erythromycin, fluconazole, itraconazole, ketoconazole: may cause CV effects. Use caution when administering together.

Dopamine agonists, levodopa: antagonized effects of these drugs. Dosage adjustment may be needed.

Lorazepam: clearance of lorazepam is reduced by 20% when given with quetiapine. Adjust dosage as necessary.

Phenytoin: increases clearance of oral quetiapine fivefold. Avoid concurrent use.

Thioridazine: increases clearance of oral quetiapine by 65%. Avoid concurrent use.

Drug-lifestyle
Alcohol use: may potentiate cognitive and motor effects. Discourage alcohol use during quetiapine therapy.

Adverse reactions
CNS: asthenia, *dizziness,* dysarthria, *headache,* hypertonia, **neuroleptic malignant syndrome,** somnolence.

CV: orthostatic hypotension, palpitations, peripheral edema, tachycardia.

EENT: ear pain, pharyngitis, rhinitis.

GI: abdominal pain, anorexia, constipation, dry mouth, dyspepsia.

Hematologic: leukopenia.

Metabolic: *weight gain.*

Musculoskeletal: back pain.

Respiratory: dyspnea, increased cough.

Skin: diaphoresis, rash.

Other: fever, flulike syndrome.

Overdose and treatment
Overdose typically causes an exaggeration of pharmacologic effects: drowsiness, sedation, tachycardia, hypotension. Hypokalemia and first-degree heart block also may occur.

For acute overdose, treatment includes establishing and maintaining an airway to ensure adequate oxygenation and ventilation. Consider gastric lavage and administration of activated charcoal with a laxative. Begin CV and ECG monitoring immediately. If the patient needs an antiarrhythmic, don't give disopyramide, procainamide, quinidine, or bretylium because of the theoretical risk of QT-interval prolongation that could add to the effects of quetiapine. Give I.V. fluids or sympathomimetic drugs (not epinephrine or dopamine) to treat hypotension and circulatory collapse. For severe extrapyramidal symptoms, administer anticholinergics.

Special considerations
■ To detect possible cataract formation, make sure patient has an examination of his ocular lenses before therapy begins or shortly thereafter and also at 6-month intervals during long-term treatment.

■ Total and free T_4 may decrease during therapy, but the change usually isn't clinically significant. Although rare, some patients experience increased thyroid-stimulating hormone and require thyroid replacement.

■ Cholesterol and triglyceride levels may increase during therapy.

■ Asymptomatic, transient, reversible increases in serum transaminases (primarily ALT) may occur. These increases usually occur during the first 3 weeks of therapy and return to pretreatment levels as therapy continues.

■ Watch for evidence of neuroleptic malignant syndrome, a potentially fatal syndrome that may be caused by antipsychotic drugs.

Reactions may be *common,* uncommon, *life-threatening,* or COMMON AND LIFE-THREATENING.

Evidence includes hyperpyrexia, muscle rigidity, altered mental status, and autonomic instability.
- To minimize the risk of tardive dyskinesia, give the smallest effective dose for the shortest effective duration.
- Closely supervise schizophrenic patients during therapy because of their increased risk of suicide.

Breast-feeding patients
- Breast-feeding isn't recommended during quetiapine therapy.

Pediatric patients
- Safety and effectiveness in children haven't been established.

Patient teaching
- Teach elderly patients about the increased risk of falls during therapy.
- Caution patient to avoid hazardous activities until the full CNS effects of the drug are known—especially during the first 3 to 5 days of therapy and during dosage increases or resumption of suspended therapy.
- Tell patient not to become overheated or dehydrated during therapy.
- Advise patient to avoid alcohol during therapy.
- Remind patient to have an eye examination at the start of therapy and every 6 months during therapy to check for cataract formation.
- Tell patient not to take other prescribed drugs, OTC medications, or herbal remedies without consulting the prescriber.
- Urge women to notify prescriber about planned, suspected, or known pregnancy.

- Advise women not to breast-feed during therapy.

---

risperidone
Risperdal

Pharmacologic classification: benzisoxazole derivative

Therapeutic classification: antipsychotic

Pregnancy risk category C

How supplied
Available by prescription only
Oral solution: 1 mg/ml
Tablets: 0.25 mg, 0.5 mg, 1 mg, 2 mg, 3 mg, 4 mg

Indications and dosages
Psychosis
Adults: initially, 1 mg P.O. b.i.d. Increase by 1 mg b.i.d. on days 2 and 3 of treatment to a target of 3 mg b.i.d. Slower adjustment may be warranted and better tolerated. Wait at least 1 week before adjusting dosage again. Dosages above 6 mg/day haven't been found more effective than lower dosages, but they were more likely to cause extrapyramidal effects.
▶ DOSAGE ADJUSTMENT. Elderly or debilitated patients, hypotensive patients, or patients with severe renal or hepatic impairment should start with 0.25 to 0.5 mg P.O. once daily to b.i.d. Increase by 0.5 mg b.i.d. on days 2 and 3 to a target of 1.5 mg P.O. b.i.d. Wait at least 1 week before increasing dosage again.

Pharmacodynamics

Antipsychotic action: Risperidone's exact mechanism of action is unknown. Its antipsychotic activity may be mediated through a combination of dopamine type 2 (D_2) and serotonin type 2 (5-HT_2) antagonism. Antagonism at receptors other than D_2 and 5-HT_2 may explain the drug's other effects.

Pharmacokinetics

Absorption: Drug is well absorbed after oral administration. Absolute oral bioavailability is 70%. Food does not affect rate or extent of absorption.

Distribution: Plasma protein binding is about 90% for drug and 77% for its major active metabolite, 9-hydroxyrisperidone.

Metabolism: Drug is extensively metabolized in the liver to 9-hydroxyrisperidone, which is the predominant circulating metabolite and appears about equally as effective as risperidone with respect to receptor binding activity. (About 6% to 8% of whites and a low percentage of Asians show little or no activity of the enzyme responsible for conversion of the drug to its active metabolite; they are termed "poor metabolizers.")

Excretion: Metabolite is excreted in urine by the kidneys. Clearance of drug and its metabolite is reduced in renally impaired patients.

Contraindications and precautions

Contraindicated in patients hypersensitive to drug and in breastfeeding patients.

Use cautiously in patients with prolonged QT interval, CV disease, cerebrovascular disease, dehydration, hypovolemia, a history of seizures, or exposure to extreme heat or conditions that could affect metabolism or hemodynamic responses.

Interactions

Drug-drug

Antihypertensives: may increase hypotensive effects. Monitor patient's blood pressure, and adjust dosage as needed.

Carbamazepine: may increase risperidone clearance, thereby decreasing its effectiveness. Monitor patient closely, and adjust dosage as needed.

Clozapine: may decrease risperidone clearance, increasing the risk of toxicity. Monitor patient closely, and adjust dosage as needed.

CNS depressants: may cause additive CNS depression. Administer concurrently with caution.

Dopamine agonists, levodopa: effects are antagonized by risperidone. Monitor patient, and adjust dosages as needed.

Drug-lifestyle

Sun exposure: may cause photosensitivity reactions. Urge patient to avoid prolonged or unprotected sun exposure.

Adverse reactions

CNS: aggressiveness, *agitation, anxiety, dizziness, extrapyramidal symptoms, headache, insomnia,* **neuroleptic malignant syndrome,** *somnolence,* tardive dyskinesia.
CV: chest pain, orthostatic hypotension, **prolonged QT interval,** tachycardia.

Reactions may be *common,* uncommon, *life-threatening,* or COMMON AND LIFE-THREATENING.

EENT: abnormal vision, pharyngitis, *rhinitis,* sinusitis.
GI: *constipation, dyspepsia, increased salivation, nausea, vomiting.*
Musculoskeletal: arthralgia, back pain.
Respiratory: cough, upper respiratory infection.
Skin: dry skin, photosensitivity, rash.
Other: fever.

Overdose and treatment

Overdose typically causes an exaggeration of pharmacologic effects: drowsiness, sedation, tachycardia, hypotension, and extrapyramidal symptoms. Hyponatremia, hypokalemia, prolonged QT interval, widened QRS complex, and seizures also may occur.

There is no specific antidote to risperidone overdose. Provide appropriate supportive care. Establish and maintain an airway, and ensure adequate ventilation. Consider gastric lavage (after intubation, if the patient is unconscious) and administration of activated charcoal with a laxative. Cardiac monitoring is essential to detect possible arrhythmias. If the patient needs an antiarrhythmic, don't give disopyramide, procainamide, or quinidine because of the theoretical risk of QT-interval prolongation that could add to the effects of risperidone. Also, avoid bretylium because its alpha-blocking properties could add to those of risperidone and cause hypotension.

Special considerations

■ Risperidone and 9-hydroxyrisperidone may lengthen the QT interval in some patients, although it causes no average increase even at 12 to 16 mg/day (well above the recommended dose). Even so, other drugs that prolong the QT interval have been linked to torsades de pointes, a life-threatening arrhythmia. This risk may rise if the patient takes such drugs or has bradycardia, an electrolyte imbalance, or congenital prolongation of the QT interval.
■ Drug may have an antiemetic effect that could mask evidence of overdose, intestinal obstruction, Reye's syndrome, or brain tumor.
■ Tardive dyskinesia may occur after prolonged risperidone therapy. It may not appear until months or years later, and it may disappear spontaneously or persist for life despite discontinuation of drug.
■ Neuroleptic malignant syndrome is rare, but in many cases fatal. It doesn't necessarily stem from the length of drug use or type of neuroleptic. Monitor patient closely for hyperpyrexia, muscle rigidity, altered mental status, irregular pulse, altered blood pressure, and diaphoresis.
■ When resuming therapy after an interruption, follow the typical 3-day initiation schedule.
■ When switching the patient from another antipsychotic to risperidone, immediately discontinue the other drug when risperidone therapy begins, if appropriate.

Breast-feeding patients
■ Breast-feeding should be discontinued during drug therapy.

Pediatric patients
■ Safety and efficacy in children haven't been established.

Geriatric patients
- Low-dose risperidone may help in treating behavioral problems, particularly aggression, in elderly patients with dementia.
- Elderly patients may have an increased risk of falls (from orthostatic hypotension) and movement disorders.

Patient teaching
- Caution patient to rise slowly from a lying or sitting position to minimize the effects of orthostatic hypotension.
- Warn patient to avoid hazardous activities until the full CNS effects of the drug are known.
- Advise patient to avoid alcohol during drug therapy.
- Tell patient not to take other prescribed drugs, OTC medications, or herbal remedies without consulting prescriber.
- Urge women to notify prescriber about planned, suspected, or known pregnancy.

---

thioridazine
Mellaril-S

thioridazine hydrochloride
Apo-Thioridazine◇, Mellaril, Novo-Ridazine◇, PMS Thioridazine◇

Pharmacologic classification: phenothiazine (piperidine derivative)

Therapeutic classification: antipsychotic

Pregnancy risk category C

How supplied
Available by prescription only
Oral concentrate: 30 mg/ml, 100 mg/ml (3% to 4.2% alcohol)
Suspension: 25 mg/5 ml, 100 mg/ 5 ml
Tablets: 10 mg, 15 mg, 25 mg, 50 mg, 100 mg, 150 mg, 200 mg

Indications and dosages
Psychosis
Adults: initially, 50 to 100 mg P.O. t.i.d., increasing in gradual increments to 800 mg daily in divided doses, if needed. Dosage varies.

Dysthymic disorder, behavioral disturbances in geriatric patients with dementia, behavioral problems in children
Adults: initially, 25 mg P.O. t.i.d. Maintenance dosage is 20 to 200 mg daily.
Children over age 2: usually, 0.5 to 3 mg/kg/day P.O. in divided doses. Give 10 mg b.i.d. or t.i.d. to children with moderate disorders and 25 mg b.i.d. or t.i.d. to severely disturbed hospitalized children.
▷ DOSAGE ADJUSTMENT. Elderly patients tend to require lower doses, adjusted to individual response.

Pharmacodynamics
Antipsychotic action: Thioridazine is thought to exert antipsychotic effects by postsynaptic blockade of CNS dopamine receptors, which inhibits dopamine-mediated effects.
Other actions: Thioridazine has many other central and peripheral effects as well: It produces both alpha and ganglionic blockade and counteracts histamine- and serotonin-mediated activity.

Pharmacokinetics

Absorption: Rate and extent of absorption vary with administration route. Absorption of oral tablets is erratic and variable, with onset ranging from 30 minutes to 1 hour. Absorption of oral concentrates and suspensions is much more predictable.

Distribution: Drug is distributed widely into the body, including breast milk. Effects peak in 2 to 4 hours; steady state serum level occurs in 4 to 7 days. Drug is 91% to 99% protein-bound.

Metabolism: Drug is metabolized extensively by the liver and forms the active metabolite mesoridazine; duration of action is 4 to 6 hours.

Excretion: Drug is mostly excreted as metabolites in urine; some is excreted in feces via the biliary tract.

Contraindications and precautions

Contraindicated in patients hypersensitive to drug and in patients with coma, CNS depression, or severe hypertensive or hypotensive cardiac disease.

Use cautiously in elderly or debilitated patients and in those with hepatic disease, renal disease, CV disease, respiratory disorders, seizure disorders, glaucoma, prostatic hypertrophy, hypocalcemia, severe reactions to insulin, severe reactions to electroconvulsive therapy, and exposure to extreme cold, extreme heat, or organophosphate insecticides.

Interactions
Drug-drug

Antacids that contain aluminum or magnesium, antidiarrheals: decreased thioridazine absorption. Separate administration times.

Antiarrhythmics (disopyramide, procainamide, quinidine): increased risk of arrhythmias and conduction defects. Avoid concurrent administration.

Anticholinergics (such as atropine), antidepressants, antihistamines, antiparkinsonians, MAO inhibitors, meperidine, phenothiazines: may cause oversedation, paralytic ileus, visual changes, and severe constipation. Monitor patient for adverse reactions and adjust dosage as needed.

Appetite suppressants, sympathomimetics (including ephedrine, epinephrine, phenylephrine, phenylpropanolamine): may decrease stimulatory and pressor effects. Dosage adjustment may be needed.

Beta blockers: may inhibit thioridazine metabolism, increasing plasma levels and the risk of toxicity. Monitor blood levels closely.

Bromocriptine: may antagonize the therapeutic effect of bromocriptine on prolactin secretion. Avoid concurrent use.

Carbamazepine oral suspension: causes rubbery orange precipitate when mixed with thioridazine oral liquid. Avoid concurrent use.

Central-acting antihypertensives, such as clonidine, guanabenz, guanadrel, guanethidine, methyldopa, reserpine: may inhibit blood pressure response. Adjust dosage according to blood pressure response.

CNS depressants, such as analgesics, barbiturates, narcotics, parenteral magnesium sulfate, tranquilizers, and general, spinal, or epidural anesthetics: may have added effects. Monitor patient for oversedation, respiratory depression, and hypotension, and adjust dosage as needed.

Dopamine: decreased vasoconstricting effects of dopamine. Avoid concurrent use.

Epinephrine: thioridazine may cause epinephrine reversal. Avoid concurrent use.

Levodopa: possible decreased effectiveness of levodopa and loss of therapeutic effect caused by dopamine blockade. Adjust dosage as needed.

Lithium: may result in severe neurologic toxicity, an encephalitis-like syndrome, and decreased therapeutic response to thioridazine. Avoid concurrent use.

Metrizamide: increases the risk of seizures. Avoid use in patients with seizure disorders.

Nitrates: may cause hypotension. Monitor patient's blood pressure and adjust dosage as needed.

Phenobarbital: increased renal excretion of thioridazine causes decreased therapeutic response. Monitor blood levels and adjust the dose as needed.

Phenytoin: altered phenytoin metabolism of, which increases the risk of toxicity or underdosing. Monitor patient's blood phenytoin levels and adjust dosage as needed.

Propylthiouracil: increases the risk of agranulocytosis. Monitor patient's CBC with differential regularly.

Drug-food
Caffeine: increased metabolism may cause decreased response to mesoridazine and may require dosage adjustment. Discourage foods and beverages that contain caffeine.

Drug-lifestyle
Alcohol use: may cause additive effects. Discourage concomitant use.

Heavy smoking: increased metabolism may cause decreased response to mesoridazine and may require dosage adjustment. Recommend smoking cessation.

Sun exposure: increased risk of photosensitivity reactions. Discourage prolonged or unprotected sun exposure.

Adverse reactions
CNS: dizziness, EEG changes, extrapyramidal symptoms, ***neuroleptic malignant syndrome,*** sedation, *tardive dyskinesia.*
CV: ECG changes, *orthostatic hypotension,* tachycardia.
EENT: *blurred vision, ocular changes,* retinitis pigmentosa.
GI: *constipation, dry mouth.*
GU: dark urine, *erectile dysfunction,* gynecomastia, inhibited ejaculation, menstrual irregularities, *sexual dysfunction, urine retention.*
Hematologic: *agranulocytosis, transient leukopenia.*
Hepatic: cholestatic jaundice, elevated liver enzymes.
Metabolic: increased appetite, weight gain.
Skin: allergic reactions, *mild photosensitivity.*
Other: hyperprolactinemia.

Overdose and treatment
Overdose causes CNS depression characterized by deep, unarousable sleep, possible coma, hypotension, hypertension, extrapyramidal symptoms, abnormal involuntary

---

Reactions may be *common,* uncommon, ***life-threatening,*** or COMMON AND LIFE-THREATENING.

muscle movements, agitation, seizures, arrhythmias, ECG changes, hypothermia or hyperthermia, autonomic nervous system dysfunction, and possible respiratory and vasomotor collapse.

Treatment is symptomatic and supportive. Maintain the patient's vital signs, airway, body temperature, and fluid and electrolyte balance. Don't induce vomiting because drug inhibits cough reflex, and aspiration may occur. Perform gastric lavage, and then give activated charcoal and saline cathartics. Dialysis doesn't help.

Regulate patient's body temperature as needed. Treat hypotension with I.V. fluids; don't give epinephrine. Give parenteral diazepam or barbiturates for seizures. Give parenteral phenytoin (1 mg/kg adjusted to blood pressure) for arrhythmias. Give benztropine (1 to 2 mg) or parenteral diphenhydramine (10 to 50 mg) for extrapyramidal symptoms. Contact a local or regional poison information center for specific instructions.

Special considerations

■ Oral drug forms may cause stomach upset. Administer with food or fluid.

■ Keep liquid forms from contacting skin; a rash could result.

■ Dilute concentrate in 60 to 120 ml (2 to 4 oz) of liquid, preferably water, a noncaffeinated carbonated drink, fruit juice, tomato juice, milk, or pudding.

■ All liquid forms must be protected from light.

■ Doses above 300 mg/day are usually reserved for adults with severe psychosis. Don't exceed 800 mg daily because of ophthalmic toxicity.

■ Drug can cause pink to brown discoloration of patient's urine.

■ Thioridazine commonly causes sedation, anticholinergic effects, orthostatic hypotension, photosensitivity reactions, and delayed or absent ejaculation. It has the lowest risk of extrapyramidal symptoms of all the phenothiazines.

■ Check patient at least every 6 months for abnormal body movements.

■ Thioridazine causes false-positive results on tests for urinary porphyrins, urobilinogen, amylase, and 5-hydroxyindoleacetic acid because metabolites darken patient's urine. It also causes false-positive results on urine pregnancy tests that use human chorionic gonadotropin. And it may cause false-positive results on tests for phenylketonuria.

■ After abrupt withdrawal of long-term therapy, patient may experience gastritis, nausea, vomiting, dizziness, tremor, a feeling of warmth or cold, diaphoresis, tachycardia, headache, or insomnia.

Breast-feeding patients

■ Thioridazine may enter breast milk. Make sure potential benefits to mother outweigh potential harm to infant.

Pediatric patients

■ Drug isn't recommended for patients under age 2.

Geriatric patients

■ Elderly patients have a higher risk of adverse reactions, especially tardive dyskinesia and other extrapyramidal effects. They also face a higher risk of falling in response to the effects of orthostatic hypotension and movement disorders.

Patient teaching
■ Urge patient to take drug exactly as prescribed and not to change the dosage or double the dose after missing one.
■ Explain the dropper technique used to accurately measure a dose, and explain which fluids are appropriate for diluting the concentrate.
■ Tell patient to avoid hazardous activities until the full CNS effects of the drug are known. Reassure patient that sedative effects typically subside after several weeks.
■ Warn patient not to get liquid form on his skin because rash and irritation may result.
■ To prevent photosensitivity reactions, urge patient to minimize sun exposure, to wear sunscreen when going outdoors, and to avoid heat lamps and tanning beds.
■ Tell patient to avoid temperature extremes (such as hot or cold baths, sunlamps, or tanning beds) because drug may alter thermoregulation.
■ Urge patient to maintain adequate hydration.
■ If patient develops a dry mouth, suggest sugarless gum, sugarless candy, ice chips, or artificial saliva to help relieve the symptoms.
■ Caution patient not to drink alcohol or take sedating medications during therapy.
■ Tell patient not to take other prescribed drugs, OTC medications, or herbal remedies without consulting prescriber.

■ Caution patient not to stop therapy without consulting prescriber.
■ Tell patient to notify prescriber about difficult urination, sore throat, dizziness, or fainting.

---

thiothixene, thiothixene hydrochloride
Navane

Pharmacologic classification: thioxanthene

Therapeutic classification: antipsychotic

Pregnancy risk category C

How supplied
Available by prescription only
Capsules: 1 mg, 2 mg, 5 mg, 10 mg, 20 mg
Injection: 2 mg/ml, 5 mg/ml
Oral concentrate: 5 mg/ml (7% alcohol)

Indications and dosages
Acute agitation
Adults: 4 mg I.M. b.i.d. to q.i.d. Maximum, 30 mg I.M. daily. Change to P.O. form as soon as possible because I.M. dose form is irritating.

Mild to moderate psychosis
Adults: initially, 2 mg P.O. t.i.d. May increase gradually to 15 mg daily.

Severe psychosis
Adults: initially, 5 mg P.O. b.i.d. May increase gradually to 20 to 30 mg daily. Maximum recommended dosage, 60 mg daily.

Reactions may be *common,* uncommon, *life-threatening,* or COMMON AND LIFE-THREATENING.

▶ **Dosage adjustment.** Elderly patients tend to require lower doses, adjusted to individual response.

Pharmacodynamics

Antipsychotic action: Thiothixene is thought to exert antipsychotic effects by postsynaptic blockade of CNS dopamine receptors, which inhibits dopamine-mediated effects.

Other actions: Thiothixene has many other central and peripheral effects; it also acts as an alpha-blocking agent.

Pharmacokinetics

Absorption: Drug is rapidly absorbed. Action begins 10 to 30 minutes after I.M. administration.

Distribution: Drug is widely distributed into the body. Effects peak 1 to 6 hours after I.M. administration. Drug is 91% to 99% protein-bound.

Metabolism: Drug is metabolized in the liver.

Excretion: Thiothixene is mostly excreted as parent drug in feces via the biliary tract.

Contraindications and precautions

Contraindicated in patients hypersensitive to drug and in those with circulatory collapse, coma, CNS depression, or blood dyscrasia.

Use cautiously in elderly or debilitated patients, in patients undergoing alcohol withdrawal, and in patients who have renal disease, hepatic disease, CV disease, glaucoma, prostatic hyperplasia, a history of seizure disorders, or exposure to extreme heat, extreme cold, or organophosphate insecticides.

Interactions
Drug-drug

Antacids that contain aluminum or magnesium, antidiarrheals: decreased thiothixene absorption. Separate administration times.

Antiarrhythmics (disopyramide, procainamide, quinidine): increased risk of arrhythmias and conduction defects. Avoid concurrent administration.

Anticholinergics (such as atropine), antidepressants, antihistamines, antiparkinsonians, MAO inhibitors, meperidine, phenothiazines: may cause oversedation, paralytic ileus, visual changes, and severe constipation. Monitor patient for adverse reactions and adjust dosage as needed.

Appetite suppressants, sympathomimetics (including ephedrine, epinephrine, phenylephrine, phenylpropanolamine): may decrease stimulatory and pressor effects. Dosage adjustment may be needed.

Beta blockers: may inhibit thiothixene metabolism, increasing plasma levels and the risk of toxicity. Monitor blood levels closely.

Bromocriptine: may antagonize the therapeutic effect of bromocriptine on prolactin secretion. Avoid concurrent use.

Central-acting antihypertensives, such as clonidine, guanabenz, guanadrel, guanethidine, methyldopa, reserpine: may inhibit blood pressure response. Adjust dosage according to blood pressure response.

CNS depressants, such as analgesics, barbiturates, narcotics, parenteral magnesium sulfate, tranquilizers, and general, spinal, or epidural anesthetics: may have added effects. Monitor patient for oversedation,

respiratory depression, and hypotension, and adjust dosage as needed.
Dopamine: decreased vasoconstricting effects of dopamine. Monitor patient for lack of therapeutic effect.
Epinephrine: thiothixene may cause epinephrine reversal. Avoid concurrent use.
Levodopa: possible decreased effectiveness of levodopa and loss of therapeutic effect caused by dopamine blockade. Adjust dosage as needed.
Lithium: may result in severe neurologic toxicity, an encephalitis-like syndrome, and decreased therapeutic response to thiothixene. Avoid concurrent use.
Metrizamide: increases the risk of seizures. Use cautiously in patients with seizure disorders.
Nitrates: may cause hypotension. Monitor patient's blood pressure and adjust dosage as needed.
Phenobarbital: increased renal excretion of thiothixene causes decreased therapeutic response. Monitor blood levels and adjust the dose as needed.
Phenytoin: altered phenytoin metabolism of, which increases the risk of toxicity of underdosing. Monitor patient's blood phenytoin levels and adjust dosage as needed.
Propylthiouracil: increases the risk of agranulocytosis. Monitor patient's CBC with differential regularly.

Drug-herb
Nutmeg: may cause a loss of symptom control or interfere with psychiatric drug therapy. Urge avoidance of nutmeg.

Drug-lifestyle
Alcohol use: may cause increased CNS depression. Discourage concomitant use.
Heavy smoking: increased metabolism may cause decreased response to thiothixene and may require dosage adjustment. Recommend smoking cessation.
Sun exposure: increased risk of photosensitivity reactions. Discourage prolonged or unprotected sun exposure.

Adverse reactions
CNS: agitation, dizziness, drowsiness, EEG changes, *extrapyramidal reactions,* insomnia, **neuroleptic malignant syndrome,** pseudoparkinsonism, restlessness, sedation, **seizures,** *tardive dyskinesia.*
CV: ECG changes, *hypotension,* tachycardia.
EENT: *blurred vision,* nasal congestion, ocular changes.
GI: *constipation, dry mouth.*
GU: erectile dysfunction, gynecomastia, inhibited ejaculation, menstrual irregularities, *sexual dysfunction, urine retention.*
Hematologic: *agranulocytosis,* leukocytosis, **transient leukopenia.**
Hepatic: elevated liver enzymes, jaundice.
Metabolic: weight gain.
Skin: allergic reactions, *mild photosensitivity,* pain at I.M. injection site, sterile abscess.

Overdose and treatment
Overdose causes CNS depression characterized by deep, unarousable sleep, possible coma, hypotension, hypertension, extrapyramidal symptoms, abnormal involuntary muscle movements, agitation, sei-

---

Reactions may be *common,* uncommon, *life-threatening,* or COMMON AND LIFE-THREATENING.

zures, arrhythmias, ECG changes, hypothermia or hyperthermia, autonomic nervous system dysfunction, and possible respiratory and vasomotor collapse.

Treatment is symptomatic and supportive. Maintain the patient's vital signs, airway, body temperature, and fluid and electrolyte balance. Don't induce vomiting because drug inhibits cough reflex, and aspiration may occur. Perform gastric lavage, and then give activated charcoal and saline cathartics. Dialysis doesn't help.

Regulate patient's body temperature as needed. Treat hypotension with I.V. fluids; don't give epinephrine. Give parenteral diazepam or barbiturates for seizures. Give parenteral phenytoin (1 mg/kg adjusted to blood pressure) for arrhythmias. Give benztropine (1 to 2 mg) or parenteral diphenhydramine (10 to 50 mg) for extrapyramidal symptoms.

Special considerations
- Measure patient's blood pressure before and after parenteral administration.
- Don't give drug by I.V. route; extravasation can cause necrosis.
- Give I.M. injection deep into upper outer quadrant of the buttock. Massage the area afterward may help prevent abscesses.
- Solution for injection may be slightly discolored. Contact pharmacist if it's excessively discolored or a precipitate develops.
- After reconstitution, drug is stable for 48 hours at room temperature.
- Protect liquid form from light.

- Avoid contact between skin and liquid or injectable drug forms; a rash could develop.
- Dilute oral concentrate in 60 to 120 ml (2 to 4 oz) of liquid, preferably water, carbonated drinks, fruit juice, tomato juice, milk, or pudding.
- Shake oral concentrate before administration.
- To help minimize stomach upset, give oral form with food or fluid.
- Check patient at least once every 6 months for abnormal body movements.
- Extrapyramidal effects are common.
- Protect patient from exposure to sunlight or heat lamps because photosensitivity reactions may occur.
- Provide sugarless gum, sugarless hard candy, or ice if patient complains of a dry mouth.
- Drug causes false-positive results on tests for urinary porphyrins, urobilinogen, amylase, and 5-hydroxyindoleacetic acid because metabolites darken patient's urine. Drug also causes false-positive results on urine pregnancy tests that use human chorionic gonadotropin.
- After abrupt withdrawal of long-term therapy, patient may develop gastritis, nausea, vomiting, dizziness, tremor, a feeling of warmth or cold, diaphoresis, tachycardia, headache, and insomnia.

Breast-feeding patients
- Thiothixene may enter breast milk. Make sure potential benefits to mother outweigh potential harm to infant.

Pediatric patients
- Drug isn't recommended for children under age 12.

Geriatric patients
- Elderly patients have a higher risk of adverse reactions, especially tardive dyskinesia, other extrapyramidal effects, and falls caused by the effects of orthostatic hypotension and movement disorders.

Patient teaching
- Explain the risk of dystonic reactions and possible permanent tardive dyskinesia, and urge the patient to notify prescriber about abnormal body movements.
- Explain the dropper technique used to accurately measure a dose, and explain which fluids are appropriate for diluting the concentrate.
- Tell patient to shake concentrate before administration.
- Urge patient to take drug exactly as prescribed and not to change the dosage or double the dose after missing one.
- Warn patient not to get liquid form on his skin because rash and irritation may result.
- Tell patient to avoid hazardous activities until the full CNS effects of drug are known. Reassure patient that sedation typically subsides after a few weeks.
- To prevent photosensitivity reactions, tell patient to minimize sun exposure, to wear sunscreen when going outdoors, and to avoid heat lamps and tanning beds.
- Tell patient to avoid temperature extremes (such as hot or cold baths, sunlamps, or tanning beds) because drug may alter thermoregulation.

- If patient develops a dry mouth, suggest sugarless gum, sugarless candy, ice chips, or artificial saliva to help relieve the symptoms.
- Caution patient not to drink alcohol or take sedating medications.
- Caution patient not to take other prescribed drugs, OTC medications, or herbal remedies without consulting prescriber.
- Tell patient not to stop therapy abruptly or without consulting prescriber.
- Tell patient to notify prescriber about difficult urination, sore throat, dizziness, or fainting.

trifluoperazine hydrochloride
Apo-Trifluoperazine◊, Novo-Flurazine◊, Solazine◊, Stelazine, Terfluzine◊

Pharmacologic classification: phenothiazine (piperazine derivative)

Therapeutic classification: antiemetic, antipsychotic

Pregnancy risk category C

How supplied
Available by prescription only
Injection: 2 mg/ml
Oral concentrate: 10 mg/ml
Tablets (regular and film-coated): 1 mg, 2 mg, 5 mg, 10 mg

Indications and dosages
Anxiety states
Adults: 1 to 2 mg P.O. or I.M. b.i.d. Increase dosage p.r.n., but don't exceed 6 mg/day.

Schizophrenia and other psychotic disorders

Adults: For outpatients, 1 to 2 mg P.O. b.i.d., increased p.r.n. For hospitalized patients, 2 to 5 mg P.O. b.i.d. May increase gradually to 40 mg daily. For I.M. injection, 1 to 2 mg q 4 to 6 hours p.r.n. Maximum, 10 mg/24 hours.

Children ages 6 to 12 (hospitalized or under close supervision): 1 mg P.O. daily or b.i.d. May increase gradually to 15 mg daily. Alternatively, 1 mg I.M. once or twice daily.

▶ Dosage adjustment. Elderly patients tend to require lower doses, adjusted to individual effect.

Pharmacodynamics

Antiemetic action: Antiemetic effects are attributed to dopamine receptor blockade in the medullary chemoreceptor trigger zone.

Antipsychotic action: Trifluoperazine is thought to exert antipsychotic effects by postsynaptic blockade of CNS dopamine receptors, which inhibits dopamine-mediated effects.

Other actions: Trifluoperazine has many other central and peripheral effects; it produces alpha and ganglionic blockade and counteracts histamine- and serotonin-mediated activity.

Pharmacokinetics

Absorption: Rate and extent of absorption vary with route of administration. Absorption of oral tablets is erratic and variable. Onset of action ranges from 30 minutes to 1 hour. Absorption of oral concentrate is much more predictable.

Drug is absorbed rapidly when given by I.M. route.

Distribution: Drug is distributed widely throughout the body, including breast milk. It's 91% to 99% protein-bound. Effect peak in 2 to 4 hours; steady state serum levels occur in 4 to 7 days.

Metabolism: Drug is metabolized extensively by the liver, but no active metabolites are formed; duration of action is about 4 to 6 hours.

Excretion: Drug is mostly excreted in urine via the kidneys; some is excreted in feces via the biliary tract.

Contraindications and precautions

Contraindicated in patients hypersensitive to phenothiazines and in patients experiencing coma, CNS depression, bone marrow suppression, or liver damage.

Use cautiously in elderly or debilitated patients; in patients exposed to extreme heat, extreme cold, or organophosphate insecticides; and in patients with renal disease, hepatic disease, CV disease, a seizure disorder, glaucoma, or prostatic hyperplasia.

Interactions

Drug-drug

Antacids that contain aluminum or magnesium, antidiarrheals: decreased trifluoperazine absorption. Separate administration times.

Antiarrhythmics (disopyramide, procainamide, quinidine): increased risk of arrhythmias and conduction defects. Avoid concurrent administration.

Anticholinergics (such as atropine), antidepressants, antihistamines, an-

tiparkinsonians, MAO inhibitors, meperidine, phenothiazines: may cause oversedation, paralytic ileus, visual changes, and severe constipation. Monitor patient for adverse reactions and adjust dosage as needed.

Appetite suppressants, sympathomimetics (including ephedrine, epinephrine, phenylephrine, phenylpropanolamine): may decrease stimulatory and pressor effects. Dosage adjustment may be needed.

Beta blockers: may inhibit trifluoperazine metabolism, increasing plasma levels and the risk of toxicity. Monitor blood levels closely.

Bromocriptine: may antagonize the therapeutic effect of bromocriptine on prolactin secretion. Avoid concurrent use.

Central-acting antihypertensives, such as clonidine, guanabenz, guanadrel, guanethidine, methyldopa, reserpine: may inhibit blood pressure response. Adjust dosage according to blood pressure response.

CNS depressants, such as analgesics, barbiturates, narcotics, parenteral magnesium sulfate, tranquilizers, and general, spinal, or epidural anesthetics: may have added effects. Monitor patient for oversedation, respiratory depression, and hypotension, and adjust dosage as needed.

Dopamine: decreased vasoconstricting effects of dopamine. Monitor patient for lack of therapeutic effect.

Epinephrine: trifluoperazine may cause epinephrine reversal. Avoid concurrent use.

Levodopa: possible decreased effectiveness of levodopa and loss of therapeutic effect caused by dopamine blockade. Adjust dosage as needed.

Lithium: may result in severe neurologic toxicity, an encephalitis-like syndrome, and decreased therapeutic response to trifluoperazine. Avoid concurrent use.

Metrizamide: increases the risk of seizures. Use cautiously in patients with seizure disorders.

Nitrates: may cause hypotension. Monitor patient's blood pressure and adjust dosage as needed.

Phenobarbital: increased renal excretion of trifluoperazine causes decreased therapeutic response. Monitor blood levels and adjust the dose as needed.

Phenytoin: possible inhibition of phenytoin metabolism, which increases the risk of toxicity. Monitor patient's blood phenytoin levels and adjust dosage as needed.

Propylthiouracil: increases the risk of agranulocytosis. Monitor patient's CBC with differential regularly.

Drug-food
Caffeine: increased drug metabolism leads to decreased therapeutic effects. Discourage consumption of caffeine-containing foods and beverages.

Drug-lifestyle
Alcohol use: may cause increased CNS depression. Discourage concomitant use.

Heavy smoking: increased metabolism may cause decreased response to trifluoperazine and may require dosage adjustment. Recommend smoking cessation.

Sun exposure: increased risk of photosensitivity reactions.

Discourage prolonged or unprotected sun exposure.

Adverse reactions

CNS: dizziness, drowsiness, *extrapyramidal symptoms,* fatigue, headache, insomnia, **neuroleptic malignant syndrome,** pseudoparkinsonism, *tardive dyskinesia.*
CV: ECG changes, *orthostatic hypotension,* tachycardia.
EENT: *blurred vision,* ocular changes.
GI: *dry mouth, constipation,* nausea.
GU: erectile dysfunction, gynecomastia, inhibited lactation, menstrual irregularities, *sexual dysfunction, urine retention.*
Hematologic: *agranulocytosis, transient leukopenia.*
Hepatic: cholestatic jaundice, elevated results of liver function tests.
Metabolic: weight gain.
Skin: allergic reactions, pain at I.M. injection site, *photosensitivity,* sterile abscess, rash.

Overdose and treatment

Overdose causes CNS depression characterized by deep, unarousable sleep, possible coma, hypotension, hypertension, extrapyramidal symptoms, dystonia, abnormal involuntary muscle movements, agitation, seizures, arrhythmias, ECG changes, hypothermia or hyperthermia, autonomic nervous system dysfunction, and possible respiratory and vasomotor collapse.

Treatment is symptomatic and supportive. Maintain the patient's vital signs, airway, body temperature, and fluid and electrolyte balance. Don't induce vomiting because drug inhibits cough reflex, and aspiration may occur. Perform gastric lavage, and then give activated charcoal and saline cathartics. Dialysis doesn't help.

Regulate patient's body temperature as needed. Treat hypotension with I.V. fluids; don't give epinephrine. Give parenteral diazepam or barbiturates for seizures. Give parenteral phenytoin (1 mg/kg adjusted to blood pressure) for arrhythmias. Give benztropine (1 to 2 mg) or parenteral diphenhydramine (10 to 50 mg) for extrapyramidal symptoms.

Special considerations

■ Some clinicians recommend using trifluoperazine only for psychosis. And other drugs, such as benzodiazepines, usually make a better choice for treating anxiety. However, if you give trifluoperazine for anxiety, don't exceed 6 mg daily for 12 weeks.
■ Measure patient's blood pressure before and after parenteral administration.
■ Give I.M. injection deep into upper outer quadrant of the buttock. Massage the area afterward may help prevent abscesses. Extravasation can cause skin necrosis.
■ Solution for injection may be slightly discolored. Contact pharmacist if it's excessively discolored or a precipitate develops.
■ Protect liquid form from light.
■ Avoid contact between skin and liquid or injectable drug forms; a rash could develop.
■ Dilute oral concentrate in 60 to 120 ml (2 to 4 oz) of liquid, preferably water, carbonated drinks, fruit juice, tomato juice, milk, or pudding.

- Shake oral concentrate before administration.
- To help minimize stomach upset, give oral form with food or fluid.
- Drug may cause pink to brown discoloration of urine or blue-gray skin.
- Drug commonly causes extrapyramidal symptoms and photosensitivity reactions. It has less sedative and autonomic activity than aliphatic and piperidine phenothiazines.
- Check patient at least once every 6 months for abnormal body movements.
- Protect patient from exposure to sunlight or heat lamps.
- Drug causes false-positive results on tests for urinary porphyrins, urobilinogen, amylase, and 5-hydroxyindoleacetic acid because metabolites darken patient's urine. Drug also causes false-positive results on urine pregnancy tests that use human chorionic gonadotropin. And it may cause false-positive results on tests for phenylketonuria.
- For some patients, angina may worsen during trifluoperazine therapy; however, ECG changes are less common than with other phenothiazines.
- After abrupt withdrawal of long-term therapy, patient may develop gastritis, nausea, vomiting, dizziness, tremor, a feeling of warmth or cold, diaphoresis, tachycardia, headache, insomnia, anorexia, muscle rigidity, altered mental status, and evidence of autonomic instability.

Breast-feeding patients
- Trifluoperazine may enter breast milk. Make sure potential benefits to mother outweigh potential harm to infant.

Pediatric patients
- Drug isn't recommended for children under age 6.

Geriatric patients
- Elderly patients have an increased risk of adverse reactions, especially tardive dyskinesia, other extrapyramidal effects, and falls caused by the effects of orthostatic hypotension and movement disorders.

Patient teaching
- Explain the risk of dystonic reactions, akathisia, and possible permanent tardive dyskinesia, and urge the patient to notify prescriber about abnormal body movements.
- Urge patient to take drug exactly as prescribed and not to change the dosage or double the dose after missing one.
- Tell patient to avoid hazardous activities until the full CNS effects of drug are known. Reassure patient that sedation typically subsides after a few weeks.
- To prevent photosensitivity reactions, tell patient to minimize sun exposure, to wear sunscreen when going outdoors, and to avoid heat lamps and tanning beds.
- Tell patient to avoid temperature extremes (such as hot or cold baths, sunlamps, or tanning beds) because drug may alter thermoregulation.
- If patient develops a dry mouth, suggest sugarless gum, sugarless

---

Reactions may be *common,* uncommon, *life-threatening,* or COMMON AND LIFE-THREATENING.

candy, ice chips, or artificial saliva
to help relieve the symptoms.
- Caution patient not to drink alcohol or take sedating medications.
- Caution patient not to take other prescribed drugs, OTC medications, or herbal remedies without consulting prescriber.
- Tell patient not to stop therapy abruptly or without consulting prescriber.
- Tell patient to notify prescriber about difficult urination, sore throat, dizziness, fainting, or inhibited ejaculation.

CHAPTER 10

Central nervous system stimulants

343 ■ **Introduction**

348 ■ **Generic drugs**

■ amphetamine sulfate

■ caffeine

■ dextroamphetamine sulfate

■ diethylpropion hydrochloride

■ doxapram hydrochloride

■ methamphetamine hydrochloride

■ methylphenidate hydrochloride

■ modafinil

■ pemoline

■ selegiline hydrochloride (See Chapter 8, ANTIPARKINSONIANS)

Central nervous system (CNS) stimulants are used mainly to treat attention deficit hyperactivity disorder (ADHD) and, to a lesser extent, narcolepsy. Some drugs in this class—such as diethylpropion (Tenuate), and amphetamine sulfate—are sometimes used to help manage obesity, although this use is controversial. CNS stimulants are also sometimes used as adjunctive treatments for depression, particularly in patients with serious illnesses, frail elderly patients, patients who need opiates for pain control, and apathetic patients with dementia. (See *Central nervous system stimulants: A growing role?*, page 344.)

UNDERSTANDING ATTENTION DEFICIT HYPERACTIVITY DISORDER

ADHD is one of the most common psychiatric problems among children of diverse cultural backgrounds and geographic regions. Experts estimate that this disorder affects 3% to 6% of all school-age children, although it accounts for nearly half of clinic visits. It usually surfaces during the first few years of grade school. Currently, this disorder is diagnosed 4 to 9 times more often in boys than girls, but some evidence suggests that this imbalance may be changing.

Symptoms of ADHD include varying degrees of inattention, hyperactivity, and impulsivity. Symptoms may occur from preschool age into adulthood. Usually, they diminish by about half every 5 years between ages 10 and 25. Hyperactivity diminishes more rapidly than impulsivity and trouble concentrating. For a significant percentage of children, symptoms persist into adulthood.

ADHD can cause mild to severe deficits in academic, social, and occupational performance. Children affected by this disorder have an increased risk of developing other psychiatric conditions as well, such as antisocial behavior, substance abuse, mood disorders, and anxiety disorders. As many as 65% of children with ADHD also have autism, Tourette syndrome, mental retardation, or fragile X syndrome. Thus, treating this disorder can be complex and commonly requires multiple therapeutic approaches (environmental, educational, psychotherapeutic) along with drug therapy.

No one knows precisely what causes ADHD (See *Physiology of attention deficit hyperactivity disorder*, page 345.) The diagnosis is based on the child's early behavior patterns, the persistence of symptoms over time, the presence of symptoms in varied settings, and impairments in school, social, and occupational performance.

Attaining a diagnosis requires a comprehensive work-up that includes interviews of the child's adult caregivers and teachers, a medical and neurological examination, a mental status examination, and an assessment of the child's cognitive ability. The examination must include assessment of the child's height, weight, vital signs, sleeping habits, eating habits, any involuntary movements or tics, and possibly liver function tests. Also, find out if the patient has a family history of tics or Tourette syndrome.

Central nervous system stimulants: A growing role?

For some patients, central nervous system (CNS) stimulants may prove helpful for treating conditions other than attention deficit hyperactivity disorder (ADHD) or narcolepsy. For instance, methylphenidate, amphetamine, and dextroamphetamine may help in treating resistant depression, especially when added to existing therapy with a tricyclic antidepressant.

Because so many effective antidepressants are currently available, the practice of combining a CNS stimulant and a tricyclic antidepressant isn't common. Even so, a brief trial may be worthwhile for selected patients with resistant conditions.

CNS depressants may be helpful for other patients as well, such as medically frail elderly patients, patients who have had a cerebrovascular accident, and patients with severe medical illnesses, severe cardiac disease, or a combination of AIDS and depression, which may increase the risk of adverse effects from typical antidepressant therapy.

Finally, methylphenidate may help treat apathy in patients with dementia, and it may improve pain control when given together with opiates. For most of the unconventional uses described here, methylphenidate is the CNS stimulant of choice—at much lower dosages than those typically used for ADHD or narcolepsy.

Treating attention deficit hyperactivity disorder

Once a diagnosis of ADHD has been established, the child will start treatment with a CNS stimulant. About 70% to 90% of children with this disorder respond to CNS stimulants. First-line drugs include methylphenidate and dextroamphetamine. Although pemoline has proven just as effective, its increased risk of hepatotoxicity disqualifies it from first-line status. And although methamphetamine is also approved for treating the disorder, little evidence exists to support its use over first-line drugs. What's more, it may carry a higher risk of abuse and a greater likelihood of adverse peripheral effects than other CNS stimulants.

Methylphenidate, dextroamphetamine, and pemoline seem to have similar rates of efficacy among children of wide-ranging demographic and ethnic characteristics; however, individual children may have varying responses to each of these drugs. In other words, despite their similar efficacy profiles, a child may respond better to one drug than another; the child may even respond differently to a generic version than to a trade name version of a drug. Giving an immediate-release form of methylphenidate or dextroamphetamine as a single daily test dose after breakfast can help determine tolerability and response.

Typically, treatment with a CNS stimulant improves the child's ability to pay attention and decreases the tendency toward impulsivity, hyperactivity, and distractibility. Cognitive effects include improvements in vigilance, reaction times, short-term memory, and learning of verbal and nonverbal material. CNS stimulants also can improve

Physiology of attention deficit hyperactivity disorder

So far, we don't know much about what happens in attention deficit hyperactivity disorder (ADHD), and we've found no biological markers for the disorder or its component symptoms. However, advances in neuroimaging and functional studies have revealed that the core symptoms of ADHD—inattention and hyperactivity—involve frontosubcortical pathways in the brain.

What's more, recent genetic research points to a possible genetic component. These studies have implicated the D_4 dopamine receptor, dopamine transporter, and D_2 receptor genes in the pathophysiology of the disorder. Other studies have suggested that complications of pregnancy and delivery, environmental toxins, marital discord, family dysfunction, and low socioeconomic class also may influence the development of ADHD.

classroom and interpersonal relationships by decreasing oppositional and aggressive behavior. In general, however, treatment affects academic performance less than it affects behavior patterns.

All CNS stimulants have a rapid onset of action, and immediate and sometimes dramatic results may occur with only a few doses. Likewise, when therapy ends, drug effects may dissipate rapidly.

Drug effects

Because the pathophysiology of ADHD is unclear, the mechanism by which CNS stimulants exert their therapeutic effects is unclear as well. However, these drugs probably improve symptoms by facilitating catecholaminergic transmission (dopamine, norepinephrine, serotonin). Because methylphenidate and amphetamine both affect primarily dopamine, most experts suspect that dopamine plays the most prominent role in the disorder's pathophysiology.

As a group, CNS stimulants cause both central and peripheral sympathomimetic effects, including mild cardiovascular effects (increased heart rate and blood pressure) and CNS effects (arousal, wakefulness, euphoria, and increased energy).

UNDERSTANDING NARCOLEPSY

Narcolepsy is a serious, lifelong neurologic disorder characterized mainly by excessive daytime sleepiness and recurrent daily sleep attacks. Other symptoms may occur as well, such as cataplexy, sleep paralysis, certain types of hallucinations, and disrupted nighttime sleep. (See *Elements of narcolepsy,* page 346.) The disorder probably results from decreased monoaminergic and increased cholinergic activity.

For most people with narcolepsy, excessive daytime sleepiness is usually constant. The person typically takes repeated short naps (10 to 20 minutes), but finds them only partially refreshing. Within 2 or 3 hours, the person may again feel sleepy and need to take another nap. Although sleep usually oc-

Elements of narcolepsy

Besides excessive daytime sleepiness and recurrent daily sleep attacks, people with narcolepsy may experience cataplexy, sleep paralysis, hallucinations, and disrupted sleep.

Cataplexy

This sudden, bilateral loss of muscle tone is commonly provoked by a strong emotion, such as laughter, and usually lasts less than 5 minutes. The patient maintains a normal level of consciousness during the attack, which may range from mild to severe. A mild attack may cause nothing more than facial weakness; a severe attack can cause the patient to physically collapse.

At least 60% of patients with narcolepsy have cataplexy; up to 75% of affected patients have one or more attacks each day. Recovery from an attack of cataplexy typically is rapid and complete.

Sleep paralysis

Between 30% and 50% of narcoleptics experience sleep paralysis, which is the inability to move or speak while awake, while falling asleep (hypnogogic sleep paralysis), or while waking up (hypnopompic sleep paralysis). Sleep paralysis usually lasts less than 10 minutes, and it may include eye fluttering, moaning, and tingling or numbness of the limbs.

Hallucinations

Hypnogogic hallucinations or, less commonly, hypnopompic hallucinations occur in 20% to 40% of patients with narcolepsy. Because some elements of normal wakefulness remain, these hallucinations are unlike dreams; they represent a change in the person's state of consciousness. Visual hallucinations are the most common type of hallucination. Many patients report seeing someone near, over, or under the bed.

Disrupted sleep

In healthy people, sleep takes place in gradual stages. In contrast, people with narcolepsy may enter directly into rapid eye movement (REM) sleep—called a sleep-onset REM period—or they may have a sharply reduced time before REM sleep starts (called REM latency). In fact, cataplexy is the intrusion of REM sleep into an awake or a drowsy state.

About 60% to 80% of patients with narcolepsy also have disrupted nighttime sleep, especially late in the course of the disorder when the person reaches 40 to 50 years old.

curs passively, as in these short naps, it may also occur unexpectedly while the person is eating, standing up, or walking. Thus, people with narcolepsy have a significantly increased risk of accidents and injuries.

They're also more likely to experience anxiety, depression, low self-esteem, irritability, and social withdrawal. They may have increased levels of marital stress from sexual dysfunction and a decreased libido. And because most people know little about narcolepsy, people who have it may be considered lazy or careless.

About 200,000 Americans have been diagnosed with narcolepsy. Gender and race seem to have no influence on it. And although the disorder may have a genetic component (human leukocyte antigen marker DR2), no test is available for screening or diagnosis.

Usually, narcolepsy is diagnosed in a person's 20s. However, excessive daytime sleepiness typically begins during adolescence. Sleep studies, such as a nocturnal polysomnogram or the multiple sleep latency test, can confirm the diagnosis and rule out more common sleep disorders, such as sleep apnea.

Treating narcolepsy

Nondrug treatments, such as improving sleep hygiene and taking short naps throughout the day, can help to reduce the intrusion of narcolepsy into a person's life. However, most affected people also need drug treatment. A CNS stimulant can help to minimize the two main symptoms of narcolepsy: excessive daytime sleepiness and cataplexy.

Currently, methylphenidate is the drug used most often in the United States for narcolepsy, followed by dextroamphetamine. However, this pattern may change as clinicians obtain added experience with modafinil. Other drugs may help to control cataplexy and nighttime sleep disruption, such as selegiline hydrochloride, tricyclic antidepressants, and selective serotonin reuptake inhibitors.

Treatment with a CNS stimulant can improve objective measures of alertness and performance (such as driving). About 65% to 85% of patients seem to respond adequately to treatment. However, keep in mind that patients with narcolepsy may need dosages that substantially exceed the recommended maximums for treatment of ADHD. For example, narcoleptic patients may need a controversial dosage of 100 mg/day of methylphenidate.

PATIENT TEACHING

When a child has ADHD, make sure the child and her parents understand the diagnosis, the reason for drug treatment, the expected benefits of drug treatment, and the possible adverse effects of drug treatment. Explain the benefits of "drug holidays" during low-stress times, such as weekends, summers, and other school breaks.

Whether a CNS stimulant is intended to treat ADHD or narcolepsy, stress the need for strict compliance with therapy. If the patient takes methylphenidate, dextroamphetamine, or pemoline, tell the patient or parents that the drug may cause decreased appetite, insomnia, stomachache, and headache. Urge the patient to take the drug with a meal to help minimize stomachaches and altered appetite.

Also, briefly review the less common adverse effects, such as worsened moods and abnormal movements or tics. Make sure that patients and parents know that most people need a period of dosage adjustment. Urge teenage and adult patients to avoid alcohol during therapy. As needed, refer children and adults to national support groups.

amphetamine sulfate

Pharmacologic classification: amphetamine

Therapeutic classification: CNS stimulant, short-term adjunctive anorexigenic, sympathomimetic amine

Controlled substance schedule II

Pregnancy risk category C

How supplied
Available by prescription only
Tablets: 5 mg, 10 mg

Indications and dosages
Attention deficit hyperactivity disorder
Children age 6 and older: 5 mg P.O. daily or b.i.d. Increase by 5 mg weekly until desired response occurs. Dosage rarely exceeds 40 mg/day. If giving divided daily doses, give first dose upon awakening and later doses at 4- to 6-hour intervals.
Children ages 3 to 5: 2.5 mg P.O. daily. Increase by 2.5 mg weekly until desired response occurs.

Narcolepsy
Adults: 5 to 60 mg/day P.O. as a single dose or divided. Usual initial dose is 10 mg/day, increased by 10 mg weekly until desired response occurs or you reach maximum dosage of 60 mg/day.
Children over age 12: 10 mg/day P.O., increased by 10 mg weekly, p.r.n.
Children ages 6 to 12: 5 mg/day P.O., increased by 5 mg weekly, p.r.n.

Short-term adjunct treatment in exogenous obesity
Adults: 5 to 30 mg daily in divided doses of 5 to 10 mg.

Pharmacodynamics
CNS stimulant action: Amphetamine sulfate is a sympathomimetic amine with CNS stimulant activity; in hyperactive children, it has a paradoxical calming effect. The cerebral cortex and reticular activating system appear to be the primary sites of activity; amphetamine releases nerve terminal stores of norepinephrine, promoting transmission of nerve impulses. At high dosages, effects are mediated by dopamine.
Anorexigenic action: Anorexigenic effects probably occur in the hypothalamus, where decreased smell and taste acuity decreases the appetite. Amphetamine sulfate may be tried for short-term control of refractory obesity, along with calorie restriction and behavior modification.

Pharmacokinetics
Absorption: Drug is absorbed completely within 3 hours after oral administration; therapeutic effects persist for 4 to 24 hours.
Distribution: Drug is distributed widely throughout body, with high levels in the brain. Therapeutic plasma levels are 5 to 10 mcg/dl.
Metabolism: Drug is metabolized by hydroxylation and deamination in the liver.
Excretion: Drug is excreted in urine.

Reactions may be *common,* uncommon, *life-threatening,* or COMMON AND LIFE-THREATENING.

Contraindications and precautions

Contraindicated in patients with hypersensitivity or unusual reactions to sympathomimetic amines; in patients with symptomatic CV disease, hyperthyroidism, moderate to severe hypertension, glaucoma, advanced arteriosclerosis, or a history of drug abuse; in patients who took an MAO inhibitor within 14 days; and in patients who are agitated.

Use cautiously in elderly, debilitated, or hyperexcitable patients and in those with suicidal or homicidal tendencies.

Interactions

Drug-drug

Acetazolamide, antacids, sodium bicarbonate: may enhance reabsorption of amphetamine and prolong its duration of action. Consider a lower amphetamine dosage.

Ammonium chloride or ascorbic acid: enhances amphetamine excretion and shortens its duration of action. Monitor blood levels of drug and adjust dosage as needed.

Antihypertensives: may antagonize antihypertensive effects. Avoid concomitant use.

Barbiturates: counteract amphetamine by CNS depression. Avoid concomitant use.

CNS stimulants: additive effects. Carefully weigh benefits of a second CNS stimulant against risk to the patient.

Guanethidine: effectiveness decreased by amphetamines. Avoid concomitant use.

Haloperidol, phenothiazines: decreases amphetamine effects.

Monitor patient for lack of therapeutic effect.

Insulin: may alter insulin requirements. Monitor patient's blood glucose levels regularly.

MAO inhibitors or drugs with MAO-inhibiting effects, such as furazolidone: use of amphetamine sulfate within 14 days of such therapy may cause hypertensive crisis. Avoid concomitant use of amphetamine sulfate and MAO inhibitors.

Drug-food

Caffeine: produces additive effects. Avoid concomitant use.

Adverse reactions

CNS: chills, dizziness, dysphoria, euphoria, headache, *hyperactivity, insomnia,* irritability, *restlessness, talkativeness,* tremor.

CV: *arrhythmias,* hypertension, *palpitations, tachycardia.*

GI: anorexia, constipation, diarrhea, dry mouth, metallic taste, weight loss.

GU: altered libido, impotence.

Metabolic: elevated plasma corticosteroid levels.

Skin: urticaria.

Overdose and treatment

Acute overdose may cause arrhythmias, circulatory collapse, coma, confusion, delirium, diaphoresis, fever, flushing, hyperreflexia, hypertension, insomnia, irritability, mydriasis, restlessness, seizures, self-injury, tachypnea, tremor, and death.

Give symptomatic, supportive treatment. Keep patient in a cool room, monitor her temperature, and minimize external stimulation. If ingestion was recent (within 4 hours), perform gastric lavage or induce emesis. Activated charcoal, sodium chloride catharsis, and urine acidification may enhance excretion. Forced fluid diuresis may help as well. In massive ingestion, hemodialysis or peritoneal dialysis may be needed. Give haloperidol if needed for psychotic symptoms and diazepam for hyperactivity.

Special considerations
- Because drug has high abuse potential, avoid giving it to patients with a history of substance abuse, if possible.
- Don't use amphetamine capsules for initial therapy or for adjusting the dosage. Once dosage has been established, however, capsules can be used for once-daily dosing.
- To minimize insomnia, avoid giving drug after 4 p.m.
- Amphetamines may interfere with tests of urine steroids.
- Give drug as an adjunct to psychosocial measures in children with attention deficit hyperactivity disorder.
- Amphetamines aren't recommended for weight reduction in children under age 12.
- Amphetamines are contraindicated in children under age 3.

Patient teaching
- Explain that drug causes sympathomimetic activation, including tachycardia and hyperactivity.
- Tell patient to use extra caution when performing hazardous activities because drug may cause rebound drowsiness.
- If patient takes drug as an aid for weight management, refer her to a

dietician for dietary recommendations. Also, recommend that she have a physical examination before starting an exercise routine.
- Tell patient to notify prescriber about growing tolerance to the drug.

---

caffeine
Cafcit, Caffedrine, NoDoz, Quick Pep, Vivarin,

Pharmacologic classification: methylxanthine

Therapeutic classification: CNS stimulant, analeptic, respiratory stimulant

Pregnancy risk category C

How supplied
Available without a prescription
Citrate: 20 mg/ml
Tablets: 150 mg, 200 mg
Tablets (chewable): 100 mg
Available by prescription only
Injection: 250 mg/ml, 121.25 mg/ml with sodium benzoate (128.75 mg/ml)

Indications and dosages
CNS depression
Adults: 100 to 200 mg P.O. q 3 to 4 hours p.r.n. For emergencies, give 250 to 500 mg I.M. or I.V.
Infants and children: 4 mg/kg I.M., I.V., or S.C. q 4 hours p.r.n. Maximum: 2.5 g/24 hours.

Pharmacodynamics
CNS stimulant action: Caffeine is a xanthine derivative; it increases levels of cAMP by inhibiting phosphodiesterase. Thus, it stimulates

all levels of the CNS, hastens and clarifies thinking, and improves arousal and psychomotor coordination.

Respiratory stimulant action: In respiratory depression and neonatal apnea, caffeine in large doses can increase respiratory rate. It also can increase the contractile force and decrease fatigue level of skeletal muscle.

Pharmacokinetics

Absorption: Caffeine is well absorbed from the GI tract; absorption after I.M. injection may be slower.

Distribution: Caffeine is distributed rapidly throughout the body; it crosses the blood-brain barrier and placenta. About 17% is protein-bound.

Metabolism: Caffeine is metabolized by the liver; in neonates, liver metabolism is much less evident and half-life may approach 80 hours. Plasma half-life in adults is 3 to 4 hours.

Excretion: Caffeine is excreted in urine.

Contraindications and precautions

Contraindicated in patients hypersensitive to drug.

Use cautiously after an acute MI and in patients with a history of peptic ulcer, symptomatic arrhythmias, or palpitations.

Interactions

Drug-drug

Beta agonists (such as albuterol, metaproterenol, terbutaline): increases risk of cardiac effects and tremors. Avoid concomitant use.

Cimetidine, disulfiram, fluoroquinolones (such as ciprofloxacin and enoxacin), oral contraceptives: inhibit caffeine metabolism, thus increasing its effects. Avoid concomitant use.

Xanthine derivatives (such as theophylline): may increase the risk of stimulant-induced adverse reactions, such as insomnia, nervousness, tachycardia, tremor. Avoid concomitant use.

Drug-lifestyle

Smoking: may enhance caffeine elimination. Urge patient to stop smoking.

Adverse reactions

CNS: agitation, excitement, headache, *insomnia,* muscle tremor, nervousness, restlessness, twitching.

CV: extrasystoles, *palpitations, tachycardia.*

GI: diarrhea, nausea, stomach pain, vomiting.

GU: *diuresis.*

Other: tinnitus, withdrawal symptoms (headache, irritability) after abrupt discontinuation.

Overdose and treatment

Overdose may cause altered consciousness, arrhythmias, diuresis, dyspnea, fever, insomnia, muscle twitching, and seizures in adults. In infants, it may cause alternating hypotonicity and hypertonicity, bradycardia, hypotension, opisthotonoid posture, severe acidosis, and tremors.

Provide symptomatic, supportive treatment. It may include gastric lavage and activated charcoal. Carefully monitor patient's vital signs, ECG, and fluid and electrolyte balance. Give diazepam or phenobarbital for seizures; keep in mind, however, that diazepam may worsen respiratory depression.

Special considerations
■ Many clinicians strongly discourage use of caffeine for treating CNS depression.
■ Expect the following amounts of caffeine (in mg/cup) in these common beverages: 40 to 180 in brewed coffee, 30 to 120 in instant coffee, 24 to 64 in cola drinks, 20 to 110 in brewed tea, and 3 to 5 in decaffeinated coffee.
■ Many OTC pain relievers contain caffeine, and it has been used to relieve headache after lumbar puncture. However, evidence of its analgesic effects is conflicting. It also may be included in a hydrophilic base (30%) or hydrocortisone cream to treat atopic dermatitis.
■ If patient has a symptomatic arrhythmia or takes aminophylline or theophylline, limit caffeine-containing beverages.
■ Caffeine may increase blood glucose levels and cause false-positive results on tests of urate. By increasing certain urinary catecholamines, it also may cause false-positive results on tests for pheochromocytoma and neuroblastoma.

Breast-feeding patients
■ Caffeine appears in breast milk. Recommend an alternative feeding method during caffeine therapy.

Pediatric patients
■ Unlabeled uses for caffeine include neonatal apnea. To control neonatal apnea, maintain plasma caffeine level at 5 to 20 mcg/ml.
■ Adverse CNS effects are usually more severe in children.
■ For neonates, avoid caffeine products that contain sodium benzoate because they may cause kernicterus.

Geriatric patients
■ Elderly patients are more sensitive to caffeine and should take lower doses.

Patient teaching
■ Urge patient to avoid excessive caffeine consumption, and the resulting CNS stimulation, by learning the caffeine content of beverages and foods.
■ Warn patient not to exceed recommended caffeine dosage and not to substitute caffeine for sleep. Tell patient to discontinue caffeine if she develops dizziness or tachycardia.

dextroamphetamine sulfate
Adderall, Dexedrine, Ferndex

Pharmacologic classification: **amphetamine**

Therapeutic classification: **CNS stimulant, short-term adjunctive anorexigenic, sympathomimetic amine**

Controlled substance schedule II

Pregnancy risk category C

How supplied
Available by prescription only

Capsules (sustained-release): 5 mg, 10 mg, 15 mg
Elixir: 5 mg/5 ml
Tablets: 5 mg, 10 mg, 20 mg, 30 mg

Indications and dosages
Attention deficit hyperactivity disorder
Children age 6 and over: 5 mg once daily or b.i.d., increased by 5 mg weekly p.r.n. Rarely should dosage exceed 40 mg/day.
Children ages 3 to 5: 2.5 mg/day P.O., increased by 2.5 mg weekly, p.r.n.

Narcolepsy
Adults: 5 to 60 mg/day P.O. in divided doses. Sustained-release form allows once-daily dosing.
Children over age 12: 10 mg/day P.O., increased by 10 mg weekly, p.r.n.
Children ages 6 to 12: 5 mg/day P.O., increased by 5 mg weekly, p.r.n.

Short-term adjunct in exogenous obesity
Adults: 5 to 30 mg/day P.O. in divided doses of 5 to 10 mg and taken 30 to 60 minutes before meals. Alternatively, give one 10- or 15-mg sustained-release capsule daily as a single dose in the morning.

Pharmacodynamics
Anorexigenic action: Anorexigenic effects are thought to occur in the hypothalamus, where decreased smell and taste acuity decreases appetite. Dextroamphetamine may be tried for short-term control of refractory obesity, along with calorie restriction and behavior modification.

CNS stimulant action: Dextroamphetamine sulfate is a sympathomimetic amine with CNS stimulant activity; in hyperactive children, it has a paradoxical calming effect. The cerebral cortex and reticular activating system appear to be the primary sites of activity; amphetamine releases nerve terminal stores of norepinephrine, promoting transmission of nerve impulses. At high dosages, effects are mediated by dopamine.

Pharmacokinetics
Absorption: Drug is rapidly absorbed from the GI tract; peak serum levels occur 2 to 4 hours after oral administration; long-acting capsules are absorbed more slowly and have a longer duration of action.
Distribution: Drug is distributed widely throughout the body.
Metabolism: Unknown.
Excretion: Drug is excreted in urine.

Contraindications and precautions
Contraindicated in patients with hypersensitivity or unusual reactions to sympathomimetic amines; in patients with symptomatic CV disease, hyperthyroidism, moderate to severe hypertension, glaucoma, advanced arteriosclerosis, or a history of drug abuse; and in patients who took an MAO inhibitor within 14 days.

Use cautiously in agitated patients and those with Tourette syndrome or motor or phonic tics.

◇ Available in Canada only   *Unlabeled use

Interactions
Drug-drug
Acetazolamide, alkalizing drugs, antacids, sodium bicarbonate: enhanced dextroamphetamine reabsorption, which prolongs duration of action. Consider a lower dextroamphetamine dosage.

Acidifying drugs, ammonium chloride, ascorbic acid: enhanced dextroamphetamine excretion, which shortens duration of action. Monitor patient's blood levels to assess need for higher dextroamphetamine dosage.

Adrenergic blockers: effect inhibited by amphetamines. Avoid concomitant use.

Antihypertensives: may antagonize antihypertensive effects. Avoid concomitant use.

Barbiturates: CNS depression antagonizes dextroamphetamine. Avoid concomitant use.

Chlorpromazine: inhibits central stimulant effects of amphetamine and may be used to treat amphetamine poisoning.

CNS stimulants, haloperidol, phenothiazines, theophylline, tricyclic antidepressants: increased CNS effects. Avoid concomitant use.

Insulin, oral antidiabetic drugs: requirements may be altered. Monitor patient's blood glucose levels regularly.

Lithium carbonate: may inhibit antiobesity and stimulating effects of amphetamines. Evaluate patient thoroughly before combining these two therapies.

MAO inhibitors or drugs with MAO-inhibiting activity, such as furazolidone: may cause hypertensive crisis within 14 days of such therapy. Avoid concomitant use.

Meperidine: analgesic effect is potentiated by amphetamines. Reduced meperidine dosage may be needed.

Methenamine: increased urinary excretion of amphetamines, which leads to reduced efficacy. Avoid concomitant use.

Norepinephrine: adrenergic effect enhanced by amphetamines. Reduced norepinephrine dosage may be needed.

Phenobarbital, phenytoin: possible synergistic anticonvulsant action. Don't administer concurrently with dextroamphetamine.

Drug-food
Caffeine: may increase effects of dextroamphetamine and related amines. Avoid concomitant use.

Adverse reactions
CNS: chills, dizziness, dysphoria, euphoria, headache, *insomnia,* overstimulation, *restlessness,* tremor.
CV: *arrhythmias,* hypertension, *palpitations, tachycardia.*
GI: anorexia, constipation, diarrhea, dry mouth, GI upset, unpleasant taste, weight loss.
GU: altered libido, impotence.
Skin: urticaria.

Overdose and treatment
Overdose may cause widely varied individual responses. Toxic symptoms may occur at 15 to 30 mg and can cause severe reactions; however, doses of 400 mg or more have not always been fatal. Evidence of overdose may include aggressiveness, confusion, hallucinations, hyperreflexia, panic, restlessness, tachypnea, and tremor. Fatigue and

depression usually follow this excitement stage. Other symptoms may include abdominal cramps, arrhythmias, changes in blood pressure, diarrhea, nausea, shock, and vomiting. Death is usually preceded by seizures and coma.

Treat a dextroamphetamine overdose symptomatically and supportively. If ingestion was within 4 hours, perform gastric lavage or induce emesis. Sedate the patient with a barbiturate. Monitor her vital signs and fluid and electrolyte balance. Urine acidification may enhance excretion, and saline catharsis with magnesium citrate may hasten evacuation of unabsorbed sustained-release drug from the GI tract.

Special considerations
■ When administering drug for narcolepsy, give daily dose when patient awakens in the morning.
■ When administering drug for anorexigenic effects, give doses 30 to 60 minutes before meals. To minimize insomnia, avoid giving drug within 6 hours of bedtime.
■ Check patient's vital signs regularly during therapy, and watch for evidence of excessive stimulation.
■ When patient develops tolerance to anorexigenic effect, discontinue drug; don't increase dosage.
■ Monitor diabetic patient's blood and urine glucose levels because drug may alter insulin requirement.
■ Drug may interfere with tests of urine steroids and may elevate plasma corticosteroid levels.

Breast-feeding patients
■ Safety of breast-feeding during dextroamphetamine therapy hasn't been established. Recommend an alternative feeding method during therapy.

Pediatric patients
■ Drug isn't recommended for treatment of obesity in children under age 12.
■ Drug isn't recommended for treatment of attention deficit hyperactivity disorder (ADHD) in children under age 3.

Geriatric patients
■ Use lower dosage in elderly patients, and avoid giving drug to elderly patients with CV, CNS, or GI disturbances.

Patient teaching
■ Instruct patient to take drug early in the day to minimize insomnia.
■ Tell patient not to crush sustained-release forms or to increase the dosage without consulting prescriber.
■ Instruct parents to provide drug-free periods for children with ADHD, especially during periods of reduced stress.
■ Caution patient to avoid caffeine-containing foods and beverages during therapy.
■ Warn patient to avoid hazardous activities until drug's full CNS effects are known.

diethylpropion hydrochloride
Tenuate, Tenuate Dospan

Pharmacologic classification: amphetamine

Therapeutic classification: short-term adjunctive anorexigenic, sympathomimetic amine

Controlled substance schedule IV

Pregnancy risk category B

How supplied
Available by prescription only
Tablets: 25 mg
Tablets (controlled-release): 75 mg

Indications and dosages
Short-term adjunct in exogenous obesity
Adults: 25 mg P.O. t.i.d. before meals. Another 25-mg dose may be given in the evening to control nighttime hunger. Alternatively, give 75 mg controlled-release tablet P.O. at midmorning.

Pharmacodynamics
CNS stimulant action: The cerebral cortex and reticular activating system appear to be the primary sites of activity; amphetamines release nerve terminal stores of norepinephrine, promoting nerve impulse transmission.
Anorexigenic action: The precise mechanism of appetite control is unknown; anorexigenic effects are thought to occur in the hypothalamus, where decreased smell and taste acuity decreases appetite.

Pharmacokinetics
Absorption: Drug is readily absorbed after oral administration; therapeutic effects persist for 4 hours with regular tablets, longer with controlled-release form.
Distribution: Drug is widely distributed throughout the body.
Metabolism: Drug is metabolized in the liver.
Excretion: Drug is excreted in urine.

Contraindications and precautions
Contraindicated in patients with hypersensitivity or unusual reactions to sympathomimetic amines; in patients with hyperthyroidism, severe hypertension, glaucoma, advanced arteriosclerosis, or a history of drug abuse; and in patients who took an MAO inhibitor within 14 days.

Use cautiously in patients with mild to moderate hypertension, symptomatic CV disease (including arrhythmias), or seizure disorders.

Interactions
Drug-drug
Antidepressants: may have increased effectiveness. Decreased antidepressant dosage may be needed.
Barbiturates: CNS depression may antagonize diethylpropion and decrease its effects. Don't administer concurrently.
Guanethidine: antihypertensive effects may be decreased by diethylpropion. Don't administer concurrently.
Insulin: weight loss may decrease insulin requirements in diabetic

patients. Check blood glucose levels frequently during therapy.
MAO inhibitors or drugs with MAO-inhibiting effects, such as furazolidone: may cause hypertensive crisis if diethylpropion administered within 14 days of such therapy. Avoid concomitant use.

Drug-food
Caffeine: causes additive CNS stimulation. Discourage concomitant use.

Adverse reactions
CNS: anxiety, drowsiness, fatigue, headache, insomnia, *nervousness.*
CV: *arrhythmias,* ECG changes, elevated blood pressure, *palpitations,* **pulmonary hypertension,** *tachycardia.*
EENT: blurred vision, mydriasis.
GI: abdominal cramps, constipation, diarrhea, dry mouth, nausea, unpleasant taste, vomiting.
GU: altered libido, changes in menstruation, impotence.
Metabolic: decreased blood glucose levels.
Skin: urticaria, rash.

Overdose and treatment
Acute overdose may cause aggressive behavior, arrhythmias, blood pressure changes, confusion, cramps, diarrhea, hallucinations, hyperreflexia, nausea, restlessness, tachypnea, tremor, and vomiting. Fatigue and depression usually follow initial stimulation; seizures and coma may result.

Provide symptomatic, supportive treatment. If ingestion was within 4 hours, perform gastric lavage or induce emesis. If needed, give a sedative. If acute hypertension develops, give phentolamine I.V. Monitor patient's vital signs and fluid and electrolyte balance.

Special considerations
■ Obtain an ECG before starting therapy; avoid giving drug if patient has a history of mitral valve prolapse or other CV problems.
■ Give drug adjunctively with caloric restriction and behavior modification for a patient with exogenous obesity.
■ Drug can be used to stop nighttime overeating and rarely causes insomnia.
■ Drug is considered the safest of the sympathomimetic amines for patients who have mild to moderate hypertension.
■ Don't crush controlled-release form of drug.

Breast-feeding patients
■ Drug appears in breast milk; recommend an alternative feeding method during therapy.

Pediatric patients
■ Drug isn't recommended for weight reduction in children under age 12.

Geriatric patients
■ Lower dosages may be effective in elderly patients because of their reduced renal function.

Patient teaching
■ Warn patient against exceeding the prescribed dosage.
■ Emphasize the importance of careful adherence to the total treatment program, including diet and exercise, if weight control is to be successful. Make sure patient un-

derstands dietary restrictions that must accompany drug therapy to obtain maximum benefit.
- Urge patient to avoid foods high in tyramine, such as beer, wine, and aged cheese, because hypertensive reactions may occur when these foods are combined with drug.
- Tell patient to swallow controlled-release form whole and not to chew or crush it.
- Recommend that the patient avoid caffeine-containing beverages during therapy because they could lead to overstimulation.
- Tell patient that drug may color urine pink to brown. Explain that this effect is harmless.
- Explain that extreme fatigue and depression may occur if drug is abruptly discontinued after prolonged use.

---

doxapram hydrochloride
Dopram

Pharmacologic classification: analeptic

Therapeutic classification: CNS and respiratory stimulant

Pregnancy risk category B

How supplied
Available by prescription only
Injection: 20 mg/ml (benzyl alcohol 0.9%)

Indications and dosages
Postanesthesia respiratory stimulation
Adults: 0.5 to 1 mg/kg of body weight as a single I.V. injection (not to exceed 1.5 mg/kg) or as multiple injections q 5 minutes (not to exceed 2 mg/kg). Alternatively, infuse 250 mg of drug I.V. in 250 ml of normal saline solution or D_5W at an initial rate of 5 mg/minute until a satisfactory response occurs. Maintain infusion at 1 to 3 mg/minute. Recommended maximum total dose for I.V. infusion is 4 mg/kg (about 300 mg) for an average adult.

Drug-induced CNS depression
Adults: For I.V. injection, give a priming dose of 2 mg/kg and repeat in 5 minutes and again q 1 to 2 hours until patient awakens (and again if relapse occurs). Maximum, 3 g daily. For I.V. infusion, give a priming dose of 2 mg/kg and repeat in 5 minutes and again in 1 to 2 hours if needed. If response occurs, infuse 1 mg/ml at 1 to 3 mg/minute for up to 2 hours until patient awakens. Maximum, 3 g/day. After a rest period of 30 minutes to 2 hours, repeat I.V. infusion as needed.

Pharmacodynamics
Respiratory stimulant action: Doxapram increases the respiratory rate by directly stimulating the medullary respiratory center and possibly by indirectly acting on chemoreceptors in the carotid artery and aortic arch. Drug increases catecholamine release.

Pharmacokinetics
Absorption: After I.V. administration, action begins in 20 to 40 seconds; effect peaks in 1 to 2 minutes. Pharmacologic action persists for 5 to 12 minutes.

Distribution: Drug is distributed throughout the body.
Metabolism: Drug is 99% metabolized by the liver.
Excretion: Metabolites are excreted in urine.

Contraindications and precautions

Contraindicated in patients with seizure disorders, head injury, CV disorders, uncompensated heart failure, severe hypertension, CVA, hypoxia not linked to hypercapnia, or respiratory failure or incompetence caused by neuromuscular disorders, muscle paresis, flail chest, obstructed airway, pulmonary embolism, pneumothorax, restrictive respiratory disease, acute bronchial asthma, or extreme dyspnea. Contraindicated in newborns because product contains benzyl alcohol.

Use cautiously in patients with bronchial asthma, severe tachycardia or other arrhythmias, cerebral edema, increased CSF pressure, hyperthyroidism, pheochromocytoma, or metabolic disorders.

Interactions
Drug-drug
Anesthetics, such as cyclopropane, enflurane, halothane: sensitize the myocardium to catecholamines. Discontinue at least 10 minutes before giving doxapram.
MAO inhibitors, sympathomimetics: may produce added pressor effects. Avoid concomitant use.
Neuromuscular blockers used after anesthesia: residual effects may be temporarily masked by doxapram. Avoid concomitant use.

Adverse reactions
CNS: apprehension, bilateral Babinski's signs, disorientation, dizziness, *headache,* hyperactivity, paresthesia, *seizures.*
CV: *arrhythmias, chest pain and tightness, hypertension,* lowered T waves, *variations in heart rate.*
EENT: *laryngospasm,* sneezing.
GI: diarrhea, nausea, vomiting.
GU: albuminuria, bladder stimulation with incontinence, increased BUN levels, urine retention.
Hematologic: decreased erythrocyte and leukocyte counts, reduced hemoglobin and hematocrit levels.
Musculoskeletal: muscle spasms.
Respiratory: *bronchospasm,* cough, dyspnea, *rebound hypoventilation.*
Skin: diaphoresis, pruritus.
Other: hiccups, flushing.

Overdose and treatment
Overdose may cause dyspnea, hypertension, skeletal muscle hyperactivity, and tachycardia and other arrhythmias.

Treatment is supportive. Keep oxygen and resuscitative equipment available, but use oxygen with caution because a rapid increase in partial pressure of oxygen can suppress carotid chemoreceptor activity. Keep I.V. anticonvulsants available to treat seizures.

Special considerations
■ Doxapram should be used only in surgery or an emergency department. Use as an analeptic is strongly discouraged.
■ Establish an adequate airway before giving drug; prevent aspiration of vomitus by placing patient on his side.

- For I.V. infusion, dilute to 1 mg/ml. Don't infuse doxapram faster than recommended rate because hemolysis may occur. Drug should be used only on an intermittent basis; maximum infusion period is 2 hours.
- Don't combine doxapram, which is acidic, with alkaline solutions, such as thiopental sodium; solution is compatible with D_5W, $D_{10}W$, and normal saline solution.
- Avoid repeated injections in a single site because of risk of thrombophlebitis or local skin irritation.
- Monitor patient's blood pressure, heart rate, deep tendon reflexes, and arterial blood gas levels before giving drug and every 30 minutes afterward. Discontinue drug if arterial blood gases deteriorate or mechanical ventilation begins.
- Give oxygen cautiously if patient has COPD and receives narcotics or has just undergone surgery; doxapram-stimulated respiration increases oxygen demand.
- Besides standard uses, drug also has been given to patients with chronic pulmonary disease associated with acute hypercapnia

Breast-feeding patients
- Safe use in breast-feeding hasn't been established, and distribution of drug into breast milk is unknown.

Pediatric patients
- Safety in children under age 12 hasn't been established.

Geriatric patients
- Elderly patients may be predisposed to several illnesses that preclude drug's use.

methamphetamine hydrochloride
Desoxyn, Desoxyn Gradumets

Pharmacologic classification: amphetamine

Therapeutic classification: CNS stimulant, short-term adjunctive anorexigenic, sympathomimetic amine

Controlled substance schedule II

Pregnancy risk category C

How supplied
Available by prescription only
Tablets: 5 mg
Tablets (extended-release): 5 mg, 10 mg, 15 mg

Indications and dosages
Attention deficit hyperactivity disorder
Children age 6 and older: initially, 5 mg P.O. once daily or b.i.d., increased by 5 mg weekly, p.r.n. Usual effective dose is 20 to 25 mg/day.

Short-term adjunct in exogenous obesity
Adults: 2.5 to 5 mg P.O. b.i.d. or t.i.d. 30 minutes before meals or 10 to 15 mg P.O. daily of extended-release form in the morning. Therapy shouldn't last more than a few weeks.

Pharmacodynamics
Anorexigenic action: Anorexigenic effects are thought to occur in the hypothalamus, where decreased smell and taste acuity decrease appetite. Methamphetamine hydro-

---

chloride may be tried for short-term control of refractory obesity, along with calorie restriction and behavior modification.

CNS stimulant action: Methamphetamine is a sympathomimetic amine with CNS stimulant activity; in hyperactive children, it has a paradoxical calming effect. The cerebral cortex and reticular activating system appear to be the primary sites of activity; amphetamines release nerve terminal stores of norepinephrine, promoting nerve impulse transmission. At high dosages, effects are mediated by dopamine.

Pharmacokinetics
Absorption: Drug is rapidly absorbed from the GI tract after oral administration; effects last 6 to 12 hours. Extended-release form prolongs absorption.

Distribution: Drug is widely distributed throughout the body. It crosses the placenta and enters breast milk.

Metabolism: Drug is metabolized in the liver to at least seven metabolites.

Excretion: Drug is excreted in urine.

Contraindications and precautions
Contraindicated in patients with hypersensitivity or unusual reactions to sympathomimetic amines; in patients with symptomatic CV disease, hyperthyroidism, moderate to severe hypertension, glaucoma, advanced arteriosclerosis, or a history of drug abuse; in patients who took an MAO inhibitor with-

in 14 days; and in patients who are agitated.

Use cautiously in elderly, debilitated, asthenic, or psychopathic patients and in those with history of suicidal or homicidal tendencies.

Interactions
Drug-drug
Acetazolamide, antacids, sodium bicarbonate: enhance methamphetamine reabsorption, which prolongs duration of action. Consider reducing methamphetamine dosage.

Antihypertensives: may antagonize antihypertensive effects. Don't administer concurrently.

Ascorbic acid: enhances methamphetamine excretion, which shortens duration of action. Consider increasing methamphetamine dosage.

Barbiturates: CNS depression antagonizes methamphetamine. Don't administer concurrently.

CNS stimulants (including caffeine): additive effects. Avoid concomitant use.

General anesthesia: increased risk of arrhythmias. If possible, wean patient from methamphetamine hydrochloride for a few weeks before administration of general anesthesia.

Haloperidol, phenothiazines: decreased methamphetamine effects. Monitor patient closely for lack of therapeutic effect.

Insulin: methamphetamine hydrochloride may alter insulin requirements in diabetic patient. Monitor patient's blood glucose levels frequently.

Melatonin: enhances monoaminergic effects of methamphetamine and may worsen insomnia. Avoid concomitant use.

MAO inhibitors or drugs with MAO-inhibiting effects, such as furazolidone: use of methamphetamine hydrochloride within 14 days of such therapy may cause hypertensive crisis. Avoid concomitant use of methamphetamine hydrochloride and MAO inhibitors.

Adverse reactions

CNS: dizziness, euphoria, headache, hyperexcitability, *insomnia, irritability, nervousness,* talkativeness, tremor.
CV: *arrhythmias,* hypertension, *palpitations, tachycardia.*
EENT: blurred vision, mydriasis.
GI: anorexia, constipation, diarrhea, dry mouth, metallic taste.
GU: altered libido, impotence.
Skin: urticaria.

Overdose and treatment

Overdose may cause aggressiveness, confusion, hallucinations, hyperreflexia, panic, restlessness, tachypnea, and tremor. Fatigue and depression usually follow the excitement stage. Other symptoms may include abdominal cramps, arrhythmias, changes in blood pressure, diarrhea, nausea, shock, and vomiting. Death is usually preceded by seizures and coma.

Treat overdose symptomatically and supportively. If ingestion was within 4 hours, perform gastric lavage or induce emesis. Sedate the patient with a barbiturate. Monitor patient's vital signs and fluid and electrolyte balance. Give phentolamine I.V. for severe acute hypertension. Give chlorpromazine to decrease CNS stimulation and sympathomimetic effects. Urine acidification may enhance excretion, and saline catharsis with magnesium citrate may hasten evacuation of unabsorbed long-acting drug from the GI tract. Hemodialysis or peritoneal dialysis may be helpful in severe cases.

Special considerations

■ Amphetamines may be used for adjunctive, short-term control of refractory obesity together with calorie restriction and behavior modification. Methamphetamine isn't recommended as first-line treatment of obesity.
■ Don't use the extended-release form to start treatment or until the daily dose equals or exceeds the strengths available in this form.
■ Don't crush extended-release dosage forms.
■ Rapid withdrawal after prolonged use may lead to depression, increased appetite, and somnolence.

Breast-feeding patients

■ Amphetamines appear in breast milk. Recommend an alternative method of feeding during therapy.

Pediatric patients

■ Amphetamines may be used as an adjunctive treatment to psychosocial measures in children with attention deficit hyperactivity disorder.
■ When treating behavioral disorders in children, consider discontinuing methamphetamine periodically to evaluate its effectiveness and the need for continued therapy.
■ Drug isn't recommended for weight reduction in children under age 12.

Reactions may be *common,* uncommon, *life-threatening,* or COMMON AND LIFE-THREATENING.

Geriatric patients
■ Use caution when giving drug to elderly or debilitated patients because they may be especially sensitive to the drug's effects.

Patient teaching
■ Warn patient that drug has a high risk of abuse. Urge her not to take drug to combat fatigue.
■ Tell patient to avoid caffeine-containing beverages and alcohol.
■ Instruct patient to take drug 1 hour before meals, and to take the last daily dose at least 6 hours before bedtime to prevent insomnia.
■ If patient takes extended-release form, tell her to do so at the start of the day.
■ Caution patient to avoid hazardous activities until drug's full CNS effects are known.
■ Warn patient not to increase dosage without consulting prescriber.

---

methylphenidate hydrochloride
Concerta, Methylin, Methylin ER, Ritalin, Ritalin-SR

Pharmacologic classification: piperidine CNS stimulant

Therapeutic classification: CNS stimulant

Controlled substance schedule II

Pregnancy risk category C

How supplied
Available by prescription only
Tablets: 5 mg, 10 mg, 20 mg
Tablets (sustained-release): 20 mg
Tablets (extended release): 10 mg, 18 mg, 20 mg, 36 mg

Indications and dosages
Attention deficit hyperactivity disorder (Ritalin, Methylin)
Children age 6 and older: initially, 5 mg P.O. b.i.d., before breakfast and lunch. Increase by 5 to 10 mg weekly, p.r.n., until an optimum dosage of 2 mg/kg/day. Don't exceed 60 mg/day.
Attention deficit hyperactivity disorder (Concerta)
Children age 6 and older not currently using methylphenidate: initially, 18 mg P.O. once daily in the morning.
Children age 6 and older also using methylphenidate: if previous methylphenidate daily dose is 5 mg b.i.d. or t.i.d. or 20 mg sustained-release, give 18 mg P.O. every morning. If previous methylphenidate daily dose is 10 mg b.i.d. or t.i.d. or 40 mg sustained-release, give 36 mg P.O. every morning. If previous methylphenidate dose is 15 mg b.i.d. or t.i.d. or 60 mg sustained-release, give 54 mg P.O. every morning. Adjust dosages in 18 mg-increments weekly p.r.n. Don't exceed 54 mg/day.

Narcolepsy
Adults: 10 mg P.O. b.i.d. or t.i.d., 30 to 45 minutes before meals. Some patients may need up to 60 mg daily. For sustained-release form, calculate dosage with regular tablets in q 8-hour intervals and administer as such.

Pharmacodynamics
CNS stimulant action: The cerebral cortex and reticular activating sys-

tem appear to be the primary sites of activity; methylphenidate releases nerve terminal stores of norepinephrine, promoting nerve impulse transmission. Like amphetamines, it has a paradoxical calming effect in hyperactive children. At high doses, effects are mediated by dopamine.

Pharmacokinetics
Absorption: Drug is absorbed rapidly and completely after oral administration; plasma levels peak in 1 to 2 hours. Duration of action is usually 4 to 6 hours but varies widely; sustained-release tablets may act for up to 8 hours.
Distribution: Unknown.
Metabolism: Methylphenidate is metabolized by the liver.
Excretion: Drug is excreted in urine.

Contraindications and precautions
Contraindicated in patients hypersensitive to drug, patients with glaucoma or motor tics, patients with a family history or diagnosis of Tourette syndrome, and patients with a history of agitation, marked anxiety, or tension.

Use cautiously in patients with a history of drug abuse, EEG abnormalities, hypertension, or seizures.

Interactions
Drug-drug
Anticoagulants, anticonvulsants, coumarin, phenylbutazone, tricyclic antidepressants: inhibited metabolism and increased serum levels of these drugs when given with methylphenidate. If patient needs concurrent therapy, watch laboratory values closely to help maintain control of seizures.
Bretylium, guanethidine: hypotensive effects may be decreased. Monitor patient's blood pressure closely.
MAO inhibitors or drugs with MAO-inhibiting activity: may cause severe hypertension. Don't use within 14 days of methylphenidate.

Drug-lifestyle
Caffeine: may enhance CNS stimulation and decrease methylphenidate effectiveness in treating attention deficit hyperactivity disorder (ADHD). Avoid concomitant use.

Adverse reactions
CNS: akathisia, dizziness, drowsiness, dyskinesia, headache, insomnia, nervousness, *seizures,* Tourette syndrome.
CV: angina, *arrhythmias,* changes in blood pressure and pulse rate, palpitations, tachycardia.
GI: abdominal pain, anorexia, nausea, vomiting (Concerta).
Hematologic: anemia, *leukopenia, thrombocytopenia,* thrombocytopenic purpura.
Metabolic: weight loss.
Respiratory: (Concerta) upper respiratory infection, cough.
Skin: *erythema multiforme, exfoliative dermatitis,* rash, urticaria.

Overdose and treatment
Overdose may cause agitation, arrhythmias, coma, confusion, delirium, diaphoresis, dry mouth, euphoria, fever, flushing, headache, hyperreflexia, hypertension, muscle twitching, mydriasis, palpitations, seizures, self-injury, tachy-

---

Reactions may be *common,* uncommon, *life-threatening,* or COMMON AND LIFE-THREATENING.

cardia, toxic psychosis, tremors, and vomiting.

Treat overdose symptomatically and supportively. Place patient in a cool room, monitor her temperature, minimize stimulation, and protect her from injury. Perform gastric lavage or, if she has an intact gag reflex, induce emesis. Maintain her airway and circulation. Closely monitor her vital signs and fluid and electrolyte balance. Apply external cooling blankets if needed.

Special considerations
- Keep in mind that drug has abuse potential, and that some abusers dissolve tablets and inject drug.
- Drug may decrease seizure threshold in patients with seizure disorders.
- During long-term therapy, monitor patient's CBC, differential, and platelet counts.
- Drug has also been used to treat apathetic or withdrawn senile behavior and mild depression.
- After high-dose, long-term use, abrupt withdrawal may unmask severe depression. Taper the dosage gradually to prevent acute rebound depression.
- Concerta tablets shouldn't be chewed, divided, or crushed.
- Concerta shouldn't be administered to patients with preexisting severe GI narrowing.

Pediatric patients
- Methylphenidate is the drug of choice for treating ADHD. Therapy usually stops after puberty.

- Drug isn't recommended for treating ADHD in children under age 6.
- Sustained-release form allows once daily, at-home dosing.
- To minimize insomnia, avoid late-day or evening dosing, especially with sustained-release form.
- Check patient's vital signs regularly for increased blood pressure or other signs of excessive stimulation.
- Because drug may suppress growth, monitor patient's height and weight during therapy.
- Because drug may cause Tourette syndrome, monitor patient carefully early in therapy.
- If drug causes paradoxical aggravation of symptoms, reduce dosage or discontinue therapy.
- Intermittent drug-free periods during low-stress times, such as weekends and school holidays, may help prevent tolerance to drug and may allow decreased dosage when therapy resumes.

Patient teaching
- Explain the reason for therapy and the risks and benefits the patient can expect.
- Advise a narcoleptic patient to take first dose on awakening in the morning. Advise parent of child with ADHD to give last dose several hours before bedtime to avoid insomnia.
- Warn patient against using drug to mask fatigue. Also, urge patient to get adequate rest during therapy and to notify prescriber if excessive CNS stimulation occurs.
- Caution patient to avoid hazardous activities until drug's full effects are known.

■ Tell patient that the shell of the tablet may appear in stool.
■ Warn patient not to alter dosage without consulting prescriber.
■ Tell patient not to chew, divide, or crush sustained-release form.

---

modafinil
Provigil

Pharmacologic classification: benzhydryl sulfinylacetamide derivative

Therapeutic classification: CNS stimulant

Controlled substance schedule IV

Pregnancy risk category C

How supplied
Tablets: 100 mg, 200 mg

Indications and dosages
Excessive daytime sleepiness from narcolepsy
Adults: 200 mg/day P.O., given as a single dose in the morning.
▶ **DOSAGE ADJUSTMENT.** In patients with severe hepatic impairment, give 100 mg/day P.O. as a single dose in the morning.

Pharmacodynamics
CNS stimulant action: The exact mechanism of action by which modafinil promotes wakefulness is unknown. It has actions similar to sympathomimetics, including amphetamines, but modafinil differs structurally from amphetamines and doesn't seem to produce CNS stimulation by altering the release of dopamine or norepinephrine.

Pharmacokinetics
Absorption: Absorption is rapid; plasma levels peak in 2 to 4 hours.
Distribution: Modafinil is well distributed in body tissue. It's moderately bound (about 60%) to plasma protein, mainly albumin.
Metabolism: Drug is primarily metabolized (about 90%) in the liver, with renal elimination of metabolites.
Excretion: Less than 10% is renally excreted as unchanged drug.

Contraindications and precautions
Contraindicated in patients hypersensitive to drug and in patients with a history of left ventricular hypertrophy, ischemic ECG changes, chest pain, arrhythmias, or other clinically significant signs of mitral valve prolapse with CNS stimulant use.

Use cautiously in patients with a recent MI, unstable angina, or a history of psychosis. Use cautiously, and in reduced dosages, in patients with severe hepatic impairment, with or without cirrhosis. Also, use cautiously in patients who take MAO inhibitors.

Interactions
Drug-drug
Carbamazepine, phenobarbital, rifampin or other inducers of CYP3A4: altered modafinil levels. Monitor patient closely.
Cyclosporine: serum cyclosporine levels may be reduced. Use together cautiously, and monitor blood drug levels.
Diazepam, phenytoin, propranolol, and other drugs metabolized by CYP2C19: possible increase in

---

serum levels of these drugs because modafinil is a reversible inhibitor of the cytochrome P-450 isoenzyme. Use together cautiously, and adjust dosage as necessary.

Itraconazole, ketoconazole, or other inhibitors of CYP3A4: altered modafinil levels. Monitor patient closely.

Methylphenidate: may delay modafinil absorption by about 1 hour. Separate administration times.

Oral, depot, and implanted contraceptives: reduced contraceptive serum level and possible reduced contraceptive effectiveness. Recommend alternative or additional method of contraception during modafinil therapy and for 1 month after drug is discontinued.

Phenytoin, warfarin: may increase serum levels of these drugs because modafinil may inhibit CYP2C9 activity, especially at higher dosages. Monitor patient closely for evidence of toxicity, and adjust dosage as needed.

Tricyclic antidepressants, such as clomipramine, desipramine: levels increased by modafinil. Reduce tricyclic antidepressant dosage as needed.

Adverse reactions

CNS: amnesia, anxiety, ataxia, cataplexy, confusion, depression, dizziness, dyskinesia, emotional lability, *headache,* hypertonia, insomnia, nervousness, paresthesia, syncope, tremor.

CV: arrhythmias, chest pain, hypertension, hypotension, vasodilation.

EENT: abnormal vision, amblyopia, epistaxis, gingivitis, laryngitis, mouth ulcer, pharyngitis, *rhinitis,* thirst.

GI: anorexia, diarrhea, dry mouth, *nausea,* vomiting.

GU: abnormal ejaculation, abnormal urine, albuminuria, urine retention.

Hematologic: eosinophilia.

Hepatic: abnormal liver function.

Metabolic: hyperglycemia.

Musculoskeletal: joint disorder, neck pain, rigid neck.

Respiratory: asthma, dyspnea, lung disorder.

Skin: dry skin, herpes simplex.

Other: chills, fever.

Overdose and treatment

Overdose may cause agitation or excitation, insomnia, and increased heart rate and blood pressure. Most patients recover fully by the next day.

Provide supportive care as appropriate, including CV monitoring. If there are no contraindications, perform gastric lavage or induce emesis as appropriate. Data aren't available to support the use of dialysis or urine acidification or alkalinization in enhancing drug elimination.

Special considerations

■ Food has no effect on overall bioavailability, but modafinil absorption may be delayed by about one hour if drug is given with food.

■ Safety and efficacy haven't been established among patients with severe renal impairment.

■ Patients have tolerated dosages up to 400 mg daily as a single dose, but no consistent evidence exists to sug-

gest that this dosage confers benefits above standard dosage levels.
■ Although not considered significant, modafinil may lead to elevated gamma-glutamyl transpeptidase levels and abnormal eosinophil counts.
■ No specific withdrawal symptoms have occurred for up to 14 days after 9 months of therapy.

Breast-feeding patients
■ No data exists to show whether modafinil appears in breast milk. Because many drugs are, however, give modafinil cautiously to a breast-feeding woman.

Pediatric patients
■ Safety and efficacy haven't been established in patients under age 16.

Geriatric patients
■ Safety and efficacy in patients over age 65 haven't been established.
■ Consider a reduced dosage for elderly patients because elimination of the drug and its metabolites may be reduced.

Patient teaching
■ Warn patient not to take any other prescribed drugs, OTC medications, or herbal remedies during therapy without consulting prescriber.
■ Urge patient to avoid alcohol while taking modafinil.
■ Tell patient to notify prescriber about a rash, hives, or a related allergic reaction.
■ Caution patient to avoid hazardous activities until drug's full CNS effects are known.

■ Warn woman that modafinil therapy raises the risk of pregnancy with oral, depot, and implanted contraceptives. Suggest using a different or additional method of contraception during therapy and for 1 month afterward.
■ Tell women to notify prescriber if they intend to breast-feed.

---

pemoline
Cylert

Pharmacologic classification: oxazolidinedione derivative

Therapeutic classification: CNS stimulant

Controlled substance schedule IV

Pregnancy risk category B

How supplied
Available by prescription only
Tablets: 18.75 mg, 37.5 mg, 75 mg
Tablets (chewable and containing povidone): 37.5 mg

Indications and dosages
Attention deficit hyperactivity disorder
Children age 6 and older: initially, 37.5 mg P.O. given in the morning, increased by 18.75 mg/day at weekly intervals, p.r.n. Effective dosage, 56.25 to 75 mg/day. Maximum, 112.5 mg/day.

Narcolepsy*
Adults: 50 to 200 mg/day, divided and given after breakfast and lunch.

Pharmacodynamics

CNS stimulant action: Pemoline differs structurally from methylphenidate and amphetamines; however, like those drugs, it has a paradoxical calming effect on children with attention deficit hyperactivity disorder (ADHD). Its mechanism of action is unknown, but it may be mediated by dopamine. The drug's CNS stimulant effect has been studied in adults with narcolepsy, in fatigue, in depressed and schizophrenic patients, and in elderly patients.

Pharmacokinetics

Absorption: Drug is well absorbed after oral administration. Therapeutic effects peak within 4 hours and persist for about 8 hours.
Distribution: Distribution is unknown. Drug is 50% protein-bound.
Metabolism: Pemoline is metabolized by the liver to active and inactive metabolites.
Excretion: Drug and its metabolites are excreted in urine; 75% of an oral dose is excreted within 24 hours.

Contraindications and precautions

Contraindicated in patients with hepatic dysfunction and hypersensitivity or unusual reactions to drug.

Use cautiously in patients with impaired renal or hepatic function.

Interactions

Drug-food
Caffeine: may decrease pemoline efficacy in ADHD. Avoid concurrent use.

Adverse reactions

CNS: abnormal oculomotor function, dizziness, drowsiness, dyskinetic movements, fatigue, hallucinations, headache, *insomnia,* irritability, mild depression, **seizures,** *Tourette syndrome.*
GI: abdominal pain, anorexia, nausea.
Hematologic: *aplastic anemia.*
Hepatic: elevated liver enzymes, HEPATIC FAILURE.
Skin: rash.

Overdose and treatment

Overdose may cause agitation, excitement, hallucinations, hyperreflexia, irregular respirations, restlessness, and tachycardia.

Provide symptomatic, supportive treatment. Place patient in a cool room, monitor her temperature, minimize stimulation, and protect her from injury. Perform gastric lavage if symptoms aren't severe. Monitor patient's vital signs and fluid and electrolyte balance. Consider giving chlorpromazine or haloperidol to reverse CNS stimulation. Hemodialysis may help.

Special considerations

■ Keep in mind that drug has abuse potential; discourage its use for analeptic effect because CNS stimulation superimposed on CNS depression may cause neuronal instability and seizures.
■ Determine patient's baseline liver function, and obtain liver function tests periodically. If abnormalities arise, discontinue therapy.
■ To minimize insomnia and provide maximum daytime benefit, give drug in a single morning dose.

■ Because drug may precipitate Tourette syndrome, monitor patient closely during the start of therapy.

■ Check patient's vital signs regularly for increased blood pressure or other signs of excessive CNS stimulation.

■ Monitor patient's CBC, differential, and platelet counts during long-term therapy.

■ Measure blood and urine glucose levels in diabetic patients because drug may alter insulin requirements.

■ Avoid abrupt withdrawal after high-dose, long-term use because it may unmask severe depression. Instead, taper the dosage gradually to prevent acute rebound depression.

■ Make sure patient gets adequate rest; fatigue may result as drug wears off.

■ Although pemoline has been used to treat narcolepsy, depression, and schizophrenia, these uses are controversial.

Pediatric patients
■ Because it raises the risk of life-threatening hepatic failure, avoid using pemoline as first-line therapy for children with ADHD.

■ Drug isn't recommended for treating ADHD in children under age 6.

■ Drug has been linked to growth suppression; check patient's height and weight during therapy.

Patient teaching
■ Explain the need for therapy and the anticipated risks and benefits. Review the signs and symptoms of adverse reactions, and urge patient or parent to report them.

■ Explain that therapeutic effects may not appear for 3 to 4 weeks.

■ Caution patient to avoid hazardous activities until drug's full CNS effects are known.

■ Tell patient to avoid caffeine-containing beverages because they can increase CNS stimulation.

■ Caution patient or parent not to alter dosage without consulting prescriber.

■ Suggest intermittent drug-free periods during such low-stress times as weekends and school holidays. These periods can help to establish patient's condition, prevent drug tolerance, and allow a decreased dosage when therapy resumes.

■ Warn patient not to use drug to relieve fatigue. Urge patient to get adequate rest and to report excessive CNS stimulation.

■ Instruct diabetic patient to monitor blood glucose levels carefully because drug may alter insulin needs.

CHAPTER 11

Drugs for treating alcoholism and substance abuse

373 ■ **Introduction**

385 ■ **Generic drugs**

■ bupropion hydrochloride

■ chlordiazepoxide, chlordiazepoxide hydrochloride (See Chapter 4, ANTIANXIETY DRUGS)

■ clonidine hydrochloride

■ clorazepate dipotassium (See Chapter 4, ANTIANXIETY DRUGS)

■ diazepam (See Chapter 4, ANTIANXIETY DRUGS)

■ disulfiram

■ flumazenil

■ mesoridazine besylate (See Chapter 9, ANTIPSYCHOTICS)

■ methadone hydrochloride

■ naloxone hydrochloride

■ naltrexone hydrochloride

■ nicotine

■ nicotine polacrilex

■ oxazepam (See Chapter 4, ANTIANXIETY DRUGS)

Alcoholism and other substance disorders affect more than 25% of American adults at some point in their lives. For some people, the term *substance abuse* is most applicable to their condition. For others, the term *substance dependence* is more appropriate. Criteria for these two substance disorders appear in the *Diagnostic and Statistical Manual of Mental Disorders*, 4th edition. In general, the criteria that define abuse and dependence are the same across all substances. (See *Defining substance abuse and dependence*, page 374.) Typically, substance dependence is the focus of professional treatment; substance abuse isn't.

For some substance disorders, such as cocaine dependence, no drugs are available to aid in treatment. For dependence on alcohol, nicotine, and opioids, however, drugs of several different types may be helpful, such as benzodiazepines, antidepressants, opioid antagonists, opioid agonists, anticonvulsants, and antihypertensives.

UNDERSTANDING ALCOHOLISM

Alcohol (ethanol) dependence affects about 20% of men and 11% of women at some point in their lives. Alcohol is a central nervous system (CNS) depressant that probably potentiates the receptor function of the inhibitory amino acid gamma-aminobutyric acid (GABA) and inhibits the receptor function of the excitatory amino acid N-methyl-D-aspartate (NMDA). Alcohol also acts on noradrenergic, dopaminergic, serotonergic, and opioid pathways.

Long-term exposure to alcohol most likely decreases synthesis of GABA and increases synthesis of NMDA. When alcohol use abruptly stops, the relative lack of GABA and relative excess of NMDA probably play a role creating the symptoms of alcohol withdrawal.

Another possible mechanism for alcohol withdrawal is that of neuronal sensitization, or "kindling." Kindling is a process by which repeated exposure to electrical or chemical stimuli causes progressively exaggerated neuronal responses to those stimuli. With alcohol, repeated withdrawal syndromes may lead to increased CNS excitability and progressively severe withdrawal symptoms. That's why antikindling drugs are sometimes used to treat alcohol withdrawal.

Treating alcoholism

Treatment of alcohol dependence involves several steps. The first is to address the symptoms of acute withdrawal. (See *Elements of alcohol withdrawal*, page 375.) Once the patient successfully navigates withdrawal, the next step is to maintain abstinence and prevent a relapse back to alcohol dependence.

Also, look for medical problems that may have been caused by or worsened by long-term alcohol consumption. Medical complications of alcoholism are common and varied; it affects virtually all organ systems. Common examples of medical complications of alcoholism include liver disease, gastrointestinal (GI) disease, anemia, malnutrition, and CNS disturbances.

Defining substance abuse and dependence

The terms *substance abuse* and *substance dependence* refer to two different conditions, one more serious than the other. Substance abuse includes the following characteristics:

- continued use of a substance despite persistent social or work problems that stem from its use
- recurrent substance-related legal problems
- recurrent use of a substance in situations where it's physically hazardous to do so (such as drinking while driving).

Substance dependence is a more severe disorder characterized by at least three of the following during a single 12-month period:

- having physical tolerance to the substance
- having withdrawal symptoms after abruptly stopping the substance
- using increasing amounts of the substance or using the substance over a longer period of time
- having a persistent desire to cut down on use of the substance or making unsuccessful efforts to stop using it
- spending large amounts of time to obtain the substance or to recover from its effects
- restricting or giving up important social or work activities because of substance use
- using the substance despite knowing that persistent or recurrent physical or psychological problems probably result from it or are worsened by it.

Managing withdrawal

In theory, any CNS depressant that's cross-tolerant to alcohol could be used to treat alcohol withdrawal, including benzodiazepines, barbiturates, even alcohol itself. Benzodiazepines are the drugs of choice because they're safer in high doses and have fewer adverse effects than the others. Those used most commonly include chlordiazepoxide, clorazepate dipotassium, diazepam, lorazepam (unlabeled), and oxazepam.

Longer-acting drugs—such as chlordiazepoxide, clorazepate dipotassium, and diazepam—effectively control alcohol withdrawal with few rebound effects when therapy stops. However, shorter-acting drugs, such as lorazepam and oxazepam, have no active metabolites and may be better for patients with alcoholic liver disease.

The most common way to treat alcohol withdrawal with benzodiazepines is to give an amount that tapers gradually over 3 to 7 days. Various benzodiazepines may be used at equipotent doses (See *Alcohol withdrawal treatment: Comparing benzodiazepines*, page 376.) You can determine a benzodiazepine dosage from the score of an alcohol withdrawal assessment scale, such as the Clinical Institute Withdrawal Assessment for Alcohol. This tool and the shorter revised version each produce an

Elements of alcohol withdrawal

Alcohol withdrawal is a progressive, occasionally life-threatening condition. Symptoms may begin within hours after the patient stops drinking, and they may last 3 to 7 days. Usually, they're mild to moderate even if the patient receives no treatment to minimize them. They typically include the following:

- anxiety
- autonomic hyperactivity, which may cause tachycardia, diaphoresis, and increased blood pressure
- depression
- insomnia
- nausea
- tremor
- vomiting.

Usually, these symptoms subside on their own over a few days. However, in a small number of patients, symptoms progress to a more serious level. For example, some patients develop hallucinations (primarily visual or auditory). About 10 to 15% develop seizures (usually the tonic-clonic type). And less than 1% develop delirium tremens.

Delirium tremens is a syndrome of acute autonomic hyperactivity that includes severe hyperthermia and delirium. About 20% of patients who progress to this stage of withdrawal die, usually from cerebrovascular accident or cardiovascular collapse.

Because you have no way of knowing which patients will have mild, self-limiting symptoms and which will progress to seizures or delirium tremens, your best course of action for any patient undergoing alcohol withdrawal is to assess him closely and begin supportive treatment quickly if needed.

---

objective score of the severity of a patient's alcohol withdrawal. The benzodiazepine dosage can be derived from that score.

Other drugs show promise in treating alcohol withdrawal as well. One is the antikindling drug carbamazepine, which may be as effective as oxazepam at treating alcohol withdrawal in inpatient alcoholics. The typical dosage is 200 mg three to four times daily for 5 to 7 days. Another is the centrally acting antihypertensive clonidine.

Because chronic alcohol ingestion can cause nutritional deficits, it's important to provide nutritional supplementation as well as drug treatment during alcohol withdrawal. Alcoholics are commonly deficient in thiamine (vitamin B_1), which may lead to Wernicke's encephalopathy. Folic acid also may be diminished. During withdrawal, the patient should take 100 mg of thiamine daily, along with a multivitamin and folic acid. Maintenance of fluid and electrolyte balance is also important during alcohol withdrawal.

Preventing relapse

Two drugs can be used to help prevent a relapse into alcohol depen-

Alcohol withdrawal treatment: Comparing benzodiazepines

DRUG	METABOLITES	EQUIVALENT DOSE (MG)
chlordiazepoxide	■ desmethylchlordiazepoxide ■ desmethyldiazepam ■ demoxepam	10
clorazepate	■ desmethyldiazepam	7.5
diazepam	■ desmethyldiazepam ■ nordiazepam	5
lorazepam	■ inactive glucuronide conjugate	1
oxazepam	■ inactive glucuronide conjugate	15

dence: disulfiram or naltrexone. Disulfiram is an aversive drug that makes the patient physically ill when he drinks alcohol during drug treatment. The prospect of this unpleasant (possibly life-threatening) reaction may help to decrease the patient's alcohol cravings. Naturally, your frank descrpition of this reaction also helps to reduce the patient's cravings.

Perhaps the biggest problem in using disulfiram to prevent relapse is that it requires the patient to comply with drug therapy—which many patients don't. That's why many clinicians require that someone watch the patient take his medication at least three days each week. The observer may be a clinic staff member or a friend or family member.

Naltrexone seems to reduce the craving for alcohol and the number of drinking days, particularly when drug treatment is combined with psychosocial treatment. Unlike disulfiram, naltrexone isn't an aversive drug. Instead, it seems to block some of the reinforcing properties of alcohol, thereby decreasing the desire to drink. Despite its promising effects, however, naltrexone is rarely used in community settings, possibly because of its cost. It also does nothing to dissuade the patient from relapsing into dependence if he takes another drink.

Therapy with disulfiram or naltrexone can help to decrease alcohol craving and decrease the amount of alcohol consumed if a relapse does occur. However, preventing relapse commonly involves much more than just drug therapy. Supportive programs, such as Alcoholics Anonymous, can be crucial in maintaining a patient's recovery. For some patients, combined psychotherapy and drug therapy offer the best chance at continued recovery.

Drug effects

Benzodiazepines help patients weather alcohol withdrawal by enhancing GABA, thereby blocking the compensatory CNS excitation caused by alcohol withdrawal.

Carbamazepine, which isn't cross-tolerant with alcohol, seems to improve membrane stabilization through its antikindling effects. The drug not only blocks the seizures that can occur with alcohol withdrawal, but it also improves some of the psychiatric symptoms of alcohol withdrawal, such as anxiety and agitation

Clonidine probably decreases withdrawal symptoms (including diaphoresis, hypertension, tremor, pulse, and agitation) by decreasing noradrenergic outflow from the locus ceruleus. It has no anticonvulsant activity and doesn't seem to affect withdrawal seizures.

Disulfiram produces its unpleasant reaction by inhibiting aldehyde dehydrogenase, which blocks oxidation of alcohol at the acetaldehyde stage. This action significantly increases acetaldehyde levels in the blood, which in turn produces the unpleasant disulfiram reaction that occurs after alcohol ingestion. The disulfiram reaction persists for as long as alcohol is being metabolized. (See *Elements of a disulfiram reaction*.)

Naltrexone is a pure opioid receptor antagonist that blocks the pharmacologic effects of opioid analgesics. By blocking opioid receptors, it also seems to decrease the pleasurable feelings a person receives from drinking.

UNDERSTANDING NICOTINE DEPENDENCE

Although the percentage of American adults who smoke has dropped sharply, smoking remains the single

> ### Elements of a disulfiram reaction
>
> Exposure to alcohol (either ingested or applied topically) while taking disulfiram results in a highly unpleasant reaction that, at its most severe, may be life-threatening. The intensity of a disulfiram reaction varies with the amount of alcohol consumed; the reaction may last from 30 minutes to several hours. A typical disulfiram reaction causes these symptoms:
> - chest pains
> - confusion
> - dyspnea
> - flushing
> - hypotension
> - nausea
> - severe vomiting
> - sweating
> - tachycardia
> - throbbing in the head and neck
> - vertigo.
>
> A severe disulfiram reaction may cause acute heart failure, arrhythmias, cardiovascular collapse, myocardial infarction, respiratory depression, seizures, unconsciousness, and death.

most preventable cause of death in our society. An increasing percentage of smokers are considered heavy smokers, and one of every six deaths in the United States can be attributed to smoking.

Because nicotine produces psychoactive effects and reinforces drug-taking behavior, most people find it exceedingly hard to stop smoking. Indeed, a 1990 Gallup poll found that 74% of smokers wanted to quit but were unable to do so because of their dependence. Of the 46 million current smokers in the United States, 34% try to quit each year, but only 2.5% succeed. For many smokers, drug treatment known as nicotine replacement therapy can help them succeed.

Treating nicotine dependence

Two forms of therapy are available for patients who wish to stop smoking: nicotine replacement therapy and the antidepressant bupropion hydrochloride. Nicotine replacement therapy helps people stop smoking by reducing withdrawal symptoms and partially satisfying the craving for cigarettes. Encourage this form of therapy for all people who smoke except for those in whom it may be contraindicated, such as pregnant women and people with cardiovascular (CV) disease.

Several forms of nicotine replacement therapy are available: transdermal patches, chewing gum, nasal spray, and inhaler. Nicotine gum and two types of patches are available in over-the-counter (OTC) forms. Although each form has advantages and disadvantages, all forms of nicotine replacement therapy improve cessation rates. (See *Comparing nicotine replacement therapies*.) Under strict medical supervision, patients who combine therapies (using both a patch and nicotine gum, for example) may be even more likely to quit smoking.

For patients who use a single form of nicotine replacement therapy, the proper dosage can do much to foster cessation. Encourage patients to use an adequate amount of the chosen nicotine replacement form without exceeding the manufacturer's recommendations. This is especially important early in therapy.

When tested against a placebo, bupropion hydrochloride has doubled patients' ability to stop smoking. This drug was originally marketed as the antidepressant Wellbutrin, but it seems to have similar smoking cessation effects in all patients, whether or not they have a history of depression. Combining bupropion with a nicotine patch may produce higher quit rates than either treatment used alone.

Drug effects

The addictive properties of nicotine stem from its effects on the release of several neurotransmitters, including serotonin, norepinephrine, dopamine, and GABA. By sharply increasing neurotransmitter levels, nicotine causes reward sensations, such as stimulation and pleasure. After chronic stimulation from long-term nicotine use, however, the person develops tolerance to these neurotransmitter effects. The continuous presence of nicotine in the brain then becomes necessary for the person to maintain normal functioning.

Nicotine replacement products provide a way to attain this neurotransmitter stimulation without tobacco. Likewise, bupropion may cause a surge of dopamine similar to the one that follows nicotine administration. Bupropion may reduce withdrawal symptoms (which probably result from increased norepinephrine release) by reduc-

Comparing nicotine replacement therapies

PRODUCT	ADVANTAGES	DISADVANTAGES
nicotine polacrilex Nicorette	■ Available without a prescription ■ Patient-controlled nicotine level	■ Unappealing flavor, jaw fatigue, jaw and mouth soreness, and headache ■ Provides a low nicotine dose, especially the 2-mg strength ■ Hasn't been proven more effective than placebo after 1 year of treatment in a primary care setting
nicotine transdermal systems Habitrol, NicoDerm CQ, Nicotrol, ProStep	■ Available without a prescription ■ Once-a-day dosing ■ Provides a steady level of nicotine, which spares patient from having to respond to nicotine cravings ■ Low abuse potential	■ Local skin reactions in half of patients, although reactions can be minimized by rotating application sites and applying corticosteroid cream ■ Risk of sleep disturbances with 24-hour patches ■ Patient can't control amount of nicotine received ■ Low morning nicotine coverage with 16-hour patches
nicotine nasal spray Nicotrol NS	■ Patient-controlled nicotine level ■ Nicotine levels that peak 15 minutes after using spray, which mimics the action of nicotine after smoking	■ Requires a prescription ■ Nasal and throat irritation in most patients, although it typically diminishes in a few days ■ Greater risk of dependence than with other nicotine replacement therapies
nicotine inhaler Nicotrol Inhaler	■ Patient-controlled nicotine level ■ May satisfy behavioral aspects of smoking (hand-to-mouth ritual)	■ Requires a prescription ■ Possible local irritation, such as burning in throat, coughing, sneezing, hiccups

(continued)

Comparing nicotine replacement therapies (continued)

PRODUCT	ADVANTAGES	DISADVANTAGES
bupropion Zyban	■ More successful than nicotine patch in one large trial ■ May be used safely with the nicotine patch ■ Reduces nicotine cravings without providing nicotine	■ May cause dry mouth and insomnia ■ Not suitable for patients with a history of eating disorders or seizures

ing noradrenergic firing in the locus ceruleus.

Pharmacokinetics

Because nicotine undergoes extensive first-pass metabolism in the liver, nicotine replacement therapies must bypass the liver. Nicotine gum and the nicotine inhaler rely primarily on buccal absorption. The nasal spray form is absorbed through nasal mucosa. And the transdermal patch uses percutaneous absorption. The time needed for nicotine levels to peak varies with the delivery form used:
- nasal spray: 4 to 15 minutes
- inhaler: 15 to 30 minutes
- chewing gum: 25 to 30 minutes
- transdermal patch: 2 to 10 hours.

Nicotine is less than 5% bound to plasma proteins and is eliminated in a biphasic manner with a terminal half-life of 1 to 4 hours. Keep in mind, however, that residual absorption after removal of a transdermal patch may keep nicotine in the patient's system for 12 to 18 hours.

The liver metabolizes nicotine into more than 20 inactive metabolites. The major one is cotinine, which has a plasma half-life of 10 to 40 hours. Nicotine and its metabolites are excreted in urine, with about 20% of an absorbed nicotine dose excreted unchanged.

UNDERSTANDING OPIOID DEPENDENCE

Opioid is a broad term that refers to opium-derived drugs, such as morphine and codeine, as well as synthetic substances, such as hydrocodone and meperidine. All of these products exert their effects by binding with opioid receptors, and all are antagonized by naloxone, an opioid antagonist.

At least five types of opioid receptors exist: μ (mu, two subtypes), K (kappa, three subtypes), Δ (delta, two subtypes), E (epsilon), and Σ (sigma). Analgesia probably results from activation of μ_1, K, and Δ receptors, and possibly E and Σ receptors. Some adverse effects of opioid analgesics—such as sedation, respiratory depression, and decreased GI motility—may stem from activation of μ_2 receptors.

The risk of physical dependence on opioids also may be related to activation of μ_2 receptors. In fact, about 25% of people who use opioids on a sporadic basis become dependent on them. Commonly abused opioids include heroin, hydromorphone, codeine, meperidine, butorphanol, and hydrocodone. Heroin abuse in particular has risen in recent years, with 1996 estimates of more than 340,000 people using heroin during the previous month.

In a person physically dependent on opioids, abrupt discontinuation leads to an opioid withdrawal syndrome. Symptoms usually include sweating, rhinorrhea, nausea, flu-like symptoms, agitation, flushing, diarrhea, muscle cramps, hallucinations, stomach cramps, and sleep disturbances. The time it takes for symptoms to develop depends on the half-life of the drug being used. In general terms, symptoms begin two to three half-lives after the last opioid dose. Half-life also determines how long the withdrawal syndrome may last. For example, for such short-acting opioids as morphine and heroin, withdrawal begins in 6 to 12 hours, peaks in 48 to 72 hours, and may last 7 to 14 days.

Treating opioid dependence

Although opioid withdrawal isn't life-threatening, it may be uncomfortable enough that the addicted person continues to use opioids rather than weather the withdrawal. That's why the goal of detoxification is to limit patient discomfort by reducing withdrawal symptoms as much as possible. Drugs commonly used to accomplish that purpose include cyclobenzaprine to reduce muscle cramps, dicyclomine to reduce GI symptoms, and clonidine to decrease tremors, diaphoresis, and agitation. Another option is to convert the patient to an equivalent dose of another opioid and then gradually reduce the dose to minimize withdrawal. (Because withdrawal can harm a developing fetus, pregnant women addicted to opioids should switch to methadone maintenance instead of undergoing withdrawal.)

If the goal is to speed withdrawal, giving an opioid antagonist such as naloxone or naltrexone (along with clonidine, cyclobenzaprine, and dicyclomine) will precipitate it. The advantage of using an opioid antagonist is that, although the withdrawal may be more severe, it will take much less time than an unassisted withdrawal, especially for a long-acting opioid. A newer process known as ultra-rapid opioid detoxification involves the use of general anesthesia or heavy sedation for patients undergoing detoxification; however, the long-term efficacy and safety of this procedure has yet to be proven.

Using methadone maintenance

The goal of opioid maintenance is to substitute an opioid with a long half-life—usually methadone—for the opioid being abused. (See *An alternative to methadone maintenance,* page 382.)

With a half-life of 24 to 36 hours and good oral bioavailability, methadone can prevent the onset of opioid withdrawal symptoms for 24 hours or more. It also can reduce or eliminate cravings for opioids, and it blocks the effects of

An alternative to methadone maintenance

In some states, methadone may not be the only drug available for treating patients with opioid addiction. The other alternative is levo-alpha-acetyl-methadol (LAAM). Like methadone, LAAM is a long-acting opioid. Unlike methadone, it can prevent the onset of opioid withdrawal for more than 72 hours. LAAM may be the drug of choice for patients who can't come to a clinic each day for their methadone or for patients who have persistent withdrawal symptoms while taking methadone.

Pharmacokinetics

LAAM is well absorbed from the GI tract. It's highly bound to tissue protein, which may contribute to its long duration of action. It hasn't been widely studied in pregnant or breast-feeding women.

The drug undergoes hepatic N-demethylation to nor-levomethadyl acetate (called nor-LAAM). Nor-LAAM is then demethylated to form dinor-levomethadyl acetate (dinor-LAAM). These metabolites are more potent opioid agonists than the parent compound.

Up to about one-third of LAAM and its metabolites undergo renal excretion, and a significant amount is excreted in bile. Enterohepatic recirculation may occur. In patients with severe liver dysfunction, methadone is probably a better choice than LAAM.

Adverse effects

The adverse effects caused by LAAM are similar to those of other opioids. They may include respiratory depression, sedation, constipation, and sexual dysfunction. This drug also may raise the risk of hepatotoxicity.

LAAM may accumulate after repeated doses, especially among patients with impaired renal or hepatic function. However, because of its long half-life, it can accumulate even in healthy patients if given more often than every 48 hours.

Overdose

An overdose of LAAM can be fatal, producing central nervous system depression, respiratory depression, hypothermia, bradycardia, and hypotension. Begin supportive measures immediately, especially to ensure respiration. Parenteral naloxone can help to reverse some of the opioid-induced respiratory depression. Keep in mind, however, that a physically dependent patient may develop withdrawal symptoms that can't by suppressed while naloxone works.

illicitly used opioids, such as heroin. Of the roughly 600,000 opioid-dependent Americans, 115,000 are enrolled in methadone maintenance treatment programs.

Ideally, these programs combine methadone administration with counseling and rehabilitative services. They not only help to manage opioid dependence, but they also cut drug-related crime, the transmission of human immunodeficiency virus from shared needles, and the death rate for opioid-addicted patients.

Preventing relapse

After a patient is completely detoxified from opioids, taking naltrexone can help to prevent relapse, especially in combination with counseling and a 12-step program. Patients typically take either 50 mg/day or 100 to 150 mg two to three times a week.

PATIENT TEACHING

Your teaching topics will differ somewhat based on whether you're treating a patient for alcoholism, nicotine dependence, or opioid dependence.

Alcoholism

- Urge the patient to avoid hazardous activities during therapy because the drug may make him drowsy.
- Caution the patient not to stop the drug abruptly and not to change the dosage without consulting the prescriber.
- Tell him to avoid alcohol and other CNS depressants during therapy because they could cause additive CNS depression.
- If the patient takes disulfiram, describe the reaction that will develop if he drinks alcohol. Explain that he must avoid all sources of alcohol, including alcoholic beverages, vinegars, many liquid cough and cold medications (both prescription and OTC), foods cooked with alcohol, and such topical products as aftershave lotions, colognes, and liniments.
- Tell the patient not to take disulfiram within 12 hours after drinking alcohol.

- If necessary, tell the patient that he may crush disulfiram tablets and mix them with liquid.
- Urge the patient to wear or carry medical identification that documents his use of disulfiram or naltrexone.
- If the patient takes naltrexone, explain that opioid analgesics will have no effect. Stress that taking enough opioid analgesic to overcome the effects of naltrexone can result in coma, serious injury, or death.
- Because naltrexone raises the risk of liver injury, tell the patient to stop taking the drug and to notify the prescriber about white bowel movements, dark urine, yellowing of the eyes, or abdominal pain that lasts longer than a few days.

Nicotine dependence

- If your patient has underlying CV disease, uncontrolled hypertension, insulin-dependent diabetes, or peptic ulcer disease, urge him to consult a physician before self-medicating with nicotine replacement therapy.
- Warn any patient who receives nicotine replacement therapy to avoid cigarettes and other products that contain nicotine during nicotine replacement therapy.
- Because smoking induces hepatic enzymes that can increase the clearance of some drugs (such as theophylline, imipramine, oxazepam, and propranolol), inform patients who take these drugs that their dosages may need adjustment when smoking stops.
- If the patient uses nicotine gum, tell him to chew it on a fixed schedule (about 1 piece every 1 to 2 hours for 1 to 3 months) rather

than an as-needed schedule because doing so typically yields better results.

■ If the patient uses transdermal patches, tell him to apply a patch in the morning on the day he quits and to replace it with a new one every succeeding morning. Make sure he knows how and where to apply it, and how to discard it safely.

■ If the patient takes bupropion, tell him not to exceed the recommended dosage because of the risk of seizures. Also, tell him not to take Wellbutrin with Zyban because they contain the same active ingredient.

■ Tell the patient to avoid alcohol while taking bupropion.

Opioid dependence

■ If your patient takes methadone, make sure he understands the danger of overdose if he takes it more often than prescribed or together with other opioid agonists.

■ Explain that additive sedative effects can result if he combines methadone with benzodiazepines, antidepressants, alcohol, or any other CNS depressant.

■ If the patient has take-home privileges for his opioid replacement doses, urge him to keep them locked up to prevent accidental poisoning of children or other household members.

■ If the patient takes naltrexone, make sure he knows that it will cause withdrawal if he's opioid-dependent.

■ Warn the patient about the risk of taking enough opioid to overcome the effects of naltrexone.

■ Urge the patient to wear or carry medical identification that documents his use of methadone or naltrexone.

bupropion hydrochloride
Zyban

Pharmacologic classification:
aminoketone

Therapeutic classification:
nonnicotine smoking cessation aid

Pregnancy risk category B

How supplied
Available by prescription only
Tablets (sustained-release): 150 mg

Indications and dosages
Smoking cessation treatment
Adults: 150 mg/day P.O. for 3 days.
Increase to maximum of 300 mg/
day P.O., given as two equal doses
taken at least 8 hours apart.

Pharmacodynamics
Smoking cessation action: Drug is a
relatively weak inhibitor of the
neuronal uptake of norepinephrine, serotonin, and dopamine. It
doesn't inhibit MAO. The mechanism by which it enhances the ability to stop smoking is unknown.

Pharmacokinetics
Absorption: After oral use, plasma
levels peak within 3 hours.
Distribution: Volume of distribution from a single 150-mg dose is
estimated to be 1,950 L. Bupropion
is about 80% bound to plasma
proteins at concentrations up to
200 mcg/ml.
Metabolism: Drug is extensively
metabolized in the liver, mainly by
the P-450 2B6 isoenzyme system,
to three active metabolites.
Excretion: Mean elimination half-
life is thought to be about 21

hours. After oral administration,
87% of a dose can be recovered in
urine and 10% in feces. About
0.5% of the dose is excreted unchanged.

Contraindications and precautions
Contraindicated within 14 days of
taking an MAO inhibitor, during
therapy with other drugs that contain bupropion (such as Wellbutrin
and Wellbutrin SR), in patients hypersensitive to drug or its components, and in patients with seizure
disorders or a current or previous
diagnosis of bulimia nervosa or
anorexia nervosa.

Use cautiously in patients with
recent MI, unstable heart disease,
or renal or hepatic impairment.

Interactions
Drug-drug
*Antidepressants, antipsychotics, sys-
temic corticosteroids, theophylline:*
reduced seizure threshold. Use extreme caution when administering
concomitantly.
Benzodiazepines: abrupt benzodiazepine withdrawal lowers seizure
threshold. Use extreme caution
when administering concomitantly.
*Carbamazepine, phenobarbital,
phenytoin:* may induce bupropion
and decrease effects. Increased
bupropion dosage may be needed.
Cimetidine: inhibits bupropion
metabolism and increases effects.
Decreased bupropion dosage may
be needed.
Cyclophosphamide, orphenadrine:
may affect enzyme CYP2B6 metabolism. Since Bupropion is metabolized to hydroxybupropion by this

---

isoenzyme, it may cause an inter-action. Avoid concomitant use.
Levodopa: may increase risk of adverse reactions. Avoid concomitant use if possible. If necessary, give small initial doses of bupropion and increase gradually.
MAO inhibitors, phenelzine: may increase risk of acute bupropion toxicity. Don't administer concurrently.

Drug-herb
St. John's wort: increased risk of serotonin syndrome. Avoid concomitant use.

Adverse reactions
CNS: agitation, dizziness, hot flashes, *insomnia,* somnolence, tremor.
CV: ***complete AV block***, hypertension, hypotension, tachycardia.
EENT: *dry mouth,* taste perversion.
GI: anorexia, dyspepsia, increased appetite.
GU: impotence, polyuria, urinary frequency and urgency.
Metabolic: edema, weight gain.
Musculoskeletal: arthralgia, leg cramps and twitching, myalgia, neck pain.
Respiratory: bronchitis, ***bronchospasm.***
Skin: dry skin, pruritus, rash, urticaria.
Other: allergic reactions.

Overdose and treatment
Overdose may cause labored breathing, salivation, an arched back, ptosis, ataxia, and seizures.
   If patient is conscious and ingestion occurred within 12 hours, perform gastric lavage or induce emesis with syrup of ipecac, as ap-propriate. If the patient is stuporous, comatose, or having seizures, he may need intubation before gastric lavage. Also, give activated charcoal every 6 hours for the first 12 hours. Maintain ECG and EEG monitoring for the first 48 hours. Give a benzodiazepine I.V. for seizures, if needed. Ensure adequate fluid intake, and obtain baseline blood tests. No data are available regarding the benefits of dialysis, hemoperfusion, or diuresis.

Special considerations
■ Make sure the patient isn't taking Wellbutrin, which is bupropion packaged under a different trade name for depression treatment.
■ Because of dose-dependent risk of seizures, don't exceed 300 mg/day for smoking cessation.
■ After patient sets a target date for smoking cessation, start drug therapy about 1 week beforehand, while patient is still smoking. This pattern allows drug to reach steady-state in the patient's blood before the cessation attempt.
■ Therapy usually lasts 7 to 12 weeks. Stop therapy after 7 weeks if patient has made no progress towards abstinence.
■ Dose need not be tapered when stopping treatment.

Breast-feeding patients
■ Drug and its metabolites are secreted in breast milk. Because of possible serious adverse effects in infants, don't combine breast-feeding and bupropion therapy.

Pediatric patients
■ Safety and efficacy in children haven't been established.

Reactions may be *common,* uncommon, ***life-threatening,*** or COMMON AND LIFE-THREATENING.

Geriatric patients
■ Safety and efficacy in patients age 60 and older haven't been established.

Patient teaching
■ Stress the importance of combining behavioral interventions, counseling, and support services with drug therapy to achieve smoking cessation.
■ Instruct patient to separate doses by at least 8 hours.
■ Explain that therapy usually lasts 7 to 12 weeks.
■ Caution patient that smoking during therapy reduces the chance of successful cessation.
■ Warn patient not to take St. John's wort during therapy.
■ Caution patient about an increased risk of seizures if he has a seizure disorder or an eating disorder, if he exceeds the recommended dose, or if he takes other forms of bupropion.
■ Tell patient not to use both drug and nicotine patch unless prescriber approves; concurrent use may increase blood pressure.

---

clonidine hydrochloride
Catapres, Catapres-TTS, Dixarit ◇

Pharmacologic classification:
central-acting alpha agonist, antiadrenergic

Therapeutic classification:
antihypertensive

Pregnancy risk category C

How supplied
Available by prescription only

Tablets: 0.1 mg, 0.2 mg, 0.3 mg
Transdermal: TTS-1 (releases 0.1 mg/24 hours), TTS-2 (releases 0.2 mg/24 hours), TTS-3 (releases 0.3 mg/24 hours)

Indications and dosages
Adjunctive therapy in nicotine withdrawal*
Adults: initially, 0.15 mg/day P.O., gradually increased to 0.4 mg/day P.O. as tolerated. Alternatively, apply transdermal patch (0.2 mg/24 hours) and replace weekly for the first 2 or 3 weeks after smoking cessation.

Adjunctive therapy in opiate withdrawal*
Adults: 5 to 17 mcg/kg/day P.O. in divided doses for up to 10 days. Adjust dosage to avoid hypotension and excessive sedation, and withdraw drug slowly.

Pharmacodynamics
Antihypertensive action: Clonidine decreases peripheral vascular resistance by stimulating central alpha-adrenergic receptors, thus decreasing cerebral sympathetic outflow. Drug may also inhibit renin release. Initially, clonidine may stimulate peripheral alpha-adrenergic receptors, producing transient vasoconstriction.
Smoking cessation and opioid cessation actions: Actions probably involve noradrenergic and dopaminergic effects. The CNS effects of dopamine may influence the reinforcement properties of addictive drugs. Nicotine withdrawal may involve the absence of CNS effects of norepinephrine. Bupropion's weak inhibition of neuronal uptake

---

of norepinephrine and dopamine may play a role.

Pharmacokinetics
Absorption: Clonidine is absorbed well from the GI tract when administered orally. Blood pressure begins to decline in 30 to 60 minutes. Maximum effect occurs in 2 to 4 hours. After topical application, transdermal clonidine is absorbed well; plasma levels reach therapeutic range 2 to 3 days after initial application.
Distribution: Clonidine is distributed widely into the body.
Metabolism: Drug is metabolized in the liver, where nearly 50% is transformed to inactive metabolites.
Excretion: About 65% of a dose is excreted in urine; 20% is excreted in feces. Half-life ranges from 6 to 20 hours in patients with normal renal function.

Contraindications and precautions
Contraindicated in patients hypersensitive to drug. Transdermal form is contraindicated in patients hypersensitive to any component of the adhesive layer.

Use cautiously in patients with severe coronary disease, recent MI, cerebrovascular disease, and impaired hepatic or renal function.

Interactions
Drug-drug
Barbiturates, sedatives: may increase CNS depressant effects of clonidine. Avoid concomitant use.
Beta blockers, such as propranolol: may have additive effects, raising the risk of bradycardia and rebound hypertension with withdrawal. Administer cautiously with clonidine.
MAO inhibitors, tolazoline, tricyclic antidepressants: may inhibit antihypertensive effects of clonidine. Increased clonidine dosage may be needed.

Drug-herb
Capsicum: may reduce antihypertensive effects. Avoid concurrent use.

Drug-lifestyle
Alcohol use: may increase CNS depressant effects of alcohol. Discourage concurrent use.

Adverse reactions
CNS: agitation, depression, *dizziness, drowsiness,* fatigue, malaise, *sedation, weakness.*
CV: *bradycardia,* orthostatic hypotension, *severe rebound hypertension.*
GI: anorexia, *constipation, dry mouth,* nausea, vomiting.
GU: impotence, loss of libido, urine retention.
Metabolic: slightly increased serum glucose levels, weight gain.
Skin: *dermatitis with transdermal patch, pruritus,* rash.

Overdose and treatment
Overdose may cause agitation, apnea, bradycardia, CNS depression, diarrhea, hypertension, hypotension, hypothermia, irritability, lethargy, respiratory depression, and seizures.

Don't induce emesis after an overdose of oral clonidine because rapid onset of CNS depression raises the risk of aspiration. After en-

---

Reactions may be *common,* uncommon, *life-threatening,* or COMMON AND LIFE-THREATENING.

suring an adequate airway, empty the patient's stomach by gastric lavage; follow with activated charcoal. If overdose occurs from transdermal therapy, remove patch and provide symptomatic, supportive treatment.

Special considerations
■ Drug reduces symptoms of withdrawal, such as irritability, frustration, anger, anxiety, difficulty concentrating, restlessness, and a depressed mood.
■ Monitor patient's weight daily at the start of therapy to detect possible fluid retention.
■ Monitor patient's pulse and blood pressure frequently, and adjust dosage according to patient's response and tolerance.
■ Patients with renal impairment may respond to smaller doses of drug.
■ Give drug 4 to 6 hours before scheduled surgery.
■ Don't stop drug abruptly; instead, reduce dosage gradually over 2 to 4 days to prevent severe rebound hypertension.
■ Clonidine may decrease urine excretion of vanillylmandelic acid and catecholamines. It may slightly increase blood or serum glucose levels, and it may cause a weakly positive Coombs' test.
■ Clonidine may be used to lower blood pressure quickly in some hypertensive emergencies.
■ Remove transdermal patch during defibrillation or synchronized cardioversion because of its electrical conductivity.
■ Drug is also used to diagnose pheochromocytoma and to treat delayed growth in children, diabet-ic diarrhea, hypertension, menopausal symptoms, neuralgia, ulcerative colitis, and vascular headache.

Breast-feeding patients
■ Clonidine appears in breast milk. Recommend an alternate feeding method during therapy.

Pediatric patients
■ Safety and efficacy in children haven't been established; make sure potential benefits outweigh possible risks.

Geriatric patients
■ Elderly patients may be more sensitive to the hypotensive effects of clonidine and, consequently, may need lower doses.
■ Monitor patient's renal function closely during therapy.

Patient teaching
■ Explain the reason for therapy; emphasize the importance of follow-up visits in establishing therapeutic regimen.
■ Discuss the value of adjunctive therapies to increase the likelihood of smoking cessation, such as behavioral therapies, counseling, and support services.
■ To minimize the effects of orthostatic hypotension, caution patient to avoid sudden position changes.
■ Warn patient to avoid hazardous activities until he develops tolerance to sedation, drowsiness, and other CNS effects.
■ If patient develops a dry mouth, suggest using ice chips or sugar-free hard candy or gum.
■ Review possible adverse effects and the need to report them. Urge patient to notify prescriber about a

weight gain of more than 5 pounds (2.27 kg) in a single week.

■ Tell patient not to stop drug suddenly because rebound hypertension may develop.

■ If patient uses a transdermal patch, tell him to rotate the application site weekly. Remind him to remove the old patch before applying a new one.

■ Warn patient not to take other prescribed drugs, OTC medications, or herbal remedies without consulting prescriber.

■ To ensure nighttime blood pressure control, tell patient to take last dose at bedtime.

■ Advise women of childbearing age to use effective birth control and to notify prescriber about intended, suspected, or known pregnancy.

---

disulfiram
Antabuse

Pharmacologic classification:
aldehyde dehydrogenase inhibitor

Therapeutic classification: alcohol deterrent

Pregnancy risk category NR

How supplied
Available by prescription only
Tablets: 250 mg, 500 mg

Indications and dosages
Chronic alcoholism (adjunctive therapy)
Adults: 500 mg P.O. (maximum) as a single dose in the morning for 1 to 2 weeks. Then 125 to 500 mg daily (average, 250 mg) until patient achieves permanent self-control. Treatment may continue for months or years.

Pharmacodynamics
Antialcoholic action: Disulfiram irreversibly inhibits aldehyde dehydrogenase, which prevents the oxidation of alcohol after the acetaldehyde stage. Drug interacts with ingested alcohol to produce acetaldehyde levels five to 10 times higher than those produced by normal alcohol metabolism. Excess acetaldehyde produces a highly unpleasant reaction (nausea, vomiting, and other symptoms) to even a small quantity of alcohol. Tolerance to disulfiram doesn't develop; rather, sensitivity to alcohol increases as therapy continues.

Pharmacokinetics
Absorption: Disulfiram is absorbed completely after oral administration, but effects may not occur for 3 to 12 hours. Toxic reactions to alcohol may occur up to 2 weeks after taking the last dose.
Distribution: Drug is highly lipid-soluble and is initially localized in adipose tissue.
Metabolism: Drug is mostly oxidized in the liver and excreted in urine as free drug and metabolites, such as carbon disulfide, diethylamine, and diethyldithiocarbamate.
Excretion: Most of drug is excreted in urine; 5% to 20% is unabsorbed and eliminated in feces. A small amount is eliminated through the lungs. Total elimination may take several days.

Reactions may be *common,* uncommon, *life-threatening,* or COMMON AND LIFE-THREATENING.

Contraindications and precautions

Contraindicated in patients intoxicated by alcohol or within 12 hours of alcohol ingestion (including alcohol-containing medicines and other products). Contraindicated in patients receiving metronidazole or paraldehyde and in patients with psychoses, myocardial disease, coronary occlusion, or hypersensitivity to disulfiram or to other thiuram derivatives used in pesticides and rubber vulcanization.

Use with extreme caution in patients who are receiving phenytoin or who have diabetes mellitus, hypothyroidism, seizure disorders, cerebral damage, nephritis, or hepatic cirrhosis or insufficiency. Don't give drug during pregnancy.

Interactions
Drug-drug

Alfentanil: may prolong disulfiram duration of effect. Reduced disulfiram dosage may be needed.

Bacampicillin: may precipitate disulfiram reaction. Don't administer together.

Barbiturates, chlordiazepoxide, CNS depressants, coumarin anticoagulants, diazepam, midazolam, paraldehyde, phenytoin: disulfiram may decrease metabolism of these drugs and increase their blood levels. Monitor their levels when giving them concurrently, and adjust dosages as needed.

Isoniazid: may produce ataxia, unsteady gait, or marked behavioral changes. Avoid concomitant use.

Metronidazole: increased risk of psychosis or confusion. Avoid concomitant use.

Tricyclic antidepressants, especially amitryptiline: may cause transient delirium. Monitor patient for this complication if concurrent use is necessary.

Drug-herb

Passion flower, pill-bearing spurge, pokeweed, squaw vine, squill, sundew, sweet flag, tormentil, valerian, yarrow: may cause disulfiram reaction if herbal form contains alcohol. Don't use together.

Drug-food

Caffeine: metabolism is inhibited by disulfiram, which greatly increases its half-life and may cause exaggerated or prolonged caffeine effects. Avoid concomitant use.

Drug-lifestyle

Alcohol use (including all sources, such as cough syrups, liniments, shaving lotions, back-rub preparations): may cause a disulfiram reaction for up to 2 weeks after single disulfiram dose. The longer disulfiram therapy lasts, the more sensitive the patient becomes to alcohol. Avoid alcohol for 2 weeks after disulfiram therapy stops.

Marijuana: possible synergistic CNS stimulation. Avoid concomitant use.

Adverse reactions

CNS: delirium, depression, drowsiness, fatigue, headache, neuritis, peripheral neuritis, polyneuritis, psychotic reactions, restlessness.

EENT: optic neuritis.

GI: garlic or metallic aftertaste.

GU: impotence.

Metabolic: elevated serum cholesterol.

Skin: acneiform or allergic dermatitis, occasional eruptions.
Other: *disulfiram reaction* (from alcohol use), which may include anxiety, arthropathy, blurred vision, chest pain, confusion, copious vomiting, diaphoresis, dyspnea, flushing, hyperventilation, hypotension, nausea, palpitations, syncope, thirst, throbbing headache, and weakness. A severe reaction may cause *acute heart failure, arrhythmias, CV collapse, MI, respiratory depression, seizures, unconsciousness, or death.*

Overdose and treatment
Overdose may cause abnormal EEG findings, altered consciousness, coma, drowsiness, GI upset, hallucinations, incoordination, speech impairment, and vomiting.

Treat an overdose with gastric aspiration or lavage and supportive therapy.

Special considerations
■ Disulfiram therapy requires close medical supervision. Patient must clearly understand the consequences of disulfiram use and must give informed consent before therapy starts.
■ Administer drug only if patient is cooperative, motivated, and receiving supportive psychiatric therapy.
■ A complete physical examination and laboratory studies (including CBC, electrolytes, transaminases) should precede therapy and be repeated regularly.
■ Don't start disulfiram until at least 12 hours have passed since alcohol ingestion.

■ If morning dose causes drowsiness, allow patient to take drug in the evening.
■ Disulfiram may decrease urinary vanillylmandelic acid excretion and increase urine levels of homovanillic acid. Rarely, it may decrease ^{131}I uptake or protein-bound iodine levels.
■ Treatment of alcohol-induced disulfiram reaction is supportive and symptomatic. Although the reaction usually isn't life-threatening, keep emergency equipment and drugs available because arrhythmias and severe hypotension may occur. Treat severe reactions as you would treat shock, by giving plasma or electrolyte solutions as needed. Large I.V. doses of ascorbic acid, iron, and antihistamines have been used but are of uncertain value. Hypokalemia has been reported; it requires careful monitoring and potassium supplements.

Patient teaching
■ Explain that disulfiram helps to discourage alcohol use but doesn't cure alcoholism.
■ Describe the seriousness of a disulfiram reaction and the consequences of alcohol use during therapy.
■ Warn patient to avoid all sources of alcohol, including some prescribed and herbal preparations, cough syrups, and foods made with wine, sherry, cooking wine, or liqueur. Even external use of alcohol, as in after-shave lotions or liniments, may cause a disulfiram reaction.
■ Tell patient that alcohol reaction may occur for up to 2 weeks after a single dose of disulfiram. The

---

Reactions may be *common,* uncommon, *life-threatening,* or COMMON AND LIFE-THREATENING.

longer the disulfiram therapy, the more sensitive the patient will be to alcohol.
■ Warn patient that drug may cause drowsiness.
■ Instruct patient to carry medical identification that identifies his use of disulfiram and includes the phone number of the prescriber or clinic to contact if a reaction occurs.
■ Advise women of childbearing age to use effective birth control and to immediately notify prescriber about planned, suspected, or known pregnancy.

flumazenil
Romazicon

Pharmacologic classification: benzodiazepine antagonist

Therapeutic classification: antidote

Pregnancy risk category C

How supplied
Available by prescription only
Injection: 0.1 mg/ml in 5-ml and 10-ml multiple-dose vials

Indications and dosages
Complete or partial reversal of benzodiazepine sedative effects (conscious sedation) after anesthesia or short diagnostic procedures
Adults: initially, 0.2 mg I.V. over 15 seconds. If patient fails to reach desired level of consciousness after 45 seconds, repeat dose at 1-minute intervals until you've given a cumulative dose of 1 mg (the first

dose plus four more doses). Most patients respond after receiving 0.6 to 1 mg. If resedation occurs, dosage may be repeated after 20 minutes, but patient should receive no more than 1 mg at one time and 3 mg/hour.

Suspected benzodiazepine overdose
Adults: initially, 0.2 mg I.V. over 30 seconds. If patient fails to reach desired level of consciousness after 30 seconds, give 0.3 mg over 30 seconds. If response still isn't adequate, give 0.5 mg over 30 seconds and repeat 0.5-mg doses at 1-minute intervals until you've given a cumulative dose of 3 mg. Most patients with benzodiazepine overdose respond to cumulative doses of 1 and 3 mg; rarely, patients who respond partially after 3 mg may require additional doses. Don't give more than 5 mg over 5 minutes initially; sedation that persists after this amount is unlikely to be caused by benzodiazepines. If resedation occurs, dosage may be repeated after 20 minutes, but patient should receive no more than 1 mg at one time and 3 mg/hour.

Pharmacodynamics
Antidote action: Flumazenil competitively inhibits the actions of benzodiazepines on the gamma-aminobutyric acid-benzodiazepine receptor complex.

Pharmacokinetics
Absorption: Action begins 1 to 2 minutes after injection. An 80% response occurs within 3 minutes; effects peak in 6 to 10 minutes.

Distribution: Initial distribution half-life is 7 to 15 minutes, and drug redistributes rapidly. It's about 50% bound to plasma proteins.

Metabolism: Drug is rapidly extracted from the blood and metabolized by the liver. Metabolites that have been identified are inactive. Ingestion of food during an I.V. infusion enhances extraction of drug from plasma, probably by increasing hepatic blood flow.

Excretion: About 90% to 95% of drug appears in urine as metabolites; the rest is excreted in the feces. Plasma half-life is about 54 minutes.

Contraindications and precautions

Contraindicated in patients hypersensitive to drug or to benzodiazepines, in patients who show evidence of serious tricyclic antidepressant overdose, and in those who received a benzodiazepine to treat a potentially life-threatening condition (such as status epilepticus). Mixed overdoses should not receive flumazenil, especially if seizures (from any cause) are likely to occur.

Use cautiously in alcohol-dependent or psychiatric patients, in those at high risk for developing seizures, and in those with head injuries, signs of seizures, or a recent therapeutic use of high benzodiazepine doses (as in the ICU).

Interactions
Drug-drug

Antidepressants, drugs that can cause seizures or arrhythmias: increased risk of seizures or arrhythmias after flumazenil removes the effects of benzodiazepine overdose. Monitor the patient closely for seizures or arrhythmias.

Adverse reactions

CNS: agitation, *dizziness,* emotional lability, *headache,* insomnia, *seizures,* tremor.
CV: *arrhythmias,* cutaneous vasodilation, palpitations.
EENT: *abnormal or blurred vision.*
GI: nausea, vomiting.
Respiratory: dyspnea, hyperventilation.
Skin: *diaphoresis.*
Other: *pain* (at injection site).

Overdose and treatment

In clinical trials, large doses of flumazenil I.V. given to volunteers who had no benzodiazepine agonist produced no serious adverse reactions, clinical signs or symptoms, or altered laboratory tests. In patients with benzodiazepine overdose, large flumazenil doses may cause agitation or anxiety, hyperesthesia, increased muscle tone, or seizures. Seizures may be treated with barbiturates, phenytoin, or benzodiazepines.

Special considerations

■ Flumazenil may be given by direct injection or diluted with compatible solution. After 24 hours, discard unused drug that has been drawn into a syringe or diluted.
■ To minimize pain at injection site, give drug through a freely flowing I.V. solution running into a large vein. Compatible solutions include D_5W, lactated Ringer's injection, and normal saline solution.

Reactions may be *common,* uncommon, *life-threatening,* or COMMON AND LIFE-THREATENING.

- Take safety precautions because drug may cause agitation,
- Because flumazenil has a shorter duration of action than benzodiazepines, resedation may occur after initial reversal of benzodiazepine effect. Monitor patient for resedation according to duration of drug being reversed, particularly long-acting benzodiazepines (such as diazepam) or high doses of shorter-acting benzodiazepines (such as 10 mg of midazolam). Usually, serious resedation is unlikely if patient has no sign of it 2 hours after a 1-mg dose of flumazenil.
- If patient is physically dependent on benzodiazepines, watch closely for seizures.
- If patient has a history of panic disorder, expect flumazenil to cause an increased risk of panic attacks.

Breast-feeding patients
- Because no data are available regarding excretion of drug into breast milk, use drug cautiously in breast-feeding women.

Pediatric patients
- Because no data are available regarding risks, benefits, or dosage range in children, drug isn't recommended for children.

Patient teaching
- Because of the risk of resedation, urge patient to avoid hazardous activities, alcohol, CNS depressants, and OTC drugs for 24 hours after treatment.

methadone hydrochloride
Dolophine, Methadose

Pharmacologic classification: opioid

Therapeutic classification: analgesic, narcotic detoxification adjunct

Controlled substance schedule II

Pregnancy risk category C

How supplied
Available by prescription only
Injection: 10 mg/ml
Oral solution: 5 mg/5 ml, 10 mg/ 5 ml, 10 mg/ml (concentrate)
Tablets: 5 mg, 10 mg, 40 mg for oral solution (for narcotic abstinence syndrome)

Indications and dosages
Narcotic abstinence syndrome
Adults: 15 to 20 mg P.O. daily (highly individualized). Maintenance dosage is 20 to 120 mg P.O. daily. Adjust dose, p.r.n. Daily doses above 120 mg require special state and federal approval. If patient feels nauseated, give 25% of total P.O. dose in two injections, S.C. or I.M.

Pharmacodynamics
Analgesic action: Methadone is an opiate agonist with analgesic activity caused by an affinity for opiate receptors similar to that of morphine. It is recommended for severe, chronic pain and is also used in detoxification and maintenance of patients with opiate abstinence syndrome.

Pharmacokinetics
Absorption: Methadone is well absorbed from the GI tract. Compared to parenteral administration, oral administration delays onset and prolongs duration of action. Action begins and effects peak in 30 to 60 minutes.
Distribution: Drug is highly bound to tissue protein, which may explain its cumulative effects and slow elimination.
Metabolism: Methadone is metabolized primarily in the liver by N-demethylation.
Excretion: Duration of action is 4 to 6 hours, increasing to 22 to 48 hours with multiple dosing. Half-life is prolonged (7 to 11 hours) in patients with hepatic dysfunction. Excretion in urine, the major route, is dose-dependent. Methadone metabolites are also excreted in feces via bile.

Contraindications and precautions
Contraindicated in patients hypersensitive to drug.

Use cautiously in elderly or debilitated patients and in those with acute abdominal conditions, Addison's disease, asthma or other respiratory disorders, head injury, hypothyroidism, increased intracranial pressure, prostatic hyperplasia, severe renal or hepatic impairment, or urethral stricture.

Interactions
Drug-drug
CNS depressants, such as *antidepressants, antihistamines, barbiturates, benzodiazepines, general anesthetics, muscle relaxants, narcotic analgesics, phenothiazines,* and

sedative-hypnotics: increased respiratory and CNS depression, sedation, and hypotensive effects. Avoid concomitant use.
Cimetidine: may increase respiratory and CNS depression, causing confusion, disorientation, apnea, or seizures. Reduced methadone dosage may be needed.
Opioid antagonist: may cause acute withdrawal syndrome in patients physically dependent on methadone. Use with caution, and monitor closely.
Rifampin: may reduce methadone blood level. Dosage adjustment may be needed.

Drug-lifestyle
Alcohol use: increased respiratory and CNS depression, sedation, and hypotensive effects. Discourage alcohol consumption during methadone treatment.

Adverse reactions
CNS: agitation, *choreic movements, clouded sensorium, dizziness, euphoria,* headache, insomnia, *lightheadedness, sedation,* **seizures** (with large doses), *somnolence,* syncope.
CV: **bradycardia, cardiac arrest,** edema, *hypotension,* palpitations, *shock.*
EENT: visual disturbances.
GI: *anorexia, biliary tract spasm, constipation, dry mouth, ileus, nausea, vomiting.*
GU: *decreased libido, urine retention.*
Respiratory: **respiratory arrest, respiratory depression.**
Skin: *diaphoresis,* induration (after S.C. injection), pruritus, tissue irritation, urticaria.

Other: pain at injection site, physical dependence.

Overdose and treatment

Overdose commonly causes CNS depression, respiratory depression, and miosis (pinpoint pupils). It also may cause apnea, bradycardia, cardiopulmonary arrest, circulatory collapse, hypotension, hypothermia, pulmonary edema, seizures, and shock. Toxicity may result from an accumulation of drug over several weeks.

To treat acute overdose, ensure a patent airway, and provide ventilation as needed. If the patient has clinically significant respiratory or CV depression, give naloxone. Because methadone has a longer duration of action than naloxone, be prepared to give repeated naloxone doses if necessary. Monitor patient's vital signs closely.

If oral overdose occurred within 2 hours, empty patient's stomach immediately by inducing emesis with ipecac syrup or performing gastric lavage. Follow with activated charcoal via nasogastric tube. Use caution because of the risk of aspiration. Provide continued respiratory support, and correct fluid or electrolyte imbalance. Monitor patient's laboratory values, vital signs, and neurologic status closely.

Special considerations

■ A patient addicted to heroin or opiates who starts a methadone maintenance program may develop acute withdrawal that includes coldlike symptoms, body aches, abdominal cramps, nausea, irritability, depression, and diarrhea. Patient probably will need another analgesic if pain control is necessary.

■ At the start of methadone maintenance, patient must be observed taking drug each day. At-home doses will increase as program continues without incident.

■ Before giving methadone, verify patient's participation in a methadone maintenance program, and confirm correct dosage.

■ Oral liquid form (not tablets) is legally required and is the only form available in drug maintenance programs.

■ Dispersible tablets may be dissolved in 4 oz (120 ml) of water or fruit juice; oral concentrate must be diluted to at least 3 oz (90 ml) with water before administration.

■ Drug may also be used to treat severe, chronic pain. Regimented, round-the-clock scheduling is most beneficial. Tolerance may develop with long-term use, and patient may need a higher dosage to achieve the same degree of analgesia.

■ Physical and psychological dependence may occur. Be aware of potential for abuse.

■ Respiratory depression, hypotension, profound sedation, or coma may result from concomitant use with alcohol, general anesthetics, hypnotics, MAO inhibitors, sedatives, tranquilizers, or tricyclic antidepressants. Use extreme caution, and monitor patient's response.

■ Methadone increases plasma amylase levels.

Breast-feeding patients

■ Methadone appears in breast milk and may cause physical dependence in breast-feeding infants.

Pediatric patients
- Drug is not recommended for use in children.
- Safe use as a maintenance drug in adolescent addicts hasn't been established.

Geriatric patients
- Because elderly patients may be more sensitive to therapeutic and adverse effects of methadone, they usually need lower doses.

Patient teaching
- As appropriate, tell patient that methadone maintenance can cause severe constipation. Recommend using a stool softener or other laxative.
- Caution patient to avoid hazardous activities because of drug's tendency to cause drowsiness.

---

naloxone hydrochloride
Narcan

Pharmacologic classification:
narcotic (opioid) antagonist

Therapeutic classification:
narcotic antagonist

Pregnancy risk category B

How supplied
Available by prescription only
Injection: 0.02 mg/ml, 0.4 mg/ml, 1 mg/ml with preservatives, 1 mg/ml paraben-free

Indications and dosages
Known or suspected narcotic-induced respiratory depression, including that caused by natural and synthetic narcotics, methadone, nalbuphine, pentazocine, and propoxyphene
Adults: 0.4 to 2 mg I.V., S.C., or I.M., repeated q 2 to 3 minutes, p.r.n. If no response is observed after 10 mg have been given, diagnosis of narcotic-induced toxicity should be questioned.
Children: 0.01 mg/kg I.V., repeated once if needed. Dosage for continuous infusion is 0.024 to 0.16 mg/kg/hour. If I.V. route isn't available, give divided doses by I.M. or S.C. route.

Postoperative narcotic depression
Adults: 0.1 to 0.2 mg I.V. q 2 to 3 minutes p.r.n. until desired response occurs.
Children: 0.005 to 0.01 mg/kg I.M., I.V., or S.C., repeated q 2 to 3 minutes p.r.n. until desired degree of reversal occurs.
Neonates (asphyxia neonatorum): 0.01 mg/kg I.V. into umbilical vein repeated q 2 to 3 minutes for three doses. Drug level for use in neonates and children is 0.02 mg/ml.

Naloxone challenge for diagnosing opiate dependence
Adults: 0.16 mg I.M. If no signs of withdrawal occur in 20 to 30 minutes, give a second dose of 0.24 mg I.V.

Pharmacodynamics
Narcotic (opioid) antagonist action: The precise mechanism of action is unknown, but it probably involves

---

Reactions may be *common,* uncommon, *life-threatening,* or COMMON AND LIFE-THREATENING.

competitive antagonism of more than one opiate receptor in the CNS. Naloxone is essentially a pure antagonist. In patients who have received an opioid agonist or other analgesic with narcotic-like effects, naloxone antagonizes most opioid effects, especially respiratory depression, sedation, and hypotension. Because opioids typically have a longer duration of action than naloxone, opioid effects may return as naloxone effects dissipate. Naloxone doesn't produce tolerance or physical or psychological dependence.

Pharmacokinetics

Absorption: Naloxone is rapidly inactivated after oral administration; therefore, it is given parenterally. Its onset of action is 1 to 2 minutes after I.V. administration and 2 to 5 minutes after I.M. or S.C. administration.
Distribution: Drug is rapidly distributed into body tissues and fluids.
Metabolism: Naloxone is rapidly metabolized in the liver, primarily by conjugation.
Excretion: Drug is excreted in urine. Duration of action is about 45 minutes, but is longer after I.M. use and higher doses as compared with I.V. use and lower doses. Plasma half-life has been reported as 60 to 90 minutes in adults, 3 hours in neonates.

Contraindications and precautions

Contraindicated in patients hypersensitive to drug.
    Use cautiously in patients with cardiac irritability and opiate ad-

diction. When given to a narcotic addict, naloxone may produce an acute abstinence syndrome. Use with caution, and monitor closely.

Interactions
Drug-drug
Cardiotoxic drugs: may have serious CV effects. Avoid concurrent use.

Adverse reactions
CNS: *seizures.*
CV: *cardiac arrest,* hypertension (higher-than-recommended doses), hypotension, tachycardia, *ventricular fibrillation.*
GI: nausea, vomiting (higher-than-recommended doses).
Respiratory: pulmonary edema.
Skin: diaphoresis.
Other: tremors, withdrawal symptoms (narcotic-dependent patients at higher-than-recommended doses).

Overdose and treatment
No serious adverse reactions have been observed with naloxone overdose except those of acute abstinence syndrome in narcotic-dependent persons.

Special considerations
■ Take a careful drug history to rule out narcotic addiction, which would cause withdrawal symptoms with naloxone administration.
■ Naloxone is the safest drug to use when cause of respiratory depression is uncertain. Don't use it for respiratory depression known to result from nonopioid drugs.
■ Naloxone may be administered by continuous I.V. infusion, which is necessary in many cases to con-

trol the adverse effects of epidurally administered morphine. Usual dose is 2 mg in 500 ml of D_5W or normal saline solution. Use solution within 24 hours after preparing it.

■ Before administration, visually inspect all parenteral products for particulates and discoloration.

■ Because naloxone has a shorter duration of action than most narcotics, vigilance and repeated doses are usually needed when managing an acute narcotic overdose in a nonaddicted patient.

■ Avoid relying too much on naloxone. Monitor patient's airway, breathing, and circulation closely. Maintain adequate respiratory and CV status at all times. Watch for respiratory overshoot, in which respiratory rate becomes higher after naloxone administration than it was before narcotic overdose. Respiratory rate increases in 1 to 2 minutes, and effect lasts 1 to 4 hours.

■ Unlabeled uses for naloxone include reversal of alcoholic coma and improvement of circulation in patients with refractory CV shock.

Breast-feeding patients
■ No data are available to demonstrate whether drug appears in breast milk.

Pediatric patients
■ Take a careful drug history to rule out narcotic addiction in the mother to avoid inducing withdrawal symptoms in the neonate.

Geriatric patients
■ Elderly patients typically receive a reduced dosage because they may be more sensitive to therapeutic and adverse effects of drug.

Patient teaching
■ Reassure family that patient will be closely monitored during and after drug administration to assess effectiveness of treatment.

---

naltrexone hydrochloride
ReVia

Pharmacologic classification:
narcotic (opioid) antagonist

Therapeutic classification:
narcotic detoxification adjunct

Pregnancy risk category C

How supplied
Available by prescription only
Tablets: 50 mg

Indications and dosages
Adjunct to maintenance of opioid-free state in detoxified patient
Adults: if naloxone challenge is negative and patient has been opioid-free for 7 to 10 days, give 25 mg P.O. If no withdrawal symptoms occur within 1 hour, give another 25 mg. Average dosage is 50 mg/day, but flexible maintenance schedule of 50 to 150 mg/day may be used, depending on schedule.

Alcoholism
Adults: 50 mg/day P.O.

Pharmacodynamics
Opioid antagonist action: The precise mechanism of action is unknown, but it probably involves

competitive antagonism of more than one opiate receptor in the CNS. Naltrexone is essentially a pure antagonist. In patients who have received single or repeated large opiate doses, naltrexone attenuates or completely but reversibly blocks the pharmacologic effects of the narcotic. Naltrexone doesn't produce physical or psychological dependence; patients reportedly develop no tolerance to its antagonist activity.

Other actions: In patients who haven't recently received an opiate, naltrexone has little or no pharmacologic effect. At oral doses of 30 to 50 mg daily, it produces minimal analgesia, only slight drowsiness, and no respiratory depression. However, in some patients, it may cause psychotomimetic effects, increased systolic or diastolic blood pressure, respiratory depression, and decreased oral temperature, which suggest opiate agonist activity.

Pharmacokinetics

Absorption: Naltrexone is well absorbed after oral administration. Plasma levels peak after 1 hour, although drug undergoes extensive first-pass hepatic metabolism (only 5% to 20% of an oral dose reaches systemic circulation unchanged). Effects peak within 1 hour.

Distribution: Drug is about 21% to 28% protein-bound. The extent and duration of antagonist activity relate directly to plasma and tissue drug levels. Drug is widely distributed throughout the body, but considerable individual variation exists.

Metabolism: Oral naltrexone undergoes extensive first-pass hepatic metabolism. Its major metabolite is believed to be a pure antagonist also, and may contribute to its efficacy. Drug and hepatic metabolites may undergo enterohepatic recirculation.

Excretion: Naltrexone is excreted primarily by the kidneys. Elimination half-life is about 4 hours; that of its major active metabolite is about 13 hours.

Contraindications and precautions

Contraindicated in patients receiving opioid analgesics, in those whose urine screens positive for opioids, in opioid-dependent patients, and in patients in acute opioid withdrawal. Also contraindicated in patients hypersensitive to drug and patients with acute hepatitis or liver failure.

Use cautiously in patients with mild hepatic disease or a history of hepatic impairment.

Interactions
Drug-drug

Drugs that alter hepatic metabolism: may increase or decrease serum naltrexone levels by altering drug metabolism. Adjust naltrexone dose as needed.

Opioid-containing drugs, such as antidiarrheals, cough and cold preparations, and opioid analgesics: attenuated opioid activity. Because naltrexone can cause potentially severe opiate withdrawal, don't give it to patients receiving opiates or in nondetoxified patients physically dependent on opiates.

Thioridazine: increased lethargy and somnolence. Adjust dosages of both drugs as needed.

Adverse reactions
CNS: *anxiety,* depression, dizziness, fatigue, *headache, insomnia, nervousness,* somnolence, **suicidal ideation**.
GI: *abdominal pain,* anorexia, constipation, increased thirst, *nausea, vomiting.*
GU: decreased potency, delayed ejaculation.
Hematologic: lymphocytosis.
Hepatic: *hepatotoxicity.*
Musculoskeletal: *muscle and joint pain.*
Skin: rash.
Other: chills.

Overdose and treatment
Naltrexone overdose has not been documented. In one study, subjects who received 800 mg/day (16 tablets) for up to 1 week showed no evidence of toxicity. In case of overdose, provide symptomatic and supportive treatment in a closely supervised environment. Contact the local or regional poison control center for further information.

Special considerations
■ Don't give naltrexone unless naloxone challenge is negative. To perform it, give 0.2 mg I.V. If no signs of opiate withdrawal appear after 30 seconds, give 0.6 mg I.V. (Or give 0.8 mg S.C. and observe patient for 20 minutes for signs of withdrawal.) If no withdrawal signs appear, test result is negative.
■ Don't give naltrexone until patient has been opioid-free for at least 7 days. Verify abstinence from opioids by urinalysis.
■ Before giving naltrexone, perform liver function tests to establish a baseline and check for possible drug-induced hepatotoxicity.
■ Drug can cause hepatocellular injury if given at higher-than-recommended doses.
■ In an emergency, if a patient receiving naltrexone requires analgesia that can only be achieved with opiates, the patient may need a higher-than-usual narcotic dose, and the resulting respiratory depression may be deeper and more prolonged.
■ Besides standard indications, naltrexone has also been used to treat eating disorders and post-concussional syndrome that fails to respond to other treatments.

Breast-feeding patients
■ No data exist to show whether drug is excreted into breast milk. Use caution when giving drug to breast-feeding women, especially because of its known hepatotoxicity.

Pediatric patients
■ Safe use of naltrexone in patients under age 18 hasn't been established.

Geriatric patients
■ Elderly patients probably need a reduced dosage.

Patient teaching
■ Inform patient that opioid medications, such as cough and cold preparations, antidiarrheal products, and narcotic analgesics may not be effective when taking nal-

trexone. Recommend a nonnarcotic alternative, if available.

■ Warn patient not to take narcotics during naltrexone therapy because doing so may lead to serious injury, coma, or death.

■ Explain that no tolerance or dependence develops as a result of naltrexone therapy.

■ Tell patient to report evidence of withdrawal, such as tremors, vomiting, bone or muscle pains, sweating, abdominal cramps.

■ Caution women of childbearing age to use birth control and to immediately report planned, suspected, or known pregnancy.

■ Tell patient to wear or carry medical identification that documents his use of naltrexone.

---

nicotine
Habitrol, Nicoderm CQ, Nicotrol, Nicotrol NS, ProStep

Pharmacologic classification:
nicotinic cholinergic agonist

Therapeutic classification:
smoking cessation aid

Pregnancy risk category D

How supplied
Available with or without a prescription
Transdermal system: designed to release nicotine at a fixed rate
Habitrol: 21 mg/day, 14 mg/day, 7 mg/day
Nicoderm: 21 mg/day, 14 mg/day, 7 mg/day
Nicotrol: 15 mg/day, 10 mg/day, 5 mg/day
ProStep: 22 mg/day, 11 mg/day

Available by prescription only
Nasal spray: metered spray pump
Nicotrol NS: 0.5 mg/ metered spray
Nicotrol inhaler: 10 mg cartridge that supplies 4 mg of nicotine

Indications and dosages
Relief of nicotine withdrawal symptoms in patients attempting smoking cessation
Habitrol, Nicoderm
Adults: initially, one 21-mg/day patch applied to a hairless part of upper trunk or upper outer arm each day for 6 weeks. After 24 hours, patch should be removed and replaced with a new one at a different site. Then, taper to 14 mg/ day for 2 to 4 weeks. Finally, taper to 7 mg/day if necessary. Nicotine substitution and gradual withdrawal typically take 8 to 12 weeks.
▶ DOSAGE ADJUSTMENT. Patients who weigh less than 100 lb (45 kg), have CV disease, or smoke less than half a pack of cigarettes daily should start therapy at 14-mg/day.
Nicotrol
Adults: initially, one 15-mg/day patch applied to a hairless part of upper trunk or upper outer arm each day for 12 weeks, applied upon awakening and removed h.s. Then, taper to 10 mg/day for 2 weeks. Finally, taper to 5 mg/day for 2 weeks if necessary. Alternatively, it patient has abstained from smoking for 2 to 4 weeks, dosage may be reduced until 5-mg/day dose has been used for 2 weeks. Nicotine substitution and gradual withdrawal typically take 14 to 20 weeks.

Nicotrol NS
Adults: initially, 1 or 2 doses/hour (dose equals two sprays, one in each nostril). Urge patient to use at least the recommended minimum of 8 doses/day. Maximum recommended dose is 40 mg or 80 sprays/day. Duration of treatment should not exceed 3 months.

ProStep
Adults: initially, one 22-mg/day patch applied to a hairless part of upper trunk or upper outer arm each day for 4 to 8 weeks. After 24 hours, patch should be removed and a new one applied to a different site. Patients who stop smoking during this period may discontinue drug, or treatment may continue for 2 to 4 more weeks at 11 mg/day. If patient weighs less than 100 lb (45 kg), start with 11 mg/day. Nicotine substitution and gradual withdrawal typically take 6 to 12 weeks.

Nicotrol inhaler
Adults: initially, 6 to 16 cartridges daily. Best effect is achieved with continuous puffing. Recommended treatment lasts up to 3 months with gradual reduction over another 6 to 12 weeks, as needed.

Pharmacodynamics
Nicotinic cholinergic action: Transdermal system and nasal spray provide nicotine, the chief stimulant alkaloid found in tobacco products, which stimulates nicotinic acetylcholine receptors in the CNS, neuromuscular junction, autonomic ganglia, and adrenal medulla.

Pharmacokinetics
Absorption: Drug is rapidly absorbed.
Distribution: Plasma protein binding is below 5%.
Metabolism: Drug is metabolized by the liver, kidney, and lung. More than 20 metabolites have been identified. Primary metabolites are cotinine (15%) and trans-3-hydroxycotinine (45%).
Excretion: Drug is excreted primarily in the urine as metabolites; about 10% is excreted unchanged. With high urine flow rates or acidified urine, up to 30% can be excreted unchanged.

Contraindications and precautions
Contraindicated in patients hypersensitive to nicotine or its components, in nonsmokers, and in patients with recent MI, life-threatening arrhythmias, and severe or worsening angina pectoris.

Use cautiously in patients with hyperthyroidism, pheochromocytoma, insulin-dependent diabetes, or peptic ulcer disease.

Interactions
Drug-drug
Acetaminophen, imipramine, oxazepam, pentazocine, propranolol, theophylline: smoking cessation may decrease induction of hepatic enzymes that metabolize these drugs. Dosage reduction of these drugs may be needed.
Adrenergic agonists, such as isoproterenol, phenylephrine: influenced by levels of circulating catecholamines. Increased dosage may be needed to maintain therapeutic effects.

Adrenergic antagonists, such as labetalol, prazosin: influenced by lower levels of circulating catecholamines. Decreased dosage may be needed.

Insulin: smoking cessation increases insulin absorption. Reduced insulin dosage may be needed. Tell patient to check blood glucose frequently.

Drug-herb

Blue cohosh: increases effects of nicotine. Don't use together.

Drug-food

Caffeine: smoking cessation may decrease induction of hepatic enzymes that metabolize caffeine. Caffeine reduction may be needed

Adverse reactions

CNS: abnormal dreams, dizziness, *headache, insomnia,* nervousness, paresthesia, somnolence.
CV: hypertension.
EENT: pharyngitis, sinusitis.
GI: abdominal pain, constipation, diarrhea, dry mouth, dyspepsia, nausea, vomiting.
GU: dysmenorrhea.
Musculoskeletal: back pain, myalgia.
Respiratory: increased cough.
Skin: *burning at application site,* cutaneous hypersensitivity, diaphoresis, *local or widespread erythema, pruritus,* rash.

Overdose and treatment

Overdose may cause symptoms of acute nicotine poisoning, including diarrhea, hypotension, nausea, respiratory failure, seizures, vomiting, and weakness.

Treat symptomatically. Give barbiturates or benzodiazepines for seizures and atropine to reduce excessive salivation or diarrhea. Give fluids to treat hypotension and increase urine flow, which enhances drug elimination.

Special considerations

■ Minimize your exposure to nicotine in transdermal patches. After contact, wash your hands with plain water because soap can enhance absorption.
■ Don't give Nicotrol NS to patients with chronic nasal disorders or severe reactive airway disease.
■ Use of the inhaler commonly causes increased coughing.
■ Patients unable to stop smoking during the first 4 weeks of therapy probably won't benefit from continued therapy. They may benefit from counseling to identify reasons for their lack of success.

Breast-feeding patients

■ Nicotine passes freely into breast milk and is readily absorbed after oral administration. Weigh the infant's risk of exposure to nicotine against his risk of exposure from the mother's continued smoking.

Pediatric patients

■ Safety and efficacy in children have not been established.
■ The amount of nicotine in a single patch is enough to kill a child if ingested; even used patches contain a substantial amount of residual nicotine.

Patient teaching

- Make sure that patient reads and understands the information packaged with the product.
- Explain that nicotine can evaporate from a transdermal patch once it's removed from the package. Tell patient to apply it promptly after exposing it to air.
- Urge patient not to alter patch in any way (by folding or cutting it, for example) before applying it.
- Urge patient not to smoke during therapy; explain that adverse effects could result from increased nicotine levels.
- Tell patient not to store patch at temperatures above 86° F (30° C).
- Discourage use of transdermal system for longer than 3 months. Long-term nicotine consumption by any route can be habit-forming and dangerous.
- Tell patient to remove patch and to immediately notify prescriber about a generalized rash or persistent or severe local skin reactions, such as pruritus, edema, or erythema.
- Teach patient how to dispose of a patch properly by folding it in half, bringing the adhesive sides together. If the patch came in a protective pouch, tell him to place the used patch in the pouch from which he removed the new patch.
- Stress that new and used patches and inhalers are dangerous to children and pets. Urge patient to store them and dispose of them safely.
- Explain that continued use of Nicotrol NS probably will cause nasal irritation.
- If patient fails to stop smoking, encourage him to identify and minimize the influences that contributed to his failure. Suggest that he try the therapy again, possibly after an appropriate interval.
- Advise women of childbearing age to use birth control and to immediately report planned, suspected, or known pregnancy.

nicotine polacrilex (nicotine resin complex)
Nicorette, Nicorette DS

Pharmacologic classification: nicotinic agonist

Therapeutic classification: smoking cessation aid

Pregnancy risk category X

How supplied

Available with and without a prescription
Chewing gum: 2 mg, 4 mg of nicotine resin complex per square

Indications and dosages
Smoking cessation (temporary adjunct to medically supervised behavior modification)
Adults: One piece of gum chewed slowly and intermittently for 30 minutes whenever the urge to smoke occurs. Gum is parked between cheek and gum when not being chewed.
▶ DOSAGE ADJUSTMENT. Patients who smoke less than 25 cigarettes/day or have a Fagerstrom Tolerance Questionnaire (FTQ) score below 7 should use the 2-mg strength and shouldn't exceed 30 pieces of gum daily. Patients who smoke more than 25 cigarettes/day or have an FTQ score above 7

should use the 4-mg strength and shouldn't exceed 20 pieces of gum daily. Most patients need about 10 pieces daily in the first month.

Pharmacodynamics
Nicotine replacement action: Nicotine is an agonist at the nicotinic receptors in the peripheral nervous system and CNS and produces both behavioral stimulation and depression. It acts on the adrenal medulla to aid in overcoming physical dependence on nicotine during withdrawal from habitual smoking.

Pharmacokinetics
Absorption: Nicotine is bound to ion-exchange resin and is released only during chewing. Blood level depends on vigor of chewing.
Distribution: Distribution of nicotine into tissues hasn't been fully described. Drug crosses the placenta and appears in breast milk.
Metabolism: Drug is metabolized mainly by the liver, less so by the kidneys and lungs. The main metabolites are cotinine and nicotine-19-N-oxide.
Excretion: Nicotine and its metabolites are excreted in urine, with about 10% to 20% excreted unchanged. Excretion of nicotine is increased with acid urine and high urine output.

Contraindications and precautions
Contraindicated in nonsmokers, in pregnant patients, and in patients with recent MI, life-threatening arrhythmias, severe or worsening angina pectoris, or active temporomandibular joint disease.

Use cautiously in patients with hyperthyroidism, pheochromocytoma, insulin-dependent diabetes, peptic ulcer disease, a history of esophagitis, oral or pharyngeal inflammation, or dental conditions that could be worsened by chewing gum.

Interactions
Drug-drug
Adrenergic agonists, adrenergic blockers: altered by levels of circulating catecholamines. Dosage adjustment may be needed.
Catecholamines, cortisol: increased circulating levels with smoking and use of gum. Monitor levels, and adjust dosage accordingly.
Imipramine, pentazocine, and theophylline: metabolism of these drugs increased by smoking, an effect that's decreased by smoking cessation with or without nicotine substitutes. Monitor blood levels, and adjust dosage accordingly.
Insulin: absorption may be increased by smoking cessation. Monitor blood glucose, and adjust insulin dosage accordingly.

Drug-herb
Blue cohosh: may increase effects of nicotine. Don't use together.

Drug-food
Caffeine: metabolism increased by smoking. Avoid using together.

Adverse reactions
CNS: dizziness, headache, insomnia, irritability, light-headedness, paresthesia.
CV: atrial fibrillation.
EENT: sore throat.

GI: anorexia, eructation, excessive salivation, indigestion, nausea, vomiting.
Musculoskeletal: aching jaw muscle (from chewing).
Skin: diaphoresis.
Other: hiccups.

Overdose and treatment

The risk of overdose is small because nausea and vomiting arise soon after excessive nicotine intake. Poisoning may cause abdominal pain, cold sweats, confusion, diarrhea, disturbed hearing and vision, dizziness, headache, nausea, salivation, vomiting, and weakness.

Treatment includes induced emesis with ipecac syrup (if patient hasn't already vomited). A saline cathartic will speed passage of gum through the GI tract. If patient is unconscious, perform gastric lavage and follow with activated charcoal. Provide supportive treatment for respiratory paralysis and CV collapse as needed.

Special considerations

■ Patients most likely to benefit from therapy are smokers with a high physical dependence. Typically, they smoke more than 15 cigarettes daily, they prefer cigarettes with high nicotine levels, they usually inhale the smoke, they smoke their first cigarette within 30 minutes of awakening, and they find the first morning cigarette the hardest to give up.
■ Nicotine's CV effects are usually dose-dependent. In nonsmokers, even a small dose may cause CNS-mediated symptoms, such as hiccups, nausea, and vomiting. In smokers, chewing a 2-mg piece of gum every hour usually doesn't cause adverse CV effects.
■ Advise women of childbearing age to use birth control and to immediately report planned, suspected, or known pregnancy.

Breast-feeding patients

■ Nicotine passes freely into breast milk and is readily absorbed after oral administration. Weigh the infant's risk of exposure to nicotine against his risk of exposure from continued smoking by the mother.

Patient teaching

■ Instruct patient to chew one piece of gum instead of having a cigarette whenever he feels the urge to smoke. Most patients need about 10 pieces of gum daily during first month of treatment.
■ Tell patient to chew gum slowly and intermittently for about 30 minutes to promote slow and even buccal absorption of nicotine. After about 15 chews, advise patient to park gum between the cheek and gum for a few minutes. Fast chewing produces faster absorption and more adverse effects.
■ Inform patient that gum is sugar-free and usually doesn't stick to dentures.
■ Cola, coffee, juices, and other beverages (especially acidic ones) and foods can decrease salivary pH. Instruct patient not to eat or drink for 15 minutes before or after chewing nicotine gum.
■ If patient can successfully abstain from cigarettes after 3 months of therapy, tell him to gradually stop chewing the gum. Urge him not to use the gum for more than 6 months.

Reactions may be *common,* uncommon, ***life-threatening,*** or COMMON AND LIFE-THREATENING.

CHAPTER 12

Sedative-hypnotics

411 ■ **Introduction**

416 ■ **Generic drugs**

■ amobarbital, amobarbital sodium

■ butabarbital sodium

■ chloral hydrate

■ diazepam (See Chapter 4, ANTIANXIETY DRUGS)

■ diphenhydramine hydrochloride (See Chapter 8, ANTIPARKINSONIANS)

■ droperidol

■ estazolam

■ flurazepam hydrochloride

■ lorazepam (See Chapter 4, ANTIANXIETY DRUGS)

■ pentobarbital sodium

■ phenobarbital, phenobarbital sodium

■ promethazine hydrochloride

■ secobarbital sodium

■ temazepam

■ triazolam

■ zaleplon

■ zolpidem tartrate

Sedative-hypnotic drugs are used primarily to treat insomnia. They include certain benzodiazepines, nonbenzodiazepine hypnotics, antihistamines, chloral hydrate, and barbiturates.

UNDERSTANDING INSOMNIA

Over the course of a year, about 35% of adults develop insomnia. About half of them have severe insomnia; it tends to affect older women who have multiple medical problems, stressful lives, and anxiety. Usually, insomnia lasts several days to several weeks, although occasionally it may become chronic. The cause of insomnia may be physical, psychiatric, drug-related, or a combination of these problems. (See *What causes insomnia?*, page 412.)

Because insomnia may reflect an underlying physical or mental problem, careful assessment is crucial before starting a patient on a drug treatment. Prescription quantities should be limited to a 1-month supply.

Continued assessment is crucial as well, especially if therapy lasts longer than 3 weeks. Indeed, if the patient still has insomnia after 7 to 10 days of drug therapy—or if the condition worsens or the patient develops new or worsened abnormal behaviors—the problem almost certainly stems from an unrecognized physical or psychiatric ailment that needs attention.

TREATING INSOMNIA

Treating an underlying medical or psychiatric problem or adjusting the drugs already being used commonly relieves insomnia. If not, then the patient may benefit from nondrug treatments for insomnia. If necessary, the patient may benefit from short-term drug treatment as well.

Nondrug treatments

One of the best nondrug methods for treating insomnia involves sleep hygiene: a routine set of activities that prepare the body for sleep. Sleep hygiene includes these activities and others particular to the patient:

- setting regular times for going to bed and getting up
- making the sleep environment as comfortable as possible
- avoiding alcohol in the afternoon and evening
- avoiding caffeine in the afternoon and evening
- avoiding heavy meals close to bedtime
- avoiding exercise close to bedtime
- using the bedroom only for sleep, not for watching television or reading.

Relaxation techniques also can help to prepare the patient for sleep. They include listening to relaxing music, progressively tightening and relaxing muscle groups throughout the body, and using a "white noise" or sound machine.

If insomnia continues despite the patient's use of good sleep hygiene and relaxation techniques, she may benefit from one of sever-

What causes insomnia?

Insomnia typically results from a physical, psychiatric, or drug-related problem.

Physical causes
- asthma
- cardiovascular disease
- chronic obstructive pulmonary disease
- disruption in circadian rhythm
- fever
- infection
- nocturia
- pain
- pruritus
- restless leg syndrome
- sleep apnea

Psychiatric causes
- alcohol abuse
- anxiety
- bipolar disorder
- depression
- drug abuse
- reaction to a stressful event
- schizophrenia

Drug-related causes
- alcohol
- antidepressants
- beta agonists
- caffeine
- central nervous system stimulants
- corticosteroids
- decongestants
- nicotine
- theophylline
- thyroid replacement hormones

al sedative-hypnotic drugs used to treat insomnia.

Drug treatments

The drugs used most often to treat insomnia are benzodiazepines, such as temazepam and flurazepam. Newer classes of nonbenzodiazepine hypnotics (imidazopyridines and pyrazolopyrimidines) are becoming popular as well and include such drugs as zaleplon and zolpidem. Over-the-counter antihistamines, particularly diphenhydramine, can also be used. Drugs once used to treat insomnia that have dropped in popularity include chloral hydrate and barbiturates.

Benzodiazepines

The mainstay of drug therapy for insomnia, benzodiazepines are still considered by many clinicians to be the drugs of choice for this condition. In general, benzodiazepines are effective and fast-acting.

The choice of a particular benzodiazepine depends on the patient's symptoms. If the patient's main problem is an inability to fall asleep, then the best choice is a drug with a fast onset of action. In contrast, if the patient's main problem is early-morning awakening, then the best choice is a drug with a slightly longer duration of action, such as temazepam.

Keep in mind that long-acting benzodiazepines, such as flurazepam, may accumulate after the patient receives several doses. This accumulation tends to produce more adverse effects. Consequently, these drugs aren't recommended, particularly for elderly patients.

As a group, benzodiazepines have several disadvantages. For one, they have a relatively high risk of dependence. For another, abrupt discontinuation of a benzodiazepine can produce withdrawal symptoms. What's more, tolerance develops with continued use, creating a need for increasing doses. Finally, some patients exhibit drug-seeking behavior.

Drug effects

Benzodiazepines work by potentiating gamma-aminobutyric acid (GABA), a inhibitory neurotransmitter in the brain. Two different benzodiazepine receptors (BZD_1 and BZD_2) have recently been identified. Binding with BZD_1 appears to produce hypnotic effects. Binding with BZD_2 seems to cause anxiolytic, muscle relaxant, and anticonvulsant effects. Benzodiazepines bind to varying degrees with both receptors, which explains their range of effects.

Besides their sedative-hypnotic effects, benzodiazepines also have anxiolytic, muscle relaxant, and anticonvulsant effects.

Nonbenzodiazepine hypnotics

The nonbenzodiazepine hypnotics zaleplon and zolpidem are becoming increasingly popular as a treatment for insomnia. These relatively new drugs are short-acting with a quick onset of action. They lack active metabolites, so drug accumulation isn't likely. Plus, they seem to be less addicting than benzodiazepines and less likely to produce tolerance.

The difference between zaleplon and zolpidem lies in their kinetics. Zaleplon has a slightly faster onset than zolpidem, but zolpidem has a longer duration of action. In fact, its effects last all night. Zaleplon has such a short duration of action that patients may experience early-morning awakening; however, even if they take a second zaleplon dose during the night, residual effects still aren't likely in the morning.

The main disadvantage of these drugs is cost; they're more expensive than benzodiazepines. Their adverse effects appear to be dose-related, so always use the smallest effective dose possible, especially in elderly patients.

Drug effects

Zaleplon and zolpidem aren't benzodiazepines (they belong to the imidazopyridines and the pyrazolopyrimidines) and they have a chemical structure unrelated to benzodiazepines, barbiturates, and other hypnotics. However, they interact with the GABA-BZD receptors through which benzodiazepines cause some of their effects, such as sedation.

They induce sleep by selectively binding the GABA-BZD receptor at the BZ_1 site. Thus, they possess only hypnotic properties, and they lack anxiolytic, muscle relaxant, and anticonvulsant properties.

Antihistamines

The antihistamine diphenhydramine may be used to treat insomnia. It induces sleep by nonselectively binding with peripheral and central histamine receptor

Disadvantages of barbiturates

Although barbiturates reliably produce sedation and hypnosis, they aren't favored as a treatment for insomnia. That's because they have several serious disadvantages:

■ They're highly addictive. In fact, continuous use commonly leads to drug-seeking behavior.

■ They induce cytochrome P-450 isoenzyme pathways in the liver, which means that they may interact with many common drugs.

■ An overdose can be fatal.

sites. Its advantage over benzodiazepines is that it produces neither physical dependence nor tolerance. It's typically contraindicated in elderly patients, however, because of the anticholinergic effects to which elderly patients are especially sensitive.

Chloral hydrate

Chloral hydrate is about as effective as benzodiazepines at treating insomnia, but it's no longer considered a first-line treatment. That's in part because patients who take it tend to develop dependence, tolerance, and possible toxicity in overdose.

Another problem with chloral hydrate is that it interacts with such drugs as warfarin, phenytoin, and others. Chloral hydrate typically is reserved for patients who can't tolerate benzodiazepines. The mechanism by which chloral hydrate affects the central nervous system (CNS) isn't known. Hypnotic doses produce mild cerebral depression and quiet, deep sleep.

Barbiturates

Barbiturates can produce all levels of CNS mood alteration: excitation, sedation, hypnosis, and coma.

They also possess anticonvulsant effects and can produce respiratory depression. They work by depressing the sensory cortex, decreasing motor activity, and altering cerebellar function.

Rarely are barbiturates used to treat insomnia. Even such short-acting barbiturates as pentobarbital and secobarbital, although still on the market, aren't widely used for insomnia. That's because these drugs have certain disadvantages that make them less than desirable for treating a relatively minor problem such as insomnia. (See *Disadvantages of barbiturates*.)

PATIENT TEACHING

For all sedative-hypnotics, make sure you provide thorough patient teaching. Start by explaining that these drugs act quickly, and that the patient should receive relief from her insomnia after a single dose.

Add that these drugs tend to work effectively for a limited time. Tell the patient that the effects of the drug will decline if she takes it continuously. Urge her to take a sleeping aid only when she clearly needs it. Stress that she shouldn't exceed the prescribed dosage; instead, if drug effects seem to be declining, she should talk to the prescriber.

Explain that abruptly stopping a sleeping aid after taking it continuously can lead to withdrawal symptoms. To avoid that problem, urge her to talk with the prescriber about decreasing the drug on a schedule.

If the patient takes chloral hydrate or a barbiturate, warn her to tell the prescriber right away if she has any thoughts of suicide. Also, warn her that an overdose could be fatal. Urge her to avoid alcohol during therapy and to avoid hazardous activities during the hours just after she takes the drug. For some drugs, this caution may apply to the next day as well. Make sure to caution elderly patients about the increased risk of falls when taking a sedative-hypnotic drug.

amobarbital

amobarbital sodium
Amytal

Pharmacologic classification:
barbiturate

Therapeutic classification:
anticonvulsant, sedative-hypnotic

Controlled substance schedule II

Pregnancy risk category D

How supplied
Available by prescription only
Capsules: 200 mg
Powder for injection: 250-mg,
500-mg vials
Tablets: 30 mg

Indications and dosages
To produce sedation
Adults: usually 30 to 50 mg P.O.
b.i.d. or t.i.d. Range, 15 to 120 mg
b.i.d. to q.i.d.
Children: 2 mg/kg/day P.O., divided into four equal doses.

Insomnia
Adults: 65 to 200 mg P.O. or deep
I.M. h.s. Don't exceed 5 ml I.M.
in any one site. Maximum dose,
500 mg.
Children over age 6: 2 to 3 mg/kg
deep I.M. h.s.

To produce anticonvulsant effects
Adults: 65 to 500 mg by slow I.V.
injection (not exceeding 100
mg/minute). Maximum dose,
1 g.

Pharmacodynamics
Anticonvulsant action: The exact
cellular site and mechanism of action are unknown. Parenteral amobarbital suppresses the spread of
seizure activity produced by epileptogenic foci in the cortex, thalamus, and limbic systems by enhancing the effect of GABA. Both
presynaptic and postsynaptic excitability are decreased.
Sedative-hypnotic action: Drug acts
throughout the CNS as a nonselective depressant with an intermediate onset and duration of action.
Particularly sensitive to this drug is
the mesencephalic reticular activating system, which controls CNS
arousal. Amobarbital decreases
both presynaptic and postsynaptic
membrane excitability by facilitating the action of GABA.

Pharmacokinetics
Absorption: Amobarbital is absorbed well after oral administration. Absorption after I.M. administration is 100%. Onset of action
is 45 to 60 minutes.
Distribution: Drug is distributed
well throughout body tissues and
fluids.
Metabolism: Amobarbital is metabolized in the liver by oxidation
to a tertiary alcohol.
Excretion: Less than 1% of a dose
is excreted unchanged in the urine;
the rest is excreted as metabolites.
The half-life is biphasic, with a first
phase half-life of about 40 minutes
and a second phase of about 20
hours. Duration of action is 6 to 8
hours.

Reactions may be *common*, uncommon, *life-threatening*, or COMMON AND LIFE-THREATENING.

Contraindications and precautions

Contraindicated in patients hypersensitive to barbiturates and in patients with porphyria or bronchopneumonia or other severe pulmonary insufficiency.

Use cautiously in patients with suicidal tendencies, acute or chronic pain, a history of drug abuse, hepatic or renal impairment, or pulmonary or CV disease.

Interactions
Drug-drug

Antidepressants, antihistamines, MAO inhibitors, narcotics, sedative-hypnotics, tranquilizers: amobarbital may add to or potentiate CNS and respiratory depressant effects. Monitor patient's respiratory status closely.

Corticosteroids, digitoxin (not digoxin), doxycycline, oral contraceptives, other estrogens, theophylline, other xanthines: amobarbital enhances hepatic metabolism. Dosage adjustment may be needed.

Disulfiram, MAO inhibitors, valproic acid: decreased amobarbital metabolism and increased risk of toxicity. Avoid concurrent use.

Griseofulvin: amobarbital impairs griseofulvin effectiveness by decreasing absorption from the GI tract. Dosage adjustment may be needed.

Phenytoin: amobarbital may cause unpredictable fluctuations in serum phenytoin levels. Dosage adjustment may be necessary.

Rifampin: may decrease amobarbital levels by increasing metabolism. Monitor drug levels.

Warfarin and other oral anticoagulants: amobarbital enhances enzymatic degradation of anticoagulant. Increased anticoagulant dosage may be needed.

Drug-food

Food: decreases drug absorption. Give drug before meals or on an empty stomach to enhance absorption rate.

Drug-lifestyle

Alcohol use: amobarbital may add to or potentiate CNS and respiratory depressant effects of alcohol. Avoid concurrent use.

Adverse reactions

CNS: *drowsiness, hangover, lethargy,* paradoxical excitement, somnolence.
CV: *bradycardia,* hypotension, syncope.
GI: nausea, vomiting.
Hematologic: exacerbation of porphyria.
Respiratory: *apnea, respiratory depression.*
Skin: pain and irritation at injection site, rash, sterile abscess at injection site, *Stevens-Johnson syndrome,* urticaria.
Other: *angioedema,* physical and psychological dependence.

Overdose and treatment

Overdose may cause areflexia, coma, confusion, pulmonary edema, respiratory depression, slurred speech, somnolence, sustained nystagmus, and an unsteady gait. Fever, hypothermia, jaundice, oliguria, and shock with tachycardia and hypotension also may occur.

To treat overdose, support the patient's ventilation as needed. Give vasopressors and I.V. fluids to support circulation as needed. If ingestion was recent and patient is conscious with a functioning gag reflex, induce emesis with ipecac syrup. If emesis is inappropriate and patient has a cuffed endotracheal tube in place to prevent aspiration, perform gastric lavage. Follow with activated charcoal or a sodium chloride cathartic. Measure patient's fluid intake and output, vital signs, and laboratory values. Maintain her body temperature. Alkalinization of urine may be helpful in removing amobarbital from the body; hemodialysis may be useful in severe overdose.

Special considerations
- Amobarbital isn't commonly used as a sedative or a sleeping aid; safer benzodiazepines have replaced barbiturates for such uses.
- Give drug orally before meals or on an empty stomach to enhance the rate of absorption.
- Reconstitute powder for injection with sterile water for injection. Roll vial between hands rather than shaking it. Use 2.5 or 5 ml (for 250 or 500 mg of amobarbital) to make 10% solution. For I.M. use, prepare 20% solution by using 1.25 or 2.5 ml of sterile water for injection.
- Administer reconstituted parenteral solution within 30 minutes after opening the vial.
- Don't give amobarbital solution that's cloudy or contains precipitate 5 minutes after reconstitution.
- Administer I.M. dose deep into large muscle mass, giving no more than 5 ml in any one injection site. Sterile abscess or tissue damage may result from inadvertent superficial I.M. or S.C. injection.

- Give I.V. dose at no more than 100 mg/minute in adults or 60 mg/m^2/minute in children to minimize the risk of hypotension and respiratory depression. Keep emergency resuscitative equipment available.
- Giving full loading doses over short periods of time to treat status epilepticus in an adult may require ventilatory support.
- Assess patient's cardiopulmonary status frequently and monitor her blood counts to detect adverse reactions.
- Assess renal and hepatic laboratory studies to ensure adequate drug removal.
- Monitor patient's PT carefully when anticoagulant therapy begins or ends during amobarbital therapy. Anticoagulant dosage may need to be adjusted.
- Amobarbital may cause false-positive results on the phentolamine test. Physiologic effects of drug may impair absorption of cyanocobalamin ^{57}Co and may decrease serum bilirubin levels in neonates, epileptic patients, and patients with congenital non-hemolytic unconjugated hyperbilirubinemia. It also may change EEG patterns, specifically low-voltage, fast-activity; changes persist for a time after therapy stops.
- Besides standard uses, amobarbital has been used for preanesthetic sedation.

Breast-feeding patients
- Give drug cautiously to breast-feeding women because it passes into breast milk and may make infant drowsy. If so, dosage adjust-

---

ment or discontinuation of drug or breast-feeding may be needed.

Pediatric patients
- Safe use in children under age 6 hasn't been established.
- Amobarbital may cause paradoxical excitement in some children.

Geriatric patients
- Confusion, disorientation, and excitability may occur in elderly patients. Give drug cautiously.
- Elderly patients usually require lower dosages.

Patient teaching
- Warn patient of possible physical and psychological dependence with prolonged use.
- Tell patient to avoid alcohol during therapy.
- Urge women of childbearing age to use birth control and to immediately report planned, suspected, or known pregnancy.

butabarbital sodium
Butisol

Pharmacologic classification: barbiturate

Therapeutic classification: sedative-hypnotic

Controlled substance schedule III

Pregnancy risk category D

How supplied
Available by prescription only
Elixir: 30 mg/5 ml
Tablets: 15 mg, 30 mg, 50 mg, 100 mg

Indications and dosages
To produce sedation
Adults: 15 to 30 mg P.O. t.i.d. or q.i.d.

Insomnia
Adults: 50 to 100 mg P.O. h.s. for a maximum of 2 weeks.

Pharmacodynamics
Sedative-hypnotic action: The exact cellular site and mechanism of action are unknown. Butabarbital acts throughout the CNS as a nonselective depressant with an intermediate onset and duration of action. Particularly sensitive to the drug is the reticular activating system, which controls CNS arousal. Butabarbital decreases both presynaptic and postsynaptic membrane excitability by facilitating the action of GABA.

Pharmacokinetics
Absorption: Butabarbital is well absorbed after oral administration. Action begins in 45 to 60 minutes; levels peak in 3 to 4 hours. Serum levels needed for sedation and hypnosis are 2 to 3 mcg/ml and 25 mcg/ml, respectively.
Distribution: Drug is distributed well throughout body tissues and fluids.
Metabolism: Drug is metabolized extensively in the liver by oxidation. Its duration of action is 6 to 8 hours.
Excretion: Inactive metabolites of butabarbital are excreted in urine. Only 1% to 2% of an oral dose is excreted in urine unchanged. Terminal half-life ranges from 30 to 40 hours.

Contraindications and precautions

Contraindicated in patients hypersensitive to barbiturates and in patients with porphyria, bronchopneumonia, or other severe pulmonary insufficiency.

Use cautiously in patients with renal or hepatic impairment, acute or chronic pain, or a history of drug abuse.

Interactions
Drug-drug

Antidepressants, antihistamines, narcotics, sedative-hypnotics, tranquilizers: amobarbital may add to or potentiate CNS and respiratory depressant effects. Monitor patient's respiratory status closely.
Corticosteroids, digitoxin (not digoxin), doxycycline, oral contraceptives, other estrogens, theophylline, other xanthines: butabarbital enhances hepatic metabolism. Dosage adjustment may be needed.
Disulfiram, MAO inhibitors, valproic acid: decreased butabarbital metabolism and increased risk of toxicity. Monitor patient closely.
Griseofulvin: butabarbital impairs griseofulvin effectiveness by decreasing absorption from the GI tract. Monitor patient for lack of effectiveness, and adjust dosage as needed.
Rifampin: may decrease butabarbital levels by increasing hepatic metabolism. Monitor patient closely.
Warfarin and other oral anticoagulants: butabarbital enhances enzymatic degradation of anticoagulant. Increased anticoagulant dosage may be needed.

Drug-lifestyle
Alcohol use: butabarbital may add to or potentiate CNS and respiratory depressant effects of alcohol. Avoid concurrent use.

Adverse reactions
CNS: *drowsiness, hangover, lethargy,* paradoxical excitement in elderly patients, somnolence.
GI: nausea, vomiting.
Hematologic: decreased serum bilirubin levels in neonates, epileptic patients, and patients with congenital nonhemolytic unconjugated hyperbilirubinemia; exacerbation of porphyria.
Respiratory: *apnea, respiratory depression.*
Skin: rash, *Stevens-Johnson syndrome,* urticaria.
Other: *angioedema,* physical and psychological dependence.

Overdose and treatment
Overdose may cause areflexia, coma, confusion, pulmonary edema, respiratory depression, slurred speech, somnolence, sustained nystagmus, and an unsteady gait. Fever, hypothermia, jaundice, oliguria, and shock with tachycardia and hypotension also may occur.

To treat overdose, support the patient's ventilation as needed. Give vasopressors and I.V. fluids to support circulation as needed. If ingestion was recent and patient is conscious with a functioning gag reflex, induce emesis with ipecac syrup. If emesis is inappropriate and patient has a cuffed endotracheal tube in place to prevent aspiration, perform gastric lavage. Follow with activated charcoal. Measure patient's fluid intake and

---

output, vital signs, and laboratory values. Maintain her body temperature. Alkalinization of urine may be helpful in removing butabarbital from the body; hemodialysis may be useful in severe overdose.

Special considerations

■ Tablet may be crushed and mixed with food or fluid if patient has trouble swallowing it. Likewise, capsule may be opened and contents mixed with food or fluids.
■ Assess patient's cardiopulmonary status frequently; monitor her vital signs for significant changes.
■ Monitor patient for possible allergic reaction from tartrazine sensitivity.
■ Periodically evaluate patient's blood counts and renal and hepatic studies for abnormalities and adverse effects.
■ Assess PT and INR carefully when patient taking butabarbital starts or ends anticoagulant therapy. Anticoagulant dosage may need adjustment.
■ Watch for signs of barbiturate toxicity, such as clammy skin, constricted pupils, coma, cyanosis, and hypotension. Overdose can be fatal.
■ Prolonged administration isn't recommended because drug hasn't been proven effective after 14 days. Allow a drug-free interval of at least 1 week between dosing periods.
■ Butabarbital may cause false-positive results on the phentolamine test. Physiologic effects of drug may impair absorption of cyanocobalamin ^{57}Co. It also may change EEG patterns, specifically low-voltage, fast-activity; changes persist for a time after therapy stops. Drug also may increase sulfobromophthalein retention.
■ Besides standard indications, drug has also been used for preoperative sedation.

Breast-feeding patients
■ Drug appears in breast milk; avoid use in breast-feeding women.

Pediatric patients
■ Butabarbital may cause paradoxical excitement in children.
■ Pediatric dosage varies with age and weight of child and degree of sedation required. Give cautiously.

Geriatric patients
■ Elderly patients are more susceptible to the CNS depressant effects of butabarbital. Confusion, disorientation, and excitability may occur.
■ Elderly patients usually require lower dosages.

Patient teaching
■ Warn patient that prolonged use can result in physical or psychological dependence.
■ Emphasize the danger of combining drug with alcohol. An excessive depressant effect is possible, even if drug is taken the evening before alcohol ingestion.
■ Caution patient to avoid hazardous activities during therapy because drug may cause drowsiness.
■ Advise women of childbearing age to use birth control and to immediately report planned, suspected, or known pregnancy.

chloral hydrate
Aquachloral Supprettes, Noctec

Pharmacologic classification:
general CNS depressant

Therapeutic classification:
sedative-hypnotic

Controlled substance schedule IV

Pregnancy risk category C

How supplied
Available by prescription only
Capsules: 250 mg, 500 mg
Syrup: 250 mg/5 ml, 500 mg/5 ml
Suppositories: 325 mg, 500 mg,
650 mg

Indications and dosages
Sedation
Adults: 250 mg P.O. t.i.d. after
meals.
Children: 8 mg/kg P.O. t.i.d.
Maximum, 500 mg t.i.d.

Management of alcohol
withdrawal symptoms
Adults: 500 to 1,000 mg. May
repeat q 6 hours, p.r.n.

Insomnia
Adults: 500 mg to 1 g P.O. or P.R.
15 to 30 minutes before bedtime.
Children: 50 mg/kg P.O. or P.R.
single dose. Maximum dose, 1 g.

Pharmacodynamics
Sedative-hypnotic action: Chloral
hydrate has CNS depressant activities similar to those of the barbiturates. Nonspecific CNS depression
occurs at hypnotic doses; however,
respiratory drive is only slightly affected. Drug's primary site of action is the reticular activating system, which controls arousal. The
cellular site of action isn't known.

Pharmacokinetics
Absorption: Chloral hydrate is absorbed well after oral or rectal administration. Sleep occurs 30 to 60
minutes after a 500-mg to 1-g
dose.
Distribution: Drug and its active
metabolite, trichloroethanol, are
distributed throughout the body in
tissue and fluids. Trichloroethanol
is 35% to 41% protein-bound.
Metabolism: Drug is metabolized
rapidly and nearly completely in
the liver and erythrocytes to the
active metabolite trichloroethanol.
It is further metabolized in the
liver and kidneys to trichloroacetic
acid and other inactive metabolites.
Excretion: Inactive metabolites of
drug are excreted primarily in
urine. Minor amounts are excreted
in bile. Half-life of trichloroethanol is 8 to 10 hours.

Contraindications and
precautions
Contraindicated in patients with
impaired hepatic or renal function,
severe cardiac disease, or hypersensitivity to drug. Oral administration contraindicated in patients
with gastric disorders.
   Use with extreme caution in patients who have mental depression,
suicidal tendencies, or a history of
drug abuse.

Interactions
Drug-drug
CNS depressants, such as antihista-
mines, narcotics, sedative-hypnotics,

---

tranquilizers, tricyclic antidepressants: added or potentiated CNS depression. Use together with extreme caution.

Furosemide I.V.: increased risk of hypermetabolic state from displacement of thyroid hormone from binding sites. Patient develops sweating, hot flashes, tachycardia, and variable blood pressure. Use together with extreme caution.

Phenytoin: elimination may be increased. Monitor patient's serum drug levels.

Warfarin and other oral anticoagulants: chloral hydrate may displace oral anticoagulants from protein-binding sites, causing increased hypoprothrombinemic effects. Monitor patient's PT and INR values.

Drug-lifestyle
Alcohol use: may cause vasodilation, tachycardia, sweating, and flushing in some patients. Avoid concurrent use.

Adverse reactions
CNS: ataxia, confusion, delirium, disorientation, dizziness, drowsiness, hallucinations, hangover, light-headedness, malaise, nightmares, paradoxical excitement, somnolence, vertigo.
GI: *diarrhea,* flatulence, *nausea, vomiting.*
Hematologic: eosinophilia, *leukopenia.*
Other: hypersensitivity reactions (rash, urticaria), physical and psychological dependence.

Overdose and treatment
Overdose may cause coma, hypotension, hypothermia, pinpoint pupils, respiratory depression, and stupor. Esophageal stricture may follow gastric necrosis and perforation. GI hemorrhage has also been reported. Hepatic damage and jaundice may occur.

Treatment supports respiration (including mechanical ventilation if needed), blood pressure, and body temperature. If patient is conscious, induce emesis or perform gastric lavage. Hemodialysis will remove drug and its metabolite. Peritoneal dialysis may be effective as well.

Special considerations
■ Chloral hydrate isn't a first-line drug because of the risk of adverse or toxic effects.
■ Some brands of chloral hydrate contain tartrazine, which may cause allergic reactions in susceptible people.
■ Assess patient's level of consciousness before giving drug to ensure appropriate baseline level.
■ Give capsules with a full glass (8 oz [240 ml]) of water to lessen GI upset; dilute syrup in a half glass of water or juice before administration to improve taste.
■ Monitor patient's vital signs frequently.
■ Store drug in a dark container away from heat and moisture to prevent breakdown. Refrigerate suppositories.
■ Drug may cause false-positive results on urine glucose tests that use cupric sulfate, such as Benedict's reagent and possibly Clinitest. It doesn't interfere with Chemstrip uG, Diastix, or glucose enzymatic test strip results.

- Drug interferes with fluorometric tests for urine catecholamines; withhold it for 48 hours before the test. Drug may also interfere with Reddy-Jenkins-Thorn test for urinary 17-hydroxycorticosteroids. It also may cause false-positive results on phentolamine test.

Breast-feeding patients
- Small amounts appear in breast milk and may cause drowsiness in breast-fed infant; avoid use in breast-feeding women.

Pediatric patients
- Drug is safe and effective in children as a premedication for EEG and other procedures.

Geriatric patients
- Elderly patients may be more susceptible to CNS depressant effects because of decreased elimination. Give a reduced dosage as needed.

Patient teaching
- Teach patient how to properly take the prescribed drug form.
- Advise patient to take drug with a full glass (8 oz) of water and to dilute syrup with juice or water before taking it.
- Caution patient to avoid hazardous activities until full CNS effects of drug are known.
- Tell patient to avoid alcohol and other CNS depressants during therapy.
- Urge patient not to take other prescribed drugs, OTC medications, or herbal remedies without consulting prescriber.

- Warn patient not to increase dose or stop drug without consulting prescriber.

---

droperidol
Inapsine

Pharmacologic classification: butyrophenone derivative

Therapeutic classification: tranquilizer

Pregnancy risk category C

How supplied
Available by prescription only
Injection: 2.5 mg/ml

Indications and dosages
Anesthetic premedication
Adults: 2.5 to 10 mg I.M. 30 to 60 minutes before induction of general anesthesia.
Children ages 2 to 12: 0.088 to 0.165 mg/kg I.V. or I.M.

Adjunct for induction of general anesthesia
Adults: 0.22 to 0.275 mg/kg I.V. (preferably) or I.M. with an analgesic or general anesthetic.
Children: 0.088 to 0.165 mg/kg I.V. or I.M.

Adjunct for maintaining general anesthesia
Adults: 1.25 to 2.5 mg I.V.

For use without a general anesthetic during diagnostic procedures
Adults: 2.5 to 10 mg I.M. 30 to 60 minutes before the procedure. Give

---

additional doses of 1.25 to 2.5 mg
I.V. p.r.n.

Adjunct to regional anesthesia
Adults: 2.5 to 5 mg I.M. or slow I.V.
injection.

Antiemetic effects during chemotherapy*
Adults: 6.25 mg I.M. or by slow I.V.
injection.

Pharmacodynamics
Tranquilizer action: Droperidol
produces marked sedation by directly blocking subcortical receptors. It also blocks CNS receptors
at the chemoreceptor trigger zone,
producing an antiemetic effect.

Pharmacokinetics
Absorption: Drug is well absorbed
after I.M. injection. Sedation begins in 3 to 10 minutes, peaks at 30
minutes, and lasts for 2 to 4 hours.
Some alteration of consciousness
may persist for 12 hours.
Distribution: Not well understood.
Drug crosses the blood-brain barrier and is distributed in the CSF.
It also crosses the placenta.
Metabolism: Droperidol is metabolized by the liver to *p*-fluoro-
phenylacetic acid and *p*-hydroxy-
piperidine.
Excretion: Drug and its metabolites are excreted in urine and feces.

Contraindications and precautions
Contraindicated in patients hypersensitive or intolerant to drug.
   Use cautiously in patients with
hypotension and other CV disease
because of its vasodilatory effects,
patients with hepatic or renal disease in whom drug clearance may
be impaired, and patients who take
other CNS depressants, including
alcohol, opiates, and sedatives, because droperidol may potentiate
the effects of these drugs.

Interactions
Drug-drug
*CNS depressants, such as antidepressants, barbiturates, sedative-
hypnotics, tranquilizers:* additive or
potentiated effects. Concurrent use
may require reduced dosages of
both drugs.
Fentanyl citrate: may cause hypertension and respiratory depression.
Monitor patient's respirations and
blood pressure closely.
Opiate or other analgesics: droperidol potentiates CNS depressant effects. Concurrent use may require
reduced dosages of both drugs.

Drug-lifestyle
Alcohol use: potentiates CNS depressant effects. Avoid concurrent
use.

Adverse reactions
CNS: altered consciousness, extrapyramidal symptoms (including
dystonia, akathisia, fine tremors of
limbs), postoperative hallucinations, respiratory depression, *sedation,* temporarily altered EEG
pattern.
CV: *bradycardia,* decreased
pulmonary artery pressure, *hypotension with rebound tachycardia.*

Overdose and treatment
Overdose may cause extension of
drug's pharmacologic actions.
Treat it symptomatically and supportively.

Special considerations
- If patient needs an opiate during recovery from anesthesia, give a reduced amount initially (one-fourth to one-third the usual dosage) to prevent potentiation of respiratory depression.
- Observe patient for postoperative hallucinations or emergence delirium and drowsiness.
- Be prepared to treat severe hypotension.
- Droperidol is related to haloperidol and has an increased risk of causing extrapyramidal symptoms. Monitor patient's vital signs and watch carefully for these symptoms.
- Droperidol has been used for antiemetic effects during chemotherapy, especially with cisplatin.
- Stop drug if patient develops hypersensitivity, severe persistent hypotension, respiratory depression, paradoxical hypertension, or dystonia.
- In patients who are withdrawing from alcohol, drug may raise the risk of sudden death from cardiac arrythmias.

Breast-feeding patients
- No data exist to demonstrate whether droperidol appears in breast milk.

Pediatric patients
- Safety and efficacy in children under age 2 haven't been established.

Geriatric patients
- Give drug cautiously to elderly patients because they have an increased risk of extrapyramidal symptoms, CNS disturbances, and adverse CV effects.

Patient teaching
- Tell patient about possible postoperative effects of drug.

estazolam
ProSom

Pharmacologic classification:
benzodiazepine

Therapeutic classification:
hypnotic

Controlled substance schedule IV

Pregnancy risk category X

How supplied
Available by prescription only
Tablets: 1 mg, 2 mg

Indications and dosages
Short-term management of insomnia characterized by difficulty in falling asleep, frequent nocturnal awakening, or early-morning awakening
Adults: initially, 1 mg P.O. h.s. May increase to 2 mg as needed and tolerated.
▶ DOSAGE ADJUSTMENT. In small or debilitated older adults, start with 0.5 mg P.O. h.s. Carefully increase to 1 mg if needed.

Pharmacodynamics
Hypnotic action: Estazolam depresses the CNS at the limbic and subcortical levels of the brain. It produces a sedative-hypnotic effect by potentiating GABA at its receptor in the ascending reticular activating system, which increases in-

hibition and blocks cortical and limbic arousal.

Pharmacokinetics

Absorption: Estazolam is rapidly and completely absorbed through the GI tract in 1 to 3 hours. Levels usually peak within 2 hours (range is 30 minutes to 6 hours).
Distribution: Estazolam is 93% protein-bound.
Metabolism: Drug is extensively metabolized in the liver.
Excretion: Metabolites are excreted primarily in urine, less than 5% as unchanged drug. About 4% of a 2-mg dose is excreted in feces. Elimination half-life ranges from 10 to 24 hours; clearance is accelerated in smokers.

Contraindications and precautions

Contraindicated in pregnant patients or patients hypersensitive to drug.

Use cautiously in patients with depression, suicidal tendencies, and hepatic, renal, or pulmonary disease.

Interactions

Drug-drug

Antihistamines, barbiturates, general anesthetics, MAO inhibitors, narcotics, phenothiazines, tricyclic antidepressants: potentiated CNS depressant effects. Monitor patient closely.
Cimetidine, disulfiram, isoniazid, oral contraceptives: possible diminished hepatic metabolism of estazolam, resulting in increased plasma levels and increased CNS depressant effects. Monitor patient closely.

Digoxin, phenytoin: increased phenytoin and digoxin levels, possibly resulting in toxicity. Dose adjustment may be needed.
Probenecid: speeds and lengthens benzodiazepine effect. Dosage adjustment may be needed.
Rifampin: increases clearance and decreases half-life of estazolam. Dosage adjustment may be needed.
Theophylline: antagonizes estazolam's pharmacologic effects. Monitor patient closely.

Drug-lifestyle

Alcohol use: may cause excessive respiratory and CNS depression. Avoid concomitant use.
Heavy smoking: accelerates estazolam's metabolism, resulting in diminished clinical efficacy. Avoid concomitant use, and discourage smoking.

Adverse reactions

CNS: *abnormal thinking, asthenia,* fatigue, *daytime drowsiness,* dizziness, *hypokinesia, somnolence.*
GI: abdominal pain, dyspepsia.
Hepatic: increased AST levels.
Musculoskeletal: back pain, stiffness.

Overdose and treatment

Benzodiazepine overdose may cause apnea, coma, confusion, hypotension, impaired coordination, reduced or absent reflexes, respiratory depression, seizures, slurred speech, or somnolence.

Provide symptomatic and supportive care. Maintain patient's airway, and give fluids. If excitation occurs, don't give barbiturates. Especially because the patient may have ingested more than one drug, perform gastric lavage immediately. Monitor patient's respiration, pulse rate, and blood pressure. Flumazenil, a specific benzodiazepine antagonist, may be useful.

Special considerations
- Drug should be taken until sleep pattern is established and then slowly tapered.
- Remove all safety hazards, such as cigarettes, from patient's reach.
- Regularly obtain blood counts, urinalysis, and blood chemistry analyses.
- Withdraw drug slowly after prolonged use.

Breast-feeding patients
- Drug appears in breast milk; avoid use in breast-feeding patients.

Pediatric patients
- Safety and efficacy in children haven't been established.

Geriatric patients
- Elderly patients may be more susceptible to CNS depressant effects of estazolam. Use with caution, and reduce dosage as needed.
- To prevent injury from dizziness and falls, supervise elderly patients during daily activities, especially at the start of treatment and after dosage increases.

Patient teaching
- Tell patient to notify prescriber about other drugs and herbal remedies she takes and about her usual alcohol consumption.
- Encourage good sleep habits and regular exercise during therapy.

- Urge patient to avoid caffeine and other stimulants, especially late in the day.
- Tell patient to avoid alcohol and other CNS depressants during therapy. Also, tell her to avoid alcohol the day after taking drug in the evening.
- Caution patient to avoid hazardous activities until full CNS effects of drug are known.
- Warn patient not to stop drug abruptly after taking it daily for a prolonged period and not to vary or increase dosage without consulting prescriber.
- Inform patient that she may have rebound insomnia for 1 or 2 nights after therapy stops. Explain that insomnia may indicate a serious medical condition; encourage follow-up care if it persists.
- Advise women to immediately notify prescriber about planned, suspected, or known pregnancy.

---

flurazepam hydrochloride
Apo-Flurazepam◇, Dalmane, Novoflupam◇

Pharmacologic classification: benzodiazepine

Therapeutic classification: sedative-hypnotic

Controlled substance schedule IV

Pregnancy risk category X

How supplied
Available by prescription only
Capsules: 15 mg, 30 mg

Indications and dosages
Insomnia
Adults: 15 to 30 mg P.O. h.s.
▶ DOSAGE ADJUSTMENT. In patients over age 65, give 15 mg P.O. h.s.

Pharmacodynamics
Sedative action: Flurazepam depresses the CNS at the limbic and subcortical levels of the brain. It produces sedation by potentiating the effect of GABA on its receptor in the ascending reticular activating system, which increases inhibition and blocks cortical and limbic arousal.

Pharmacokinetics
Absorption: When given orally, flurazepam is absorbed rapidly through the GI tract. Action begins within 20 minutes, peaks in 1 to 2 hours, and lasts 7 to 10 hours.
Distribution: Drug is distributed widely throughout the body. About 97% of a dose is bound to plasma protein.
Metabolism: Drug is metabolized in the liver to the active metabolite desalkylflurazepam.
Excretion: Desalkylflurazepam is excreted in urine; half-life is 50 to 100 hours.

Contraindications and precautions
Contraindicated in pregnant patients and those hypersensitive to drug.

Use cautiously in patients with impaired renal or hepatic function, chronic pulmonary insufficiency, mental depression, suicidal tendencies, or a history of drug abuse.

Interactions
Drug-drug
Antidepressants, antihistamines, barbiturates, general anesthetics, MAO inhibitors, narcotics, phenothiazines: flurazepam potentiates CNS depressant effects. Monitor patient closely.
Cimetidine, disulfiram, isoniazid, oral contraceptives, ritonavir: may decrease benzodiazepine metabolism, leading to toxicity. Monitor patient closely.
Digoxin: serum levels may increase, resulting in toxicity. Monitor patient's serum levels closely.
Haloperidol: benzodiazepines may decrease plasma haloperidol levels. Monitor serum levels closely.
Levodopa: flurazepam may decrease therapeutic effects of levodopa. Dosage adjustment may be needed.
Phenytoin: may increase phenytoin levels. Monitor serum levels closely.
Rifampin: may enhance benzodiazepine metabolism. Dosage adjustment may be needed.
Theophylline: may antagonize flurazepam. Dosage adjustment may be needed.

Drug-lifestyle
Alcohol use: may cause excessive CNS and respiratory depression. Avoid use together.
Heavy smoking: accelerated flurazepam metabolism and possible reduced effectiveness. Discourage concurrent use.

Adverse reactions
CNS: altered EEG pattern, *coma,* confusion, *daytime sedation,* disorientation, *disturbed coordination, dizziness, drowsiness,* hallucina-

tions, *headache,* lethargy, light-headedness, nervousness, staggering ataxia.
GI: abdominal pain, diarrhea, heartburn, nausea, vomiting.
Hepatic: elevated liver enzymes.
Other: physical or psychological dependence.

Overdose and treatment
Overdose may cause bradycardia, confusion, dyspnea, hypoactive reflexes, hypotension, impaired coordination, labored breathing, slurred speech, somnolence, unsteady gait, and eventual coma.

Monitor patient's vital signs and support blood pressure and respiration until drug effects subside. Provide mechanical ventilatory assistance via endotracheal tube if needed to maintain a patent airway and support oxygenation. Give I.V. fluids to promote diuresis. Give vasopressors, such as dopamine and phenylephrine, to treat hypotension as needed. If ingestion was recent and patient is conscious, induce emesis. If patient has an endotracheal tube in place, perform gastric lavage. After emesis or lavage, give activated charcoal with a cathartic as a single dose. Dialysis has limited value. If excitation occurs, don't give barbiturates; doing so may worsen the excitatory state or potentiate CNS depressant effects. Flumazenil, a specific benzodiazepine antagonist, may be useful as an adjunct to supportive therapy.

Special considerations
■ Studies have demonstrated a "carryover effect." Drug is most effective after 3 or 4 nights of use because of long half-life. Don't increase dose more frequently than every 5 days.
■ Monitor patient's hepatic function, AST, ALT, bilirubin, and alkaline phosphatase levels.
■ Drug is useful for patients who have trouble falling asleep and who awaken frequently at night and early in the morning.
■ Although prolonged use is not recommended, this drug has proven effective for up to 4 weeks of continuous use.
■ Rapid withdrawal after prolonged use can cause withdrawal symptoms.
■ Lower doses are effective in patients with renal or hepatic dysfunction.

Breast-feeding patients
■ Drug appears in breast milk and may cause sedation, feeding difficulties, and weight loss in a breast-fed infant. Avoid giving drug to breast-feeding women.

Pediatric patients
■ Use of flurazepam during labor may cause flaccidity in neonate.
■ If mother took drug during pregnancy, observe neonate closely for withdrawal symptoms.
■ Neonates have increased sensitivity to flurazepam because of their slower metabolism. Thus, the risk of toxicity is greatly increased.
■ Drug isn't recommended for children under age 15.

Geriatric patients
■ Drug typically isn't recommended for elderly patients.

Reactions may be *common,* uncommon, *life-threatening,* or COMMON AND LIFE-THREATENING.

- Because of decreased elimination, elderly patients typically receive reduced dosages.
- Elderly patients are more susceptible to CNS depressant effects of flurazepam. Provide assistance with walking and daily activities at the start of therapy and after dosage increases.

Patient teaching
- Advise patient not to exceed prescribed dosage.
- Warn patient to avoid alcohol during therapy. Stress the risk of excessive CNS depression from concurrent use, even if drug is taken the evening before alcohol ingestion.
- Warn patient not to discontinue drug abruptly after prolonged use.
- Inform patient that rebound insomnia may occur when therapy ends.
- Urge women to stop taking drug and to immediately notify prescriber about suspected or known pregnancy.

---

pentobarbital sodium
Nembutal

Pharmacologic classification:
barbiturate

Therapeutic classification:
anticonvulsant, sedative-hypnotic

*Controlled substance schedule II
(III for suppositories)*

Pregnancy risk category D

How supplied
Available by prescription only
Capsules: 50 mg, 100 mg

Elixir: 18.2 mg/5 ml
Injection: 50 mg/ml, 1-ml, and 2-ml disposable syringes; 2-ml, 20-ml, and 50-ml vials
Suppositories: 30 mg, 60 mg, 120 mg, 200 mg

Indications and dosages
Sedation
Adults: 20 to 40 mg P.O. b.i.d., t.i.d., or q.i.d.
Children: 2 to 6 mg/kg/day P.O.in divided doses. Maximum, 100 mg/dose.

Insomnia
Adults: 100 mg P.O. h.s. or 150 to 200 mg deep I.M. or 120 to 200 mg P.R.
Children: 2 to 6 mg/kg I.M. to maximum of 100 mg/dose. Or 30 mg P.R. (ages 2 months to 1 year), 30 to 60 mg P.R. (ages 1 to 4), 60 mg P.R. (ages 5 to 12), 60 to 120 mg P.R. (ages 12 to 14).

Anticonvulsant effects
Adults: initially, 100 mg I.V. After 1 minute, additional doses may be given. Maximum, 500 mg/dose.
Children: initially, 50 mg. After 1 minute, additional small doses may be given until desired effect occurs.

Pharmacodynamics
Sedative-hypnotic action: Exact cellular site and mechanism of action are unknown. Pentobarbital acts throughout the CNS as a nonselective depressant with a fast onset of action and short duration of action. Particularly sensitive to this drug is the reticular activating system, which controls CNS arousal. Pentobarbital decreases both presynaptic and postsynaptic mem-

brane excitability by facilitating the action of GABA.

Anticonvulsant action: Pentobarbital suppresses the spread of seizure activity produced by epileptogenic foci in the cortex, thalamus, and limbic systems by enhancing the effect of GABA. Both presynaptic and postsynaptic excitability are decreased, and the seizure threshold is raised.

Pharmacokinetics

Absorption: Drug is absorbed rapidly after oral or rectal administration. Action begins in 10 to 15 minutes. Serum levels peak 30 to 60 minutes after oral administration, 10 to 15 minutes after I.M. administration, and immediately after I.V. administration. Serum levels needed for sedation and hypnosis are 1 to 5 mcg/ml and 5 to 15 mcg/ml, respectively. After oral or rectal administration, hypnosis lasts 1 to 4 hours.

Distribution: Drug is distributed widely throughout the body. About 35% to 45% is protein-bound. Drug accumulates in fat with long-term use.

Metabolism: Drug is metabolized in the liver by penultimate oxidation.

Excretion: 99% of pentobarbital is eliminated as glucuronide conjugates and other metabolites in the urine. Terminal half-life ranges from 35 to 50 hours. Duration of action is 3 to 4 hours.

Contraindications and precautions

Contraindicated in patients hypersensitive to barbiturates and in patients with porphyria or severe respiratory disease with dyspnea or obstruction.

Use cautiously in elderly or debilitated patients and in those with acute or chronic pain, mental depression, suicidal tendencies, a history of drug abuse, or impaired hepatic function.

Interactions
Drug-drug

Antidepressants, antihistamines, narcotics, sedative-hypnotics, tranquilizers: pentobarbital may add to or potentiate CNS and respiratory depressant effects. Use together with extreme caution.

Corticosteroids, digitoxin (not digoxin), doxycycline, oral contraceptives, other estrogens, theophylline, other xanthines: pentobarbital enhances hepatic metabolism. Dosage adjustment may be needed.

Disulfiram, MAO inhibitors, valproic acid: decreased pentobarbital metabolism and increased risk of toxicity. Monitor patient closely.

Griseofulvin: pentobarbital impairs griseofulvin effectiveness by decreasing absorption from the GI tract. Monitor patient for lack of effectiveness, and adjust dosage adjustment as needed.

Rifampin: may decrease pentobarbital levels by increasing hepatic metabolism. Monitor patient closely.

Warfarin and other oral anticoagulants: pentobarbital enhances enzymatic degradation of anticoagulant. Increased anticoagulant dosage may be needed.

Drug-lifestyle

Alcohol use: pentobarbital may add to or potentiate CNS and respiratory depressant effects of alcohol. Avoid concurrent use.

Adverse reactions

CNS: *drowsiness,* hallucinations, *hangover, lethargy,* paradoxical excitement in elderly patients, somnolence.

CV: *bradycardia,* hypotension, syncope.

GI: nausea, vomiting.

Hematologic: exacerbation of porphyria.

Respiratory: *respiratory depression.*

Skin: rash, *Stevens-Johnson syndrome,* urticaria.

Other: *angioedema,* myasthenia gravis, nystagmus, physical and psychological dependence.

Overdose and treatment

Overdose may cause areflexia, coma, confusion, fever, hypothermia, jaundice, oliguria, pulmonary edema, respiratory depression, slurred speech, somnolence, sustained nystagmus, and an unsteady gait. Shock with tachycardia and hypotension may occur as well. Serum levels above 10 mcg/ml may produce profound coma; levels above 30 mcg/ml may be fatal.

To treat overdose, support patient's ventilation and pulmonary function as needed. Give vasopressors and I.V. fluids to support cardiac function and circulation. If ingestion was recent and patient is conscious and has an intact gag reflex, induce emesis with ipecac syrup. If emesis is contraindicated and patient has a cuffed endotracheal tube in place to prevent aspiration, perform gastric lavage. Follow with activated charcoal. Measure patient's intake and output, vital signs, and laboratory parameters. Maintain her body temperature. Alkalinization of urine may help to remove drug from the body. Hemodialysis may be useful in severe overdose.

Special considerations

■ Use I.V. route only for emergency treatment, and don't give more than 50 mg/minute to prevent hypotension and respiratory depression. Be prepared to perform emergency resuscitative measures.

■ Give I.M. dose deep into large muscle mass. Don't give more than 5 ml into any one site.

■ Discard solution that's discolored or contains precipitate.

■ To ensure accurate doses, don't divide suppositories.

■ Drug has no analgesic effect and may cause restlessness or delirium in patients with pain.

■ Nembutal tablets contain tartrazine dye, which may cause allergic reactions in susceptible persons.

■ Adults who receive full loading doses over short periods of time for status epilepticus will need ventilatory support.

■ To prevent rebound of REM sleep after prolonged therapy, stop drug gradually over 5 to 6 days.

■ Pentobarbital may cause false-positive results on the phentolamine test. Physiologic effects of drug may impair absorption of cyanocobalamin [57]Co and may decrease serum bilirubin levels in neonates, epileptic patients, and patients with congenital non-

hemolytic unconjugated hyper-bilirubinemia.. It also may change EEG patterns, specifically low-voltage, fast-activity; changes persist for a time after therapy stops.
■ Besides standard indications, drug is also used for preoperative sedation, intracranial hypertension, and hypothermia caused by near drowning (unlabeled).

Breast-feeding patients
■ Pentobarbital appears in breast milk. Don't give drug to breast-feeding women.

Pediatric patients
■ Barbiturates may cause paradoxical excitement in children. Use with caution.

Geriatric patients
■ Elderly patients typically have increased susceptibility to drug's CNS depressant effects. Give a reduced dosage as needed.
■ Confusion, disorientation, and excitability may occur in elderly patients. Use drug cautiously.

Patient teaching
■ Tell patient not to take drug continuously for longer than 2 weeks.
■ Emphasize the dangers of combining drug with alcohol. An excessive depressant effect may occur even after taking drug the evening before alcohol ingestion.
■ Tell patient not to stop drug abruptly without consulting prescriber.
■ Advise pregnant patient that pentobarbital taken late in pregnancy may harm fetus or neonate. Explain that withdrawal symptoms may occur.

phenobarbital
Barbita, Solfoton

phenobarbital sodium
Luminal

Pharmacologic classification:
barbiturate

Therapeutic classification:
anticonvulsant, sedative-hypnotic

Controlled substance schedule IV

Pregnancy risk category D

How supplied
Available by prescription only
Capsules: 16 mg
Elixir: 15 mg/5 ml, 20 mg/5 ml
Injection: 30 mg/ml, 60 mg/ml, 65 mg/ml, 130 mg/ml
Tablets: 15 mg, 16 mg, 30 mg, 60 mg, 100 mg

Indications and dosages
All forms of epilepsy except absence seizures, febrile seizures in children
Adults: 60 to 100 mg/day P.O., divided t.i.d. or given as a single dose h.s. Alternatively, 200 to 300 mg I.M. or I.V., repeated q 6 hours p.r.n.
Children: 1 to 6 mg/kg/day P.O., usually divided q 12 hours, although drug may be given once daily. Alternatively, give 4 to 6 mg/kg/day I.V. or I.M. and monitor patient's blood levels.

Status epilepticus
Adults and children: 10 to 20 mg/kg I.V. over 10 to 15 minutes. Maximum, 60 mg/minute. Repeat if necessary.

To produce sedation
Adults: 30 to 120 mg/day P.O., I.M., or I.V. in two or three divided doses. Maximum, 400 mg/24 hours.
Children: 8 to 32 mg/day P.O.

Insomnia
Adults: 100 to 200 mg P.O. or 100 to 320 mg I.M.

▷ DOSAGE ADJUSTMENT. Patients with hepatic dysfunction may need a reduced dosage.

Pharmacodynamics
Anticonvulsant action: Drug suppresses the spread of seizure activity produced by epileptogenic foci in the cortex, thalamus, and limbic systems by enhancing the effect of GABA. Both presynaptic and postsynaptic excitability are decreased, raising the seizure threshold.
Sedative-hypnotic action: Drug acts throughout the CNS as a nonselective depressant with a slow onset of action and a long duration of action. Particularly sensitive to this drug is the reticular activating system, which controls CNS arousal. Phenobarbital decreases both presynaptic and postsynaptic membrane excitability by facilitating the action of GABA. The exact cellular site and mechanism of action are unknown.

Pharmacokinetics
Absorption: Drug is well absorbed after oral and rectal administration, with 70% to 90% reaching the bloodstream. Absorption after I.M. administration is 100%. After oral administration, serum levels peak in 1 to 2 hours; CNS levels peak in 1 to 3 hours. Action begins 20 to 60 minutes or longer after an oral dosing, 5 minutes after an I.V. dose. A serum level of 10 mcg/ml is needed to produce sedation; 40 mcg/ml usually produces sleep. Levels of 20 to 40 mcg/ml are considered therapeutic for anticonvulsant therapy.
Distribution: Drug is distributed widely throughout the body and is about 25% to 30% protein-bound.
Metabolism: Drug is metabolized by the hepatic microsomal enzyme system.
Excretion: 25% to 50% of a phenobarbital dose is eliminated unchanged in urine. The rest is excreted as metabolites of glucuronic acid. Half-life is 5 to 7 days.

Contraindications and precautions
Contraindicated in patients hypersensitive to barbiturates and patients with hepatic dysfunction, respiratory disease with dyspnea or obstruction, nephritis, and a history of manifest or latent porphyria.

Use cautiously in elderly or debilitated patients and in those with acute or chronic pain, depression, suicidal tendencies, a history of drug abuse, blood pressure alterations, CV disease, shock, or uremia.

Interactions
Drug-drug
Antidepressants, antihistamines, narcotics, phenothiazines, sedative-hypnotics, tranquilizers: phenobarbital may add to or potentiate CNS and respiratory depressant effects. Use together with extreme caution.

Cholestyramine: decreased phenobarbital absorption. Separate administration times by at least 2 hours.

Corticosteroids, digitoxin (not digoxin), doxycycline, oral contraceptives, other estrogens, theophylline, other xanthines: phenobarbital enhances hepatic metabolism. Dosage adjustment may be needed.

Disulfiram, MAO inhibitors, valproic acid: decreased phenobarbital metabolism and increased risk of toxicity. Monitor patient closely.

Felodipine, metoprolol, nimodipine, verapamil: possible decreased effectiveness of these drugs. Dosage adjustment may be needed.

Griseofulvin: phenobarbital impairs griseofulvin effectiveness by decreasing absorption from the GI tract. Monitor patient closely.

Influenza vaccine: phenobarbital decreases effectiveness of vaccine.

Rifampin: may decrease phenobarbital levels by increasing hepatic metabolism. Monitor serum levels.

Warfarin and other oral anticoagulants: phenobarbital enhances enzymatic degradation of anticoagulant. Increased anticoagulant dosage may be needed.

Drug-lifestyle
Alcohol use: phenobarbital may add to or potentiate CNS and respiratory depressant effects of alcohol. Avoid concurrent use.

Adverse reactions
CNS: *drowsiness, hangover, lethargy,* paradoxical excitement in elderly patients, somnolence.
CV: *bradycardia,* hypotension.
EENT: miosis.
GI: constipation, hepatotoxicity, nausea, vomiting.
Hematologic: *agranulocytosis,* exacerbation of porphyria, *leukopenia, megaloblastic anemia.*
Metabolic: hypocalcemia.
Respiratory: *apnea, respiratory depression.*
Skin: *erythema multiforme,* nerve injury at injection site, pain and swelling at injection site, rash, *Stevens-Johnson syndrome,* thrombophlebitis and necrosis at injection site, urticaria.
Other: *angioedema,* physical and psychological dependence.

Overdose and treatment
Overdose may cause areflexia, chills, coma, confusion, fever, pulmonary edema, respiratory depression, jaundice, slurred speech, somnolence, sustained nystagmus, oliguria, and an unsteady gait. Shock with tachycardia and hypotension may occur as well.

To treat overdose, support patient's ventilation and pulmonary function as needed. Give vasopressors and I.V. fluids to support cardiac function and circulation. If ingestion was recent and patient is conscious and has an intact gag reflex, induce emesis with ipecac syrup. If emesis is contraindicated and patient has a cuffed endotracheal tube in place to prevent aspiration, perform gastric lavage. Follow with activated charcoal. (Oral activated charcoal may enhance phenobarbital elimination regardless of drug's route of administration.) Measure patient's intake and output, vital signs, and laboratory parameters. Maintain her body temperature. Alkalinization of

---

urine may help to remove drug from the body.

Special considerations
- Reconstitute powder for injection with 2.5 to 5 ml sterile water for injection. Roll vial in hands rather than shaking it.
- Don't use injectable solution if it contains a precipitate.
- Administer parenteral dose within 30 minutes of reconstitution because phenobarbital hydrolyzes in solution and on exposure to air.
- Keep emergency resuscitation equipment on hand when administering phenobarbital I.V.
- Use a large vein for I.V. administration to prevent extravasation.
- Avoid I.V. administration at more than 60 mg/minute to prevent hypotension and respiratory depression. Maximum effect may not occur for up to 30 minutes after I.V. administration.
- Administer I.M. dose deep into a large muscle mass to prevent tissue injury.
- Oral solution may be mixed with water or juice to improve taste.
- Don't crush or break extended-release form because doing so will impair drug action.
- Therapeutic serum level is 10 to 40 mcg/ml.
- Besides standard indications, drug is also used for preoperative sedation, as an anticonvulsant for patients with head injuries, and as a treatment for alcohol withdrawal (unlabeled).
- Phenobarbital may cause false-positive results on the phentolamine test. Physiologic effects of drug may impair absorption of cyanocobalamin [57]Co and may decrease serum bilirubin levels in neonates, epileptic patients, and patients with congenital non-hemolytic unconjugated hyper-bilirubinemia. It also may increase sulfobromophthalein retention. And it may change EEG patterns, specifically low-voltage, fast-activity; changes persist for a time after therapy stops.

Breast-feeding patients
- Phenobarbital appears in breast milk; avoid giving drug to breast-feeding women.

Pediatric patients
- Paradoxical hyperexcitability may occur in children. Use drug cautiously.
- Phenobarbital extended-release capsules aren't recommended for children under age 12.

Geriatric patients
- Elderly patients are more sensitive to drug effects and usually need a reduced dosage.
- Confusion, disorientation, and excitability may occur in elderly patients.

Patient teaching
- Advise patient that prolonged use of drug may cause physical and psychological dependence.
- Warn patient to avoid alcohol and other CNS depressants during therapy. An excessive depressant effect is possible even after taking drug the evening before alcohol ingestion.
- Caution patient not to stop taking drug suddenly because doing so could cause a withdrawal reaction.

■ Tell patient to avoid hazardous activities until full CNS effects of drug are known.

---

promethazine hydrochloride
Anergan 25, Anergan 50, Histantil◇, Pentazine, Phencen-50, Phenergan, Phenergan Fortis, Phenergan Plain, Phenoject-50, Promet, Prorex-25, Prorex-50, Prothazine, Prothazine Plain, V-Gan-25, V-Gan-50

Pharmacologic classification: phenothiazine derivative

Therapeutic classification: antihistamine (H$_1$-receptor antagonist); antiemetic; antivertigo; preoperative, postoperative, or obstetric sedative and adjunct to analgesics

Pregnancy risk category C

How supplied
Available by prescription only
Injection: 25 mg/ml, 50 mg/ml
Suppositories: 12.5 mg, 25 mg, 50 mg
Syrup: 6.25 mg/5 ml, 25 mg/5 ml
Tablets: 12.5 mg, 25 mg, 50 mg

Indications and dosages
Sedation
Adults: 25 to 50 mg P.O. or I.M. h.s., or p.r.n.
Children: 12.5 to 25 mg P.O., I.M., or P.R. h.s.

Pharmacodynamics
Antiemetic and antivertigo actions: The central antimuscarinic actions of antihistamines probably are responsible for their antivertigo and antiemetic effects; promethazine probably also inhibits the medullary chemoreceptor trigger zone.
Antihistamine action: Drug competes with histamine for H$_1$-receptors, thereby suppressing allergic rhinitis and urticaria. It doesn't prevent histamine release.
Sedative action: CNS depressant mechanism of promethazine is unknown; phenothiazines probably cause sedation by reducing stimuli to the brainstem reticular system.

Pharmacokinetics
Absorption: Promethazine is well absorbed from the GI tract. Action begins 20 minutes after P.O., P.R., or I.M. administration and 3 to 5 minutes after I.V. administration. Effects usually last 4 to 6 hours but may persist for 12 hours.
Distribution: Drug is distributed widely throughout the body and is highly protein-bound. It crosses the placenta.
Metabolism: Drug is metabolized in the liver.
Excretion: Drug's metabolites are excreted in urine and feces.

Contraindications and precautions
Contraindicated in acutely ill or dehydrated children; in newborns, premature neonates, and breast-feeding patients; in patients hypersensitive to drug or to sulfites; and in patients with bladder neck obstruction, CNS depression, coma, intestinal obstruction, prostatic hyperplasia, seizure disorders, and stenosing peptic ulcers.

Reactions may be *common*, uncommon, *life-threatening*, or COMMON AND LIFE-THREATENING.

Use cautiously in patients with asthma, sleep apnea, or cardiac, pulmonary, or hepatic disease.

Interactions
Drug-drug
Antihistamines, CNS depressants (such as antianxiety drugs, barbiturates, sleeping aids, tranquilizers): additive CNS depression may occur. Use together with extreme caution.
Epinephrine: increased hypotension. Don't use together.
Levodopa: promethazine may block antiparkinsonian action. Monitor patient closely.
MAO inhibitors: by interfering with detoxification of antihistamines and phenothiazines. MAO inhibitors prolong and intensify sedative and anticholinergic effects. Don't use together.

Drug-lifestyle
Alcohol use: additive CNS depression may occur. Discourage alcohol use during therapy.
Sun exposure: may cause photosensitivity reactions. Urge precautions.

Adverse reactions
CNS: confusion, disorientation, dizziness, *drowsiness,* extrapyramidal symptoms, *sedation,* sleepiness.
CV: hypertension, hypotension.
EENT: blurred vision.
GI: constipation, *dry mouth,* nausea, vomiting.
GU: urine retention.
Hematologic: *agranulocytosis, leukopenia, thrombocytopenia.*
Skin: photosensitivity, rash.

Overdose and treatment
Overdose may cause either CNS depression (sedation, reduced mental alertness, apnea, and CV collapse) or CNS stimulation (insomnia, hallucinations, tremors, or seizures). Atropine-like signs and symptoms, such as dry mouth, flushed skin, fixed and dilated pupils, and GI symptoms, are common, especially in children.

Perform gastric lavage to empty patient's stomach; don't induce vomiting. Give vasopressors (but not epinephrine) for hypotension. Give diazepam or phenytoin for seizures. Correct acidosis and electrolyte imbalance as needed. Urine acidification promotes drug excretion. Don't give stimulants. Dialysis isn't helpful.

Special considerations
■ Pronounced sedative effects may limit use of this drug in some ambulatory patients.
■ The 50-mg/ml form is for I.M. use only; inject it deep into a large muscle mass.
■ Don't give drug by S.C. route because doing so may cause chemical irritation and necrosis.
■ Drug may be given by I.V. route at no more than 25 mg/ml and a rate no higher than 25 mg/minute. When using I.V. drip, wrap drug container in aluminum foil to protect drug from light.
■ Promethazine and meperidine (Demerol) may be mixed in the same syringe.
■ Drug may prevent, reduce, or mask response to diagnostic skin tests; stop therapy 4 days before such tests. Promethazine also may cause hyperglycemia. It may cause

false-positive or false-negative results on pregnancy test. And it may interfere with ABO blood grouping tests.
■ Besides standard indications, drug is also used for motion sickness, nausea and rhinitis, allergy symptoms.

Breast-feeding patients
■ Antihistamines such as promethazine shouldn't be used during breast-feeding. Many of these drugs are secreted in breast milk, raising the risk of unusual excitability in infants, especially premature infants and other neonates, who may develop seizures.

Pediatric patients
■ Use cautiously in children who have respiratory dysfunction.
■ Safety and efficacy in children under age 2 haven't been established.
■ Don't give promethazine to infants under age 3 months.

Geriatric patients
■ Elderly patients are usually more sensitive to adverse effects of antihistamines and are especially likely to experience more dizziness, sedation, hyperexcitability, dry mouth, and urine retention than younger patients. Symptoms usually respond to dosage reduction.

Patient teaching
■ Warn patient about possible photosensitivity and ways to avoid it.
■ Caution patient to avoid hazardous activities until full sedative effects of drug are known.
■ When treating motion sickness, tell patient to take first dose 30 to 60 minutes before travel and then, on succeeding days, upon arising and with evening meal.

---

secobarbital sodium
Novosecobarb◊, Seconal

Pharmacologic classification:
barbiturate

Therapeutic classification:
anticonvulsant, sedative-hypnotic

Controlled substance schedule II

Pregnancy risk category D

How supplied
Available by prescription only
Capsules: 50 mg, 100 mg
Injection: 50 mg/ml in 2-ml disposable syringe

Indications and dosages
Insomnia
Adults: 100 mg P.O., 100 to 200 mg I.M., or 50 to 250 mg I.V.

Status epilepticus
Adults: 250 to 350 mg I.M. or I.V.
Children: 15 to 20 mg/kg I.V. over 15 minutes.

Pharmacodynamics
Sedative-hypnotic action: Secobarbital acts throughout the CNS as a nonselective depressant with a rapid onset and short duration of action. Particularly sensitive to this drug is the reticular activating system, which controls CNS arousal. Secobarbital decreases both presynaptic and postsynaptic membrane excitability by facilitating the action of GABA. The exact cellular

site and mechanism of action are unknown.

Pharmacokinetics
Absorption: After oral administration, 90% of secobarbital is absorbed within 2 hours. After rectal administration, secobarbital is nearly 100% absorbed. Serum levels peak 2 to 4 hours after oral or rectal administration. Action begins within 15 minutes after oral administration. Effects peak 15 to 30 minutes after oral or rectal administration, 7 to 10 minutes after I.M. administration, and 1 to 3 minutes after I.V. administration. Levels of 1 to 5 mcg/ml are needed to produce sedation, 5 to 15 mcg/ml to produce hypnosis. Hypnosis lasts for 1 to 4 hours after an oral dose of 100 to 150 mg.
Distribution: Drug is distributed rapidly throughout body tissues and fluids; about 30% to 45% is protein-bound.
Metabolism: Drug is oxidized in the liver to inactive metabolites. Duration of action is 3 to 4 hours.
Excretion: 95% of a dose is eliminated as glucuronide conjugates and other metabolites in urine. Drug has an elimination half-life of about 30 hours.

Contraindications and precautions
Contraindicated in patients hypersensitive to barbiturates and in patients with porphyria or respiratory disease with dyspnea or obstruction.

Use cautiously in patients with acute or chronic pain, depression, suicidal tendencies, a history of drug abuse, or impaired hepatic or renal function.

Interactions
Drug-drug
Antidepressants, antihistamines, narcotics, tranquilizers: secobarbital may add to or potentiate CNS and respiratory depressant effects. Use together with extreme caution.
Corticosteroids, digitoxin (not digoxin), doxycycline, oral contraceptives, other estrogens, theophylline, other xanthines: secobarbital enhances hepatic metabolism. Dosage adjustment may be needed.
Disulfiram, MAO inhibitors, valproic acid: decreased secobarbital metabolism and increased risk of toxicity. Monitor patient closely.
Griseofulvin: secobarbital impairs griseofulvin effectiveness by decreasing absorption from the GI tract. Dosage adjustment may be needed.
Rifampin: may decrease secobarbital levels by increasing hepatic metabolism. Monitor serum levels.
Warfarin and other oral anticoagulants: secobarbital enhances enzymatic degradation of anticoagulant. Increased anticoagulant dosage may be needed.

Drug-lifestyle
Alcohol use: secobarbital may add to or potentiate CNS and respiratory depressant effects of alcohol. Avoid concurrent use.

Adverse reactions
CNS: altered EEG patterns, *drowsiness, hangover, lethargy,* paradoxical excitement in elderly patients, somnolence.
CV: hypotension with I.V. use.

GI: nausea, vomiting.
Respiratory: *respiratory depression.*
Skin: pain at injection site, rash, *Stevens-Johnson syndrome,* tissue reactions, urticaria.
Other: *angioedema,* physical and psychological dependence.

Overdose and treatment
Overdose may cause areflexia, chills, coma, confusion, fever, jaundice, oliguria, pulmonary edema, respiratory depression, slurred speech, somnolence, sustained nystagmus, and an unsteady gait. Shock with tachycardia and hypotension may occur as well.

To treat overdose, support patient's ventilation and pulmonary function as needed. Give vasopressors and I.V. fluids to support cardiac function and circulation. If ingestion was recent (within 4 hours) and patient is conscious and has an intact gag reflex, induce emesis with ipecac syrup. If emesis is contraindicated and patient has a cuffed endotracheal tube in place to prevent aspiration, perform gastric lavage. Follow with activated charcoal. Measure patient's intake and output, vital signs, and laboratory parameters. Maintain her body temperature. Roll her from side to side every 30 minutes to avoid pulmonary congestion. Alkalinization of urine may be helpful in removing drug from her body; hemodialysis may be useful in severe overdose.

Special considerations
■ Dilute secobarbital injection with sterile water for injection,
normal saline injection, or Ringer's injection solution.
■ Don't use a solution that's discolored or that contains precipitate.
■ Use I.V. route only in an emergency or when other routes aren't available. Total I.V. dose shouldn't exceed 500 mg.
■ To prevent hypotension and respiratory depression, avoid I.V. administration at more than 50 mg/ 15 seconds. Keep emergency resuscitative equipment on hand.
■ Administer I.M. dose deep into large muscle to prevent tissue injury.
■ Inject no more than 250 mg (5 ml) into any one I.M. site.
■ Secobarbital sodium injection, diluted with lukewarm tap water to 10 to 15 mg/ml, may be administered rectally in children. Administer a cleansing enema before the secobarbital enema.
■ Monitor patient's hepatic and renal studies frequently to prevent possible toxicity.
■ Secobarbital may cause false-positive results on the phentolamine test. Physiologic effects of the drug may impair absorption of cyanocobalamin ^{57}Co.
■ Besides standard uses, drug is also used for preoperative sedation.

Breast-feeding patients
■ Because drug enters breast milk, don't give it to breast-feeding women.

Pediatric patients
■ Drug may cause paradoxical excitement in children; use it cautiously.

Geriatric patients
- Elderly patients are more susceptible to drug effects and usually require lower doses.
- Confusion, disorientation, and excitability are more likely among elderly patients.

Patient teaching
- Emphasize the danger of combining drug with alcohol. An excessive depressant effect is possible even if drug is taken the evening before alcohol ingestion.
- Tell patient to avoid hazardous activities until full effects of drug are known.

---

temazepam
Restoril

Pharmacologic classification: benzodiazepine

Therapeutic classification: sedative-hypnotic

Controlled substance schedule IV

Pregnancy risk category X

How supplied
Available by prescription only
Capsules: 7.5 mg, 15 mg, 30 mg

Indications and dosages
Insomnia
Adults: 7.5 to 30 mg P.O. 30 minutes before bedtime.

▶ **DOSAGE ADJUSTMENT.** For elderly or debilitated patients, start with 7.5 mg P.O. h.s until individual response is known.

Pharmacodynamics
Sedative-hypnotic action: Drug depresses the CNS at the limbic and subcortical levels of the brain. It produces a sedative-hypnotic effect by potentiating the effect of GABA on its receptor in the ascending reticular activating system, which increases inhibition and blocks cortical and limbic arousal.

Pharmacokinetics
Absorption: When administered orally, drug is well absorbed through the GI tract. Levels peak in 72 to 96 minutes (mean, 90 minutes). Action begins in 30 to 60 minutes.
Distribution: Drug is widely distributed throughout the body and is 96% protein-bound.
Metabolism: Drug is metabolized in the liver, primarily to inactive metabolites.
Excretion: Metabolites are excreted in urine as glucuronide conjugates. Half-life of drug is 4 to 20 hours.

Contraindications and precautions
Contraindicated in pregnant patients and patients hypersensitive to drug or to other benzodiazepines.

Use cautiously in patients with impaired renal or hepatic function, chronic pulmonary insufficiency, severe or latent mental depression, suicidal tendencies, or a history of drug abuse.

Interactions
Drug-drug
Antidepressants, antihistamines, barbiturates, general anesthetics, MAO inhibitors, narcotics, and phe-

---

nothiazines: temazepam potentiates CNS depressant effects. Use together with extreme caution.
Haloperidol: temazepam may decrease plasma haloperidol levels. Dosage adjustment may be needed.
Levodopa: benzodiazepines block therapeutic levodopa effects. Dosage adjustment may be needed.

Drug-lifestyle
Alcohol use: may increase CNS depression. Avoid concurrent use.
Heavy smoking: accelerates temazepam metabolism, thus lowering clinical effectiveness. Discourage concurrent use.

Adverse reactions
CNS: amnesia, anxiety, confusion, daytime sedation, disturbed coordination, depression, *dizziness, drowsiness,* euphoria, fatigue, headache, *lethargy,* minor changes in EEG patterns, nervousness, nightmares, weakness, vertigo.
EENT: blurred vision.
GI: diarrhea, dry mouth, nausea.
Hepatic: elevated liver enzymes.
Other: physical and psychological dependence.

Overdose and treatment
Overdose may cause bradycardia, confusion, dyspnea, hypoactive or absent reflexes, hypotension, impaired coordination, labored breathing, slurred speech, somnolence, and unsteady gait and, ultimately, coma.

Monitor patient's vital signs, and support her blood pressure and respiration until drug effects subside. Provide mechanical ventilatory assistance via endotracheal tube if needed to maintain a patent airway and support adequate oxygenation. Give fluids and vasopressors, such as dopamine and phenylephrine I.V., to treat hypotension as needed. If ingestion was recent and patient is conscious and has an intact gag reflex, induce emesis with ipecac syrup. If patient has a cuffed endotracheal tube, perform gastric lavage. After emesis or lavage, give activated charcoal with a cathartic as a single dose. Flumazenil, a specific benzodiazepine antagonist, may be useful, but weigh the possibility of causing withdrawal in a benzodiazepine-dependent patient against possible benefits. Don't give barbiturates if excitation occurs. Dialysis is of limited value.

Special considerations
- Evaluate the cause of patient's insomnia because it commonly suggests an underlying disorder, such as depression.
- Drug is useful for patients who have trouble falling asleep or who awaken repeatedly during the night.
- Prolonged use isn't recommended, but drug has proven effective for up to 4 weeks of continuous use.
- Remove all safety hazards, such as cigarettes, from patient's reach.
- Impose safety measures, such as raising side rails and placing call bell within easy reach, to minimize the risk of injury.
- Monitor patient's hepatic function tests for early signs of toxicity; patients with hepatic dysfunction should receive a reduced dosage.
- Don't stop drug abruptly after long-term use; instead, taper dosage gradually.

Reactions may be *common,* uncommon, *life-threatening,* or COMMON AND LIFE-THREATENING.

- Store drug in a cool, dry place protected from light.

Breast-feeding patients
- Avoid use of temazepam in breast-feeding women because drug appears in breast milk and may cause sedation, feeding difficulties, or weight loss in infant.

Pediatric patients
- Safe use in patients under age 18 hasn't been established.

Geriatric patients
- Elderly patients are more susceptible to CNS depressant effects of temazepam. Use with caution.
- Lower dosages are usually effective in elderly patients because of their decreased elimination.
- Elderly patients may need assistance with ambulation and activities of daily living at the start of therapy and after dosage increases.

Patient teaching
- Inform patient that long-term use of drug may cause physical and psychological dependence.
- As needed, teach patient safety measures to prevent injury, such as gradual position changes and assisted ambulation.
- Tell patient to avoid hazardous activities until full sedative effects of drug are known. Explain that drug may cause extreme tiredness.
- Discourage use of alcohol during therapy; stress the risk of excessive CNS depression with concurrent use.
- Tell patient not to change dosage without consulting prescriber.

- Tell patient that rebound insomnia may occur after stopping drug.
- Advise women to immediately notify prescriber about planned, suspected, or known pregnancy.

---

triazolam
Halcion

Pharmacologic classification:
benzodiazepine

Therapeutic classification:
sedative-hypnotic

Controlled substance schedule IV

Pregnancy risk category X

How supplied
Available by prescription only
Tablets: 0.125 mg, 0.25 mg

Indications and dosages
Insomnia (short-term treatment)
Adults: 0.125 to 0.25 mg P.O. h.s. for up to 10 days. If patient fails to respond, increase to maximum of 0.5 mg P.O. h.s.
▶ DOSAGE ADJUSTMENT. For elderly patients, give 0.125 mg P.O. h.s., increased as needed to 0.25 mg.

Pharmacodynamics
Sedative-hypnotic action: Triazolam depresses the CNS at the limbic and subcortical levels of the brain. It produces a sedative-hypnotic effect by potentiating the effect of GABA on its receptor in the ascending reticular activating system, which increases inhibition and blocks cortical and limbic arousal.

Pharmacokinetics

Absorption: Drug is well absorbed through the GI tract after oral administration. Action starts in 15 to 30 minutes. Levels peak in 1 to 2 hours.

Distribution: Drug is distributed widely throughout the body and is 78% to 89% protein-bound.

Metabolism: Drug is metabolized in the liver, primarily to inactive metabolites.

Excretion: Metabolites of triazolam are excreted in urine. Half-life of ranges from about 1½ to 5½ hours.

Contraindications and precautions

Contraindicated in pregnant patients, patients hypersensitive to benzodiazepines, and patients taking ketoconazole, itraconazole, nefazodone, or any other drug that impairs oxidative metabolism of triazolam by cytochrome P-450 3A.

Use cautiously in patients who have impaired renal or hepatic function, chronic pulmonary insufficiency, sleep apnea, mental depression, suicidal tendencies, or a history of drug abuse.

Interactions
Drug-drug

Antidepressants, antihistamines, barbiturates, general anesthetics, MAO inhibitors, narcotics, and phenothiazines: triazolam potentiates CNS depression. Use together with extreme caution.

Cimetidine, isoniazid, oral contraceptives, and possibly disulfiram: decreased hepatic metabolism of triazolam and increase plasma levels. Monitor patient closely.

Digoxin: increased digoxin levels and increased risk of toxicity. Monitor patient and serum levels closely.

Erythromycin: decreases triazolam clearance. Monitor patient closely.

Haloperidol: triazolam may decrease serum haloperidol levels. Dosage adjustments may be needed.

Levodopa: benzodiazepines may decrease therapeutic effects of levodopa. Dosage adjustments may be needed.

Drug-food

Grapefruit juice: increases triazolam levels. Avoid concurrent use.

Drug-lifestyle

Alcohol use: potentiates CNS depressant effects and enhances amnestic effects even in small amounts. Avoid concurrent use.

Heavy smoking: accelerates triazolam metabolism, thus reducing effectiveness. Avoid concurrent use.

Adverse reactions

CNS: amnesia, ataxia, confusion, depression, *dizziness, drowsiness, headache,* lack of coordination, light-headedness, minor changes in EEG patterns, nervousness, rebound insomnia.

GI: nausea, vomiting.

Hepatic: elevated liver enzymes.

Other: physical or psychological dependence.

Overdose and treatment

Overdose may cause bradycardia, confusion, dyspnea, hypoactive reflexes, hypotension, impaired coordination, labored breathing, slurred speech, somnolence, an unsteady gait and, ultimately, coma.

Monitor patient's vital signs, and support her blood pressure and respiration until drug effects subside. Provide mechanical ventilatory assistance via endotracheal tube if needed to maintain a patent airway and support adequate oxygenation. Give fluids and vasopressors, such as dopamine and phenylephrine I.V., to treat hypotension as needed. If ingestion was recent and patient is conscious and has an intact gag reflex, induce emesis with ipecac syrup. If patient has a cuffed endotracheal tube, perform gastric lavage. After emesis or lavage, give activated charcoal with a cathartic as a single dose. Flumazenil, a specific benzodiazepine antagonist, may be useful, but weigh the possibility of causing withdrawal in a benzodiazepine-dependent patient against possible benefits. Don't give barbiturates if excitation occurs. Dialysis is of limited value.

Special considerations
- Monitor patient's liver function studies to detect early toxicity.
- Keep patient in bed when giving drug; sedation or hypnosis begins rapidly.
- Store drug in a cool, dry place away from light.

Breast-feeding patients
- Avoid use of triazolam in breast-feeding women because drug is excreted in breast milk and may cause sedation, feeding difficulties, or weight loss in infant.

Pediatric patients
- Safe use in patients under age 18 hasn't been established.

Geriatric patients
- Elderly patients are more susceptible to CNS depressant effects of triazolam. Use with caution.
- Elderly patients who receive triazolam need assistance with ambulation and activities of daily living when therapy starts and dosages increase.

Patient teaching
- Inform patient that drug may cause physical and psychological dependence.
- Instruct patient not to take other prescribed drugs, OTC medications, or herbal remedies without consulting prescriber.
- Tell patient not to change triazolam dosage without consulting prescriber.
- Suggest other measures to promote sleep, such as drinking warm fluids, listening to quiet music, avoiding alcohol near bedtime, exercising regularly, and maintaining a regular sleep pattern.
- Caution patient to avoid hazardous activities until full sedative effects of drug are known. Explain that drug may cause drowsiness.
- To minimize the risk of injuries, teach safety measures at the start of therapy, including gradual position changes and avoidance of cigarette smoking after taking drug.
- Caution patient not to take triazolam when a full night's sleep (and clearance of drug from the body) won't occur before normal daily activities resume.

- Advise patient that rebound insomnia may occur after therapy stops.
- Urge patient to notify prescriber if insomnia continues because it could indicate a serious medical condition.
- Tell women to immediately notify prescriber about planned, suspected, or known pregnancy.

---

zaleplon
Sonata

Pharmacologic classification:
pyrazolopyrimidine

Therapeutic classification:
hypnotic

Controlled substance schedule IV

Pregnancy risk category C

How supplied
Available by prescription only
Capsules: 5 mg, 10 mg

Indication and dosages
Insomnia (short-term treatment)
Adults: 10 mg/day P.O. just before bedtime. Increase to 20 mg if needed. Low-weight adults may respond to 5 mg.

▶ DOSAGE ADJUSTMENT. For elderly or debilitated patients, patients with mild to moderate hepatic failure, or patients receiving cimetidine, start with 5 mg/day P.O. given just before bedtime. Doses over 10 mg aren't recommended.

Pharmacodynamics
Hypnotic action: Although zaleplon is a hypnotic with a chemical structure unrelated to benzodiazepines, it interacts with the GABA BZ receptor complex in the CNS. Benzodiazepines may cause sedative, anxiolytic, muscle relaxant, and anticonvulsant effects by modulating this complex.

Pharmacokinetics
Absorption: Rapidly and almost completely absorbed. Levels peak within 1 hour. Taking drug after a high-fat or heavy meal delays peak by about 2 hours.
Distribution: Distributed substantially into extravascular tissues. Plasma protein-binding is about 60%.
Metabolism: Extensively metabolized to inactive metabolites, primarily by aldehyde oxidase and to a lesser extent by CYP3A4. Less than 1% of dose is excreted unchanged in urine.
Excretion: Rapidly excreted, with a mean half-life of about 1 hour.

Contraindications and precautions
Contraindicated in patients with severe hepatic impairment.
Use cautiously in elderly and debilitated patients, in those with compromised respiratory function, and in those with evidence of depression.

Interactions
Drug-drug
Carbamazepine, phenobarbital, phenytoin, rifampin, other CYP3A4 inducers: may reduce bioavailability and peak levels of zaleplon by about 80%. Consider a different hypnotic.

Cimetidine: increases zaleplon bioavailability and peak levels by 85%. Patient taking cimetidine should start with 5 mg of zaleplon. *CNS depressants, such as imipramine, thioridazine:* may produce additive CNS effects. Use cautiously together.

Drug-food
High-fat foods, heavy meals: possible delay of sleep onset from prolonged absorption and 2-hour delay in peak zaleplon levels. Separate administration from meals.

Drug-lifestyle
Alcohol use: may increase CNS effects. Avoid concurrent use.

Adverse reactions
CNS: amnesia, anxiety, asthenia, depersonalization, depression, difficulty concentrating, dizziness, hallucinations, *headache,* hypertonia, hypoesthesia, malaise, migraine, nervousness, paresthesia, somnolence, tremor, vertigo.
CV: chest pain, peripheral edema.
EENT: abnormal vision, conjunctivitis, eye pain, ear pain, hyperacusis, epistaxis, parosmia.
GI: constipation, dry mouth, anorexia, dyspepsia, nausea, abdominal pain, colitis.
GU: dysmenorrhea.
Musculoskeletal: arthritis, back pain, myalgia.
Respiratory: bronchitis.
Skin: photosensitivity, pruritus, rash.
Other: fever.

Overdose and treatment:
Overdose usually causes exaggerated CNS depressant effects ranging from drowsiness to coma. Immediately perform gastric lavage when appropriate, and provide general supportive measures to manage symptoms.

Special considerations
■ Because of the risk of abuse and dependence, don't give more than a 1-month supply of drug.
■ Start treatment only after evaluating patient carefully because sleep disturbances may indicate an underlying physical or psychiatric disorder.
■ Because zaleplon works rapidly, it should be taken immediately before bed or after patient goes to bed and has trouble falling asleep.
■ Don't give drug with or after a high-fat or heavy meal.
■ Therapy typically lasts 7 to 10 days. Reevaluate patient if hypnotics are to be taken for more than 2 to 3 weeks.
■ Closely monitor elderly or debilitated patients and patients with compromised respiratory function from preexisting illness.
■ Adverse reactions are usually dose-related. Use the lowest effective dose.

Breast-feeding patients
■ A small amount of drug appears in breast milk. Don't give drug during breast-feeding because effects on infants are unknown.

Pediatric patients
■ Safety and effectiveness haven't been established in children.

Patient teaching

- Tell patient that drug may cause dependence and is recommended only for short-term use.
- Explain that zaleplon works rapidly. Caution patient to take it immediately before bed or after going to bed and having trouble falling asleep.
- Tell patient not to take drug after a high-fat or heavy meal.
- Advise patient to take drug only if she can sleep for at least 4 undisturbed hours.
- Warn patient that drowsiness, dizziness, light-headedness, and lack of coordination commonly occur within 1 hour after taking drug.
- Caution patient to avoid hazardous activities until full CNS effects of drug are known.
- Urge patient to avoid alcohol during therapy.
- Tell patient not to take other prescribed drugs, OTC medications, or herbal remedies without consulting prescriber.
- Inform patient that zaleplon may cause changes in behavior and thinking, including outgoing or aggressive behavior, loss of personal identity, confusion, strange behavior, agitation, hallucinations, worsening of depression, or suicidal thoughts. Tell patient to notify prescriber immediately if any of these symptoms occur.
- Advise patient to report continued sleep problems.
- Warn patient not to abruptly stop drug because withdrawal symptoms may occur, including unpleasant feelings, stomach and muscle cramps, vomiting, sweating, shakiness, and seizures.

- Inform patient that insomnia may recur for a few nights after stopping drug, but that it should resolve on its own.

---

zolpidem tartrate
Ambien

Pharmacologic classification: **imidazopyridine**

Therapeutic classification: **hypnotic**

Controlled substance schedule IV

Pregnancy risk category B

How supplied
Available by prescription only
Tablets: 5 mg, 10 mg

Indications and dosages
Insomnia (short-term treatment)
Adults: 10 mg P.O. immediately before bedtime.
▶ **DOSAGE ADJUSTMENT.** For elderly or debilitated patients, start with 5 mg/day P.O. given just before bedtime. Doses over 10 mg aren't recommended.

Pharmacodynamics
Hypnotic action: Zolpidem that interacts with benzodiazepine-GABA or omega-receptor complex and shares some pharmacologic properties of benzodiazepines. However, its chemical structure is unrelated to benzodiazepines, barbiturates, or other hypnotic drugs and it has no muscle relaxant or anticonvulsant effects.

Pharmacokinetics
Absorption: Drug is absorbed rapidly from the GI tract with a mean peak time of 1½ hours. Food delays drug absorption.
Distribution: About 92.5% of drug is protein-bound.
Metabolism: Zolpidem is converted to inactive metabolites in the liver.
Excretion: Drug is primarily eliminated in urine; elimination half-life is about 2½hours.

Contraindications and precautions
No known contraindications. Use cautiously in patients with conditions that could affect metabolism or hemodynamic response and in patients with a decreased respiratory drive, depression, or a history of alcohol or drug abuse.

Interactions
Drug-drug
CNS depressants: enhanced CNS depression. Don't use together.

Drug-lifestyle
Alcohol use: may cause excessive CNS depression. Urge caution with concurrent use.

Adverse reactions
CNS: abnormal dreams, amnesia, anxiety, asthenia, daytime drowsiness, depression, dizziness, hangover, *headache,* lethargy, lightheadedness, nervousness, sleep disorder.
CV: chest pain, palpitations.
EENT: dry mouth, pharyngitis, rhinitis, sinusitis.

GI: abdominal pain, anorexia, constipation, diarrhea, dyspepsia, nausea, vomiting.
Musculoskeletal: arthralgia, back pain, myalgia.
Skin: rash.
Other: flulike symptoms, *hypersensitivity reactions.*

Overdose and treatment
Overdose may cause symptoms ranging from somnolence to light coma. CV and respiratory compromise also may occur.

To treat an overdose, provide general symptomatic and supportive measures along with immediate gastric lavage when appropriate. Give I.V. fluids as needed. Flumazenil may be useful. Treat hypotension and CNS depression as needed. Don't give sedatives after zolpidem overdose even if excitation occurs.

Special considerations
- Carefully evaluate the cause of patient's insomnia before starting treatment because it may indicate a physical or psychiatric disorder.
- Zolpidem has CNS depressant effects similar to other sedative-hypnotics. Because of its rapid onset, drug should be given immediately before bed.
- Therapy should last only 7 to 10 days. Reevaluate patient if therapy will last more than 2 weeks.
- If patient takes other CNS depressants, dosage adjustment may be needed because of additive effects.
- Monitor patients who have a history of addiction or drug or alcohol abuse because they have an in-

creased risk of habituation and dependence.
▪ If hospitalized patient is depressed, suicidal, or known to abuse drugs, take steps to prevent hoarding and intentional overdose.

Pediatric patients
▪ Safety and effectiveness in children under age 18 haven't been established.

Geriatric patients
▪ Elderly patients may have impaired motor or cognitive performance after repeated exposure.
▪ Unusual sensitivity to sedative-hypnotics may occur in elderly patients. Recommended dose is 5 mg rather than 10 mg.

Patient teaching
▪ Tell patient not to take drug with or immediately after a meal.
▪ Urge patient to take drug exactly as prescribed and not to increase dosage if drug effects seem to decline.
▪ Inform patient that tolerance and dependence may occur if drug is taken for more than a few weeks.
▪ Warn patient not to drink alcoholic beverages or take other sleep aids during therapy to avoid serious adverse effects.
▪ Caution patient to avoid hazardous activities until full CNS effects of drug are known.

CHAPTER 13

Drugs for treating Alzheimer's disease and migraine headaches

455 ■ **Introduction**

459 ■ **Generic drugs**

■ donepezil hydrochloride

■ ergotamine tartrate

■ methysergide maleate

■ naratriptan hydrochloride

■ propranolol hydrochloride

■ rizatriptan benzoate

■ sumatriptan succinate

■ tacrine hydrochloride

■ zolmitriptan

In recent years, researchers have developed promising new drug treatments for Alzheimer's disease and for migraine headaches.

UNDERSTANDING ALZHEIMER'S DISEASE

Alzheimer's disease affects 2 to 4 million Americans and is the most common cause of dementia nationwide. Progressive and degenerative, it causes about 55% of all cases of dementia. Risk factors for this disease include advancing age, female gender, and genetic predisposition.

Alzheimer's disease is classified into three stages. Each stage is characterized by increasing dementia that results from diminished neuronal function and decreased neurotransmitters. Specifically, the disease is characterized by a decrease in the enzyme choline acetyltransferase, which is responsible for synthesizing acetylcholine. Advancing illness is also characterized by neurofibrillary tangles, neuronal plaques, and substantial neuronal death.

Treating Alzheimer's disease

For patients who have mild Alzheimer's disease—Stage I or II— two drugs may help to slow the symptoms of cognitive decline: donepezil and tacrine. These drugs are cholinesterase inhibitors; they help to reduce the breakdown of acetylcholine by inhibiting the enzyme acetylcholinesterase.

Keep in mind that neither donepezil nor tacrine can cure Alzheimer's disease or even improve its outcome. They simply delay the effects of the disease. During treatment, they improve patients' scores on the Alzheimer's disease assessment scale. Once they're discontinued, however, the test scores return to baseline within 6 weeks.

Drug effects

Donepezil and tacrine work by enhancing cholinergic function in the brain. They appear to be equally effective. However, they differ in tolerability. Tacrine has been linked to serious hepatotoxicity and requires that you test the patient's liver function every other week in the early stages of treatment. If the patient's liver function test results rise to more than five times normal, you'll need to discontinue the drug. If not, then you may be able to decrease the testing cycle to every 3 months after the first 16 weeks.

Rarely will you need to monitor the liver function of a patient who takes donepezil. As a result, treatment with donepezil is typically simpler and less costly. Another advantage is that donepezil can be given once daily rather than four times daily, as with tacrine. For these reasons, donepezil is considered the drug of choice for treating Alzheimer's disease.

UNDERSTANDING MIGRAINE HEADACHES

More than 11 million Americans have migraine headaches, primarily young women in their 30s and 40s. Indeed, women are three times more likely than men to have them.

No one knows precisely what causes migraine headaches. They seem to result from circulation changes in the brain. Researchers suspect that decreased cerebral blood flow leads to ischemia, which then leads to rebound vascular dilation and neurogenic inflammation, which in turn cause the pain and other symptoms we define as a migraine headache. Plasma serotonin levels rise during the attack as well.

Usually, a migraine starts with visual disturbances, tingling sensations, and neurologic symptoms. This aura usually lasts 15 to 20 minutes. The person then develops severe unilateral or bilateral pain, nausea, vomiting, photophobia, and odor aversion.

Treating migraine headaches

The plan for a patient who has migraine headaches typically includes both nondrug and drug treatments. Nondrug treatment focuses on teaching the patient to avoid substances or situations known to trigger or raise the risk of migraines. For instance, the patient should try to avoid noise, bright lights, extreme temperatures, smoke, chocolate, caffeine, nitrates in processed meats, and citrus. The patient also may need to avoid certain drugs, such as estrogen, nitroglycerin, and nicotine.

Drug treatment for migraines may follow one of two approaches: reducing the pain of acute attacks and preventing migraines or reducing their frequency. Drugs used to manage the pain of an acute attack include anti-inflammatory drugs (such as acetaminophen and aspirin), ergotamine derivatives, and a class of drugs known as the "triptans" (naratriptan, rizatriptan, sumatriptan, zolmitriptan). Drugs used to prevent migraines or reduce their frequency include beta blockers, calcium channel blockers, and tricyclic antidepressants.

Pain management

Over-the-counter (OTC) analgesics, such as acetaminophen and aspirin, are sometimes effective in treating mild to moderate migraines. One OTC form of Excedrin also contains caffeine; it commonly is more effective than acetaminophen or aspirin alone. Another option for mild to moderate migraines is an OTC nonsteroidal anti-inflammatory drug, such as ibuprofen or naproxen.

Ergotamine derivatives have been used for decades to treat migraines and commonly are effective for moderate to severe headaches. They relieve pain by constricting cerebral and peripheral vessels through alpha adrenergic blockade. They also have serotonergic activity. Their major disadvantage is the severe nausea, vomiting, and coronary or peripheral ischemia they cause. In fact, the patient probably should take an antiemetic as well as the ergotamine derivative to control the nausea and vomiting.

A new group of drugs, commonly called the triptans, has been widely used in recent years. Many clinicians now consider them first-line treatment for moderate to severe migraines. The triptans relieve pain by acting as serotonin agonists; they constrict cranial vessels and inhibit the release of pro-inflammatory neuropeptides. All are available in oral forms, and sumatriptan is also available as a subcutaneous injection and a nasal spray. The advantage of the latter two forms is that they begin working much faster than the typical oral forms do.

The triptans are much less likely to cause nausea and vomiting than ergotamine derivatives. However, up to 40% of the patients who take them develop a rebound headache within 24 hours of the first attack, making follow-up treatment necessary. Because any analgesic may become less effective over time, patients may need to try new treatments from time to time.

Prophylaxis

Certain patients may be better served by a prophylactic approach to migraine treatment than by the standard pain-relief approach. (See *Migraine prophylaxis: When is it warranted?*) Keep in mind that prophylactic treatment typically reduces the frequency of headaches but probably won't eliminate them. The patient should complete at least three months of prophylactic treatment before you determine whether its effects are adequate.

Usually, the first choice of drugs for prophylactic migraine therapy are beta-adrenergic receptor blockers, such as propranolol and nadolol. By antagonizing beta-adrenergic receptors, the beta blockers allow unopposed alpha adrenergic activity and prevent pain-causing vasodilation of the cerebral vasculature and meningeal arteries.

Tricyclic antidepressants, such as nortriptyline and amitriptyline, are also commonly used. They're especially helpful for patients who have symptoms of depression, although the doses used as migraine prophylaxis typically are lower than those used for treating depression. Tricyclic antidepressants probably

Migraine prophylaxis: When is it warranted?

Certain characteristics may warrant prophylactic treatment for your patient's migraines.
- The patient has severe migraines.
- The patient has more than two attacks each month.
- The patient's migraines last longer than 48 hours.
- Drugs for treating the patient's acute attacks cause unacceptable adverse effects.
- Drugs for treating the patient's acute attacks provide inadequate pain relief.

prevent migraines by inhibiting presynaptic reuptake of norepinephrine and 5-HT into neuronal terminals.

Calcium channel blockers, such as verapamil and nimodipine, offer a third choice. They interfere with calcium entry into cells, thus preventing rebound vasodilation that causes headache pain.

And methysergide offers a last resort. Although it works by a largely unknown mechanism, we do know that it antagonizes peripheral serotonin receptors. Because it has dangerous adverse effects, notably fibrosis, don't let patients take it for more than 6 continuous months. After a 3- to 4-week washout period, the patient can then begin the next treatment cycle.

PATIENT TEACHING

Your patient teaching topics will vary somewhat with your patient's drug treatment. In general, however, make sure to cover these points.

Alzheimer's disease

■ Tell the patient and family that no drug can cure Alzheimer's disease, but that drug treatment may be able to delay the progress of the disease.

■ Explain that the purpose of drug therapy is to help the patient maintain functional abilities and quality of life for as long as possible.

■ Stress that drug treatment is most effective when given early in the disease.

Migraine headaches

■ When treating a patient for acute migraine attacks, caution the patient not to exceed the prescribed drug dosage.

■ Urge the patient to call the prescriber if the drug fails to relieve the headaches.

■ Mention that the patient may experience a rebound headache within 24 hours after the first one, and that he may need to take an extra dose to relieve it.

■ If you're providing prophylactic treatment for migraines, urge the patient to take it faithfully each day.

■ Emphasize that the drug isn't meant to relieve the pain of existing headaches but to reduce their frequency or perhaps to prevent them altogether.

■ Explain that prophylactic drugs commonly take several months to achieve their full effect. Tell the patient not to expect results right away, but to expect a gradual reduction in headache frequency.

donepezil hydrochloride
Aricept

Pharmacologic classification:
acetylcholinesterase inhibitor

Therapeutic classification:
cholinomimetic

Pregnancy risk category C

How supplied
Available by prescription only
Tablets: 5 mg, 10 mg

Indications and dosages
Mild to moderate dementia of the Alzheimer's type
Adults: initially, 5 mg/day P.O. h.s. After 4 to 6 weeks, dosage may be increased to 10 mg daily.

Pharmacodynamics
Anticholinesterase action: Drug probably inhibits acetylcholinesterase in the CNS, increasing acetylcholine and temporarily improving cognitive function in patients with Alzheimer's disease. Drug doesn't alter the course of the underlying disease process.

Pharmacokinetics
Absorption: Donepezil is well absorbed with a relative bioavailability of 100%. Plasma levels peak in 3 to 4 hours. Steady state occurs within 15 days.
Distribution: Steady state volume of distribution is 12 L/kg. Donepezil is about 96% bound to plasma proteins, mainly to albumins (about 75%) and alpha$_1$-acid glycoprotein (about 21%) over the range of 2 to 1,000 ng/ml.

Metabolism: Drug is extensively metabolized to four major metabolites (two known to be active) and several minor metabolites (not all have been identified). Donepezil is metabolized by cytochrome CYP-450 isoenzymes 2D6 and 3A4 and undergoes glucuronidation.
Excretion: Drug is excreted intact in urine and extensively metabolized by the liver. Elimination half-life is about 70 hours; mean apparent plasma clearance is 0.13 L/hour/kg. About 17% of drug is eliminated by the kidneys as unchanged drug.

Contraindications and precautions
Contraindicated in patients hypersensitive to drug or to piperidine derivatives.

Use very cautiously in patients with sick sinus syndrome or other supraventricular cardiac conduction condition because drug may cause bradycardia. Also use cautiously in patients who take NSAIDs and patients with asthma, CV disease, a history of ulcer disease, or seizures.

Interactions
Drug-drug
Anticholinergics: may interfere with anticholinergic activity. Monitor patient closely.
Bethanechol, succinylcholine: may produce additive effects. Monitor patient closely.
Carbamazepine, dexamethasone, phenobarbital, phenytoin, rifampin: may increase rate of donepezil elimination. Dosage adjustment may be needed.

Cholinesterase inhibitors, choli-nomimetics: may produce synergistic effect. Monitor patient closely.

Drug-herb
Jaborandi tree, pill-bearing spurge: additive effect may occur, increasing the risk of toxicity. Urge caution when used together.

Adverse reactions
CNS: abnormal dreams, aggression, aphasia, ataxia, crying, depression, dizziness, fatigue, *headache, insomnia,* irritability, nervousness, paresthesia, restlessness, *seizures,* somnolence, tremor, vertigo.
CV: atrial fibrillation, chest pain, hypertension, hypotension, syncope, vasodilation.
EENT: blurred vision, cataract, eye irritation.
GI: anorexia, bloating, *diarrhea,* epigastric pain, fecal incontinence, GI bleeding, *nausea,* vomiting.
GU: frequent urination, hot flashes, increased libido, nocturia.
Metabolic: dehydration, weight loss.
Musculoskeletal: arthritis, bone fracture, muscle cramps, toothache.
Respiratory: bronchitis, dyspnea, sore throat.
Skin: diaphoresis, pruritus, urticaria.
Other: ecchymosis, influenza, pain.

Overdose and treatment
Overdose may cause cholinergic crisis characterized by bradycardia, collapse, hypotension, respiratory depression, salivation, seizures, severe nausea, diaphoresis, and vomiting. Increasing muscle weakness may also occur and may be fatal if respiratory muscles are involved.

Tertiary anticholinergics such as atropine may be used as an antidote. Start atropine sulfate at 1 to 2 mg I.V. and adjust subsequent doses based on patient response. Atypical responses in blood pressure and heart rate have been reported with other cholinomimetics when given with quaternary anticholinergics, such as glycopyrrolate. It isn't known whether dialysis can remove donepezil or its metabolites.

Special considerations
■ Syncope have been reported after drug use. Monitor patient's blood pressure.
■ Drug may increase gastric acid secretion from increased cholinergic activity. If patient has an increased risk of ulcer (if he has a history of ulcer disease or he takes an NSAID, for example) watch closely for symptoms of active or occult GI bleeding.
■ Anorexia, diarrhea, fatigue, insomnia, muscle cramps, nausea, and vomiting occur more often with the 10-mg dose than the 5-mg dose. These effects are mostly mild and transient, sometimes lasting 1 to 3 weeks. They usually resolve with continued therapy.
■ Drug may obstruct bladder outflow.
■ Cholinomimetics raise the risk of generalized seizures. However, keep in mind that seizure activity also may result from Alzheimer's disease.

Breast-feeding patients
■ No data are available to demonstrate presence of drug in breast

---

milk. Avoid use of donepezil in breast-feeding women.

Pediatric patients
■ Safety and efficacy in children haven't been established.

Geriatric patients
■ Mean plasma drug levels of elderly patients with Alzheimer's disease are comparable with those observed in young healthy volunteers.

Patient teaching
■ Tell caregiver to give drug in the evening, just before bed.
■ Explain to patient and caregiver that drug doesn't alter disease but may stabilize or reduce symptoms. This effect depends on drug being given at regular intervals.
■ Urge patient and caregiver to immediately report significant adverse effects or changes in patient's overall health status.
■ Urge patient and caregiver to tell all health care professionals about donezepil therapy before patient receives anesthesia.

---

ergotamine tartrate
Cafergot, Ergomar, Ergostat, Gynergen, Medihaler Ergotamine, Wigraine

Pharmacologic classification: ergot alkaloid

Therapeutic classification: vasoconstrictor

Pregnancy risk category X

How supplied
Available by prescription only

Aerosol inhaler: 360 mcg/metered spray
Suppositories: 2 mg (with 100 mg caffeine)
Tablets (S.L.): 2 mg
Tablets: 1 mg◊ (with or without 100 mg caffeine)

Indications and dosages
To prevent or abort vascular headache, including migraine and cluster headaches
Adults: initially, 2 mg S.L. or P.O. Then 1 to 2 mg S.L. or P.O. q 30 minutes. Maximum, 6 mg/attack or 24 hours, and 10 mg/week. Alternatively, give 1 inhalation; if headache continues after 5 minutes, repeat 1 inhalation. As needed, continue repeating inhalations at least 5 minutes apart up to 6 inhalations/24 hours or 15 inhalations weekly. Patient may also use 2-mg rectal suppository at onset of attack and then repeat in 1 hour p.r.n. Maximum, 2 suppositories/attack or 5 suppositories/week.
*Children:** 1 mg S.L. in older children and adolescents. If no improvement, another 1-mg dose may be given after 30 minutes.

Pharmacodynamics
Vasoconstrictor action: By stimulating alpha-adrenergic receptors, drug causes peripheral vasoconstriction if vascular tone is low. In hypertonic blood vessels, it causes vasodilation. It has minimal effects on blood pressure and stronger effects on veins and venules than on arteries and arterioles.
     At high doses, drug is a competitive alpha-adrenergic blocker. At therapeutic doses, it inhibits norepinephrine reuptake. It reduces

the increased platelet aggregation caused by serotonin.

In the treatment of vascular headaches, it probably causes direct vasoconstriction of the dilated carotid artery bed while decreasing the amplitude of pulsations. Serotonergic and catecholaminergic effects probably are involved.

Pharmacokinetics
Absorption: Drug is rapidly absorbed after inhalation and variably absorbed after oral administration. Levels peak in 30 minutes to 3 hours. Caffeine may increase the rate and extent of absorption. Drug undergoes first-pass metabolism after oral administration.
Distribution: Drug is widely distributed throughout the body.
Metabolism: Drug is extensively metabolized in the liver.
Excretion: 4% of a dose is excreted in urine within 96 hours; remainder of dose is presumably excreted in feces. Ergotamine is dialyzable.

Contraindications and precautions
Contraindicated in pregnant patients, patients hypersensitive to ergot alkaloids, and patients with coronary artery disease, hepatic dysfunction, hypertension, peripheral and occlusive vascular diseases, renal dysfunction, sepsis, or severe pruritus.

Interactions
Drug-drug
Erythromycin and other macrolides: may cause symptoms of ergot toxicity if used together. Give a vasodilator (such as nifedipine, nitro-

prusside, or prazosin) as appropriate for such a reaction.
Propranolol and other beta blockers: block natural pathway for vasodilation in patients receiving ergot alkaloids and may cause excessive vasoconstriction. Use together with extreme caution.

Drug-lifestyle
Caffeine: may increase rate and extent of absorption. Advise patient of synergistic effect.

Adverse reactions
CNS: numbness and tingling in fingers and toes.
CV: chest pain, increased arterial pressure, peripheral vasoconstriction, precordial distress and pain, transient tachycardia or bradycardia.
GI: *nausea,* vomiting.
Musculoskeletal: muscle pain in limbs, weakness in legs.
Skin: localized edema, pruritus.

Overdose and treatment
Overdose may cause adverse vasospastic effects, delirium, hypertension, hypotension, impaired mental function, lassitude, nausea, rapid or weak pulse, seizures, severe dyspnea, shock, spasms of the limbs, unconsciousness, and vomiting.

To treat an overdose, provide supportive, symptomatic care with prolonged and careful monitoring. If patient is conscious and ingestion was recent, induce emesis or perform gastric lavage. If patient is comatose, perform gastric lavage only after a cuffed endotracheal tube has been placed. Activated charcoal and a saline (magnesium sulfate) cathartic may be used as

---

Reactions may be *common,* uncommon, **life-threatening**, or COMMON AND LIFE-THREATENING.

well. Provide respiratory support. Apply warmth (not direct heat) to ischemic limbs if vasospasm occurs. As needed, give a vasodilator (nitroprusside, prazosin, or tolazoline) and diazepam I.V. for seizures. Dialysis may be helpful.

Special considerations
■ Drug is most effective when given during prodromal stage of headache or as soon as possible after it begins. Provide a quiet, dim environment to help patient relax after taking drug.
■ S.L. route is preferred during early stage of headache because drug is absorbed rapidly.
■ Store drug in light-resistant container.
■ Obtain a detailed diet history to help reveal relationships between foods and onset of headaches.
■ Rebound headache or an increase in duration or frequency may occur when drug is stopped.
■ If patient experiences severe vasoconstriction with tissue necrosis, give sodium nitroprusside I.V. or tolazoline by intra-arterial route. Heparin I.V. and 10% dextran 40 in D_5W injection also may be given to prevent vascular stasis and thrombosis.
■ Drug isn't effective for muscle contraction (tension) headaches.

Breast-feeding patients
■ Drug appears breast milk; use it cautiously during breast-feeding. Excessive amounts or prolonged use may inhibit lactation.

Pediatric patients
■ Safety and efficacy of ergotamine in children haven't been established.

Geriatric patients
■ Use caution with elderly patients.

Patient teaching
■ Teach patient how to use inhaler, if appropriate.
■ Tell patient not to eat, drink, or smoke while S.L. tablet is dissolving.
■ Caution patient to avoid alcohol because it may worsen headache.
■ Tell patient to avoid smoking; it may increase adverse drug effects.
■ If patient uses an inhaler, tell him to gargle and rinse his mouth after each dose to help prevent coughing, hoarseness, and irritation. Urge him to promptly notify prescriber if he develops mouth, throat, or lung infection.
■ Warn patient to avoid prolonged exposure to very cold temperatures because they may increase the adverse effects of drug.
■ Urge patient to notify prescriber about persistent numbness or tingling in fingers or toes, red or violet blisters on hands or feet, or chest, muscle, or abdominal pain.
■ Caution patient not to exceed recommended dosage.

methysergide maleate
Sansert

Pharmacologic classification: ergot alkaloid

Therapeutic classification: vasoconstrictor

Pregnancy risk category X

How supplied
Available by prescription only
Tablets: 2 mg

Indications and dosages
Prevention of vascular headaches, including migraine and cluster headaches
Adults: 4 to 8 mg/day P.O. in divided doses with meals. Intervals of 3 to 4 weeks must separate each 6-month course of therapy.

Pharmacodynamics
Vasoconstrictor action: Drug competitively blocks serotonin peripherally and may act as a serotonin agonist in the brainstem. Antiserotonin effects inhibit peripheral vasoconstriction and pressor effects, serotonin-induced inflammation, and platelet aggregation fostered by serotonin.

The mechanism by which drug prevents vascular headaches is unknown; however, it may result from humoral factors that affect the pain threshold, and from its central serotonin-agonist effect.

Pharmacokinetics
Absorption: Drug is rapidly absorbed from the GI tract.
Distribution: Methysergide is widely distributed in body tissues.
Metabolism: Drug is metabolized in the liver to methylergonovine and glucuronide metabolites.
Excretion: 56% of a dose is excreted in urine as unchanged drug and its metabolites. Plasma elimination half-life is 10 hours.

Contraindications and precautions
Contraindicated in pregnant patients, debilitated patients, and patients with severe hypertension or arteriosclerosis, peripheral vascular insufficiency, renal or hepatic disease, coronary artery disease, phlebitis or cellulitis of the legs, collagen diseases, fibrotic processes, or valvular heart disease.

Use cautiously in patients with peptic ulcer, suspected coronary artery disease, or aspirin or tartrazine allergies.

Interactions
Drug-drug
Beta blockers: increased risk of peripheral ischemia and possible peripheral gangrene. Use concurrently with extreme caution.
Narcotic analgesics: methysergide may reverse analgesic effect. Monitor patient closely.

Adverse reactions
CNS: *ataxia,* feelings of dissociation, drowsiness, *euphoria,* hallucinations, hyperesthesia, insomnia, lethargy, light-headedness, rapid speech, *vertigo,* weakness.
CV: bruits; cold, numb, painful limbs with or without paresthesia and diminished or absent pulses; *fibrotic thickening of heart valves, aorta, inferior vena cava, and common iliac branches (retroperitoneal fibrosis);* edema; flushing; orthostatic hypotension; peripheral murmurs; tachycardia; vasoconstriction that causes chest pain, abdominal pain, and vascular insufficiency in the legs.
GI: constipation, diarrhea, heartburn, nausea, vomiting.
Hematologic: eosinophilia, *neutropenia.*
Musculoskeletal: arthralgia, myalgia.

Reactions may be *common,* uncommon, *life-threatening,* or COMMON AND LIFE-THREATENING.

Respiratory: *pulmonary fibrosis* (dyspnea, tightness and pain in chest, pleural friction rubs, and effusion).
Skin: hair loss, rash.

Overdose and treatment

Overdose may cause dizziness, euphoria, hyperactivity, peripheral vasospasm with diminished or absent pulses, and coldness, mottling, and cyanosis of the limbs.

To treat an overdose, provide supportive, symptomatic care with prolonged and careful monitoring. If patient is conscious and ingestion was recent, induce emesis or perform gastric lavage. If patient is comatose, perform gastric lavage only after a cuffed endotracheal tube has been placed. Activated charcoal and a saline (magnesium sulfate) cathartic may be used as well. Give I.V. fluids, if needed, and monitor patient's vital signs. Apply warmth (not direct heat) to ischemic limbs if vasospasm occurs. As needed, give a vasodilator (nitroprusside, prazosin, or tolazoline). Contact a poison control center for more information.

Special considerations

■ Don't give drug for acute migraine, vascular headache, or muscle contraction headache.
■ If drug is given for cluster headaches, patient typically takes it only during the cluster.
■ Protection against headache develops after 1 to 2 days and persists for 1 to 2 days after therapy stops.
■ Adverse reactions occur in up to 50% of patients.

■ GI effects can be reduced by introducing drug gradually and by giving it with food or milk.
■ Reduce dosage gradually for 2 to 3 weeks before discontinuing drug.
■ Besides standard indications, drug has also been used to control diarrhea in patients with cancer.

Breast-feeding patients
■ Avoid breast-feeding during therapy.

Pediatric patients
■ Drug isn't recommended for use in children because of fibrosis risk.

Patient teaching
■ Tell patient to take drug with food.
■ Caution him to monitor his calorie intake to minimize weight gain.
■ Tell patient not to take drug for longer than 6 months at any one time and to wait 3 to 4 weeks before restarting it.
■ Tell patient to immediately notify prescriber about numbness or tingling in hands or feet, red or violet blisters on hands and feet, flank or chest pain, shortness of breath, leg cramps when walking, or any other evidence of impaired circulation.
■ Warn patient to avoid smoking and prolonged exposure to very cold temperatures because they may increase adverse drug effects.
■ Caution him to also avoid alcoholic beverages because alcohol may worsen his headaches.
■ Tell patient to report illness or infection because they may increase sensitivity to drug effects.
■ Advise women of childbearing age to use birth control and to no-

tify prescriber about planned, suspected, or known pregnancy.

■ Explain that after stopping drug, his body may need time to adjust depending on the amount used and the duration of time involved.

■ Inform patient that drug may cause drowsiness and to use caution when driving or performing other tasks requiring alertness.

■ Drug may contain tartrazine, which can cause allergic reaction.

---

naratriptan hydrochloride
Amerge

Pharmacologic classification:
selective 5-hydroxytryptamine$_1$
(5-HT$_1$) receptor subtype agonist

Therapeutic classification:
antimigraine drug

Pregnancy risk category C

How supplied
Available by prescription only
Tablets: 1 mg, 2.5 mg

Indications and dosages
Acute migraine headaches with or without aura
Adults: 1 or 2.5 mg P.O. as a single dose, individualized based on possible benefit of the 2.5-mg dose weighed against its greater risk of adverse effects. If headache returns or responds only partially, dose may be repeated after 4 hours. Maximum, 5 mg in 24 hours.

▶ **DOSAGE ADJUSTMENT.** In patients with mild to moderate renal or hepatic impairment, consider a lower initial dose and don't exceed the maximum 2.5 mg over 24 hours.

Don't give drug to patients with severe renal or hepatic impairment.

Pharmacodynamics
Antimigraine action: Naratriptan binds with high affinity to 5-HT$_{1D}$ and 5-HT$_{1B}$ receptors. One theory suggests that activation of these receptors on intracranial blood vessels leads to vasoconstriction, which relieves the migraine.

Another hypothesis suggests that activation of 5-HT$_{1D/1B}$ receptors on sensory nerve endings in the trigeminal system inhibits release of pro-inflammatory neuropeptides.

Pharmacokinetics
Absorption: Drug is well absorbed, with about 70% oral bioavailability. Plasma levels peak in 2 to 4 hours.
Distribution: Steady state volume of drug's distribution is 170 L. Plasma protein-binding is 28% to 31%.
Metabolism: In vitro, naratriptan is metabolized by many cytochrome P-450 isoenzymes to inactive metabolites.
Excretion: Naratriptan is eliminated mainly in urine, with 50% of dose unchanged and 30% as metabolites. Mean elimination half-life is 6 hours.

Contraindications and precautions
Contraindicated in patients hypersensitive to drug or its components, patients with severe renal (creatinine clearance below 15 ml/minute) or hepatic (Child-Pugh grade C) impairment, and patients with a history or evidence of

---

ischemic cardiac disorders, cerebrovascular disorders (such as CVA or transient ischemic attack), or peripheral vascular disorders (such as ischemic bowel disease). Also contraindicated in patients with hemiplegic or basilar migraine or with significant underlying CV diseases, including angina pectoris, MI, or silent myocardial ischemia. Drug and other 5-HT$_1$ agonists are also contraindicated in patients with risk factors for coronary artery disease, such as hypertension, hypercholesterolemia, obesity, diabetes, a strong family history of coronary artery disease, females with surgical or physiologic menopause, males over age 40, or smoking. Drug should not be given to patients with uncontrolled hypertension because of possible increase in blood pressure.

Interactions
Drug-drug
Ergot-containing or ergot-type drugs or other 5-HT$_1$ agonists: may prolong vasospastic reactions because their actions may be additive. Don't use these drugs within 24 hours of naratriptan.
Oral contraceptives: may increase naratriptan levels. Dosage adjustment may be needed.
Selective serotonin reuptake inhibitors, such as fluoxetine, fluvoxamine, paroxetine, sertraline: may (rarely) cause weakness, hyperreflexia, and incoordination when given with 5-HT$_1$ agonists. If patient needs accessory therapy with naratriptan and a selective serotonin reuptake inhibitor, monitor him carefully.

Drug-lifestyle
Smoking: increases naratriptan clearance by 30%. Discourage concurrent use.

Adverse reactions
CNS: dizziness, drowsiness, fatigue, malaise, paresthesias, vertigo.
CV: *abnormal ECG changes* (prolonged PR and QT intervals, abnormal ST segments and T waves, PVCs, atrial flutter or fibrillation), increased blood pressure, palpitations, syncope, tachyarrhythmias.
EENT: ear-nose-throat infection, photophobia.
GI: hyposalivation, nausea, vomiting.
Other: sensations of heaviness, pressure, tightness, warm or cold temperatures.

Overdose and treatment
Overdose may cause blood pressure to rise sharply 30 minutes to 6 hours after ingestion.

In some patients, blood pressure returns to normal in 8 hours; others need antihypertensive treatment. No specific antidote exists. Perform ECG monitoring for evidence of ischemia. Monitor patient for at least 24 hours after an overdose or while symptoms persist. The effect of hemodialysis or peritoneal dialysis is unknown.

Special considerations
■ Use drug only if patient has a clear diagnosis of migraine. It isn't intended for prevention of migraines or for managing hemiplegic or basilar migraine.
■ Patient should have a satisfactory CV evaluation before therapy. However, you should still give first

dose in a medical facility equipped to care for patients with coronary artery disease. Consider ECG monitoring.

■ Perform periodic cardiac reevaluation in patients who have or develop risk factors for coronary artery disease.

■ Safety and effectiveness haven't been established for cluster headaches.

Breast-feeding patients
■ Use cautiously in breast-feeding patients.

Pediatric patients
■ Safety and effectiveness in children under age 18 haven't been established.

Geriatric patients
■ Don't give drug to elderly patients.

Patient teaching
■ Tell patient that drug is intended to relieve, not prevent, migraine headaches.

■ Caution patient to tell prescriber about possible risk factors for coronary artery disease.

■ Instruct him to take a dose as soon as possible after a headache starts. If he feels no response or a partial response to the first tablet, tell him to contact the prescriber before taking a second dose. Usually, he'll need to wait at least 4 hours after the first dose before taking the second one. Tell him not to exceed 2 doses in 24 hours.

■ Tell patient to notify prescriber about sudden or severe abdominal pain following naratriptan administration.

■ Urge women not to take drug if they suspect or know that they're pregnant.

---

propranolol hydrochloride
Inderal, Inderal LA, Intensol

Pharmacologic classification: beta blocker

Therapeutic classification: adjunctive therapy for MI, antianginal, antiarrhythmic, antihypertensive, prophylactic therapy for migraine

Pregnancy risk category C

How supplied
Available by prescription only
Capsules (extended-release): 60 mg, 80 mg, 120 mg, 160 mg
Injection: 1 mg/ml
Solution: 4 mg/ml, 8 mg/ml, 20 mg/ 5 ml, 40 mg/5 ml, 80 mg/ml (concentrated)
Tablets: 10 mg, 20 mg, 40 mg, 60 mg, 80 mg, 90 mg

Indications and dosages
Prevention of frequent, severe, uncontrollable, or disabling migraine or vascular headache
Adults: initially, 80 mg/day in divided doses or one sustained-release capsule once daily. Usual maintenance dosage is 160 to 240 mg/day, divided t.i.d. or q.i.d.

Anxiety (adjunctive treatment)*
Adults: 10 to 80 mg P.O. 1 hour before anxiety-provoking activity.

Essential, familial, or senile movement tremors
Adults: 40 mg P.O. b.i.d. as conventional tablets. Response is highly individualized. Optimum suppression is usually achieved with 120 to 320 mg daily P.O. divided t.i.d.

Pharmacodynamics
Antianginal action: Propranolol decreases myocardial oxygen consumption and relieves angina by blocking catecholamine access to beta-adrenergic receptors.

Antiarrhythmic action: Through its myocardial beta-adrenergic blocking effects, drug decreases heart rate and prevents exercise-induced increases in heart rate. It also decreases myocardial contractility, cardiac output, and SA and AV nodal conduction velocity.

Antihypertensive action: Exact mechanism is unknown. Drug may reduce blood pressure by blocking adrenergic receptors (thus decreasing cardiac output), by decreasing sympathetic outflow from the CNS, and by suppressing renin release.

Migraine prophylactic action: May result from inhibited vasodilation.

MI prophylactic action: Mechanism by which propranolol decreases death rate after MI is unknown.

Pharmacokinetics
Absorption: Drug is absorbed almost completely from the GI tract. Absorption is enhanced when given with food. Plasma levels peak 60 to 90 minutes after administration of regular-release tablets. After I.V. administration, levels peak in about 1 minute. Action begins almost immediately.

Distribution: Drug is distributed widely throughout the body and is more than 90% protein-bound.

Metabolism: Hepatic metabolism is almost total. Oral dosage form undergoes extensive first-pass metabolism.

Excretion: About 96% to 99% of a dose is excreted in urine as metabolites; the rest is excreted in feces as unchanged drug and metabolites. Biologic half-life is about 4 hours.

Contraindications and precautions
Contraindicated in patients with bronchial asthma, cardiogenic shock, heart failure (unless failure results from a tachyarrhythmia responsive to propranolol), malignant hypertension, Raynaud's syndrome, or sinus bradycardia with heart block greater than first-degree.

Use cautiously in elderly patients, patients taking other antihypertensives, and patients with diabetes mellitus, impaired renal or hepatic function, nonallergic bronchospastic diseases, or thyrotoxicosis.

Interactions
Drug-drug
Aluminum hydroxide antacids: decreases GI absorption. Dosage adjustments may be needed.

Antiarrhythmics (lidocaine, procainamide, quinidine): may produce additive or toxic effects. Monitor patient closely.

Anticholinergics, tricyclic antidepressants: may antagonize propranolol-induced bradycardia. Monitor patient's heart rate closely.

Antidiabetic drugs, insulin: propranolol may alter dosage requirement in previously stable diabetic patients. Dosage adjustments may be needed.

Antihypertensives, especially catecholamine-depleting drugs such as reserpine: propranolol may potentiate antihypertensive effects. Monitor patient's blood pressure closely.

Calcium channel blockers, especially verapamil I.V.: may depress myocardial contractility or AV conduction. Concurrent I.V. use of a beta blocker and verapamil may (rarely) cause serious adverse reactions, especially in patients with severe cardiomyopathy, heart failure, or recent MI. Use together with extreme caution.

Chlorpromazine, fluoxetine: decreased propanolol clearance. Monitor patient closely.

Cimetidine: may decrease propranolol clearance by inhibiting hepatic metabolism and thus enhancing its beta-blocking effects. Monitor patient closely.

Epinephrine: causes severe vasoconstriction, bradycardia, first- and second-degree heart block. Monitor patient's ECG closely.

MAO inhibitors, sympathomimetics (such as isoproterenol): propranolol may antagonize beta-adrenergic stimulating effects. Monitor patient closely.

NSAIDs, phenothiazines: may antagonize hypotensive effects. Monitor patient's blood pressure closely.

Phenytoin, rifampin: accelerated propranolol clearance. Dosage adjustments may be needed.

Tubocurarine and related compounds: high propranolol dosage may potentiate neuromuscular blocking effect. Monitor patient closely.

Drug-herb
Betel palm: may reduce temperature-elevating effects and enhanced CNS effects. Don't use together.

Drug-lifestyle
Alcohol use: slows the rate of propranolol absorption. Dosage adjustments may be needed.

Adverse reactions
CNS: depression, *fatigue,* hallucinations, insomnia, *lethargy,* lightheadedness, vivid dreams.
CV: *bradycardia, heart failure, hypotension,* intensified AV block, intermittent claudication.
GI: abdominal cramping, constipation, diarrhea, flatus, nausea, vomiting.
Hematologic: *agranulocytosis.*
Hepatic: elevated levels of alkaline phosphatase, BUN, lactic dehydrogenase, and serum transaminase.
Respiratory: *bronchospasm.*
Skin: rash.
Other: fever.

Overdose and treatment
Overdose may cause bradycardia, bronchospasm, heart failure, and severe hypotension.

After acute ingestion, induce emesis or perform gastric lavage. Follow with activated charcoal to reduce absorption. Give symptomatic and supportive care. Give atropine (0.25 to 1 mg) for bradycardia; if no response occurs, give isoproterenol cautiously. Give cardiac glycosides and diuretics for cardiac failure. Give glucagons, vasopressors, or both for hypotension; epinephrine is preferred. Give isoproterenol and aminophylline for bronchospasm.

Special considerations
■ Drug may mask signs of hypoglycemia.
■ Drug also has been used to reduce mortality after MI and to treat aggression and rage, arrhythmias (supraventricular, ventricular, and atrial), angina, hypertension, hyperthyroidism, hypertrophic subaortic stenosis, menopausal symptoms, pheochromocytoma, preoperative pheochromocytoma, recurrent GI bleeding in cirrhotic patients, stage fright, and tachyarrhythmias from excessive catecholamine action during anesthesia.
■ Never give propranolol as an adjunct in treating pheochromocytoma unless patient has been pretreated with an alpha-adrenergic blocker.

Breast-feeding patients
■ Drug appears in breast milk; an alternative feeding method is recommended during therapy.

Pediatric patients
■ Safety and efficacy of propranolol in children haven't been established. Give drug to a child only if potential benefits outweigh risks.

Geriatric patients
■ Elderly patients may need a lower maintenance dosage because of increased bioavailability or delayed metabolism.
■ Elderly patients have an increased risk of adverse effects.

Patient teaching
■ Review proper use, dosage, and possible adverse effects.
■ Tell patient not to take other prescribed drugs, OTC medications, or herbal remedies without consulting prescriber.
■ Tell patient to avoid hazardous activities until full effects of drug are known.
■ Warn elderly patients that they may have a higher risk of adverse effects, especially falls, when they take propranolol with other drugs.
■ Warn patient not to abruptly stop taking propranolol.

rizatriptan benzoate
Maxalt, Maxalt-MLT

Pharmacologic classification:
selective 5-hydroxytryptamine ($5\text{-HT}_{1B/1D}$) receptor agonist

Therapeutic classification:
antimigraine

Pregnancy risk category C

How supplied
Tablets: 5 mg, 10 mg
Tablets (orally disintegrating): 5 mg, 10 mg

Indications and dosages
Acute migraine headaches with or without aura
Adults: initially, 5 or 10 mg P.O. If first dose is ineffective, give another dose at least 2 hours after the first. Maximum, 30 mg in 24 hours.
▷ DOSAGE ADJUSTMENT. If patient also receives propranolol, give

5 mg of rizatriptan P.O. Maximum, three doses (15 mg) in 24 hours.

Pharmocodynamics

Antimigraine action: Rizatriptan probably agonizes serotonin receptors on extracerebral, intracranial blood vessels. This action causes vasoconstriction of affected vessels, inhibition of neuropeptide release, and reduction of pain transmission in the trigeminal pathways.

Pharmacokinetics

Absorption: Bioavailablity after oral administration is 45%. Plasma levels peak in 60 to 90 minutes.
Distribution: Rizatriptan is minimally protein-bound.
Metabolism: Primary metabolism occurs via oxidative deamination by MAO-A to the indoleacetic acid metabolite, which is not active at the $5-HT_{1B/1D}$ receptor.
Excretion: 82% of drug is excreted in urine and 12% excreted in feces after oral administration.

Contraindications and precautions

Contraindicated in patients hypersensitive to drug or its components, patients who have taken an MAO inhibitor within 14 days, and patients with coronary artery vasospasm (Prinzmetal's variant angina), hemiplegic or basilar migraine, ischemic heart disease (angina pectoris, history of MI, or documented silent ischemia), or other significant underlying CV disease. Also contraindicated in patients with uncontrolled hypertension or within 24 hours of treatment with an 5-HT agonist or an ergotamine-containing or ergot-

type drug such as dihydroergotamine or methysergide.

Use cautiously in patients with hepatic or renal impairment and in patients with risk factors for coronary artery disease, such as age over 40 (men), diabetes, hypercholesterolemia, hypertension, obesity, smoking, strong family history of coronary artery disease, or surgical or physiologic menopause, unless a cardiac evaluation proves the patient is free from cardiac disease.

Interactions

Drug-drug

Ergot-containing or ergot-type drugs (dihydroergotamine, methysergide), other $5-HT_1$ agonists: may cause prolonged vasospastic reactions. Don't use within 24 hours of rizatriptan.
MAO inhibitors (moclobemide), nonselective MAO inhibitors (types A and B, isocarboxazid, phenelzine, tranylcypromine:) may increase plasma rizatriptan levels. Avoid concurrent use, and allow at least 14 days after stopping an MAO inhibitor before starting rizatriptan.
Propranolol: may increase rizatriptan levels up to 70%. Reduce rizatriptan dosage to 5 mg up to 3 times daily.
Selective serotonin reuptake inhibitors (fluoxetine, fluvoxamine, paroxetine, sertraline): may cause weakness, hyperreflexia, and incoordination. Monitor patient.

Adverse reactions

CNS: asthenia, decreased mental acuity, dizziness, euphoria, fatigue, headache, hypesthesia, paresthesia, somnolence, tremor, warm or cold sensations.

Reactions may be *common*, uncommon, *life-threatening*, or COMMON AND LIFE-THREATENING.

CV: chest pain, hot flashes, palpitations, pressure or heaviness in chest.
EENT: pain in neck, throat, and jaw.
GI: diarrhea, dry mouth, nausea, vomiting.
Musculoskeletal: pain.
Respiratory: dyspnea.
Skin: flushing.

Special considerations

- Give drug only after patient has a definite migraine diagnosis.
- Don't give drug to prevent migraines or to treat hemiplegic or basilar migraines or cluster headaches.
- If patient has cardiac risk factors but a satisfactory cardiac evaluation, monitor him closely after giving first dose.
- If patient develops cardiac risk factors during treatment, assess his CV status.
- The safety of treating more than four headaches in a 30-day period hasn't been established.
- Oral disintegrating tablets contain phenylalanine.

Breast-feeding patients

- Effects of drug on breast-feeding infant aren't known; avoid giving drug during breast-feeding.

Pediatric patients

- Safety and effectiveness in children under age 18 haven't been established.

Patient teaching

- Explain that drug doesn't prevent migraines.
- Tell patient that food may delay onset of drug action.

- If patient takes Maxalt-MLT, tell him to remove tablet from blister pack immediately before use. Explain that he shouldn't pop the tablet from the pack, but rather should carefully peel away the backing with dry hands. Tell him to place the tablet on his tongue, let it dissolve, and then swallow it with saliva. No water is needed or recommended.
- Explain that orally dissolving tablets don't work any faster than standard tablets.
- Urge patient to consult prescriber if headache returns after first dose; a second dose may be taken at least 2 hours after first dose. Caution patient not to take more than 30 mg in a 24-hour period.
- Tell patient to avoid hazardous activities until full effects of drug are known.
- Advise women to notify prescriber about planned, suspected, or known pregnancy.

---

sumatriptan succinate
Imitrex

Pharmacologic classification: **selective 5-hydroxytryptamine ($5-HT_1$)-receptor agonist**

Therapeutic classification: **antimigraine**

Pregnancy risk category C

How supplied

Available by prescription only
Tablets: 25 mg, 50 mg
Injection: 12 mg/ml (0.5 ml in 1-ml prefilled syringe), 6-mg single-dose

(0.5 ml in 2 ml) vial, and self-dose system kit

Nasal spray: 5-mg unit dose, 20-mg unit dose

Indications and dosages
Acute migraine headaches with or without aura, cluster headaches
Adults: 6 mg S.C. Maximum, two 6-mg injections in 24 hours separated by at least 1 hour. Or 25 to 100 mg P.O. initially. If response doesn't occur in 2 hours, give another 25 to 100 mg. Additional doses may be given in 2-hour or longer intervals. Maximum, 300 mg daily.

For nasal spray, give 5 mg, 10 mg, or 20 mg once in one nostril; may repeat once after 2 hours. Maximum, 40 mg daily.

Pharmacodynamics
Antimigraine action: Sumatriptan selectively binds to a 5-HT$_1$ receptor subtype found in the basilar artery and vasculature of the dura mater, where it presumably exerts its effect. Here, it activates the receptor to cause vasoconstriction, an action that correlates with relief of migraine and cluster headaches.

Pharmacokinetics
Absorption: Bioavailability via S.C. injection is 97% of that obtained via I.V. injection. After S.C. injection, levels peak in about 12 minutes. Drug is also rapidly absorbed by oral and intranasal routes. Bioavailabilty after oral and intranasal use is 15% to 17% and increases with increasing doses.

Distribution: Drug has a low protein-binding capacity (about 14% to 21%).

Metabolism: About 80% of drug is metabolized in the liver, primarily to an inactive indoleacetic acid metabolite.

Excretion: Drug is excreted primarily in urine, partly (20%) as unchanged drug and partly as the indoleacetic acid metabolite. Elimination half-life is about 2 hours.

Contraindications and precautions
Contraindicated in patients hypersensitive to drug, patients who took an MAO inhibitor within 14 days, patients who take ergotamine, and patients with hemiplegic or basilar migraine, ischemic heart disease (such as angina pectoris, Prinzmetal's angina, history of MI, or documented silent ischemia), or uncontrolled hypertension.

Use cautiously in women of childbearing age, in patients with sulfa allergy, in patients who may be at risk for coronary artery disease (such as postmenopausal women or men over age 40), and in patients with risk factors for coronary artery disease, such as diabetes, hypercholesterolemia, hypertension, obesity, smoking, or a family history of coronary artery disease.

Interactions
Drug-drug
Ergot and ergot derivatives: prolonged vasospastic effects when given with sumatriptan. Don't use these drugs within 24 hours of sumatriptan.

MAO inhibitors: increased toxic effects of sumatriptan. Don't use together.
Selective serotonin reuptake inhibitors: may cause weakness, hyperreflexia, and incoordination. Don't use together.

Drug-herb
Horehound: may enhance serotonergic effects. Don't use together.

Adverse reactions
CNS: anxiety, burning sensation, cold sensation, dizziness, drowsiness, fatigue, headache, heavy sensation, malaise, pressure or tightness, tight feeling in head, tingling, vertigo, warm or hot sensation, weakness.
CV: atrial fibrillation, ECG changes (such as ischemic ST-segment elevation), MI, pressure or tightness in chest, ventricular fibrillation, ventricular tachycardia.
EENT: altered vision, discomfort in throat, nose, sinuses, mouth, jaw, or tongue.
GI: abdominal discomfort, dysphagia.
Musculoskeletal: muscle cramps, myalgia, neck pain.
Skin: diaphoresis, flushing.
Other: injection site reaction.

Overdose and treatment
Overdose would be expected to cause ataxia, cyanosis, erythema of the limbs, inactivity, injection site reactions, mydriasis, paralysis, reduced respiratory rate, seizures, and tremor.

Monitor patient carefully while signs and symptoms persist and for at least 10 hours thereafter. Effect of hemodialysis or peritoneal dialysis on serum drug levels is unknown.

Special considerations
■ Nasal spray is typically well tolerated; however, adverse reactions caused by other forms of the drug can still occur.
■ Injection may (rarely) cause serious or life-threatening arrhythmias, such as atrial and ventricular fibrillation, ventricular tachycardia, MI, and marked ischemic ST elevations. It also may (somewhat less rarely) cause chest and arm discomfort, possibly from angina. Because coronary events may occur, consider giving the first dose in an outpatient setting to patients with a risk of coronary artery disease, such as postmenopausal women, men over age 40, and patients with diabetes, hypercholesterolemia, hypertension, obesity, smoking, or a strong family history of coronary artery disease.
■ Patient response to nasal spray may vary. Drug form and dosage must be made individually, weighing the possible benefit of the 20-mg dose against the increased risk of adverse events.
■ Don't give drug for hemiplegic or basilar migraine. Safety and effectiveness also haven't been established for cluster headache, which occurs most often among older, mostly male patients.
■ Don't give drug by I.V. route because coronary vasospasm may result.

Breast-feeding patients
■ Drug appears in breast milk; use caution when giving it to breast-feeding women.

Pediatric patients
- Safety and effectiveness in children haven't been established.

Patient teaching
- Explain that drug is intended to relieve migraines, not to prevent or reduce the number of attacks.
- Tell patient take drug as soon as possible after symptoms begin.
- If patient uses nasal form and has no response to the first dose, tell him to consult prescriber before taking another nasal dose.
- Explain that drug is available in a spring-loaded injector system that facilitates self-administration. Make sure he can load the injector, give the injection, and dispose of used syringes properly.
- A second injection may be given if symptoms recur. Tell patient not to give more than two injections in 24 hours and to allow at least 1 hour between doses. Pain or redness may occur at the injection site but usually lasts less than 1 hour.
- Tell patient to avoid hazardous activities until full effects of drug are known.
- Warn patient to stop the drug and immediately notify prescriber about persistent or severe chest pain, pain or tightness in his throat, wheezing, palpitations, or a rash, skin lumps, hives, or swollen eyelids, face, or lips.
- Tell women to notify prescriber about planned, suspected, or known pregnancy.

tacrine hydrochloride
Cognex

Pharmacologic classification: central-acting reversible cholinesterase inhibitor

Therapeutic classification: psychotherapeutic (for Alzheimer's disease)

Pregnancy risk category C

How supplied
Available by prescription only
Capsules: 10 mg, 20 mg, 30 mg, 40 mg

Indications and dosages
Mild to moderate dementia of the Alzheimer's type
Adults: initially, 10 mg P.O. q.i.d. Maintain dose for at least 4 weeks, then start monitoring ALT levels every other week. If patient tolerates treatment and ALT levels remain normal, increase to 20 mg P.O. q.i.d. After 4 more weeks, increase to 30 mg P.O. q.i.d. If still tolerated, increase to 40 mg P.O. q.i.d. after another 4 weeks.
▶ **Dosage adjustment.** If patient's ALT level is two to three times the upper limit of normal, monitor it weekly. If ALT level is three to five times the upper normal limit, decrease by 40 mg/day and monitor ALT level weekly. Resume dosage adjustment and every-other-week monitoring when ALT level returns to normal. If ALT level is more than five times the upper normal limit, stop treatment and monitor ALT level. Assess for evidence of hepatitis. Consider a rechallenge

---

when ALT level is normal, and monitor the level weekly.

Pharmacodynamics

Psychotherapeutic action: Tacrine presumably slows degradation of acetylcholine released by intact cholinergic neurons, thereby elevating acetylcholine levels in the cerebral cortex. If this theory is correct, the effects of tacrine may lessen as the disease advances and fewer cholinergic neurons remain functionally intact. No evidence suggests that tacrine alters the course of underlying dementia.

Pharmacokinetics

Absorption: Drug is rapidly absorbed after oral administration. Plasma levels peak in 1 to 2 hours. Absolute bioavailability of tacrine is about 17%. Food reduces bioavailability by about 30% to 40%; however, there is no food effect if tacrine is administered at least 1 hour before meals.
Distribution: Drug is about 55% bound to plasma proteins.
Metabolism: Tacrine undergoes dose-dependent first-pass metabolism. It's extensively metabolized by cytochrome P-450 isoenzymes to multiple metabolites, not all of which have been identified.
Excretion: Elimination half-life is about 2 to 4 hours.

Contraindications and precautions

Contraindicated in patients hypersensitive to drug or acridine derivatives, in patients with tacrine-related jaundice confirmed by a total bilirubin level above 3 mg/dl, and in patients who have hypersensitivity reactions from ALT elevations.

Use cautiously in patients at risk for peptic ulcer and in patients with asthma, bradycardia, a history of hepatic disease, Parkinson's disease, prostatic hyperplasia or other urinary outflow impairment, renal disease, seizure disorders, and sick sinus syndrome.

Interactions
Drug-drug

Anticholinergics: tacrine may interfere with anticholinergic activity. Monitor patient closely.
Cholinergic agonists (such as bethanechol), cholinesterase inhibitors, succinylcholine: synergistic effect is likely. Dosage adjustment may be needed.
Cimetidine, fluvoxamine: increases the plasma tacrine level. Dosage adjustment may be needed.
Drugs metabolized via the cytochrome P-450 pathway: interactions may occur. Monitor patient closely.
NSAIDs: may contribute to GI irritation and gastric bleeding. Monitor patient closely.
Theophylline: increases average plasma levels and elimination half-life of theophylline. Monitor plasma theophylline levels and decrease dosage as needed.

Drug-food

Food: may delay the drug absorption. Give drug 1 hour before meals.

Drug-lifestyle

Smoking: decreases plasma drug levels. Discourage concurrent use.

Adverse reactions

CNS: abnormal thinking, agitation, anxiety, ataxia, confusion, depression, *dizziness,* fatigue, *headache,* insomnia, **seizures,** somnolence, tremor.
CV: bradycardia, chest pain, hypertension, hypotension, palpitations.
GI: abdominal pain, altered stool color, anorexia, constipation, *diarrhea,* dyspepsia, flatulence, jaundice, loose stools, *nausea, vomiting.*
Hepatic: elevated liver enzymes.
Metabolic: weight loss.
Musculoskeletal: myalgia.
Respiratory: cough, rhinitis, upper respiratory tract infection.
Skin: diaphoresis, facial flushing, rash.

Overdose and treatment

Overdose may cause a cholinergic crisis characterized by bradycardia, diaphoresis, hypotension, salivation, seizures, severe nausea, and vomiting. Increasing muscle weakness may occur and can be fatal if respiratory muscles are involved.

Provide general support measures. Give tertiary anticholinergics, such as atropine, as an antidote. Also, give 1 to 2 mg of atropine sulfate I.V. and adjust it to effect. No data exist to suggest whether dialysis reduces tacrine or its metabolites.

Special considerations

■ Tacrine is likely to exaggerate succinylcholine-type muscle relaxation during anesthesia.
■ Because of its cholinomimetic action, drug may have vagotonic effects on the heart rate (such as bradycardia). This action may be particularly noteworthy if patient has sick sinus syndrome.
■ Monitor patient's serum ALT level every other week from at least week 4 to week 16 after therapy starts. Afterward, monitor level every 3 months if ALT no higher than twice the upper limit of normal. With each dosage adjustment, resume every-other-week monitoring. ALT elevations are more common among women. There are no other known predictors of risk of hepatocellular injury.
■ If patient can't tolerate the recommended adjustment schedule, slow the rate of increase.
■ If drug is discontinued for 4 weeks or more, restart the dosage adjustment and monitoring plan.
■ Cognitive function may worsen if drug is stopped abruptly or if dosage declines by 80 mg/day or more.

Patient teaching

■ Inform patient and family that drug doesn't alter the underlying course of the disease, but that it can reduce current symptoms. Stress that therapy will be effective only if drug is given on a regular schedule. Caution against abruptly stopping or decreasing drug (by 80 mg/day or more) because doing so may cause behavioral disturbances and a decline in cognitive function.
■ Tell patient and caregiver that drug should be taken between meals when possible. If GI upset occurs, drug may be taken with meals, but doing so probably will reduce plasma levels.
■ Caution patient to avoid hazardous activities until full sedative effects of drug are known.

■ Remind caregiver that planned dosage adjustments are integral to safe and effective use of the drug.

■ Advise patient and caregiver to immediately notify prescriber about significant adverse effects or status changes.

---

zolmitriptan
Zomig

Pharmacologic classification: selective 5-hydroxytryptamine (5-HT$_{1B/1D}$) receptor agonist

Therapeutic classification: antimigraine drug

Pregnancy risk category C

How supplied
Available by prescription only
Tablets: 2.5 mg, 5 mg

Indications and dosages
Acute migraine headaches with or without aura
Adults: initially, 2.5 mg or less P.O. To obtain a dose below 2.5 mg, cut the 2.5-mg tablet in half. If patient's headache returns after initial dose, a second dose may be given after 2 hours. Maximum, 10 mg in 24-hour period.

▶ DOSAGE ADJUSTMENT. Give less than 2.5 mg if patient has liver disease.

Pharmacodynamics
Antimigraine action: Zolmitriptan binds with high affinity to human recombinant 5-HT$_{1D}$ and 5-HT$_{1B}$ receptors, stopping migraine headaches by constricting cranial blood vessels and inhibiting release of pro-inflammatory neuropeptides.

Pharmacokinetics
Absorption: Drug is well absorbed after oral administration. Plasma levels peak in 2 hours. Mean absolute bioavailability is about 40%.
Distribution: Apparent volume of distribution is 7 L/kg. Plasma protein binding is 25%.
Metabolism: Drug is converted to an active N-desmethyl metabolite. Time to maximum metabolite level is 2 to 3 hours. Mean elimination half-life of zolmitriptan and the active N-desmethyl metabolite is 3 hours.
Excretion: Mean total clearance is 31.5 ml/minute/kg, of which one-sixth is renal clearance. Renal clearance exceeds glomerular filtration rate, which suggests renal tubular secretion. About 65% of the dose is excreted in urine and about 30% in feces.

Contraindications and precautions
Contraindicated within 14 days of taking an MAO inhibitor or within 24 hours of taking another 5-HT$_1$ agonist or ergot-containing drug. Also contraindicated in patients hypersensitive to drug or its components and in patients with uncontrolled hypertension, ischemic heart disease (angina, a history of MI, or documented silent ischemia), or other significant heart disease (including Wolff-Parkinson-White syndrome).

Use cautiously in patients with liver disease and in pregnant or breast-feeding women.

Interactions
Drug-drug
Cimetidine: doubles the half-life of zolmitriptan. Dosage adjustment may be needed.
Ergot-containing drugs: may cause additive vasospastic reactions. Monitor patient closely.
Fluoxetine, fluvoxamine, paroxetine, sertraline: may cause weakness, hyperreflexia, and incoordination. Monitor patient closely.
MAO inhibitors, oral contraceptives: increase plasma zolmitriptan levels. Adjust dosage as needed.

Adverse reactions
CNS: asthenia, *dizziness,* hyperesthesias, paresthesias, somnolence, vertigo.
CV: pain or heaviness in chest, *pain or tightness in neck, pain or tightness in throat or jaw,* palpitations.
GI: dry mouth, dyspepsia, dysphagia, nausea.
Musculoskeletal: myalgia.
Skin: diaphoresis.
Other: warm or cold sensations.

Overdose and treatment
Overdose may cause sedation. No specific antidote exists. If severe intoxication occurs, provide intensive care that includes establishing and maintaining an airway, ensuring adequate oxygenation and ventilation, and monitoring and supporting the CV system. The effect of hemodialysis or peritoneal dialysis on the plasma zolmitriptan levels is unknown.

Special considerations
- Don't give drug for migraine prophylalxis or for hemiplegic or basilar migraines.
- Safety hasn't been established for cluster headaches.
- If patient has liver disease, monitor his blood pressure during therapy.
- Rare but serious cardiac events may occur with use of 5-HT$_1$ agonists, such as coronary artery vasospasm, transient myocardial ischemia, MI, ventricular tachycardia, and ventricular fibrillation.

Breast-feeding patients
- No data exists to demonstrate whether drug appears in breast milk. Give drug cautiously to breast-feeding women.

Pediatric patients
- Safety and effectiveness in children haven't been established.

Patient teaching
- Tell patient that drug is intended to relieve migraine symptoms rather than to prevent migraines.
- Remind patient not to take drug with other migraine drugs.
- Urge patient to take drug only as prescribed and not to take a second dose without consulting prescriber. If prescriber suggests a second dose, tell patient to take it 2 hours after the first dose.
- Tell patient to immediately notify prescriber about pain or tightness in the chest or throat, palpitations, rash, skin lumps, or swelling of the face, lips, or eyelids.
- Tell patient to immediately notify prescriber about planned, suspected, or known pregnancy.

Reactions may be *common,* uncommon, **life-threatening,** or **COMMON AND LIFE-THREATENING.**

PART 3

Appendices and Index

483 ■ Guidelines for monitoring selected psychotropic drugs

485 ■ Herbs and dietary supplements used for psychotropic effects

487 ■ Resources

489 ■ Index

Guidelines for monitoring selected psychotropic drugs

DRUG	VALUES TO MONITOR
amitriptyline hydrochloride Elavil	Blood glucose level, ECG results before therapy starts, plasma drug level (110-250 ng/ml), serum creatinine level
chlorpromazine hydrochloride Thorazine	Blood pressure (orthostatic hypotension), cholesterol level, CBC, physical status (tremors, gait changes, abnormalities of neck, trunk, buccal area, limbs), plasma drug level (30-500 ng/ml), serum calcium level, signs of infection, such as sore throat, fever
citalopram hydrobromide Celexa	Blood pressure, CBC with continued therapy, heart rate, liver function, serum sodium level
clozapine Clozaril	Absolute neutrophil count (stop drug if below 1,500/mm^3), bilirubin level, blood pressure (hypertension and hypotension), CBC, ECG results, liver function, white blood cell count (stop drug if below 3,000/mm^3)
desipramine hydrochloride Norpramin	Blood pressure; ECG results in elderly patients, children, and patients with preexisting illness; heart rate; liver function during long-term therapy; mental status; plasma drug level (125-300 ng/ml); renal function during long-term therapy; weight
doxepin hydrochloride Sinequan	Blood pressure, heart rate, mental status, plasma drug level (100-200 ng/ml), weight
fluoxetine hydrochloride Prozac	AST level, bilirubin level, blood glucose level, cardiac enzyme levels, CBC with differential, extrapyramidal symptoms, liver function, serum creatinine level, serum calcium level, weight
fluphenazine Prolixin	Blood pressure (hypotension with I.V. or I.M. use), BUN, CBC, serum calcium level, signs of infection, such as sore throat, fever
haloperidol Haldol	Blood glucose level, blood pressure, CBC with differential, ECG results, extrapyramidal symptoms, plasma drug level (5-12 ng/ml), serum sodium level, liver function
nortriptyline hydrochloride Pamelor	Blood pressure; ECG results in elderly patients, children, and patients with preexisting illness; heart rate; liver and renal function during long-term therapy; mental status; plasma drug level (50-150 ng/ml)

(continued)

DRUG	VALUES TO MONITOR
olanzapine Zyprexa	BUN, creatine phosphokinase level, gamma-glutamyl transpeptidase level, heart rate, serum creatinine level, serum prolactin level
paroxetine hydrochloride Paxil	Blood pressure, BUN, heart rate, liver function, platelet count, renal function, serum sodium level, serum creatinine level
perphenazine Trilafon	CBC, exptrapyramidal symptoms, liver function, plasma drug level (0.8-1.2 nmol/L), serum calcium level, signs of infection, such as sore throat, fever
quetiapine fumarate Seroquel	BUN, cataract formation, cholesterol level, creatine phosphokinase, gamma-glutamyl transpeptidase level, serum creatinine level, serum prolactin level
risperidone Risperdal	Blood pressure (orthostatic hypotension for 3 to 5 days after therapy starts or dosage increases), BUN, creatine phosphokinase level, extrapyramidal symptoms, gamma-glutamyl transpeptidase level, liver function, serum creatinine
sertraline hydrochloride Zoloft	Blood pressure, BUN, cholesterol level, heart rate, liver function, platelet count, renal function, serum creatinine level, serum sodium level, triglyceride level
thioridazine Mellaril	Blood pressure, CBC, liver function, ophthalmologic status, serum calcium level, signs of infection, such as sore throat, fever
trifluoperazine hydrochloride Stelazine	CBC, serum calcium level, signs of infection, such as sore throat, fever

Herbs and dietary supplements used for psychotropic effects

HERB OR SUPPLEMENT AND REPORTED PSYCHOTROPIC USES	SPECIAL CONSIDERATIONS
Betony ■ Anxiety ■ Insomnia	■ Betony is also used for headache, diarrhea, and mouth irritation. ■ Caution patient not to take betony during pregnancy or breast-feeding.
Black cohosh ■ Premenstrual syndrome ■ Symptoms of menopause, such as anxiety, emotional lability, and hot flashes	■ Inform patient that benefits may take weeks to occur. ■ Caution patient not to take black cohosh during pregnancy.
Ginkgo biloba ■ Anxiety ■ Dementia from Alzheimer's disease and cerebrovascular accident	■ Data suggest that ginkgo is effective for dementia. Little data support its use for anxiety. ■ Recommend that patient use only standardized ginkgo biloba extract. ■ Caution against combining ginkgo with anticoagulant or antiplatelet drugs or herbs.
Ginseng ■ Stress	■ Ginseng is contraindicated in patients who have hypertension. ■ Watch for possible "ginseng abuse syndrome." ■ Urge patient to limit intake of caffeine and other stimulants. ■ Caution against combining ginseng with warfarin or MAO inhibitors.
Hops ■ Anxiety ■ Insomnia	■ Urge patient to avoid other CNS depressants, including alcohol, while taking hops.
Kava ■ Anxiety ■ Insomnia	■ Data suggest that kava is effective for anxiety. ■ Herb is contraindicated during pregnancy and breast-feeding. ■ Expect herb to have a mild euphoric effect. ■ Because herb may have abuse potential, suggest that patient take it for no more than 3 months. ■ Tell patient to avoid other CNS depressants, including alcohol, while taking kava.
Khat ■ Depression ■ Fatigue	■ Herb has potential for psychological dependence and abuse. ■ Khat is contraindicated in pregnancy. ■ Tell patient to avoid caffeine and other herbal stimulants (such as ephedra) while taking khat.

(continued)

HERB OR SUPPLEMENT AND REPORTED PSYCHOTROPIC USES	SPECIAL CONSIDERATIONS
Lavender ■ Anxiety ■ Insomnia	■ Urge patient to avoid other CNS depressants, including alcohol, while taking lavender. ■ Caution against taking lavender during pregnancy or breast-feeding.
Melatonin ■ Circadian rhythm disturbances ■ Insomnia ■ Jet lag	■ Avoid use by depressed patients. ■ Tell patient to start at a low dose and to avoid other CNS depressants. ■ Caution patient to avoid hazardous activities until full effects of melatonin are known.
Nutmeg ■ Insomnia	■ Tell patient that the adverse effects of nutmeg exceed its potential therapeutic effects. ■ Nutmeg may potentiate some psychoactive drugs, especially MAO inhibitors. ■ Tell patient to avoid medicinal use of nutmeg during pregnancy.
Passion flower ■ Anxiety ■ Insomnia	■ Passion flower may interact with MAO inhibitors, such as isocarboxazid, phenylzine sulfate, and tranylcypromine sulfate. ■ Tell patient not to take passion flower during pregnancy or breast-feeding.
St. John's wort ■ Depression	■ Herb may induce cytochrome P-450 isoenzyme activity and may raise the risk of serotonin syndrome if given with serotonergic drugs or MAO inhibitors. ■ Herb may cause mania in bipolar disorder. ■ Patient may need 300 mg P.O. t.i.d. ■ Tell patient not to take during pregnancy.
SAMe ■ Depression	■ SAMe may cause mania when taken by a patient with bipolar disorder. ■ Its safety is unknown when combined with prescribed antidepressants. ■ SAMe also has been used for osteoarthritis, fibromyalgia, and liver diseases.
Schisandra ■ Depression ■ Irritability ■ Memory loss	■ Herb is used in traditional Chinese medicine. ■ It may interfere with drug metabolism.
Valerian ■ Anxiety ■ Insomnia	■ Valerian has fewer adverse effects than benzodiazepines and little hangover effect. ■ Because extract has affinity for receptor sites, it may help with benzodiazepine withdrawal.

Resources

Academy of Psychosomatic Medicine
5824 N. Magnolia
Chicago, IL 60660
(773) 784-2025
www.apm.org

American Academy of Child and
Adolescent Psychiatry
3615 Wisconsin Ave., NW
Washington, DC 20016
(202) 966-7300
www.aacap.org

American Academy of Clinical
Psychiatrists
P.O. Box 45870
Glastonbury, CT 06033
(860) 633-5045
www.aacp.com

American Psychiatric Association
1400 K St., NW
Washington, DC 20005
(202) 682-6000
www.psych.org

American Psychiatric Nurses
Association
2025 M St., NW
Suite 800
Washington, DC 20036-3309
(202) 367-1133
www.apna.org

American Psychoanalytic Association
309 E. 49th St.
New York, NY 10017
(212) 752-0450
www.apsa.org

American Psychological Association
750 First St., NE
Washington, DC 20002
(202) 336-5500
www.apa.org

Anxiety Disorders Association
of America
11900 Parklawn Dr., Suite 100
Rockville, MD 20852-2624
(301) 231-9350
www.adaa.org

Anxiety Disorders Education
Program
National Institute of Mental Heath,
Room 7-99
5600 Fishers Lane
Rockville, MD 20857
(888) 8-ANXIETY
www.nimh.nih.gov/anxiety

Bazelon Center for Mental
Health Law
1101 15th Street, NW
Suite 1212
Washington, DC 20005-5002
(202) 467-5730
www.bazelon.org

Center for Mental Health Services
P.O. Box 42490
Washington, DC 20015
(800) 789-2647
www.mentalhealth.org

Center for Psychiatric Rehabilitation
Boston University
940 Commonwealth Ave. West
Boston, MA 02215
(617) 353-3549
www.bu.edu/sarpsych

Freedom From Fear
308 Seaview Ave.
Staten Island, NY 10305
(718) 351-1717

Louis de la Parte Florida Mental
Health Institute
University of South Florida
13301 Bruce B. Downs Blvd.
Tampa, FL 33612
(813) 974-4602
www.fmhi.usf.edu

National Alliance for the
Mentally Ill
200 N. Glebe Rd.
Suite 1015
Arlington, VA 22201
(800) 950-6264
www.nami.org

National Anxiety Foundation
3135 Custer Dr.
Lexington, KY 40517
www.lexington-on-
line.com/naf.html

National Attention Deficit Disorder
Association
1788 Second St., Suite 200
Highland Park, IL 60035
(847) 432-ADDA
www.add.org

National Council on Alcoholism and
Drug Dependence
121 West 21st St.
New York, NY 10010
(800) 622-2255
www.ncadd.org

National Depressive and
Manic-Depressive Association
730 N. Franklin St., Suite 501
Chicago, IL 60610-3526
(800) 826-3632
www.ndmda.org

National Institute of
Mental Health
6001 Executive Blvd.
Room 8184 MSC 9663
Bethesda, MD 20892-9669
(301) 443-8410
www.nimh.nih.gov

National Mental Health Association
1021 Prince St.
Alexandria, VA 22314-2971
(800) 969-6642
(703) 684-7722
www.nmha.org

National Self-Help Clearinghouse
365 5th Ave., Suite 3300
New York, NY 10016
(212) 817-1822
www.selfhelpweb.org

Society for Neuroscience
11 Dupont Circle, NW
Suite 500
Washington, DC 20036
(202) 462-6688
www.sfn.org

Substance Abuse and Mental Health
Services Administration
U.S. Dept of Health and
Human Services
5600 Fishers Lane, Room 15-99
Rockville, MD 20857
(301) 443-0001
www.samhsa.gov

Young Adults With Narcolepsy
1451 W. 31st St.
Minneapolis, MN 55408
(612) 824-1355
www.yawn.org

Index

Ability (handwritten)

A

Abbreviations, x
Absence seizures
  acetazolamide for, 101
  clonazepam for, 107
  ethosuximide for, 109
  valproic acid for, 139-140
Absorption of drug, 20
Accidental overdose, 33-36. *See also* Overdose
  in children, 35-36
  due to drug interactions, 33-35
  in elderly persons, 36
acetazolamide, 94-95, 101-103
acetazolamide sodium, 101-103
Aches, buspirone for, 60
Acute dystonic reaction, 275
  benztropine for, 235
Acute intermittent porphyria, chlorpro-
    mazine for, 273, 281
Acute psychiatric situations, haloperidol for,
    293
Adapin, 170
Adderall, 352
Adolescence, 25-26
  eating disorders in, 25
  sexual risk-taking in, 25-26
  suicide in, 25
Adverse effects, 14
  of anticonvulsants, 98-99
  of antidepressants, 57, 148-149
  of antipsychotics, 34, 274-279
Affect of patient, 6
Aggressive behavior
  assessment of, 40
  management of, 40-41
  trazodone for, 207
Agitation
  chlorpromazine for, 281
  in elderly persons, 28
  haloperidol for, 293
  lorazepam for, 75
  thiothixene for, 330
Agoraphobia, 51
  alprazolam for, 58
  trazodone for, 207
Agranulocytosis, 274-275
Akathisia, 275
Akinetic seizures, clonazepam for, 107

Akineton, 237
Alcohol withdrawal, 373-377
  benzodiazepines for, 374-376
  chloral hydrate for, 422
  chlordiazepoxide for, 63
  chlorpromazine for, 281
  clorazepate for, 65
  diazepam for, 68
  management of, 374-375
  oxazepam for, 83
  patient teaching about drugs for, 376-377,
    383
  physiology of, 373
  symptoms of, 375
Alcoholism, 373-377
  disulfiram for, 376-377, 390-393
  fluoxetine for, 173
  haloperidol for, 292
  lithium for, 222
  medical complications of, 373
  mesoridazine for, 272, 299
  naltrexone for, 400
  pathophysiology of, 373
  prevalence of, 373
  preventing relapse of, 375-376
  trazodone for, 207
  treatment of, 373
alprazolam, 56, 58-60
Alprazolam Intensol, 58
Alzheimer's disease, 28-29, 455
  donepezil for, 459
  effects of drugs for, 455
  incidence of, 455
  patient teaching about drugs for, 458
  stages of, 455
  tacrine for, 476
  treatment of, 455
amantadine hydrochloride, 230, 233-235
Ambien, 450
Amerge, 466
amitriptyline hydrochloride, 56, 150-151,
    153-156, 483
amobarbital, 416-419
amobarbital sodium, 416-419
amoxapine, 150-151, 156-160
amphetamine sulfate, 348-350
Amphetamines, overdose of, 38-39
Amytal, 416

Anafranil, 164
Anergan 25, 438
Anergan 50, 438
Anesthesia
  droperidol for, 424-425
  flumazenil after, 393
  midazolam for, 80
Angioedema, nortriptyline for, 189
Anorexia, amitriptyline for, 153
Antabuse, 390
Antianxiety drugs, 49-85. *See also* Anxiety
  antidepressants, 55-57
  antihistamines, 55
  benzodiazepines, 54
  beta blockers, 55
  buspirone, 54-55
  half-lives of, 56
  patient teaching about, 57
Anticholinergic effects
  of antidepressants, 151
  of antipsychotics, 275, 277
Anticonvulsants, 87-142. *See also* Seizures
  acute dose-related effects of, 98
  acute idiosyncratic effects of, 98
  adverse effects of, 98-99
  drug interactions with, 99
  effects of, 92-96
  long-term use of, 98-99
  overdose of, 99
  patient teaching about, 99-100
  pharmacokinetics of, 96-98
  quick guide to, 94-97
  selecting regimen for, 92
  teratogenicity of, 99
Antidepressants, 143-215. *See also*
    Depression
  adverse effects of, 57, 148-149
  for anxiety, 55-57
  categories of, 146
  comparison of, 150-151
  effects of, 147
  for elderly persons, 27-28
  overdose of, 39, 41, 57, 149, 152
  patient teaching about, 152
  pharmacokinetics of, 147-148
  switching between, 146
Antihistamines
  for anxiety, 55
  for insomnia, 413-414
Antiparkinsonian agents, 227-267. *See also*
    Parkinsonism
  choosing drug regimen, 230
  patient teaching about, 232
Antipsychotics, 269-339. *See also* Psychosis;
    Schizophrenia
  adverse effects of, 274-279
  comparing indications for, 272-273

effects of, 271, 274
  novel, 271, 274
  overdose of, 279
  patient teaching about, 280
  pharmacokinetics of, 274
  typical, 271
Anxanil, 73
Anxiety. *See also* Antianxiety drugs
  alprazolam for, 58
  antipsychotics for, 273
  buspirone for, 60
  chlordiazepoxide for, 63
  clorazepate for, 66
  diazepam for, 68
  doxepin for, 170
  hydroxyzine for, 73
  lorazepam for, 75
  maprotiline for, 182
  meprobamate for, 77
  mesoridazine for, 299
  midazolam for, 80
  oxazepam for, 83
  prochlorperazine for, 316
  propranolol for, 468
  trazodone for, 207
  trifluoperazine for, 334
  venlafaxine for, 214
Anxiety disorders, 51-57
  generalized anxiety disorder, 51
  obsessive-compulsive disorder, 52-53
  panic disorder, 51-52
  phobias, 51
  post-traumatic stress disorder, 52
  treatment of, 53-85
Apo-Alpraz, 58
Apo-Amitriptyline, 153
Apo-Diazepam, 68
Apo-Flurazepam, 428
Apo-Haloperidol, 292
Apo-Hydroxyzine, 73
Apo-Imipramine, 178
Apo-Lorazepam, 75
Apo-Meprobamate, 77
Apo-Oxazepam, 83
Apo-Perphenazine, 309
Apo-Thioridazine, 326
Apo-Trifluoperazine, 334
Apo-Trihex, 265
Appearance of patient, 6
Aquachloral Supprettes, 422
Aricept, 459
Arrhythmias
  antidepressant-induced, 149, 152
  antipsychotic-induced, 278
Artane, 265
Artane Sequels, 265
Arthritis pain, nortriptyline for, 189

Asendin, 156
Assessment, 4-10
  of aggression, 40
  laboratory tests, 10
  mental status examination, 6-8
  physical examination, 7-10
  psychiatric history, 4
  specialized tools for, 7
  of suicide risk, 4-6
Atarax, 73
Ativan, 75
Atopic eczema, nortriptyline for, 189
Atretol, 103
Attention deficit hyperactivity disorder, 343-345
  amphetamine for, 348
  dextroamphetamine for, 353
  diagnosis of, 343
  effects of drugs for, 345
  epidemiology of, 343
  fluoxetine for, 174
  methamphetamine for, 360
  methylphenidate for, 363
  pemoline for, 368
  physiology of, 345
  symptoms of, 343
  treatment of, 344-345
Attitude of patient, 6
Aventyl, 189
Axial system of DSM-IV, 11
Azapirones, 54-55

B

Barbita, 434
Barbiturates
  disadvantages of, 414
  for insomnia, 414
  overdose of, 39
Beck Depression Inventory, 7
Behavior assessment, 6
Behavioral problems
  antipsychotics for, 272
  mesoridazine for, 300
  thioridazine for, 326
Bell's palsy, phenytoin for, 129
Benadryl, 241
Benign familial tremor
  primidone for, 133
  propranolol for, 469
Benylin, 241
Benzodiazepine overdose, 38, 39, 54
  flumazenil for, 393
Benzodiazepine receptors, 54, 413
Benzodiazepines, 54
  for alcohol withdrawal, 374-376
  for anxiety, 54
  effects of, 54, 413

  flumazenil for reversal of, 393
  for insomnia, 412-413
  pharmacokinetics of, 54
  withdrawal from, 42-43, 54
benztropine mesylate, 230, 235-237
Beta blockers
  for anxiety, 55
  for migraine prophylaxis, 457
betony, 485
biperiden hydrochloride, 230, 237-239
biperiden lactate, 237-239
Bipolar disorder, 219-221. *See also* Mood stabilizing drugs
  carbamazepine for, 103
  causes of, 219
  fluoxetine for, 173
  initial treatment of, 220-221
  lithium for, 222
  mood swings in, 219-220
  ongoing treatment of, 221
  symptoms of manic and depressive phases of, 219
  types I and II, 219-220
black cohosh, 485
Borderline personality disorder, fluoxetine for, 174
Breast-feeding, 23
Bright light therapy for depression, 12
bromocriptine mesylate, 230, 239-241
Bulimia, amitriptyline for, 153
bupropion hydrochloride
  for depression, 150-151, 160-162
  for nicotine dependence, 378, 380, 385-387
BuSpar, 54, 60
buspirone hydrochloride, 54-56, 60-62
butabarbital sodium, 419-421
Butisol, 419

C

Cafcit, 350
Cafergot, 461
Caffedrine, 350
caffeine, 350-352
Calcium channel blockers, for migraine prophylaxis, 457
Cancer patients
  droperidol for, 425
  nortriptyline for, 189
carbamazepine
  for alcohol withdrawal, 375
  for seizure disorders, 94-95, 103-106
Carbatrol, 103
Carbolith, 222
Carbon monoxide intoxication, levodopa for, 246
Cardiovascular disorders, 9

Cardiovascular effects
of antidepressants, 149, 152
of antipsychotics, 278
Cataplexy
fluoxetine for, 173
in narcolepsy, 345
Catapres, 387
Catapres-TTS, 387
Celexa, 162, 483
Central nervous system depression
caffeine for, 350
doxapram for, 358
Central nervous system stimulants, 341-370
for attention deficit hyperactivity disorder, 343-345
effects of, 345
growing role for, 344
for narcolepsy, 345-347
overdose of, 38-39
patient teaching about, 347
Cerebyx, 111
Chemotherapy patients, droperidol for, 425
Children, 24
overdose in, 35-36
chloral hydrate, 414, 422-424
chlordiazepoxide
for alcohol withdrawal, 376
for anxiety, 56, 62-65
chlordiazepoxide hydrochloride, 62-65
Chlorpromanyl-5, 281
Chlorpromanyl-20, 281
chlorpromazine hydrochloride, 272-273, 276-277, 281-285, 483
Chorea, carbamazepine for, 104
Chronic brain syndrome, mesoridazine for, 300
Cibalith-S, 222
citalopram hydrobromide, 150-151, 162-164, 483
clomipramine hydrochloride, 150-151, 164-166
clonazepam, 94-95, 106-109
clonidine hydrochloride, 387-390
clorazepate dipotassium
for alcohol withdrawal, 376
for anxiety, 56, 65-68
for seizures, 94-95
clozapine, 272-273, 276-277, 285-288, 483
Clozaril, 285, 483
Cluster headaches
ergotamine for, 461
methysergide for, 464
sumatriptan for, 474
Cocaine dependence, 373
Cogentin, 235
Cognex, 476
Cognitive assessment, 7

Compazine, 316
Compazine Spansule, 316
Complex partial seizures, 90
carbamazepine for, 103
mephenytoin for, 124
primidone for, 133
Compliance with drug therapy, 13-14
Compoz, 241
Compulsions, 52-53
Comtan, 244
Concerta, 363
Cramps, buspirone for, 60
Cylert, 368

D

Dalmane, 428
Daytime sleepiness, modafinil for, 366
Dazamide, 101
Delirium tremens, 375
Dementia
Alzheimer's disease, 28-29, 455
donepezil for, 459
Parkinson's, 229
tacrine for, 476
thioridazine for, 326
Depacon, 139
Depakene, 139
Depakote, 139
Depakote Sprinkle, 139
L-Deprenyl hydrochloride, 261-263
Depression. See also Antidepressants
alprazolam for, 58
amitriptyline for, 153
amoxapine for, 156
in bipolar disorder, 219
bright light therapy for, 12
bupropion for, 160
causes of, 145
citalopram for, 162
desipramine for, 166-167
doxepin for, 170
in elderly persons, 27-28
fluoxetine for, 173
imipramine for, 179
lithium for, 222
maprotiline for, 182
mirtazapine for, 185
nefazodone for, 187
nortriptyline for, 189
paroxetine for, 193
phenelzine for, 196
in pregnancy, 23
prevalence of, 145
protriptyline for, 198
rating scales for, 7
relapses of, 146
sertraline for, 202

Depression *(continued)*
St. John's wort for, 147
symptoms of, 146
tranylcypromine for, 204
trazodone for, 207
treatment of, 145-146
trimipramine for, 210
venlafaxine for, 213-214
Dermatologic disorders, nortriptyline for, 189
desipramine hydrochloride, 150-151, 166-170, 483
Desoxyn, 360
Desoxyn Gradumets, 360
Desyrel, 207
Dexedrine, 352
dextroamphetamine sulfate, 352-355
Diabetic neuropathy
nortriptyline for, 189
paroxetine for, 193
Diagnosis, 10-11
Diagnostic and Statistical Manual of Mental Disorders (DSM-IV), 10
axial system of, 11
Diagnostic procedures
droperidol for, 424
midazolam for, 80
Diamox, 101
Diamox Sequels, 101
Diastat, 68
diazepam
for alcohol withdrawal, 376
for anxiety, 56, 68-72
for seizures, 94-95
Dietary supplements, 485-486
diethylpropion hydrochloride, 356-358
Dilantin, 129
Dilantin-30, 129
Dilantin-125, 129
Dilantin Infatab, 129
Dilantin Kapseals, 129
Diphen AF, 241
Diphenadryl, 241
diphenhydramine hydrochloride, 230, 241-244
Distribution of drug, 20
disulfiram, 376-377, 390-393
divalproex sodium, 139-142
Dixarit, 387
donepezil hydrochloride, 455, 459-461
Dopamine receptors, 271
Dopar, 246
Dopram, 358
doxapram hydrochloride, 358-360
doxepin hydrochloride, 56, 150-151, 170-173, 483

droperidol, 424-426
Drug absorption, 20
Drug distribution, 20
Drug excretion, 21
Drug interactions, 14-15
with anticonvulsants, 99
expanding knowledge about, 35
overdose due to, 33-35
proactive approach to, 33-35
Drug metabolism, 20-21
Drug overdose. *See* Overdose
Drug therapy, 13-15
adverse effects of, 14
compliance with, 13-14
drug interactions and, 14-15
pharmacokinetics of, 20-21
for special populations, 19-30
Duralith, 222
Dysarthria, clonazepam for, 107
Dyskinesia, tardive, 34, 275
Dysthymic disorder, thioridazine for, 326
Dystonia
acute, 275
benztropine for, 235
tardive, 34

E

Eating disorders
amitriptyline for, 153
among adolescents, 25
fluoxetine for, 174
Eclampsia, magnesium sulfate for, 122
Eczema, nortriptyline for, 189
Effexor, 213
Effexor XR, 213
Elavil, 153, 483
Eldepryl, 261
Elderly persons, 26-30
age categories of, 27
agitation in, 28
Alzheimer's disease in, 28-29
depression in, 27-28
Medicare coverage for psychiatric treatment of, 30
overdose in, 36
psychosis in, 29
substance abuse in, 26-27
Electroconvulsive therapy, 15
Emesis
antipsychotics for, 273
droperidol for, 425
Endep, 153
Endocrine problems, antipsychotic-induced, 279
Endoscopic procedures, midazolam for, 80
entacapone, 230, 244-246
Enuresis, imipramine for, 179

Epilepsy. *See also* Seizures
lamotrigine for, 117
oxcarbazepine for, 126
phenobarbital for, 434
Epitol, 103
Epival, 139
Equanil, 77
Ergomar, 461
Ergostat, 461
ergotamine tartrate, 456, 461-463
Eskalith, 222
Eskalith CR, 222
Essential tremor
primidone for, 133
propranolol for, 469
estazolam, 426-428
ethosuximide, 94-95, 109-110
Excretion of drug, 21
Extrapyramidal symptoms
amantadine for, 233
antipsychotic-induced, 34, 275, 276
benztropine for, 235
biperiden for, 237
trihexyphenidyl for, 266

F

Fatigue, buspirone for, 60
Febrile seizures, phenobarbital for, 434
Ferndex, 352
Fertility rates and psychotropic drugs, 22
Fetal risk of maternal drug therapy, 22
flumazenil, 393-395
fluoxetine hydrochloride, 56, 150-151, 173-176, 483
fluphenazine decanoate, 288-292
fluphenazine enanthate, 288-292
fluphenazine hydrochloride, 272-273, 276-277, 288-292, 483
flurazepam hydrochloride, 428-431
fluvoxamine maleate, 150-151, 176-178
Focal seizures, primidone for, 133
folic acid, for alcohol withdrawal, 375
Folstein Mini-Mental State Exam, 7, 8
fosphenytoin sodium, 94-95, 111-115

G

gabapentin, 94-95, 115-117
Gabitril, 135
Gastrointestinal dysfunction, 9-10
Generalized anxiety disorder, 51
venlafaxine for, 214
Generalized tonic-clonic seizures
acetazolamide for, 101
carbamazepine for, 103
clonazepam for, 107
mephenytoin for, 124
phenytoin for, 129

primidone for, 133
valproic acid for, 139-140
Genitourinary problems, antipsychotic-induced, 278
ginkgo biloba, 485
ginseng, 485
Gynergen, 461

H

Habitrol, 379, 403
Halcion, 445
Haldol, 292, 484
Haldol Concentrate, 292
Haldol Decanoate, 292
Haldol Decanoate 100, 292
Haldol Intensol, 292
Haldol LA, 292
Hallucinations, in narcolepsy, 346
haloperidol, 272-273, 276-277, 292-296, 484
haloperidol decanoate, 292-296
haloperidol lactate, 292-296
HANDS assessment tool, 7
Harvard Department of Psychiatry/National Screening Day Scale, 7
Head trauma patients, phenytoin for, 129
Headache, 9
antipsychotics for, 272
ergotamine for, 461
methysergide for, 464
migraine, 455-457
naratriptan for, 466
nortriptyline for, 189
paroxetine for, 193
phenytoin for, 129
propranolol for, 468
rizatriptan for, 471
sumatriptan for, 474
zolmitriptan for, 479
Hepatic problems, antipsychotic-induced, 278
Herbs, 485-486
Histanil, 438
History, Clinical and Risk Management tool, 7
History taking, 4
hops, 485
Hydramine, 241
Hydroxacen, 73
hydroxyzine hydrochloride, 73-74
hydroxyzine pamoate, 73-74
Hyperkinesia
haloperidol for, 273, 293
hydroxyzine for, 73
Hypomagnesemia, magnesium sulfate for, 121

Hypotension, orthostatic
   antidepressant-induced, 151
   antipsychotic-induced, 277
Hyzine-50, 73

I

imipramine hydrochloride, 56, 150-151, 178-
   182
Imitrex, 473
Impril, 178
Inapsine, 424
Inderal, 468
Inderal LA, 468
Insomnia, 411-414
   amobarbital for, 416
   assessment of, 412
   butabarbital for, 419
   causes of, 411, 412
   chloral hydrate for, 414, 422
   diphenhydramine for, 242
   drug treatments for, 412-414
   estazolam for, 426
   flurazepam for, 429
   lorazepam for, 75
   nondrug treatments for, 411-412
   pentobarbital for, 431
   phenobarbital for, 435
   prevalence of, 411
   secobarbital for, 440
   temazepam for, 443
   trazodone for, 207
   triazolam for, 445
   zaleplon for, 448
   zolpidem for, 450
Insurance coverage for psychiatric treatment,
   11
   Medicare, 30
Intensol, 468
Intentional overdose, 36-37. *See also*
      Overdose
   to obtain mood-altering effects, 36
   as suicide attempt, 36-37
Intermittent explosive disorder, carba-
      mazepine for, 103
Irritability
   buspirone for, 60
   lorazepam for, 75

K L

kava, 485
Keppra, 119
khat, 485
Kindling, 373
Kleptomania, fluoxetine for, 174
Klonopin, 106
L-deprenyl hydrochloride, 261-263
LAAM, 382

Lamictal, 117
lamotrigine, 94-95, 117-119
Largactil, 281
Larodopa, 246
lavender, 486
Leg movements during sleep
   carbamazepine for, 104
   clonazepam for, 107
Lennox-Gastaut syndrome, lamotrigine for,
   117
Levate, 153
levetiracetam, 94-95, 119-121
levo-alpha-acetylmethadol, 382
levodopa, 230, 231, 246-250
levodopa-carbidopa, 230, 250-254
levodopa-carbidopa adjunct
   entacapone as, 244
   pergolide as, 254
   selegiline as, 261
   tolcapone as, 263
Libritabs, 62
Librium, 62
Lithane, 222
lithium carbonate, 222-226
lithium citrate, 222-226
Lithizine, 222
Lithobid, 222
Lithonate, 222
Lithotabs, 222
lorazepam
   for alcohol withdrawal, 376
   for anxiety, 56, 75-77
   for seizures, 94-95
Loxapac, 296
loxapine hydrochloride, 272-273, 276-277,
   296-299
loxapine succinate, 296-299
Loxitane, 296
Loxitane C, 296
Loxitane IM, 296
Ludiomil, 182
Luminal, 434
Luvox, 176

M

magnesium sulfate, 94-95, 121-123
Manganese intoxication, levodopa for, 246
Mania, 219-220. *See also* Bipolar disorder
   clonazepam for, 107
   lithium for, 222
   valproic acid for, 140
maprotiline hydrochloride, 150-151, 182-185
Maxalt, 471
Maxalt-MLT, 471
Medicare coverage for psychiatric treatment,
   30
Medihaler Ergotamine, 461

melatonin, 486
Mellaril, 326, 484
Mellaril-S, 326
Menstrual irregularities, 10
Mental status examination, 6-8
 affect, 6
 appearance, 6
 attitude, 6
 behavior, 6
 cognition, 7
 Folstein Mini-Mental State Exam, 7, 8
 mood, 6
 special tools for, 7
 speech, 6
 thought pattern, 6
mephenytoin, 94-95, 123-126
meprobamate, 77-79
Meprospan, 77
Mesantoin, 123
mesoridazine besylate, 272-273, 276-277,
 299-303
Metabolism of drug, 20-21
methadone hydrochloride, 381-382, 395-398
methamphetamine hydrochloride, 360-363
Methylin, 363
Methylin ER, 363
methylphenidate hydrochloride, 363-366
methysergide maleate, 457, 463-466
midazolam hydrochloride, 56, 79-82
Migraine headache, 455-457
 antipsychotics for, 272
 cause of, 455-456
 ergotamine for, 461
 incidence of, 455
 methysergide for, 464
 naratriptan for, 466
 nortriptyline for, 189
 patient teaching about drugs for, 458
 phenytoin for, 129
 prophylaxis for, 457
 propranolol for, 468
 rizatriptan for, 471
 sumatriptan for, 474
 treatment of, 456-457
 zolmitriptan for, 479
Miltown, 77
Mini-Mental State Exam, 7, 8
Mirapex, 256
mirtazapine, 150-151, 185-187
Mitran, 62
Mixed seizures
 acetazolamide for, 101
 carbamazepine for, 103
 valproic acid for, 139-140
Moban, 303
modafinil, 366-368
Modecate, 288

Moditen Enanthate, 288
molindone hydrochloride, 272-273, 276-277,
 303-306
Monitoring psychotropic drugs, 483-484
Monoamine oxidase inhibitors, 146
Mood-altering drug effects, 36
Mood assessment, 6
Mood stabilizing drugs, 217-226. See also
 Bipolar disorder
 for bipolar disorder, 220-221
 initial treatment with, 220-221
 ongoing treatment with, 221
 patient teaching about, 221
Mood swings, 219-220
Motion sickness, diphenhydramine for, 242
Multipax, 73
Musculoskeletal discomfort, 10
Myidone, 133
Myoclonic seizures
 acetazolamide for, 101
 clonazepam for, 107
Myoclonus, fluoxetine for, 173
Mysoline, 133

N

naloxone hydrochloride, 398-400
naltrexone hydrochloride, 376, 400-403
naratriptan hydrochloride, 466-468
Narcan, 398
Narcolepsy, 345-347
 amphetamine for, 348
 dextroamphetamine for, 353
 elements of, 346
 fluoxetine for, 173
 methylphenidate for, 363
 modafinil for, 366
 pemoline for, 369
 treatment of, 347
Narcotic abstinence syndrome
 levo-alpha-acetylmethadol for, 382
 methadone for, 381-382, 395-398
Narcotic depression, postoperative, naloxone
 for, 398
Nardil, 195
Nausea and vomiting
 antipsychotics for, 273
 droperidol for, 425
Navane, 330
nefazodone hydrochloride, 150-151, 187-189
Nembutal, 431
Nephritis, magnesium sulfate for, 121
Nervine, 241
Nervine Nighttime Sleep-Aid, 241
Neuralgia
 amitriptyline for, 153
 carbamazepine for, 103-104
 clonazepam for, 107

Neuralgia *(continued)*
  nortriptyline for, 189
  phenytoin for, 129
Neuramate, 77
Neuroleptic malignant syndrome, 34, 279
Neurontin, 115
Neurosurgery patients
  fosphenytoin for, 111
  phenytoin for, 129
Nicoderm CQ, 379, 403
Nicorette, 379, 406
Nicorette DS, 406
nicotine, 378-380, 403-406
Nicotine dependence, 377-380
  effects of, 378
  pharmacokinetics of, 380
  treatment of, 378
nicotine inhaler, 379
nicotine nasal spray, 379
nicotine polacrilex, 379, 406-408
nicotine transdermal systems, 379
Nicotine withdrawal
  bupropion for, 378, 380, 385
  clonidine for, 387
  nicotine for, 378-380, 403-406
  nicotine polacrilex for, 406-408
  patient teaching about drugs for, 383-384
Nicotrol, 379, 403
Nicotrol Inhaler, 379
Nicotrol NS, 379, 403
Noctec, 422
NoDoz, 350
Norepinephrine blocking activity of antide-
    pressants, 151
Norpramin, 166, 483
nortriptyline hydrochloride, 150-151, 189-
    192, 484
Novo-Alprazol, 58
Novo-Chlorpromazine, 281
Novo-Flurazine, 334
Novo-Hydroxyzin, 73
Novo-Lorazem, 75
Novo-Peridol, 292
Novo-Ridazine, 326
Novoclopate, 65
Novodipam, 68
Novoflupam, 428
Novopramine, 178
Novosecobarb, 440
Novotriptyn, 153
Novoxapam, 83
nutmeg, 486
Nytol, 241

O

Obesity
  amphetamine for, 348
  dextroamphetamine for, 353
  diethylpropion for, 356
  methamphetamine for, 360
Obsessive-compulsive disorder, 52-53
  clomipramine for, 164
  fluoxetine for, 173
  fluvoxamine for, 176
  paroxetine for, 193
  sertraline for, 202
Ocular problems, antipsychotic-induced, 278
olanzapine, 272-273, 276-277, 306-308, 484
Opioid abstinence syndrome
  levo-alpha-acetylmethadol for, 382
  methadone for, 381-382, 395-398
Opioid dependence, 380-383
  naloxone challenge for diagnosis of, 398
  patient teaching about drugs for, 384
  preventing relapse of, 383
  risk of, 381
  treatment of, 381-382
Opioid depression, postoperative, naloxone
    for, 398
Opioid-detoxified patients, naltrexone for,
    400
Opioid-induced respiratory depression,
    naloxone for, 398
Opioid overdose, 39, 41
Opioid receptors, 380
Opioid withdrawal, 42, 381
  clonidine for, 387
Orap, 313
Ormazine, 281
Orthostatic hypotension
  antidepressant-induced, 151
  antipsychotic-induced, 277
Overdose, 33-41
  accidental, 33-36
  amphetamine, 38-39
  anticonvulsant, 99
  antidepressant, 39, 41, 57, 149, 152
  antipsychotic, 279
  barbiturate, 39
  benzodiazepine, 38, 39
  in children, 35-36
  due to drug interactions, 33-35
  in elderly persons, 36
  intentional, 36-37
  to obtain mood-altering effects, 36
  opiate, 39, 41
  signs and symptoms of, 39
  as suicide attempt, 36-37
  treatment of, 37-38

oxazepam
for alcohol withdrawal, 376
for anxiety, 56, 83-85
oxcarbazepine, 94-95, 126-129

P

Pain. *See also* Neuralgia
buspirone for, 60
migraine headache, 455-457
nortriptyline for, 189
Pamelor, 189, 484
Panic disorder, 51-52
alprazolam for, 58
clonazepam for, 106-107
fluoxetine for, 173
nortriptyline for, 189
paroxetine for, 193
sertraline for, 202
tranylcypromine for, 204
trazodone for, 207
Parkinsonism
amantadine for, 233
benztropine for, 235
biperiden for, 237
bromocriptine for, 239
clonazepam for, 107
diphenhydramine for, 242
entacapone for, 244
levodopa-carbidopa for, 250-251
levodopa for, 246
pergolide for, 254
pramipexole for, 256
ropinirole for, 258
selegiline for, 261
tolcapone for, 263
trihexyphenidyl for, 265
Parkinson's disease, 229-232. *See also*
Antiparkinsonian agents
causes of, 229
symptoms of, 229
treatment of, 229-232
Parlodel, 239
Parnate, 204
paroxetine hydrochloride, 56, 150-151, 193-
195, 484
Partial seizures
carbamazepine for, 103
complex, 90
gabapentin for, 115
lamotrigine for, 117
levetiracetam for, 120
mephenytoin for, 124
oxcarbazepine for, 126
primidone for, 133
simple, 90
tiagabine for, 135, 137
passion flower, 486

Patient monitoring, 483-484
Patient teaching
about antianxiety drugs, 57
about antidepressants, 152
about antiparkinsonian agents, 232
about antipsychotics, 280
about central nervous system stimulants,
347
about drugs for alcohol withdrawal, 376-
377, 383
about drugs for Alzheimer's disease, 458
about drugs for migraine headache, 458
about drugs for opioid withdrawal, 384
about mood stabilizing drugs, 221
about nicotine replacement therapy, 383-
384
about sedative-hypnotics, 414-415
Patient variables, 19-21
Paxil, 193, 484
Paxil CR, 193
pemoline, 368-370
Pentazine, 438
pentobarbital, 94-95
pentobarbital sodium, 431-434
pergolide mesylate, 230, 254-255
Peridol, 292
Peripheral neuropathy
nortriptyline for, 189
paroxetine for, 193
Permax, 254
Permitil, 288
perphenazine, 272-273, 276-277, 309-313,
484
Personality disorders, fluoxetine for, 174
Phantom limb pain, nortriptyline for, 189
Pharmacokinetics, 20-21
of anticonvulsants, 96-98
of antidepressants, 147-148
of antipsychotics, 274
of benzodiazepines, 54
of nicotine, 380
Phencen-50, 438
Phencyclidine psychosis, antipsychotics for,
272
phenelzine sulfate, 150-151, 195-198
Phenergan, 438
Phenergan Fortis, 438
Phenergan Plain, 438
phenobarbital, 96-97, 434-438
phenobarbital sodium, 434-438
Phenoject-50, 438
phenytoin, 96-97, 129-132
phenytoin sodium, 129-132
phenytoin sodium (extended), 129-132
phenytoin sodium (prompt), 129-132
Phenytoin substitution, fosphenytoin for, 111
Phobias, 51

Physical examination, 7-10
  cardiovascular disorders, 9
  gastrointestinal dysfunction, 9-10
  headache, 9
  musculoskeletal discomfort, 10
  reproductive changes, 10
  respiratory problems, 9
pimozide, 272-273, 276-277, 313-316
PMS Thioridazine, 326
Post-traumatic stress disorder, 52
  fluoxetine for, 174
  phenelzine for, 196
Postanesthesia respiratory stimulation,
    doxapram for, 358
Postherpetic neuralgia, nortriptyline for, 189
pramipexole dihydrochloride, 230, 256-258
Preeclampsia, magnesium sulfate for, 122
Pregnancy, 21-23
  depression in, 23
  fetal risk of maternal psychotropic drug
    therapy in, 22
  substance abuse in, 22-23
Premature ejaculation, paroxetine for, 193
Premenstrual syndrome
  alprazolam for, 58
  buspirone for, 60
  fluoxetine for, 174
  nortriptyline for, 189
Preoperative apprehension
  chlordiazepoxide for, 63
  midazolam for, 80
Preoperative sedation, midazolam for, 80
Primary care, 3-4
Primary generalized seizures
  convulsive, 90-91
  nonconvulsive, 91
primidone, 96-97, 133-135
prochlorperazine, 272-273, 276-277, 316-320
prochlorperazine edisylate, 316-320
prochlorperazine maleate, 316-320
Prolixin, 288, 483
Prolixin Decanoate, 288
Prolixin Enanthate, 288
Promet, 438
promethazine hydrochloride, 438-440
propranolol, 55, 56, 468-471
Prorex-25, 438
Prorex-50, 438
ProSom, 426
ProStep, 379, 403
Prothazine, 438
Prothazine Plain, 438
protriptyline hydrochloride, 150-151, 198-
    201
Provigil, 366
Prozac, 173, 483
Prozac Pulvules, 173

Pruritus, nortriptyline for, 189
Psychiatric disorders, 3-15
  assessment of, 4-10
  diagnosis of, 10-11
  management in primary care settings, 3-4
  treatment of, 11-15
Psychiatric history, 4
Psychiatric treatment, 11-15
  bright light therapy, 12
  drug therapy, 13-15
  electroconvulsive therapy, 15
  insurance coverage for, 11
  psychotherapy, 12-13
Psychoneurotic manifestations
  antipsychotics for, 273
  mesoridazine for, 299
Psychosis. *See also* Antipsychotics
  antipsychotics for, 272
  chlorpromazine for, 281
  clonazepam for, 107
  clozapine for, 285
  in elderly persons, 29
  fluoxetine for, 174
  fluphenazine for, 289
  haloperidol for, 292-293
  lithium for, 222
  loxapine for, 296
  mesoridazine for, 299
  molindone for, 303
  olanzapine for, 306
  perphenazine for, 309
  prochlorperazine for, 316
  quetiapine for, 320-321
  risperidone for, 323
  thioridazine for, 326
  thiothixene for, 330
  treatment of, 271-280
  trifluoperazine for, 335
Psychotherapy, 12-13

Q R

quetiapine fumarate, 272-273, 276-277, 320-
    323, 484
Quick Pep, 350
Quiess, 73
Remeron, 185
Reposans-10, 62
Reproductive changes, 10
  antipsychotic-induced, 279
Requip, 258
Resources, 487-488
Respiratory depression, narcotic-induced,
    naloxone for, 398
Respiratory problems, 9
Respiratory stimulation, postanesthesia,
    doxapram for, 358

Restless leg syndrome, carbamazepine for, 104
Restoril, 443
ReVia, 400
Reye's syndrome, phenytoin for, 129
Risperdal, 323, 484
risperidone, 272-273, 276-277, 323-326, 484
Ritalin, 363
Ritalin-SR, 363
Rivotril, 106
rizatriptan benzoate, 471-473
Romazicon, 393
ropinirole hydrochloride, 230, 258-260

S

SAMe, 486
Sansert, 463
schisandra, 486
Schizoaffective disorder, lithium for, 222
Schizophrenia, 271. *See also* Antipsychotics;
      Psychosis
   antipsychotics for, 272
   clonazepam for, 107
   clozapine for, 285
   fluoxetine for, 174
   lithium for, 222
   mesoridazine for, 299
   treatment of, 271-280
   trifluoperazine for, 335
secobarbital sodium, 440-443
Seconal, 440
Sedation
   amobarbital for, 416
   antidepressant-induced, 151
   antipsychotic-induced, 276
   butabarbital for, 419
   chloral hydrate for, 422
   diphenhydramine for, 242
   midazolam for, 80
   pentobarbital for, 431
   phenobarbital for, 435
   promethazine for, 438
Sedative-hypnotics, 409-452
   for insomnia, 411-414
   patient teaching about, 414-415
Seizures, 89-100. *See also* Anticonvulsants
   acetazolamide for, 101
   amobarbital for, 416
   antipsychotic-induced, 275, 278
   carbamazepine for, 103
   classification of, 89-90
   clonazepam for, 107
   clorazepate for, 66
   complex partial, 90
   diazepam for, 68-69
   ethosuximide for, 109
   fosphenytoin for, 111

gabapentin for, 115
   lamotrigine for, 117
   levetiracetam for, 120
   magnesium sulfate for, 121-122
   mephenytoin for, 124
   oxcarbazepine for, 126
   pentobarbital for, 431
   phenobarbital for, 434
   phenytoin for, 129
   primary generalized convulsive, 90-91
   primary generalized nonconvulsive, 91
   primidone for, 133
   principles of management of, 93
   secobarbital for, 440
   simple partial, 90
   tiagabine for, 135, 137
   treatment of, 91-100
   valproic acid for, 139-140
Selective serotonin reuptake inhibitors, 146
   for anxiety, 55-56
   overdose of, 39
selegiline hydrochloride, 230, 261-263
Senile movement tremor, propranolol for,
      469
Serax, 83
Serentil, 299
Seroquel, 320, 484
Serotonin blocking activity of antidepres-
      sants, 151
Sertan, 133
sertraline hydrochloride, 56, 150-151, 202-
      204, 484
Serzone, 187
Sexual dysfunction, 10
   antidepressant-induced, 148-149
Sexual risk-taking among adolescents, 25-26
Simple partial seizures, 90
Sinemet, 250
Sinemet CR, 250
Sinequan, 170, 483
Skeletal muscle relaxation, phenytoin for, 129
Skin reactions
   antipsychotic-induced, 278
   nortriptyline for, 189
Sleep-Eze 3, 241
Sleep problems
   antidepressant-induced, 148
   insomnia, 411-414
   narcolepsy, 345-347
Smoking cessation. *See also* Nicotine depen-
      dence
   bupropion for, 378, 380, 385
   clonidine for, 387
   nicotine for, 378-380, 403-406
   nicotine polacrilex for, 406-408
   patient teaching about drugs for, 383-384

Social phobia, 51
  alprazolam for, 58
  fluoxetine for, 174
  paroxetine for, 193
Solazine, 334
Solfoton, 434
Sominex, 241
Sonata, 448
Special populations, 19-30
  adolescents, 25-26
  children, 24
  elderly persons, 26-30
  patient variables, 19-21
  women, 21-23
Speech of patient, 6
St. John's wort, 147, 486
Status epilepticus, 89. *See also* Seizures
  diazepam for, 68
  fosphenytoin for, 111
  phenobarbital for, 434
  phenytoin for, 129
  secobarbital for, 440
  valproic acid for, 140
Stelazine, 334, 484
Stemetil, 316
Stimulants, 341-370
  for attention deficit hyperactivity disorder,
    343-345
  effects of, 345
  growing role for, 344
  for narcolepsy, 345-347
  overdose of, 38-39
  patient teaching about, 347
Substance abuse
  alcoholism, 373-377
  among elderly persons, 26-27
  cocaine dependence, 373
  definitions of substance dependence and,
    373, 374
  drug treatment of, 371-408
  nicotine dependence, 377-380
  opioid dependence, 380-383
  during pregnancy, 22
  prevalence of, 373
Suicide
  adolescent, 25
  assessing risk for, 4-6
  drug overdose and, 36-37
  prevention of, 37
  profile of person at risk for, 37
sumatriptan succinate, 473-476
Surgery patients
  chlordiazepoxide for, 63
  chlorpromazine for, 273
  doxapram for, 358
  droperidol for, 424-425
  fosphenytoin for, 111

  midazolam for, 80
  naloxone for, 398
  phenytoin for, 129
Surmontil, 210
Symmetrel, 233
Syncope, fluoxetine for, 174

T

tacrine hydrochloride, 455, 476-479
Tardive dyskinesia, 34, 275
Tardive dystonia, 34
Tasmar, 263
Tegretol, 103
temazepam, 443-445
Tension. *See also* Anxiety
  chlordiazepoxide for, 63
  hydroxyzine for, 73
  lorazepam for, 75
  meprobamate for, 77
  oxazepam for, 83
Tension headache, nortriptyline for, 189
Tenuate, 356
Tenuate Dospan, 356
Teratogenicity, 22
  of anticonvulsants, 99
Terfluzine, 334
Tetanus, chlorpromazine for, 273
Therapeutic procedures, midazolam for, 80
thiamine, 375
thioridazine, 272-273, 276-277, 326-330, 484
thioridazine hydrochloride, 326-330
thiothixene, 272-273, 276-277, 330-334
thiothixene hydrochloride, 330-334
Thor-Prom, 281
Thorazine, 281, 483
Thought pattern of patient, 6
tiagabine hydrochloride, 96-97, 135-137
Tic disorders
  antipsychotics for, 273
  clonazepam for, 107
  fluoxetine for, 174
  haloperidol for, 293
  pimozide for, 313
Tic douloureux, nortriptyline for, 189
Tobacco. *See* Nicotine dependence
Tofranil, 178
tolcapone, 230, 263-265
Topamax, 137
topiramate, 96-97, 137-139
Tourette syndrome
  antipsychotics for, 273
  fluoxetine for, 174
  haloperidol for, 293
  pimozide for, 313
Tranxene, 65
Tranxene-SD, 65
Tranxene-SD Half Strength, 65

tranylcypromine sulfate, 150-151, 204-207
trazodone hydrochloride, 150-151, 207-210
Treatment, psychiatric, 11-15
    bright light therapy, 12
    drug therapy, 13-15
    electroconvulsive therapy, 15
    insurance coverage for, 11
    psychotherapy, 12-13
Tremor
    primidone for, 133
    propranolol for, 469
Triadapin, 170
triazolam, 445-448
Trichotillomania, fluoxetine for, 173
Tricyclic antidepressants, 146
    for anxiety, 55-57
    for migraine prophylaxis, 457
    overdose of, 39
trifluoperazine hydrochloride, 272-273, 276-
        277, 334-339, 484
Trigeminal neuralgia
    carbamazepine for, 103-104
    phenytoin for, 129
Trihexane, 265
Trihexy-2, 265
Trihexy-5, 265
trihexyphenidyl hydrochloride, 230, 265-267
Trilafon, 309, 484
Trileptal, 126
trimipramine hydrochloride, 150-151
trimipramine maleate, 210-213
Triptans, 456-457
Triptil, 198
Tussat, 241
Twilite, 241

U V

Urticaria, nortriptyline for, 189
V-Gan-25, 438
V-Gan-50, 438
valerian, 486
Valium, 68
valproate sodium, 139-142
valproic acid, 96-97, 139-142
Vascular headache. *See also* Migraine
    ergotamine for, 461
    methysergide for, 464
    propranolol for, 468
venlafaxine hydrochloride, 56, 150-151, 213-
        215
Versed, 79
Vistacon-50, 73
Vistaril, 73
Vistazine 50, 73
Vivactil, 198
Vivarin, 350
Vivol, 68

W X Y Z

Weight gain
    antidepressant-induced, 148
    antipsychotic-induced, 277
Wellbutrin, 160
Wellbutrin SR, 160
Wernicke's encephalopathy, 375
Wigraine, 461
Withdrawal from drug, 42-44
    alcohol, 373-377
    benzodiazepines, 42-43, 54
    nicotine, 378-380, 383-384
    opioids, 42, 381
    risk factors for, 42
    symptoms of, 42
    treatment of, 42-44
Women, 21-23
    breast-feeding, 23
    pregnancy, 21-23
Xanax, 58
zaleplon, 413, 448-450
Zarontin, 109
Zetran, 68
zolmitriptan, 479-480
Zoloft, 202, 484
zolpidem tartrate, 413, 450-452
Zomig, 479
Zyban, 380, 385
Zyprexa, 306, 484